Contents

Chapter 4   Formulating the Method   61

Chapter 5   Ethical Issues in Research and Scholarship   73

PART II   Statistical and Measurement Concepts in Research   89

Chapter 6   Becoming Acquainted With Statistical Concepts   91

RESEARCH METHODS IN PHYSICAL ACTIVITY

Third Edition

Jerry R. Thomas, EdD
Iowa State University

Jack K. Nelson, EdD
Louisiana State University (Emeritus)

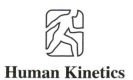

Human Kinetics

Library of Congress Cataloging-in-Publication Data

Thomas, Jerry R.
　　Research methods in physical activity / Jerry R. Thomas, Jack K.
　Nelson.--3rd ed.
　　　　p.　　cm.
　　Includes bibliographical references and index.
　　ISBN 0-88011-481-9
　　1. Physical education and training--Research.　2. Health--
Research.　3. Recreation--Research.　4. Dance--Research.
　　I. Nelson, Jack K.　II. Title.
　GV361.T47　1996
　613.7'1'072--dc20
　　　　　　　　　　　　　　　　　　　　　　　　　　　　95-25261
　　　　　　　　　　　　　　　　　　　　　　　　　　　　CIP

ISBN: 0-88011-481-9

Acquisitions Editor: Richard Frey, PhD; **Developmental Editor:** Holly Gilly; **Assistant Editor:** Kent Reel; **Editorial Assistant:** Amy Carnes; **Copyeditor:** Elaine Otto; **Proofreader:** Anne Meyer Byler; **Typesetter and Layout Artist:** Kathy Boudreau-Fuoss; **Text Designer:** Judy Henderson; **Cover Designer:** Jack Davis; **Illustrators:** Studio 2D, Craig Ronto, and Denise Lowry; **Printer:** Edwards Brothers

Interior photographs on pages 50, 64, 82, 97, 123, 148, 190, 195, 332, 405 courtesy of FPG International Corp.; pages 11, 28, 153, 253, 279, 297, 389, 418 courtesy of H. Armstrong Roberts; pages 347, 369 courtesy of Teraco's Vintage Images; page 226 courtesy of Ruth Bushman/FPG International Corp.; page 325 courtesy of John Mechling/FPG International Corp.

Printed in the United States of America　　　10　9　8　7　6　5　4

Human Kinetics
Web site: http://www.humankinetics.com/

United States: Human Kinetics, P.O. Box 5076, Champaign, IL 61825-5076
1-800-747-4457
e-mail: humank@hkusa.com

Canada: Human Kinetics, 475 Devonshire Road, Unit 100, Windsor, ON N8Y 2L5
1-800-465-7301 (in Canada only)
e-mail: humank@hkcanada.com

Europe: Human Kinetics, P.O. Box IW14, Leeds LS16 6TR, United Kingdom
(44) 1132 781708
e-mail: humank@hkeurope.com

Australia: Human Kinetics, 57A Price Avenue, Lower Mitcham, South Australia 5062
(088) 277 1555
e-mail: humank@hkaustralia.com

New Zealand: Human Kinetics, P.O. Box 105-231, Auckland 1
(09) 523 3462
e-mail: humank@hknewz.com

Preface

The first edition of this book, *Introduction to Research Methods in Health, Physical Education, Recreation, and Dance* (1985), and the second edition with a new title, *Research Methods in Physical Activity* (1990), were both well received by the graduate students and faculty at more than 150 institutions, mostly in the United States but also in several other countries. As we had anticipated (and noted in the previous prefaces), use of the book was mainly for the first graduate research methods course, which frequently is required of master's students. However, there was little use across the sometimes allied areas of health, recreation, and dance. Thus, the second edition focused directly on research methods associated with the study of physical activity as does this third edition. We intend the term *physical activity* to be inclusive and encompass exercise science, exercise and wellness, kinesiology, physical education, sport science, and sport studies to be certain that the discipline dealing with the study of physical activity and the professions frequently associated with it are reflected. We intend the contents of this book to apply conceptually to any aspect of the study of physical activity, whether in the context of exercise, sports, physical education instruction, industry, and so on.

This third edition is still designed for the beginning master's student enrolled in the first research methods course. Of course, we hope it is useful for everyone with an interest in conducting and understanding research on physical activity. Do not hesitate to buy a copy or two for your own use or as a gift for a friend (we need the money—retirement can be seen jogging toward us from the far distance; some say retirement is, or should be, running up

our backs). What a wonderful birthday, holiday, or anniversary gift a copy of this book would make. (Disclaimer: We take no responsibility for any divorce that results from using this book as an anniversary present.)

This third edition has been reorganized slightly from the first two editions. Part I provides a complete overview of the research process including developing the problem, using the library, preparing a prospectus, and understanding ethical issues in research and scholarship. Part II covers statistical and measurement concepts in research: descriptive, correlational, differences among groups, multivariate techniques, nonparametric procedures, and measurement issues associated with dependent variables. Part III presents various types of research: historical, philosophic, research synthesis, descriptive, experimental, and qualitative. Finally, Part IV provides information on preparing the research report: proposals, results and discussion, and ways of presenting the research. The appendices include statistical tables, a brief history of the field, suggested ways to deal with statistical analysis and the total process of writing research reports, and sample forms for securing permission to use human and animal subjects for research.

We have made a number of revisions to this third edition, all of which are improvements, we hope. Several individuals provided helpful reviews of the second edition in various journals; we carefully read and evaluated these, noting the positive and muttering under our breath about the negative. We can commiserate with Day (1983, p. xi), who had a reviewer describe his book "as 'both good and original.' Unfortunately, he went on to add that 'the part that is good is not original and the part that is original is not good.' " Many of you told us directly what you liked as well as things you would like to see changed, added, or deleted. (Note we have avoided the word *disliked*, as we know none of you disliked the second edition, although a few did remark disparagingly about our sense of humor or lack thereof.) Thus, in this edition we include some new jokes, funny figures and tables, and humorous sayings, as well as retaining the old ones that scored about 7 (scale 1-10) on the applause meter.

We have added more depth (and help, we hope) in chapter 2 on developing the research problem. Because of the increased need for consideration of ethical issues in research and scholarship, we have organized a new chapter (5) on that topic. Small parts and sections have been reorganized or added in the section on statistics (e.g., more on power, information on epidemiological statistics, how to establish equivalence between groups, a general means of handling nonparametric statistics). The separate part on measurement (three chapters) in the previous two editions has been integrated into a single chapter and placed in Part II.

Dr. Nancy Struna has revised her chapter on historical research (chapter 12), and Scott Kretchmar from Pennsylvania State University has contributed a new chapter on philosophic research (chapter 13). The excellent contributions of these two writers should serve to encourage more students with research interests in sport history and sport philosophy.

Much has been revised with some additions or deletions to the other chapters that were in the first and second editions and that remain in the new edition. The chapter on using the literature (chapter 2) has undergone a major revision, especially with regard to library work. We revised and updated the chapter on research synthesis (chapter 14), but we still included an example of meta-analytic procedures. We slightly revised the chapters on descriptive, experimental, and qualitative research. We no longer refer to the chapter format as the main way for organizing the thesis or dissertation; now we prefer the journal format. We advocated the journal format (called alternative in previous edition) in the earlier editions, but this has become a very popular way of organizing the thesis or dissertation. Thus, we now present the chapter format as the alternative structure.

Our approach to using statistics on the microcomputer has changed. In the first edition we supplied you with listings of statements for statistical microcomputer programs in the appendix as well as sample runs on problems in the book. In the second edition we provided statements (and sample printouts) on using SPSSPC and SPSSX. The software and hardware for statistical analysis is changing faster than we can revise this book. So in this edition, we provide a general discussion of the statistical approaches in Appendix C but no specific statements and examples. The procedures would have changed by the time the book was out and available.

We are also grateful to the Literary Executor of the late Sir Ronald A. Fisher, F.R.S., to Dr. Frank Yates, F.R.S., and to Longman Group Ltd., London for permissions to reprint Tables A.3 and A.5 from their book *Statistical Tables for Biological, Agricultural and Medical Research* (6th ed., 1974).

As we indicated in the first two editions, we have had a little help from our friends. As often as possible, we give credit through citation to the published literature. "But how about the many ideas and procedures that one has picked up from discussions with colleagues? After the passage of time, one can no longer remember who originated what idea. After the passage of even more time, it seems to me that all of the really good ideas originated with me, a proposition which I know is indefensible" (Day, 1983, p. xv).

We believe this book provides the necessary information for both the consumer and the producer of research. Although no amount of knowledge about the tools of research can replace expertise in the content area, it is unlikely that good scholars in the study of physical activity can function apart from the effective use of research tools. Researchers, teachers, technicians, counselors, and coaches need to understand the research process. If they do not, they are forced to accept information on face value or the recommendation of others. Although neither is necessarily bad, the ability to carefully evaluate and reach a valid conclusion is the mark of a professional.

We firmly believe that the topic of research need not be presented in a dry, pompous manner. As in any human enterprise, there are humorous occurrences. In fact, attempts at being overly dignified and scholarly lead to amusing and sometimes ludicrous results. Therefore, we have interjected a few anecdotes and sketches as well as some "laws" and "corollaries" to emphasize various points. We hope you will find them as enjoyable as we have in preparing them for this third edition. Our attempts at humor are designed to enliven the reading but not distract from the content. Research processes are not mysterious events that graduate students should fear. To the contrary, research processes are useful tools to which every professional should have access; they are, in fact, the very basis by which professionals make competent decisions.

Jerry R. Thomas

Jack K. Nelson

You Might Be A Graduate Student If . . .

Dear Potential Graduate Student:

Before you begin this book, it is necessary to determine if you are or have potential to be a graduate student. Score yourself one point for each of the following statements that applies to you.

YOU MIGHT BE A GRADUATE STUDENT IF

. . . your carrel is better decorated than your apartment.

. . . you have ever brought a scholarly article to a bar.

. . . you rate coffee shops by the availability of outlets for your laptop.

. . . you have ever discussed academic matters at a sporting event.

. . . you actually have a preference between microfilm and microfiche.

. . . you find the reference lists for articles more interesting than the actual text.

. . . you reflexively start analyzing those Greek letters before you realize that it's a sorority sweatshirt, not an equation.

. . . you find yourself explaining to children that you are in the "20th grade."

. . . you look forward to taking some time off to do laundry.

. . . you have more photocopy cards than credit cards.

. . . you start referring to stories like "Snow White et al."

. . . you wonder if APA style allows you to cite talking to yourself as a "personal communication."

Scoring Scale

> 5   probably a graduate student

> 8   definitely a master's student, maybe a doctoral student

>10   post-doctoral student

Humorously yours,

Professors of Research Methods

Acknowledgments

As in any work, there are numerous people who contribute and whom we should recognize. Many of these individuals are former students and colleagues who have said or done things that better developed our ideas as expressed in these pages. Also, a number of faculty who have used previous editions have either written reviews or made suggestions to us that have improved the book. While we cannot list or even recall all of these contributions, we do know you made them and we thank all of you.

In particular we thank Karen French, University of South Carolina, and Dick Magill, Louisiana State University, for allowing us to use materials that were published jointly with them. Scott Kretchmar and Nancy Struna made an invaluable contribution with their chapters on research methods in philosophy and history, topics that we simply could not write about effectively.

Finally, we thank our publisher, Rainer Martens at Human Kinetics, and Holly Gilly, our developmental editor for this edition, for their support and contributions. They have sharpened our thinking and improved our writing.

Jerry R. Thomas

Jack K. Nelson

How to Use This Book

We've included several new features in this edition in an attempt to make your life as a student easier.

 Map

There is a lot of information in this book. We've presented it in a logical order, but we do concede that while you're trying to glean all of our nuggets, you might get lost in the mine. We don't want you to lose the big picture because you're concentrating on the details. We've placed a map at the beginning of every new major section of text. It will show you how the information to follow is structured and how it relates to the rest of the information in that section.

 Key Word

Key words are defined where their first significant occurrence in the text appears. If you forget what a word means and need to refer back to the definition, use the index. Bold page numbers in the index indicate where a word is defined.

 Read

We included some suggested readings, cited alphabetically by author, at the ends of several of the chapters in our previous edition. We think giving you the citations for sources that can provide additional explanation or good examples of what we've covered is helpful. The problem with the standard end-of-chapter suggested reading list is that you often can't tell why a specific reading is suggested. In this edition, the suggested readings are signaled right next to the text that the reading will amplify.

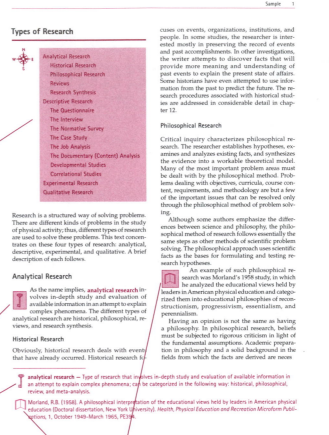

to indicate significant features. Finally, remember Thomas and Nelson's Five Laws of Oral Presentations (page 422). The way to avoid most of the problems associated with these laws is self-evident. One that may not be so obvious is practicing your presentation. We gather graduate students and faculty who are presenting papers at upcoming conferences and conduct practice sessions. Everyone presents her or his paper and has it timed. Then the audience asks questions and offers suggestions to clarify presentations and visual aids. Practice sessions improve the quality of the graduate students' presentations and strengthen their confidence.

Using a Poster Presentation to Its Best Advantage

The poster session is another way to present a conference paper. This involves the use of a large room in which presenters place summaries of their research on the wall or poster stands. The session is scheduled for a specific period, during which presenters stand by their work while anyone interested walks around, reads the material, and discusses items of interest with the presenters.

We prefer this format to oral presentations. The audience can look at the papers in which they are interested and have more detailed discussions with the authors. Within 75 minutes in a large room, 15-40 poster presentations can be made available. In contrast, 15-minute oral presentations allow only five presentations in 75 minutes. In addition, the audience must sit through several papers, often losing interest or creating a disturbance by arriving or leaving.

The presenter at a poster session should follow these guidelines:

- Know how much space is available for your materials (exact dimensions).
- Provide the necessary equipment for attaching your materials to the wall or poster board (even when the conference has indicated that supplies will be available).
- Mount your posters on contrasting backgrounds so they will be easily visible and will not blend into the backboards.
- Use figures and graphs where possible (as opposed to text and tables).
- Use large lettering for all text, numbers, and labels.

🔆 Guidelines for poster presentations

Clearly label the six parts of the poster presentation: introduction, statement of the problem, method, results (with figures and graphs), discussion and conclusions, and important references.

Summary

The journal format for theses and dissertations has the advantage of being in the form for journal publication, one of the main ways used to evaluate scholarly work. Yet it retains the essential characteristics of the complete reporting that is so valued in the thesis and dissertation. This format comprises preliminary materials (e.g., title page, abstract), the body (e.g., introduction, method, results, discussion), and a set of appendices (e.g., extended literature review, additional results). The goal of this reporting style is to promote rapid publication of quality research.

Abstracts are frequently used as a form for submitting papers to scholarly meetings so they can be evaluated for possible presentation. Usually the abstract is limited in length and form according to the format prescribed by the scholarly group to whom it is submitted. If the abstract paper is accepted for presentation, the form may be oral or poster. Oral presentations usually last 10 to 20 minutes, and poster presentations are typically limited to a specific display space.

 Check Your Understanding

1. Writing: Select a study from a journal and write a 150-word abstract in APA style (or whatever style your department uses).
2. Oral presentations: To emphasize the importance of time limits on oral presentations, we suggest that the professor organize the following presentations in class:
   a. Have each student select a published research study and present a 2-minute summary.
   b. Do the same with another study, but give a 5-minute summary.
3. Poster presentation: Have each student prepare a poster presentation of a research study

 ## Major Concept

A lightbulb signals an important concept in the text. The phrase with the lightbulb names the concept. We use these "major concept" elements to summarize lists and to highlight main ideas. Where more than one concept appears on a page, the concepts are listed in the order in which the lightbulbs appeared.

✔ Check Your Understanding

It's always a good idea to practice using the information you've learned. The problems at the ends of the chapters will help you gauge how well you understand the material. Your instructor has the answers to the questions.

After you've finished reading a chapter you can use the features to check how thoroughly you've internalized the information. Go through the maps and see if you can remember the main points of the discussion under each heading. Read the major concept phrases and try to state the information they summarize. Check yourself on the key words. Do you know what they mean? Do you need further explanation on any topic? If so, see if there is a suggested reading for it.

The *Major Concept, Key Word,* and *Read* icons appear at the beginning of some paragraphs. A corresponding icon, which outlines the major concept, defines the key word, or supplies the reference for the suggested reading, appears at the bottom of the same page. If a paragraph with an icon starts on one page but finishes on another, the corresponding icon will appear on the page on which the paragraph began. However, the actual major concept, key word, or suggested reading may appear in text on the following page. This may sound confusing now, but it will become clear as you read the book.

Chapter Introductions

We occasionally receive letters from students and faculty members concerning various aspects of research methods. Often the letters contain some humorous items that they have run across and think we would appreciate. Consequently, we thought we would introduce each chapter with a fictitious letter that relates (albeit sometimes vaguely) to that chapter. Some of the replies contain some serious comments, and some try to make a point in a lighter vein. We hope you enjoy them.

PART

Overview of the Research Process

This part provides you with an overall perspective of the research process. The introductory chapter defines and reviews the various types of research done in exercise and sport science and physical education and gives you some examples. We define science as systematic inquiry, and we discuss the steps in the scientific method. This logical method answers the following four questions (Day, 1983, p. 4), which constitute the parts of a typical thesis report:

1. What was the problem? Your answer is the Introduction.
2. How did you study the problem? Your answer is the Materials and Methods.
3. What did you find? Your answer is the Results.
4. What do these findings mean? Your answer is the Discussion.

We also present alternative approaches for doing research relative to a more philosophical discussion of science and ways of knowing. In particular, we address qualitative research, the use of field studies, and methods of introspection as strategies in answering research questions instead of relying on the traditional scientific paradigm as the only approach to research problems.

Chapter 2 suggests ways of developing a problem and using the literature to clarify the research problem, specify hypotheses, and develop the methodology. In particular, we propose a system for searching, reading, analyzing, synthesizing, organizing, and writing the review of literature.

The next two chapters in Part I present the format of the research proposal with examples. This information is typically required of the master's or doctoral student before collecting data for the thesis or dissertation. Chapter 3 defines and delimits the research problem, including the introduction, statement of the problem, research hypotheses, operational definitions, assumptions and limitations, and significance. Chapter 4 covers methodology, or how to do the research. Included are the topics of subject selection, instrumentation or apparatus, procedures, and design and analysis. We emphasize the value of pilot work conducted before the research and how cause and effect may be established.

Chapter 5 discusses ethical issues in research and scholarship. We include information on misconduct in science; ethical considerations in research writing, working with advisors, and copyright; and the use of human and animal subjects in research.

Once you have completed Part I, you should better understand the research process. Then comes the tricky part: learning all the details. We consider these details in Part II (Statistical and Measurement Concepts in Research), Part III (Types of Research), and Part IV (Writing the Research Report).

CHAPTER 1

Introduction to Research in Physical Activity

Dear Professors of Research Methods:

I don't understand why I have to buy this stupid book for my research methods class. What is there to learn about research methods anyway? I want to be a sport psychologist.

Sincerely,
I. Wanda Psycum

Dear Psycum:

The only thing you can learn from research methods books (and sport psychology books) is that you can't learn anything from research methods books, but you have to buy THIS research methods book to learn it.

Methodologically yours,
PRM

Mention the word "research" to people and, depending on their backgrounds, each will conjure up a different picture in his or her mind. One might think of going to the nearest encyclopedia; another might visualize a lab filled with test tubes, vials, and Bunsen burners. It is important, then, when beginning a text on the subject, to establish a common understanding of research. In this chapter we introduce you to the nature of research. We do this by discussing methods of problem solving and types of research. We explain the research process and relate it to the parts of a thesis. By the time you reach the end of chapter 1, you should understand what research really involves.

The Nature of Research

Research Continuum
Research for the Consumer
    Practicality and Accessibility
    Reading Research
How to Read Research
    An Example of Practical Research
    Summarizing the Nature of Research

The object of research is to determine how things are as compared to how they might be. To achieve this, research implies a careful and systematic means of solving problems and involves five characteristics (Tuckman, 1978):

• **Systematic**. Problem solving is accomplished through the identification and labeling of variables and is followed by the design of research that tests the relationships among these variables. Data are then collected that, when related to the variables, allow for the evaluation of the problem and hypotheses.

• **Logical**. Examination of the procedures used in the research process allows researchers to evaluate the conclusions drawn.

• **Empirical**. The researcher collects data on which to base decisions.

• **Reductive**. Research takes individual events (data) and uses them to establish general relationships.

• **Replicable**. The research process is recorded, enabling others to test the findings by repeating the research or to build future research on previous results.

Problems to be solved come from many sources and can entail resolving controversial issues, testing theories, and trying to improve present practice. For example, a popular topic of concern is obesity and methods of losing weight. Suppose we want to investigate this by comparing two exercise programs as to their effectiveness in reducing fat. Of course, we know that caloric expenditure will result in the loss of fat, so we will try to find out which program will do this better under specified conditions. (Note: Our approach here is to give a simple, concise overview of a research study. We do not intend it to be a model of originality or sophistication.)

This study is definitely an example of applied research (more on this in the next section). Rather than try to measure the calories expended and so on, we approach it strictly from a programmatic standpoint. Say that we are operating a health club and that we offer aerobic dance and jogging classes for people who want to lose weight. Our research question is: Which program is more effective in reducing fat?

Suppose that we have a pool of subjects to draw from and that we can randomly assign two thirds of the subjects to the two exercise programs and one third to a control group. We have their scout's honor that no one is on a drastic diet or engaging in any other strenuous activities while the study is in progress. Both the aerobic dance and the jogging classes are one hour long and are held five times a week for 10 weeks. The same enthusiastic and immensely qualified instructor teaches both classes.

Our measure of fatness is the sum of skinfold measurements taken at eight body sites. Of course, we could use other measures such as percentage of fat estimated from **hydrostatic weighing** (or total body water or some other estimate of fatness). However, we can defend our measures as valid and reliable indicators of fat-

---

Five characteristics of careful problem solving

hydrostatic weighing — Technique that measures body composition in which body density is computed by the ratio of an individual's weight in air and the loss of weight underwater.

ness, and skinfolds are functional field measures. We will measure all the subjects, including the control subjects, at the beginning and the end of the 10-week period. During the study we will try to ensure that the two programs are similar in procedural aspects such as motivational techniques and the aesthetics of the surroundings. In other words, we will not favor one group by cheering them on and not saying anything encouraging to the other; nor will we have one group exercising in an air-conditioned, cheerful, and healthful facility while the other has to sweat it out in some dingy room or parking lot. It is very important that we try to make the programs as similar as possible in every respect except the experimental treatments. The control group will not engage in any regular exercise.

So, after we have measured all the subjects on our criterion of fatness, we are ready to analyze our data. We want to see how much change in skinfold thickness has occurred and whether there are differences between the two types of exercise. Because we are dealing with samples of people (from a whole universe of similar people), we need to use some type of statistics to establish how confident we can be in our results. In other words, we need to determine the significance of our results. Suppose the mean scores for the groups are as follows:

- Aerobic dance = –21 mm
- Jogging = –25 mm
- Control = +8 mm

These values (which we made up) represent the average change in the combined skinfold thicknesses of the eight body sites. The two experimental groups lost fat, but the control group actually showed increased skinfold thicknesses over the 10-week period.

We decide to use the statistical technique of analysis of variance with repeated measures. We find a significant F ratio, indicating that significant differences exist among the three groups. Using a follow-up test procedure, we discover that both exercise groups are significantly different from the control group. But we find no significant difference between the aerobic dance and the jogging groups.

(Many of you may not have the foggiest idea what we are talking about with the statistical terms F ratio and significance, but don't worry about it. All this is explained later. This book is about these kinds of things.)

Our conclusion from this study is that both aerobic dance and jogging are effective (apparently equally so) in bringing about a loss in fatness of overweight subjects (like the ones in our study) over 10 weeks. Although these results are reasonable, please remember that this is only an example. We can also pretend that this study was published in a prestigious journal and that we won the Nobel Prize.

Research Continuum

 Research in our field can be placed on a continuum with **applied research** at one extreme and **basic research** at the opposite extreme. The research extremes have certain characteristics generally associated with them. Applied research tends to address immediate problems, to use so-called real-world settings, to use human subjects, and to have limited control over the research setting but to give results that are of direct value to practitioners. At the other extreme, basic research usually deals with theoretical problems. It uses the laboratory as the setting, frequently uses animals as subjects, carefully controls conditions, and produces results that have limited direct application. Christina (1989) suggested basic and applied forms of research were useful in informing each other as to future research directions. Table 1.1 demonstrates how research problems in motor learning might vary along a basic to applied continuum depending on their goal and approach.

 To some extent the strengths of applied research are the weaknesses of basic research, and vice versa. Considerable

---

 Applied research versus basic research

 applied research — Type of research that has direct value to practitioners but in which the researcher has limited control over the research setting.

basic research — Type of research that may have limited direct application but in which the researcher has careful control of the conditions.

 ecological validity — The extent to which research emulates the real world.

Table 1.1   Levels of Relevance of Motor Learning Research for Finding Solutions to Practical Problems in Sport

Level 1 Least direct relevance Basic research	Level 2 Moderate direct relevance Applied research	Level 3 Most direct relevance Applied research
Ultimate goal Develop theory-based knowledge appropriate for understanding motor learning in general with no requirement to demonstrate its relevance for solving practical problems.	Ultimate goal Develop theory-based knowledge appropriate for understanding the learning of sport skills in sport settings with no requirement to find immediate solutions to learning problems in sport.	Ultimate goal Find immediate solutions to learning problems in sport with no requirement to demonstrate or develop theory-based knowledge at either Level 1 or Level 2.
Main approach Test hypotheses in a laboratory setting using experimenter-designed motor tasks	Main approach Test hypotheses in a sport setting or in a laboratory setting similar to it using sport skills or motor tasks that have properties of those skills.	Main approach Test solutions to specific learning problems in sport in the settings described under the applied research at Level 2.

From "Whatever Happened to Applied Research in Motor Learning?" by R.W. Christina. In *Future Directions in Exercise and Sport Science Research* (p. 418) by J.S. Skinner et al. (Eds.), 1989, Champaign, IL: Human Kinetics. Copyright 1989 by James S. Skinner. Reprinted with permission.

controversy exists in the literature on psychology, education, and physical activity (for examples see Christina, 1989; Martens, 1979, 1987; Siedentop, 1980; Thomas, 1980) about whether research should be more basic or more applied. This issue, labeled **ecological validity**, deals with two concerns: Is the research setting perceived by the subject in the way intended by the experimenter? Does the setting have enough of the real-world characteristics to allow for generalizing to reality?

Of course, most research is neither purely applied nor purely basic but incorporates some degree of both. We believe that systematic efforts are needed in the study of physical activity to produce research that moves back and forth across Christina's (1989) levels of research (Table 1.1). Excellent summaries of this type of research and the accumulated knowledge are provided in three edited volumes representing exercise physiology, sport psychology, and motor behavior: *Physical Activity, Fitness, and Health, Handbook of Research on Sport Psychology*, and *Cognitive Issues in Motor Expertise*. An expert prepared each chapter in these recent books to summarize theories as well as basic and applied research about areas related to exercise physiology, motor expertise, and sport psychology. The novice researcher would do well to read several of these chapters as examples of how knowledge is developed and accumulated in the study of physical activity. We need more efforts to produce a related body of knowledge in the study of physical activity. Although the research base has grown tremendously in our field over the past 20 years, much remains to be done.

There is a great need to prepare proficient consumers and producers of research. To be proficient requires a thorough understanding of the appropriate knowledge base (e.g., exercise physiology, motor behavior, pedagogy, and the social and bio-

Christina, R.W. (1989). Whatever happened to applied research in motor learning? In J.S. Skinner et al. (Eds.), *Future directions in exercise and sport science research* (pp. 411-422). Champaign, IL: Human Kinetics.

Martens, R. (1979). About smocks and jocks. *Journal of Sport Psychology*, 1, 94-99.

Martens, R. (1987). Science, knowledge, and sport psychology. *Sport Psychologist*, 1, 29-55.

Bouchard, C., Shepard, R.J., & Stephens, T. (Eds.) (1994). *Physical activity, fitness, and health*. Champaign, IL: Human Kinetics.

Singer, R.N., Murphey, M., & Tennant, L.K. (Eds.) (1993). *Handbook of research on sport psychology*. New York: Macmillian.

Starkes, J.L., & Allard, F. (Eds.) (1993). *Cognitive issues in motor expertise*. Amsterdam: North Holland.

logical sciences) as well as research methods. In this book we attempt to explain the tools necessary to consume and produce research. Many of the same methods are used in the various areas of physical education, exercise science, and sports science (as well as in psychology, sociology, education, and physiology). Quality research efforts always involve some or all of the following components:

- Identification and delimitation of a problem
- Searching, reviewing, and effectively writing about relevant literature
- Specifying and defining testable hypotheses
- Designing the research to test the hypotheses
- Selecting, describing, testing, and treating the subjects
- Analyzing and reporting the results
- Discussing the meaning and implications of the findings

Research for the Consumer

We recognize that not everyone will be a researcher. Many people in our profession have little interest in research per se. In fact, some have a decided aversion to it. Researchers are sometimes viewed as strange people who deal with insignificant problems and who are out of touch with the real world (we know that none of you feel that way). In a very informative yet entertaining book on writing scientific papers, Day (1983) related the story about two men who, while riding in a hot-air balloon, encountered some cloud coverage and lost their way. When they finally descended, they did not recognize the terrain and had not the faintest idea where they were. It so happened that they were drifting over the grounds of one of our more famous scientific research institutes. When the balloonists saw a man walking alongside a road, one of them called out, "Hey, mister, where are we?" The man looked up, took in the situation, and after a few moments of reflection said, "You're in a hot-air balloon." One balloonist turned to the other and said, "I'll bet that man is a researcher." The other balloonist said, "What makes you think so?" The first replied, "His answer is perfectly accurate and totally useless" (p. 152).

Practicality and Accessibility

All kidding aside, the need for research in any profession just cannot be argued. After all, one of the primary distinctions between a discipline or profession and a trade is that the trade deals only with how to do something, whereas the discipline or profession concerns itself not only with "how" but also with "why" something should be done in a certain manner (and why it should even be done). However, even though most people in a discipline or profession recognize the need for research, most of those people do not read research results. This situation is not unique to our field. It has been reported that only 1% of chemists read research publications, fewer than 7% of psychologists read psychological research journals, and so on. The big question is why. We would guess that most professionals who do not read research believe that doing so is not necessary. The research is not practical enough or does not directly pertain to one's work. Another reason given by practitioners for not reading research publications is that they cannot understand them. The language is too technical and the terminology unfamiliar and confusing. This is a valid complaint; we could argue, however, that if the professional preparation programs were more scientifically oriented, this would not be such a problem. Nevertheless, the research literature is extremely difficult for the nonresearcher to understand.

Someone once said that a scientific paper was not meant to be read but was meant to be published. Unfortunately, we find considerable truth in that observation. We, as writers, are often guilty of trying to use language to dazzle the reader and perhaps to give the impression that our subject matter is more esoteric than it really is. We tend to write for the benefit of a rather small number of readers, that is, other researchers in our particular field. We have the problem of jargon, of course. In any field, whether it is physics, football, or cake baking, jargon confounds the outsider. The use of jargon serves as a kind of shorthand. It provides meaning to the people within the field because everyone uses those words in the same context. Research literature is famous for using a three-dollar word when a nickel word would do. As Day (1983, p. 147) asked, what self-respecting writer would use a three-letter word like "now" when one can use the elegant expression "at this point in time"? Researchers

---

 Components of quality research efforts

 Day, R.D. (1983). *How to write and publish a scientific paper* (2nd ed.). Philadelphia: ISI Press.

never "do" anything, they "perform" it; they never "start," they "initiate"; and they "terminate" instead of "end." Day further remarked that an occasional author will slip and use the word "drug," but most will salivate like Pavlov's dogs in anticipation of using "chemotherapeutic agent."

Reading Research

For years there has been a recognized need to try to bridge the gap between the researcher and the practitioner. The American Alliance for Health, Physical Education, Recreation and Dance (AAHPERD) launched a series of publications entitled *What Research Tells the Coach* [of a particular sport]. *The Journal of Physical Education, Recreation and Dance* has a feature called "Research Works," which is designed to disseminate applied research information to teachers, coaches, and fitness and recreation leaders. Yet despite these and other attempts to bridge the gap, the gap is still imposing.

It goes without saying that if one is not knowledgeable about the subject matter, one cannot read the research literature. Conversely, if you know the subject matter, you can probably wade through the researcher's jargon more effectively. For example, if you know baseball and the researcher is recommending that by shortening the radius one can increase the angular velocity, you can figure out that the researcher means to choke up on the bat.

One of the big stumbling blocks is the statistical analysis part of research reports. Even the most ardent seeker of knowledge can be turned off by such descriptions as this: "The tetrachoric correlations among the test variables were subjected to a centroid factor analysis, and orthogonal rotations of the primary axes were accomplished by Zimmerman's graphical method until simple structure and positive manifold were closely approximated." Please note that we are not criticizing the authors for such descriptions, as the reviewers and editors require them. We are just acknowledging that it is frightening to someone who is trying to read a research article and who does not know a factor analysis from a volleyball. The widespread use of computers and computerese probably compounds the mystique associated with statistics. Many people believe anything that comes out of a computer. Others are more old-fashioned and check the computer's accuracy with their calculators. A classic case of a computer mistake occurred in a high school where the computer printed the students' locker numbers in the column where their IQs were supposed to go. It is classic because no one noticed the error at the time, but at the end of the year the students with the highest locker numbers got the best grades.

How to Read Research

Despite all the hurdles that loom in the practitioner's path with regard to reading research, we contend that one can read and profit (not materially, unfortunately) from the research literature even if he or she is not well grounded in research techniques and statistical analysis. We would like to contend that after you read this book you can read any journal in any field, but the publisher would not let us. Thus, we offer the following suggestions to the practitioner on reading the research literature.

 • **Become familiar with a few publications that contain pertinent research in your field.** You might get some help on this from a professor or librarian.

• **Read only studies that are of interest to you.** That may sound too trite to mention, but some people feel obligated to wade through every article.

• **Read it as a practitioner would.** Don't look for eternal truths. Look for ideas and indications. No study is proof of anything. Only when it has been verified time and again does it constitute knowledge.

• **Read the abstract first.** This will save time by helping you determine whether you wish to read the whole thing. If you are still interested, then you can read the study to better understand the methodology and the interpretations, but do not get bogged down with details.

• **Do not be too concerned about statistical significance.** It certainly helps to understand the concept of significance, but a little common sense will serve you about as well as knowing the difference between the .02 and the .01 levels, or a one-tailed test versus a two-tailed test. Think in terms of meaningfulness. For example, if two methods of teaching bowling result in an average difference of 0.5 pins, what difference does it make whether it is significant? On the other hand, if there is a big difference that is not significant, further investigation is warranted, especially if the study involved a small number of subjects. It is certainly helpful to know the concepts of the different types of statistical analysis, but it is not crucial to being able to read a study. Just skip that part.

- **Be critical but objective.** You can usually assume that a national research journal selects studies for publication by the jury method. Two or three qualified individuals read and judge the relevance of the problem, the validity and reliability of the procedures, the efficacy of the experimental design, and the appropriateness of the statistical analysis. It is true that some studies are published that should not be. Yet if you are not an expert in research, you do not need to be suspicious about the scientific worth of a study that appears in a recognized journal. If it is too far removed from any practical application to your situation, do not read it.

You will find that the more you read, the easier it becomes to understand, simply because you become more familiar with the language and the methodology. It is like the man who was thrilled to learn he had been speaking prose all his life.

An Example of Practical Research

To illustrate our research consumer suggestions, consider the lighthearted account of a young physical education teacher and coach named Sonjia Roundball (Nelson, 1988). In a moment of weakness, Sonjia glanced through the table of contents of the *Research Quarterly for Exercise and Sport,* which had been left in her car by a graduate student friend of hers (they had used it to keep their tacos from dripping on the upholstery). She experienced a spark of interest when she noticed an article entitled "The Effects of a Season of Basketball on the Cardiorespiratory Responses of High School Girls." With some curiosity, she turned to the article and began to read. In its introductory passages, the article stated that relatively little specific information was available on the physiological changes in girls due to sport participation. A short review of literature cited a few studies on swimmers and other sport participants, and the upshot was that women athletes possess higher levels of cardiorespiratory fitness than do non-athletes. The author emphasized that no studies had tried to detect changes in girls' fitness during a season of basketball.

The next section of the study dealt with methods. It noted the length of the season, the number of games, the number of practices and their length, and the breakdown in terms of the amount of time devoted to drills, scrimmaging, and individual practice. The

subjects were 12 girls on the high school basketball team (the participants) and 14 girls in the nonparticipant group who were from physical education classes and who had similar academic and activity schedules as the participants. All subjects were tested at the beginning and end of the season on maximal oxygen consumption and various other physiological measurements dealing with ventilation, heart rate, and blood pressure. Sonjia remembered those things from her exercise physiology course a number of years ago and was willing to accept these as good indicators of cardiorespiratory fitness.

The results were then presented in tables. She did not understand these things but was willing to trust the authors as to their appropriateness. The author discovered no significant increases in any of the cardiorespiratory measures from the preseason test to the postseason test for either group. This jolted Sonjia to the quick! Surely, a strenuous sport such as basketball should produce improvements in fitness. Something must be wrong here, she thought. She further read (with small consolation) that the basketball players had higher values of maximal oxygen consumption than the nonparticipants at both the beginning and the end of the season. Sonjia then read the discussion, which mentioned things like the values being higher than similar values in other studies. (So what? Sonjia thought.) She read with more interest the observations by the authors that boys' basketball programs were more strenuous in terms of length and number of workouts. Sonjia began to think about this. The authors admitted that the number of subjects was small and that they might not detect some changes, and they offered other speculations. They concluded, however, that the training program used in this study was not strenuous enough to induce significant improvement in cardiorespiratory fitness.

Sonjia was sophisticated enough to realize the limitations of one study. Nevertheless, it was very similar to her schedule and general practice routines. She noticed in the references for the article three studies from a journal called *Medicine and Science in Sports and Exercise.* She had never read this journal, but she decided to drive over to the university the next weekend to look up this publication in the library. When she located the journal, the latest issue happened to have an article on conditioning effects of swimming on college women. Although this was a different sport and a different age-group, she reasoned that the review of literature might prove fruitful. She was right. It cited a recent study on aerobic capacity, heart rate, and energy cost during a season of girls' basketball.

Sonjia quickly located this study and now read with the excitement that comes from the personal discovery of ideas. She also was pleasantly surprised to find that it was easier reading than the first study because she was now more familiar with the terminology and the general organization of the article.

This study also reported no improvement in aerobic capacity during the season. It involved monitoring heart rates during games by telemetry, and researchers frequently observed heart rates of over 170 beats per minute (bpm). They concluded that the practice sessions were apparently too moderate in intensity and that the training should be structured to meet both the skill and the fitness demands of the sport.

Sonjia returned to her school determined to take a more scientific approach to her basketball program. To start with, she had one of her managers chart the number of minutes that players were actually engaged in movement in the practice sessions. Sonjia also had the players take their pulses at various intervals during the sessions. She was surprised to find that the heart rates rarely surpassed 130 bpm. As an outgrowth of her recent literature search, she remembered that there is an intensity threshold necessary to bring about improvement in cardiorespiratory fitness. She knew that for this age-group a heart rate of about 160 bpm was needed to provide a significant training effect. Consequently, she initiated some changes in her practice sessions (including more conditioning drills) and made the scrimmages more intensive and gamelike. To end this saga of Sonjia, you will be happy to know that Coach Roundball's team went on to win all its games, the district and the state championships, and the world games.

Summarizing the Nature of Research

Thomas Huxley wrote that science is simply common sense at its best. Moments of discovery can be very rewarding, whether that discovery is finding research that applies to your situation and can improve it, or discovering new knowledge through the research of your thesis or dissertation. Research should be viewed more as a method of problem solving than as some dark and mysterious realm inhabited by impractical people who speak and write in baffling terms. We think practitioners can

read research literature, and we are dedicated in this text to trying to facilitate the process of becoming a research consumer.

Unscientific and Scientific Methods of Problem Solving

Some Unscientific Methods of Problem Solving

Tenacity

Intuition

Authority

The Rationalistic Method

The Empirical Method

The Scientific Method of Problem Solving

Step 1: Developing the Problem (Defining and Delimiting It)

Step 2: Formulating the Hypothesis

Step 3: Gathering the Data

Step 4: Analyzing and Interpreting Results

Although there are many definitions of research, nearly all characterize research activity as some sort of structured problem solving. The word "structured" refers to the fact that a number of research techniques can be used as long as the techniques are considered acceptable by scholars in the field. Thus, research is concerned with problem solving, which then may lead to new knowledge.

 The problem-solving process involves several steps whereby the problem is developed, defined, and delimited; hypotheses are formulated; data are gathered and analyzed; and the results are interpreted with regard to the acceptance or rejection of the hypotheses. These steps are often referred to as the **scientific method of problem solving**. The steps also constitute the chapters, or sections, of the research paper, thesis, and dissertation. Consequently, we devote much of this text to the specific ways these steps are accomplished.

---

scientific method of problem solving — Method of solving problems in which the following steps are used: developing a problem, defining and delimiting the problem, forming a hypothesis, gathering data, analyzing data, and interpreting the results.

Some Unscientific Methods of Problem Solving

Before we go into more detail concerning the scientific method of problem solving, it is important to recognize some other ways by which humankind has acquired knowledge. All of us have used these methods, so they are recognizable. Helmstadter (1970) labeled the methods as tenacity, intuition, authority, the rationalistic method, and the empirical method.

Tenacity

 People sometimes cling to certain beliefs despite the lack of supporting evidence. Our superstitions are good examples of this method called **tenacity**. Coaches and athletes are notoriously superstitious. A coach may wear a particular sport coat, hat, tie, or shoes because the team won the last time he wore it. Athletes frequently have a set pattern that they consider lucky for dressing, warming up, or entering the stadium. Even though they acknowledge no logical relationship between the game's outcome and the particular routine, they are afraid to break the pattern.

Take, for example, the man who believed that black cats brought bad luck. One night when he was returning to his ranch, a black cat started to cross the road. The man swerved off onto the prairie to keep the cat from crossing in front of him and hit a hard bump that caused the headlights to go off. Unable to see the black cat in the dark night, he sped frantically over rocks, mounds, and holes until he came to a sudden stop in a ravine, wrecking his car and sustaining moderate injuries. Of course, this just confirmed his staunch belief that black cats do indeed bring bad luck. Obviously, tenacity has no place in science. It is the least reliable source of knowledge.

Intuition

Intuitive knowledge is sometimes considered to be common sense or self-evident. However, many self-evident truths are subsequently found to be false. That the earth is flat is a classic example of the intuitively obvious; that the sun is farther away in winter than in summer was once self-evident; that no one could run a mile in less than 4 minutes once was self-evident. Furthermore, for anyone to shot put more than 70 feet or pole-vault more than 18 feet or for a woman to run distances over a half-mile was impossible. One fundamental tenet of science is that we must be ever cognizant of the importance of substantiating our convictions with factual evidence.

Authority

Reference to some authority has long been used as a source of knowledge. Although this is not necessarily invalid, it does depend on the authority and on the rigidity of adherence. However, the appeal to authority has been carried to absurd lengths. Even personal observation and experience have been deemed unacceptable when they dispute authority. Supposedly, people refused to look through Galileo's telescope when he disputed Ptolemy's explanation of the world and of the heavens. Galileo was later jailed and forced to recant his beliefs. Bruno also rejected Ptolemy's theory and was burned at the stake. (Scholars read and believed Ptolemy's book on astrology and astronomy for 1,200 years after his death!) In 1543, Vesalius wrote

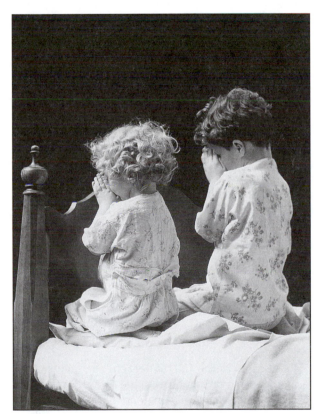

If you're going to appeal to authority, make sure the authority has impeccable qualifications.

---

tenacity — An unscientific method of problem solving in which people cling to certain beliefs regardless of the lack of supporting evidence.

a book on anatomy, much of which is still considered correct today. However, because his work clashed with Galen's theories, he met with such ridicule that he gave up his study of anatomy.

Perhaps the most crucial aspect of the appeal to authority as a means of obtaining knowledge is the right to question and to accept or reject the information. Furthermore, the authority's qualifications and the methods by which the authority acquired the knowledge also determine the validity of this source of information.

The Rationalistic Method

In the rationalistic method, we derive knowledge through reasoning. A good example is the following classic syllogism:

All men are mortal. (major premise)

The emperor is a man. (minor premise)

Therefore, the emperor is mortal. (conclusion)

Although you probably would not argue with this reasoning, the key to this method is the truth of the premises and their relationship to each other. For example,

Basketball players are tall.

Tom Thumb is a basketball player.

Therefore, Tom Thumb is tall.

In this case, however, Tom Thumb is very short. The conclusion is trustworthy only if derived from premises (assumptions) that are true. Also, the premises may not in fact be premises but rather descriptions of events or statements of fact. The statements are not connected in a cause-and-effect manner. For example,

There is a positive correlation between shoe size and mathematics performance among elementary school children (i.e., children with large shoe sizes do well in math).

Herman is in elementary school and wears large shoes.

Therefore, Herman is good in mathematics.

Of course, in the first statement the factor common to both mathematics achievement and shoe size is age. Older children tend to be bigger and thus have bigger feet than younger children. Older

children also have higher achievement scores in mathematics, but there is no cause-and-effect relationship. You must always be cognizant of this when dealing with correlation. Reasoning is fundamental in the scientific method of problem solving but cannot be used by itself to arrive at knowledge.

The Empirical Method

 The word **empirical** denotes experience and the gathering of data. Certainly, data gathering is part of the scientific method of solving problems. However, there can be pitfalls in relying too much on your own experience (or data). First, your own experience is very limited. Furthermore, your retention depends substantially on how the events agree with your past experience and beliefs, on whether things "make sense," and on your state of motivation to remember. Nevertheless, the use of data (and the empirical method) is high on the continuum of methods of obtaining knowledge as long as you are aware of the limitations of relying too heavily on this method.

The Scientific Method of Problem Solving

 The methods of acquiring knowledge previously discussed lack the objectivity and control that characterize the scientific approach to problem solving. Several basic steps are involved in the scientific method. Some authors list seven or eight steps, and others condense these steps into three or four. Nevertheless, all the authors are in general agreement as to the sequence and processes that are involved. The steps are briefly described next. Greater detail concerning the basic processes are covered in other chapters.

Step 1: Developing the Problem (Defining and Delimiting It)

This step may sound a bit contradictory, for how could the development of the problem be a part of solving it? Actually, the discussion here is not about finding a problem to study (ways of locating a problem are discussed in chapter 2); the assumption is that the researcher has already selected a topic. However, to design and execute a sound investigation, the researcher must be very specific

---

 empirical — Describes data or a study that is based on objective observations.

 Steps in the scientific method of problem solving

about what is to be studied and to what extent it will be studied.

Many ramifications constitute this step, an important one being the identification of the independent and the dependent variables. The **independent variable** is what the researcher is manipulating. If, for example, two methods of teaching a motor skill are being compared, then the teaching method is the independent variable; this is sometimes called the experimental, or treatment, variable.

The **dependent variable** is the effect of the independent variable. In the comparison of teaching methods, the measure of skill is the dependent variable. If you think of an experiment as a cause-and-effect proposition, the cause is the independent variable and the effect is the dependent variable. The latter is sometimes referred to as the yield. Thus, the researcher must define exactly what will be studied and what will be the measured effect. When this is resolved, the experimental design can be determined.

Step 2: Formulating the Hypothesis

The **hypothesis** is the expected result. When a person sets out to conduct a study, he or she generally has an idea as to what the outcome will be. This anticipated solution to the problem may be based on some theoretical construct, on the results of previous studies, or perhaps on the experimenter's past experience and observations. The last source is probably least likely or defensible because of the weaknesses of the unscientific methods of acquiring knowledge discussed previously. Regardless, the research should have some experimental hypothesis about each subproblem in the study.

We enjoy "Calvin and Hobbes," the cartoon strip by Bill Watterson. In a clever strip, Calvin is talking to his friend Susie in the lunch room:

Calvin: Curiosity is the essence of the scientific mind. For example, you know how milk comes out your nose if you laugh while drinking? Well, I'm going to see what happens when I inhale milk into my nose and laugh!

Susie (as she leaves):   Idiocy is the essence of the male mind.

Calvin: I'm guessing it will shoot out my ears. Don't you want to see??

Calvin has developed a testable hypothesis: "If I inhale milk into my nose and laugh, it will shoot out of my ears."

Susie has an untestable hypothesis (at least in our view): "Idiocy is the essence of the male mind."

One of the essential features about the hypothesis is that it be "testable." The study must be designed in such a way that the hypothesis can be either supported or refuted. It should be obvious to you, then, that the hypothesis cannot be a type of value judgment or an abstract phenomenon that cannot be observed.

For example, you might hypothesize that success in athletics is dependent solely on fate. In other words, if a team wins, it is because it was meant to be; similarly, if a team loses, it was just not meant to be. There is no way to refute this hypothesis because there is no evidence that could be obtained to test it.

Step 3: Gathering the Data

Of course, before step 2 can be accomplished, the researcher must decide on the proper methods of acquiring the necessary data to be used in testing the research hypotheses. The reliability of the measuring instruments, the controls that are employed, and the overall objectivity and precision of the data-gathering process are crucial to the problem's solution.

In terms of difficulty, gathering data may be the easiest step because in many cases it is routine. However, planning the method is one of the most difficult steps. Good methods attempt to maximize both the **internal validity** and the **external validity** of the study.

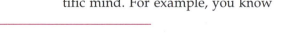

independent variable — The part of the experiment that the researcher is manipulating; also called the *experimental* or *treatment variable.*

dependent variable — The effect of the independent variable; also called the *yield.*

hypothesis — The anticipated outcome of a study or experiment.

internal validity — The extent to which the results of a study can be attributed to the treatments used in the study.

external validity — The generalizability of the results of a study.

Internal validity and external validity relate to the research design and controls that are used. Internal validity refers to the extent to which the results can be attributed to the treatments used in this study. In other words, the researcher must try to control all other variables that could influence the results. For example, Jim Nasium wants to scientifically assess the effectiveness of his exercise program in developing physical fitness in young boys. He tests his participants at the beginning and then at the end of a 9-month training program and concludes that the program brought about significant improvement in fitness. What is wrong with Jim's conclusion? His study contains several flaws. The first is that Jim gave no consideration to maturity. Nine months of maturation produced significant changes in size and in accompanying strength and endurance. Also, what else were the participants doing during this time? How do we know that their other activities were not responsible, or partly so, for the changes in their fitness levels? Chapter 16 deals with these threats to internal validity.

External validity pertains to the generalizability of the results. To what extent can the results apply to the real world? This often produces a paradox for research in the behavioral sciences because of the controls required for internal validity. In motor learning studies, for example, the task is often something novel so as to control for past experience. Furthermore, it is desirable to be able to measure the performance objectively and reliably. Consequently, the learning task is frequently a maze, a rotary pursuitmeter, or a linear position task, all of which may meet the demands for control with regard to internal validity. But then you are faced with the question of external validity: How does performance in a laboratory setting with a novel, irrelevant task apply to learning gymnastics or basketball? These questions are important and sometimes vexing, but they are not insurmountable (they will be discussed later).

Step 4: Analyzing and Interpreting Results

The novice researcher finds this step to be the most formidable for several reasons. First, this step usually involves some statistical analysis, and the novice researcher (particularly the master's student) has a limited background and a fear of statistics. Second, analysis and interpretation require considerable knowledge, experience, and insight, which the novice may lack.

That analysis and interpretation of results are the most challenging step goes without question. It is here that the researcher must provide evidence for the support or the rejection of the research hypothesis. In doing this, the researcher also compares the results with those of others and perhaps attempts to relate and integrate the results into some theoretical model. Inductive reasoning is employed in this step (whereas deductive reasoning is primarily used in the statement of the problem). The researcher attempts to synthesize the data from his or her study along with the results of other studies to contribute to the development or substantiation of a theory.

Alternative Models for Research

Normal Science
   Challenges to Normal Science
      Implications of This Discussion
Alternative Forms of Scientific Inquiry

 In the preceding section we summarized the basic steps in the scientific method of problem solving. **Science** is a way of knowing, often defined as structured inquiry. One basic goal of science is to explain things or to be able to generalize and build a theory. When a scientist develops a useful model to explain behavior, scholars often test predictions from this model using the steps of the scientific method. The model and the approaches used to test the model are called a paradigm.

Normal Science

For centuries, the scientific approaches used in studying problems in both the natural and the social sciences have been what Tho-

 science — A process of careful and systematic inquiry.

 normal science — An objective manner of study grounded in the natural sciences that is systematic, logical, empirical, reductive, and replicable.

mas Kuhn (1970), a noted science historian, has termed **normal science**. It is characterized by the elements we listed at the beginning of this chapter (i.e., systematic, logical, empirical, reductive, and replicable). Its basic doctrine is objectivity. Normal science is grounded in the natural sciences, which have long adhered to the idea of the orderliness and reality of matter, that nature's laws are absolute and discoverable by objective, systematic observations and investigations that are not influenced by (in other words, independent of) humans. The experiments are theory driven and have testable hypotheses.

Normal science received a terrific jolt with Einstein's theory of relativity and the quantum theory, which indicated that nature's laws could be influenced by humans (that is, that reality depends to a great extent on how one perceives it). Moreover, some things, such as the decay of a radioactive nucleus, happen for no reason at all. The fundamental laws that had been believed to be absolute were now considered to be statistical rather than deterministic. Phenomena could be predicted statistically but not explained deterministically (Jones, 1988).

Challenges to Normal Science

Relatively recently (since about 1960), there have been serious challenges regarding normal science's concept of objectivity (i.e., that the researcher can be detached from the instruments and conduct of the experiment). Two of the most powerful challengers to the ideal of objective knowledge have been Thomas Kuhn and Michael Polanyi (1958). They contend that objectivity is a myth. From the first inception of the idea for the hypothesis through the selection of apparatus to the analysis of the results, the observer is involved. The conduct of the experiment and the results can be considered expressions of the researcher's point of view. Polanyi has been especially opposed to the adoption of normal science for the study of human behavior.

Kuhn (1970) maintains that normal science does not really evolve in systematic steps the way that scientific writers describe it. Kuhn discusses the **paradigm crisis phenomenon**, in which researchers who have been following a particular paradigm begin to find discrepancies in it. The findings no longer agree with the pre-

dictions, and a new paradigm is advanced. Interestingly, the old paradigm does not die completely but only develops varicose veins and fades away. Many researchers with a great deal of time and effort invested in the old paradigm are reluctant to change, so it is usually a new group of researchers who propose the new paradigm. Thus, normal science progresses by revolution, with a new group of scientists breaking away and replacing the old. Kuhn and Polanyi concur that the doctrine of objectivity is simply not a reality. Nevertheless, normal science has been and will continue to be successful in the natural sciences and in certain aspects of the study of humans. However, Martens (1987) contends that it has failed miserably in the study of human behavior, especially in the more complex functions.

As a sport psychologist, Martens has asserted that laboratory experiments have limited use in answering questions about complex human behavior in sport. He considers his role as a practicing sport psychologist to have been far more productive in gaining knowledge about athletes and coaches and the solutions to their problems. Other workers in the so-called helping professions have made similar observations about both the limitations of normal science and the importance of alternative sources of knowledge in forming and shaping professional beliefs. Schein (1987), a noted scholar of social psychology, related an interesting (some might call it shocking) revelation concerning the relative impact of published research results versus practical experience. At a conference, he and a number of his colleagues were discussing what they relied on most for their classroom teaching. There seemed to be widespread agreement among these professors that the data they really believed in and used in the classroom came from personal experience and information learned in the field. Schein was making the point that different categories of knowledge can be obtained by different methods. In effect, some people are more influenced by sociological and anthropological research models than by the normal science approach.

For some time many scholars in education, psychology, sociology, anthropology, sport psychology, physical education, and other disciplines have proposed methods of studying human behavior other than those of conventional normal science. Anthropologists, sociologists, and clinical psychologists

paradigm crisis phenomenon — Development of discrepancies in a paradigm leading to proposals of a new paradigm that better explains the data.

have used in-depth observation, description, and analysis of human behavior for nearly three quarters of a century. For over 35 years, researchers in education have used participant and nonparticipant observation to obtain comprehensive, first-hand accounts of teacher and student behaviors as they occur in real-world settings. More recently, physical educators and sport psychologists have been engaged in this type of field research. A number of names given to this general form of research are ethnographic, qualitative, grounded, naturalistic, and participant observational research. Regardless of the names, the commitments, and the beliefs of the researchers, this type of research has not been well received by the adherents of normal science and the scientific method. In fact, this form of research (we will include all its forms under the name qualitative research) has often been labeled by normal scientists as superficial, lacking in rigor, and just plain unscientific. They have criticized it as being essentially subjective, which is the antithesis of objectivity, the underpinning of normal science.

Martens (1987) has referred to such adherents of normal science as the gatekeepers of knowledge because they are the research journal editors and reviewers who decide who will get published, who will serve on the editorial boards, and whose papers will be presented at conferences. Studies without internal validity do not get published, yet studies without external validity lack practical significance. Martens (p. 42) charges that normal science (in psychology) prefers publishability to practical significance.

The debates between qualitative and normal (often classified as quantitative) research have been heated and prolonged. The qualitative proponents have gained confidence and momentum in recent years, and there is no question that this point of view is to be reckoned with and recognized as a viable method of addressing problems in the behavioral sciences. Credibility is established by systematically categorizing and analyzing causal and consequential factors. The naturalistic setting of qualitative research both facilitates analysis and precludes precise control of so-called extraneous factors. The holistic interrelationship among observations and the complexity and dynamic processes of human interaction make it impossible to limit the study of human behavior to the sterile, reductionistic approach of normal science. **Reductionism**, a characteristic of normal science, assumes that complex behavior can be reduced, analyzed, and explained as parts that can then be put back together as a whole and understood. Critics of the conventional approach to research believe the central issue is the unjustified belief that normal science is the only source of true knowledge.

Implications of This Discussion

There are many implications. For example, when we study simple movements, such as linear positioning in a laboratory to reflect cognitive processing of information, do we learn anything about movements in real-world settings such as the performance of sport skills? When we evaluate EMG activity in specific muscle groups during a simple movement, does it really tell us anything about the way the nervous system controls movements in natural settings such as athletics? Can we study the association of psychological processes related to movement in laboratory settings and expect the results to apply in sport and exercise situations? When we conduct these types of experiments, are we studying nature's phenomena or laboratory phenomena?

Do not misinterpret the intent of these questions. They do not mean that nothing important can be discovered about physical activity from laboratory research. What they suggest is that these findings do not necessarily model accurately the way humans plan, control, and execute movements in natural settings associated with exercise and sport.

Kuhn's (1970) descriptions about how science advances and the limitations of applying normal science to natural settings demonstrate that scientists need to consider the various ways of knowing and that the strict application of the normal scientific method of problem solving may sometimes hinder rather than advance science. If the reductionistic approach of the scientific method has not served well the natural scientists who developed it, then certainly researchers in human behavior need to carefully assess the relative strengths and weaknesses of conventional and alternative research paradigms for their particular research questions.

---

reductionism — A characteristic of normal science that assumes that complex behavior can be reduced, analyzed, and explained as parts that can then be put back together to understand the whole.

Alternative Forms of Scientific Inquiry

Martens (1987, p. 52) has suggested that we view knowledge not as being either scientific or unscientific or reliable or unreliable but rather as existing on a continuum, such as illustrated in Figure 1.1. This continuum, labeled "DK," ranges from "Don't Know" to "Damn Konfident." Considered in this way, varying approaches to disciplined inquiry are useful in accumulating knowledge. As examples, Martens (1979, 1987) has urged sport psychologists to consider the idiographic approach, introspective methods, and field studies instead of relying on the paradigm of normal science as the only answer to research questions in sport psychology. Thomas, French, and Humphries (1986) detailed how to study children's sport knowledge and skills in games and sports. Costill (1985) discussed the study of physiological responses in practical exercise and sport settings. Locke (1989) presented a tutorial on the use of qualitative research in physical education and sport. In later chapters we give greater detail about some of these alternative strategies for research.

What we hope you gain from this section is that science is disciplined inquiry, not a set of specific procedures. Although advocates of alternative methods of research are often very persuasive, we certainly do not want you to conclude that the study of physical activity should abandon the traditional methods of normal science. We have learned much from these techniques and will continue to do so. Furthermore, we certainly do not want you to toss away this book as being pointless. We have not even begun to tell you all the fascinating things we have learned over the years (it is hard to tell whether these things should be classified as normal or abnormal science). In addition, we have many funny stories yet to tell (abnormal humor). Aside from these compelling reasons for continuing with the book, we want you to realize and appreciate that even though so-called normal science may not be the solution to all questions raised in our field, it is the recognized model for research, and it is often taught as the only ap-

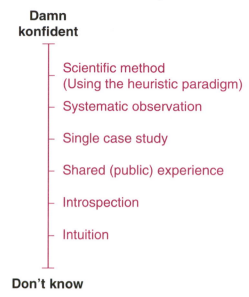

DK Theory

Damn konfident

- Scientific method (Using the heuristic paradigm)
- Systematic observation
- Single case study
- Shared (public) experience
- Introspection
- Intuition

Don't know

Figure 1.1 The degrees of knowledge theory with examples of different types of methods varying in degree of reliability.

From "Science, Knowledge, and Sport Psychology," by R. Martens, 1987, *The Sport Psychologist*, **1**(1), p. 46. Copyright 1987 by Human Kinetics. Reprinted with permission.

proach in graduate study. Furthermore, none of the alternative methods of research denounce the scientific method of problem solving. The main bones of contention are with the methods, the setting, the controls, the types of data, and the analysis.

The bottom line is that different problems require different solutions. As we said before, science is disciplined inquiry, not a set of specific procedures. We need to embrace all systematic forms of inquiry. Rather than argue about the differences, we should capitalize on the strengths of both methods to provide useful knowledge about human movement. The nature of the research questions and setting should drive the selection of approaches to acquiring knowledge. In fact, just as Christina (1989) suggested that researchers might move among levels of research (basic to applied), so researchers might move among paradigms (quantitative to qualitative) to acquire knowledge.

Thomas, J.R., French, K.E., & Humphries, C.A. (1986). Knowledge development and sport skill performance: Directions for motor behavior research. *Journal of Sport Psychology*, **8**, 259-272.

Costill, D.L. (1985). Practical problems in exercise physiology research. *Research Quarterly for Exercise and Sport*, **56**, 378-384.

Locke, L.F. (1989). Qualitative research as a form of scientific inquiry in sport and physical education. *Research Quarterly for Exercise and Sport*, **60**, 1-20.

Types of Research

Research is a structured way of solving problems. There are different kinds of problems in the study of physical activity; thus, different types of research are used to solve these problems. This text concentrates on these four types of research: analytical, descriptive, experimental, and qualitative. A brief description of each follows.

Analytical Research

As the name implies, **analytical research** involves in-depth study and evaluation of available information in an attempt to explain complex phenomena. The different types of analytical research are historical, philosophical, reviews, and research synthesis.

Historical Research

Obviously, historical research deals with events that have already occurred. Historical research fo-

cuses on events, organizations, institutions, and people. In some studies, the researcher is interested mostly in preserving the record of events and past accomplishments. In other investigations, the writer attempts to discover facts that will provide more meaning and understanding of past events to explain the present state of affairs. Some historians have even attempted to use information from the past to predict the future. The research procedures associated with historical studies are addressed in considerable detail in chapter 12.

Philosophical Research

Critical inquiry characterizes philosophical research. The researcher establishes hypotheses, examines and analyzes existing facts, and synthesizes the evidence into a workable theoretical model. Many of the most important problem areas must be dealt with by the philosophical method. Problems dealing with objectives, curricula, course content, requirements, and methodology are but a few of the important issues that can be resolved only through the philosophical method of problem solving.

Although some authors emphasize the differences between science and philosophy, the philosophical method of research follows essentially the same steps as other methods of scientific problem solving. The philosophical approach uses scientific facts as the bases for formulating and testing research hypotheses.

An example of such philosophical research was Morland's 1958 study, in which he analyzed the educational views held by leaders in American physical education and categorized them into educational philosophies of reconstructionism, progressivism, essentialism, and perennialism.

Having an opinion is not the same as having a philosophy. In philosophical research, beliefs must be subjected to rigorous criticism in light of the fundamental assumptions. Academic preparation in philosophy and a solid background in the fields from which the facts are derived are neces-

---

 analytical research — Type of research that involves in-depth study and evaluation of available information in an attempt to explain complex phenomena; can be categorized in the following way: historical, philosophical, review, and meta-analysis.

Morland, R.B. (1958). A philosophical interpretation of the educational views held by leaders in American physical education (Doctoral dissertation, New York University). *Health, Physical Education and Recreation Microform Publications*, **1**, October 1949-March 1965, PE394.

sary. Other examples and a more detailed explanation of philosophical research are given in chapter 13.

Reviews

A **review** is a critical evaluation of recent research on a particular topic. The author must be very knowledgeable about the available literature as well as the research topic and procedures. A review involves analysis, evaluation, and integration of the published literature, often leading to important conclusions concerning the research findings up to that time (for a good example of a recent review, see Blair's 1993 review of "Physical activity, physical fitness, and health").

Certain publications consist entirely of reviews, such as the *Psychological Review*, the *Annual Review of Physiology*, and the *Review of Educational Research*. A number of journals publish reviews periodically, and some occasionally devote entire issues to reviews. For example, the 50th anniversary issue of the *Research Quarterly for Exercise and Sport* (Safrit, 1980) contains some excellent reviews on various topics.

Research Synthesis

Reviews of literature are difficult to write because they require that a large number of studies be synthesized to determine common underlying findings, agreements, or disagreements. To some extent this is like trying to make sense of data collected on a large number of subjects by simply looking at the data. Glass (1977) and Glass, McGaw, and Smith (1981) proposed a quantitative means of analyzing the findings from numerous studies; this is called meta-analysis. Findings between studies are compared by changing results within studies to a common metric called effect size. Over the years many meta-analyses have been reported in the physical activity literature (Feltz & Landers, 1983; Payne & Morrow, 1993; Sparling, 1980; Thomas & French, 1985). This technique is discussed in more detail in chapter 14.

Descriptive Research

Descriptive research is concerned with status. Of the several descriptive research techniques, the most prevalent is the questionnaire. Other forms of descriptive research include the interview, the normative survey, the case study, the job analysis, the documentary analysis, developmental studies, and correlational studies. Chapter 15 provides detailed coverage of descriptive research procedures. The following paragraphs briefly identify the different types of descriptive research techniques.

The Questionnaire

The main justification for using a questionnaire is the need to obtain responses from persons from a wide geographical area. The questionnaire usually strives to secure information about present practices, conditions, and demographic data. Occasionally, a questionnaire asks for opinions or knowledge.

The Interview

The interview and the questionnaire are essentially the same technique insofar as their planning and procedures are concerned. Obviously, the interview has certain advantages over the questionnaire. The researcher can rephrase questions and ask additional ones to clarify responses and secure more

---

 review — A research paper that is a critical evaluation of research on a particular topic.

Blair, S.N. (1993). Physical activity, physical fitness, and health (1993 C.H. McCloy Research Lecture). *Research Quarterly for Exercise and Sport*, **64**, 365-376.

Safrit, M.J. (Ed.) (1980). *Research Quarterly for Exercise and Sport*, **51**(1).

Feltz, D.L., & Landers, D.M. (1983). The effects of mental practice on motor skill learning and performance: A meta-analysis. *Journal of Sport Psychology*, **5**, 25-57.

Payne, V.G., & Morrow, J.R. Jr. (1993). Exercise and $\dot{V}O_2$max in children: A meta-analysis. *Research Quarterly for Exercise and Sport*, **64**, 305-313.

Thomas, J.R., & French, K.E. (1985). Gender differences across age in motor performance: A meta-analysis. *Psychological Bulletin*. **98**, 260-282.

valid results. Becoming a skilled interviewer requires training and experience. Telephone interviewing has become increasingly more common in recent years. It costs half as much as face-to-face interviews and can cover a wide geographical area, which is generally a limitation in personal interviews. We discuss some other advantages of the telephone interview technique in chapter 15.

The Normative Survey

There have been a number of notable normative surveys in the fields of physical activity and health. The normative survey generally seeks to gather performance or knowledge data on a large sample from a population and to present the results in the form of comparative standards, or norms. The development of the norms for the AAHPERD Youth Fitness Test Manual (AAHPERD, 1958) is an outstanding example of a normative survey. Thousands of boys and girls ages 10 to 18 throughout the United States were tested on a battery of motor fitness items. Percentiles were then established to provide information for students, teachers, administrators, and parents as to comparative performances. Actually, the Youth Fitness Test was developed in response to another survey, the Kraus-Weber test, which revealed that American children scored dramatically lower on a test battery of minimum muscular fitness when compared with European children.

The Case Study

The case study is used to provide detailed information about an individual (or institution, community, etc.). It aims to determine unique characteristics about the subject or condition. This descriptive research technique is used widely in such fields as medicine, psychology, counseling, and sociology. The case study is also a technique used in qualitative research.

The Job Analysis

The objective of the job analysis is to describe in detail the various duties, procedures, responsibilities, preparations, advantages, and disadvantages of a particular job. Used widely in vocational training and counseling, the job analysis research procedures require time, attention to details, and numerous data-gathering techniques. The job analysis has not been used to a great extent in the study of physical activity, but some studies have explored the duties of the athletic director, intramural director, and physical education teacher.

The Documentary (Content) Analysis

In some respects, the **documentary** or **content analysis** could be classified under analytical research because it is used in literature reviews, historical studies, and other areas. However, the form of documentary analysis included in descriptive research is directed primarily at establishing the status of certain practices; areas of interest; and the prevalence of certain errors, usage of terms, and space counts. For example, newspapers or magazines might be studied to determine the extent of coverage (and thus public interest) devoted to certain sports or recreational activities. A study to ascertain the frequency of use of various statistical procedures in a research journal also falls under the category of documentary analysis.

Developmental Studies

In developmental research, the investigator is usually concerned with the interaction of learning or performance with maturation. For example, a researcher may wish to assess the extent to which the ability to process information about movement can be attributed to maturation as opposed to strategy, or the researcher may desire to determine the effects of growth on a physical parameter such as aerobic capacity.

Developmental research can be undertaken by what is called the longitudinal method, whereby the same subjects are studied over a period of years. Obvious logistical problems are associated with longitudinal studies, so an alternative is to select samples of subjects from different age-groups to assess the effects of maturation. This is called the cross-sectional approach.

Correlational Studies

The purpose of correlational research is to examine the relationship between certain performance variables, such as heart rate and ratings of perceived exertion; the relationship between traits such as anxiety and pain tolerance; or the correlation be-

---

documentary analysis — Type of descriptive research directed primarily at establishing the status of certain practices; areas of interest; and the prevalence of certain errors, usage of terms, and space counts.

tween attitudes and behavior, as in the attitude toward fitness and the amount of participation in fitness activities. Sometimes correlation is employed to predict performance. For example, a researcher may wish to predict percent body fat from skinfold measurements. Correlational research is descriptive in that you cannot presume a cause-and-effect relationship. All that can be established is that there is an association between two or more traits or performances.

Experimental Research

 Experimental research is usually acknowledged as being the most scientific of all the types of research because the researcher can manipulate treatments to cause things to happen (i.e., a cause-and-effect situation can be established). This contrasts with other types of research in which already existing phenomena or data from the past are observed and analyzed. For an example of an experimental study, assume that Virginia Reel, a dance teacher, hypothesizes that students would learn more effectively through the use of a videotape. First, she randomly assigns students to two sections. One section is taught by the so-called traditional method (explanation, demonstration, practice, and critique). The other section is taught in a similar manner, except the students are filmed while practicing and can thus observe themselves as the teacher critiques their performances. After 9 weeks, a panel of dance teachers evaluates both sections. In this study, method of teaching is the independent variable and dance performance (skill) is the dependent variable. After the groups' scores are compared statistically, Virginia can conclude whether her hypothesis can be supported or not.

In experimental research, the researcher attempts to control all factors except the experimental (or treatment) variable. If the extraneous factors can be successfully controlled, then the researcher can presume that the changes in the dependent variable are due to the independent variable.

Qualitative Research

 In the study of physical activity, **qualitative research** is the so-called new kid on the block. Actually, qualitative research has been used for many years in other fields, such as anthropology and sociology. Researchers in education have been engaged in qualitative methods longer than researchers in our field. As previously mentioned, several names are given to this type of research (ethnographic, naturalistic, interpretive, grounded, phenomenological, subjective, and participant observational). Some are simply name differences, whereas some have different approaches and points of focus. We have arbitrarily lumped them all under the heading of qualitative research as that seems to be the most common term used in our field.

The basic characteristics of qualitative research include the following:

- Intensive, longtime observation and extensive interviewing in a natural setting
- Precise and detailed recording of what happens in the setting through the use of field notes, audiotapes, videotapes, and other kinds of documentary evidence
- Data interpretation and analysis through the use of rich description, interpretive narratives, direct quotes, charts and tables, and sometimes statistics (usually descriptive)

Qualitative research is different from other research methods. It is a systematic method of inquiry, and it follows the scientific method of problem solving to a considerable degree; however, it deviates in certain dimensions. Qualitative research rarely establishes hypotheses at the beginning of the study. It proceeds in an inductive process in developing hypotheses and theory as the data unfold. Theory is grounded in the data (Glaser & Strauss, 1976). The researcher is the primary instrument in the data collection and analysis. Qualitative research is characterized by intensive firsthand presence. The tools of data collection are observation, interviews,

---

 experimental research — Type of research that involves the manipulation of treatments in an attempt to establish cause-effect relationships.

 qualitative research — Research method that involves intensive, long-time observation in a natural setting; precise and detailed recording of what happens in the setting; interpretation and analysis of the data using description, narratives, quotes, and charts and tables. Can also be called *ethnographic*, *naturalistic*, *interpretive*, *grounded*, *phenomenological*, *subjective*, and *participant observational*.

 Characteristics of qualitative research

and researcher-designed instruments (Goetz & LeCompte, 1984).

Research Methods Process Overview

A nice overview of the research methods course, as well as an introduction to this book, is provided in Figure 1.2. This flowchart provides a linear way to think about planning a research study. Once the problem area is identified, reading and thinking about relevant theories and concepts, as well as a careful search of the literature for relevant findings, leads to the specification of hypotheses. Operational definitions are needed in a research study so that the reader knows exactly what the researcher means by certain terms. Operational definitions are observable phenomena that enable the researcher to test empirically whether the predicted outcomes (hypotheses) can be supported. The study is designed, and the measuring devices are selected and made operational. The data are then collected and ana-

lyzed and the findings identified. Finally, the results are related back to the original hypotheses and discussed in relation to theories, concepts, and previous research findings.

The Parts of a Thesis: A Reflection on the Steps in the Research Process

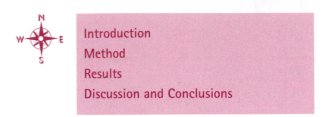

Introduction

Method

Results

Discussion and Conclusions

In this chapter, you have been introduced to the research process. The theme has been the scientific method of problem solving. Generally speaking, a thesis or research article has a standard format. This is for the purpose of expedience in that the reader

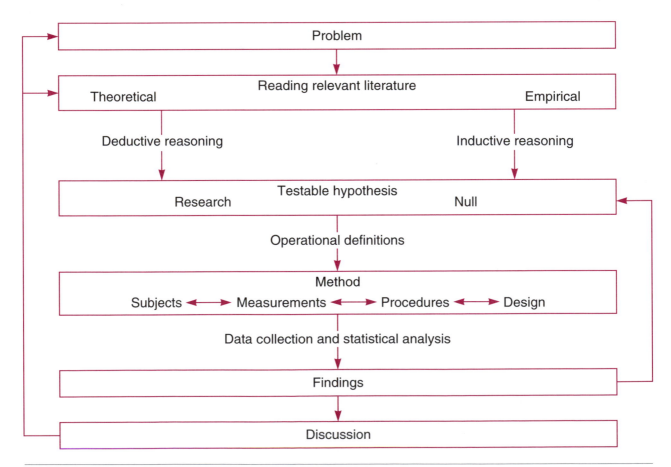

Figure 1.2   The total research setting.

knows where to find the different information, such as purpose, methods, and results. The format also reflects the steps in the scientific method of problem solving. We now look at a typical thesis format and see how the parts account for the steps in the scientific method.

Sometimes theses and dissertations are done in a chapter format where each chapter represents a separate part of the research report (e.g., Introduction). That has been a common model over the years. We believe it is more appropriate for graduate students to prepare their thesis or dissertation in a form suitable for journal publication because that is an important part of the research process. In chapter 20 we provide considerable detail about how to use journal format within a thesis or dissertation and the value of doing so. Throughout this book, we simply indicate the typical parts of a research report. These can be considered either as parts of a journal paper or as chapters depending on the format selected for the thesis or dissertation.

Introduction

Here the problem is defined and delimited. The researcher specifically identifies the problem and often states the research hypotheses. Certain terms critical to the study are operationally defined for the reader, and limitations and perhaps some basic assumptions are acknowledged.

The literature review may be in the first part, or it may warrant a separate section. When it is in the first part, it more closely adheres to the steps in the scientific method of problem solving; that is, the literature review is instrumental in the formulation of hypotheses and the deductive reasoning leading to the problem statement.

Method

As the purpose here is to make the thesis format parallel to the data-gathering steps, this part relates to the scientific method. First, the researcher explains how the data were gathered. The subjects are identified, the measuring instruments are described, the measurement and treatment procedures are presented, the experimental design

is explained, and the methods of analyzing the data are summarized. The major purpose of the method section is to describe the study in such detail and with such clarity that a reader could duplicate it.

The first two parts often comprise the **research proposal** and are presented to the student's thesis committee prior to the research being undertaken. For the proposal, these two parts are often written in future tense, then changed to past tense when the final version of the thesis is completed.

Results

The results present the pertinent findings from the data analysis and represent the contribution to new knowledge. Results correspond to the step in the scientific method in which the results are scrutinized as to their meaningfulness and reliability.

Discussion and Conclusions

In this last step in the scientific method, the **discussion**, the researcher employs inductive reasoning in an effort to analyze the findings, to compare these findings with previous studies, and to integrate them into a theoretical model. In this part, the research hypotheses are judged as to their acceptability. Then, on the basis of the analysis and discussion, conclusions are usually made. The conclusions should address the purpose and subpurposes that were specified in the first part.

Summary

Research is simply a way of solving problems. Questions are raised, and methods are devised to try to answer them. There are different ways of approaching problems (research methods). Sometimes the nature of the problem dictates the method of research. For example, if one wants to discover the origins of a sport, the historical method of research is used. Sometimes one wishes to look at a problem

---

 research proposal — A formal preparation that includes the introduction, review of literature, and proposed method for conducting the study.

 discussion — Chapter or section of a research report that explains what the results mean.

from a particular angle and selects a research method that can best answer the question.

Research on the topic of teaching effectiveness, for example, can be approached in several ways. An experimental study could be conducted in which teaching methods are compared as to their effectiveness in bringing about measurable achievement. Or a study could be designed in which teachers' behaviors are coded and evaluated using some observational instrument. Or another form of descriptive research could be used that employs the questionnaire or the interview technique to examine teachers' responses to questions concerning their beliefs or practices. Or perhaps a qualitative study could be undertaken to systematically observe and interview one teacher in one school over an extended period to portray the teacher's experiences and perceptions in the natural setting.

The point is that there isn't a single way to do research. It is true that some people do just one type of research, and, being human, some are critical of the methods used by others. However, anyone who believes his or her type of research is the only "scientific" way to solve problems is narrow and downright foolish. Science is disciplined inquiry, not a set of specific procedures.

Basic research deals primarily with theoretical problems, and the results are not intended to have immediate application. Applied research, on the other hand, strives to answer questions that have direct value to the practitioner. There is a need to prepare proficient consumers of research as well as researchers. Thus, one purpose of a book on research methods is to help the reader understand the tools necessary both to consume and to produce research.

We have presented here an overview of the nature of research. The scientific method of problem solving was contrasted with "unscientific" methods by which people acquire information. Multiple research models were discussed to emphasize that there isn't just one way to approach problems in our discipline and profession. We identified the four major types of research used in the study of physical activity: analytical, descriptive, experimental, and qualitative. These categories and the different techniques that they encompass will be covered in detail in later chapters.

 Check Your Understanding

1. Pick and read a chapter that is of interest to you from one of the references on the bottom of p. 6. Identify one basic and one applied research problem from that chapter.

2. Look through some recent issues of *Research Quarterly for Exercise and Sport*. Find and read a research article of interest that is quantitative in nature and another that is qualitative. Did you find one easier to understand than the other? Which one? Why? Surmise how difficult it might be to do each type of research.

3. Refer to and read Appendix B, "A Brief Historical Overview of Research in Physical Activity in the United States." Then read a chapter from Massengale & Swanson, *History of the Exercise and Sport Sciences*, about the history of the subfield in which you have the greatest interest. Summarize a few things about your subfield that you did not know.

CHAPTER 2

Developing the Problem and Using the Literature

Dear Professors of Research Methods:

I have been reviewing the literature on base running in baseball, specifically, the crossover start versus the slide start. There seem to be hundreds of theses already done on this subject. Do you think it is a good topic?

Sincerely,
I.M. Redundant

Dear Redundant:

Our best response is to use a quotation attributed to Mark Twain: "The researches of many commentators have already thrown much darkness on this subject, and it is probable that, if they continue, we shall soon know nothing at all about it."

Methodologically yours,
PRM

Getting started is the hardest part of almost any new venture, and research is no exception. You can't do any significant research until you have identified the area you want to investigate, learned what has been published in that area, and figured out how you are going to conduct the investigation. In this chapter, we will discuss ways by which a person can identify researchable problems, search for literature, and write the literature review.

Identifying the Research Problem

Guidelines for Finding a Topic
Using Inductive and Deductive Reasoning

Of the many major issues facing the graduate student, a primary one is the identification of a research problem. Problems may arise from real-world settings or be generated from theoretical frameworks. Regardless, a basic requirement for proposing a good research problem is in-depth knowledge about the area of interest. However, sometimes as one becomes more knowledgeable about a content area, everything seems to be already known. Thus, al-

though you want to become expert, do not become too narrow. Relating your knowledge base to other areas often provides insight into significant areas for research.

Sometimes it seems ironic that we ask students to start thinking about possible research topics in their research methods course, because they typically take the course in the first semester (or quarter) of graduate school—before they have had the opportunity to acquire the necessary in-depth knowledge. As a result, many research problems are trivial, lack a theoretical base, and replicate earlier research. Although this is a considerable shortcoming, the advantages of taking the research methods course early in the program are substantial in terms of success in other graduate courses. This is because the student learns

- to approach and solve problems in a scientific way,
- to search the literature,
- to write in a clear, scientific fashion,
- to understand basic measurement and statistical issues,
- to use an appropriate writing style,
- to be an intelligent consumer of research, and
- to appreciate the wide variety of research strategies and techniques used in an area of study.

Top 10 Problems That Have Not Been Resolved by Humankind

10. Why isn't phonetic spelled the way it sounds?

9. Why are there interstate highways in Hawaii?

8. Why do we drive on parkways and park on driveways?

7. Why is it that when you're driving and looking for an address, you turn down the volume on the radio?

6. Why are there flotation devices under plane seats instead of parachutes?

5. How does the person who drives the snowplow get to work in the mornings?

4. Why is it that when you transport something by car, it's called a shipment, but when you transport something by ship, it's called a cargo?

3. If a 7-11 is open 24 hours a day, 365 days a year, why are there locks on the doors?

2. If you tied buttered toast to the back of a cat and dropped it from a height, what would happen?

1. If a cow laughed, would milk come out of her nose?

 Advantages of taking a research methods course early in the program

Criteria in Selecting a Research Problem

Workability.   Is the contemplated study within the limits and range of your resource and time constraints? Will you have access to the necessary sample in the numbers required? Is there reason to believe you can come up with an "answer to the problem"? Is the required methodology manageable and understandable?

Critical mass.   Is the problem of sufficient magnitude and scope to fulfill the requirement that has motivated the study in the first place? Are there enough variables? enough potential results? enough to write about?

Interest.   Are you interested in the problem area, specific problem, and potential solution? Does it relate to your background? to your career interest? Does it "turn you on"? Will you learn useful skills from pursuing it?

Theoretical value.   Does the problem fill a gap in the literature? Will others recognize its importance? Will it contribute to advancement in your field? Does it improve the "state of the art"? Is it publishable?

Practical value.   Will the solution to the problem improve educational practice? Are practitioners likely to be interested in the results? Will education be changed by the outcome? Will your own educational practices be likely to change as a result?

From *Conducting Educational Research*, 2nd ed., (p. 24–25), by B.W. Tuckman, 1978, New York: Harcourt Brace Jovanovich. Copyright 1978 by Harcourt Brace Jovanovich. Reprinted with permission.

How, then, does a student without much background select a problem? It seems that the harder you try to think of a topic, the more you are inclined to think that all the problems in the field have already been solved. Adding to this frustration is the pressure of time. To assure you that important questions still wait to be addressed, we have provided a list of 10 such provocative questions on page 26.

Guidelines for Finding a Topic

 To help alleviate the topic-finding problem, we offer the following suggestions. First, be aware of the research being done at your institution, for research spawns other research ideas. Often, a researcher will have a series of studies planned. Second, be alert for any controversial issues in some area of interest. Lively controversy prompts research in efforts to resolve the issue. In any case, be sure to talk to professors and advanced graduate students in your area of interest and to use their suggestions to focus on a topic. Third, read a review paper (possibly in a review journal, research journal, or recent textbook). From there, read several research studies in the reference lists and locate other current research papers on the topic. Using all this information, make a list of either research questions that appear unanswered or logical extensions of the material you have read. Try to pick problems that are neither too hard nor too easy. The hard ones will take you forever, and you'll never get your thesis done. No one cares about the easy ones.

Of course, no single problem will necessarily meet all the criteria perfectly. For example, some theoretical problems may have limited direct application; however, theoretical problems should be directed toward issues that may ultimately prove useful to practitioners. By honestly answering the questions at the top of this page, a practical evaluation of the selected problem is possible.

An intriguing way to develop a research problem is to see how experts develop problems. Snyder and Abernethy (1992) orga-

Loehle, C. (1990). A guide to increased creativity in research—inspiration or perspiration? *BioScience*, **40**, 123–129.

Snyder, C.W. Jr., & Abernethy, B. (Eds.) (1992). *The creative side of experimentation.* Champaign, IL: Human Kinetics.

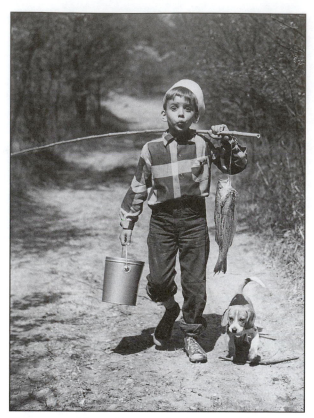

If the research problem you're interested in has been "fished out," try a different fishing hole.

nized *The Creative Side of Experimentation*, in which they had well-established scholars in motor control, motor development, and sport psychology give first-person accounts of factors that influenced their career research programs. In addition, the editors have deduced themes that seem to run through these scholars' research programs. Their analysis focuses on such questions as:

- What are common personal and professional characteristics of expert researchers?
- What types of experimentation do expert researchers perform?
- What strategies do expert experimenters use to enhance their ability to ask important questions?

Using Inductive and Deductive Reasoning

The means for identifying specific research problems comes from two methods of reasoning: in-

ductive and deductive. Figure 2.1 provides a schema of the inductive reasoning process. Individual observations are tied together into specific hypotheses, which are grouped into more general explanations that are united into theory. To move from the level of observations to that of theory requires many individual studies that test specific hypotheses. But even beyond the individual studies, someone must see how all the findings relate and then offer a theoretical explanation that encompasses all the individual findings.

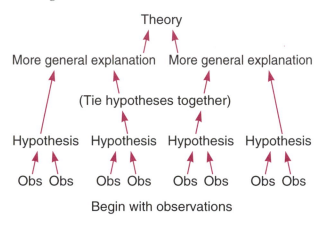

Figure 2.1   Inductive reasoning.

From *A Student Guide for Educational Research* (p. 22), by R.L. Hoenes and B.S. Chissom, 1975, Statesboro, GA: Vog Press. Copyright 1975 by Vog Press.

An example of this process can be found in the motor learning and control area. Adams (1971) proposed a **closed-loop theory** of motor skill learning. Basically, a closed-loop theory is one in which information received as feedback from a movement is compared to some internal reference of correctness (assumed to be stored in memory). Then the discrepancies between the movement and the intended movement are noted. Finally, the next attempt at the movement is adjusted to more nearly approximate the movement goal. Adams's theory ties together many previous observations about movement response. The theory was tightly reasoned but limited to slow-positioning responses. This limitation really makes it a "more general explanation," according to Figure 2.1.

---

closed–loop theory — Theory of motor skill learning advanced by Adams (1971) in which information received as feedback from a movement is compared to some internal reference of correctness.

Schmidt (1975) proposed a **schema theory**, which extended Adams's reasoning to include more rapid types of movements, frequently called ballistic tasks. (Schema theory also deals with several other limitations of Adams's theory that are not important to this discussion.) The point is that schema theory proposed to unify two general explanations, one about slow movements and the other about ballistic (rapid) movements, under one theoretical explanation—clearly an example of inductive reasoning.

Reasoning must be careful, logical, and causal; otherwise, one of our examples of inappropriate induction may result (Thomas, 1980):

> A researcher spent several weeks training a cockroach to jump. The bug became well trained and would leap high in the air on the command "Jump." The researcher then began to manipulate his independent variable, which was to remove the bug's legs one at a time. Upon removing the first leg, the researcher said "Jump," and the bug did. He then removed the second, third, fourth, and fifth leg and said "Jump" after each leg was removed, and the bug jumped every time. Upon removing the sixth leg and giving the "Jump" command, the bug just lay there. The researcher's conclusion from this research was: "When all the legs are removed from a cockroach, the bug becomes deaf." (p. 267)

Figure 2.2 presents a model of deductive reasoning. Deductive reasoning moves from a theoretical explanation of events to specific hypotheses that are tested against (or compared to) reality to evaluate whether the hypotheses are correct. Using the previously presented notions from his schema theory (to avoid explaining another theory), Schmidt advanced a hypothesis frequently called **variability of practice**. Essentially, this hypothesis (reasoned or deduced from the theory) says that practice of a variety of movement experiences (within a movement class), when compared to practicing a single movement, facilitates transfer to a new movement (but still within the same class). Several researchers have tested this hypothesis, identified by deductive reasoning, and found it viable. In fact, within any given study, both induc-

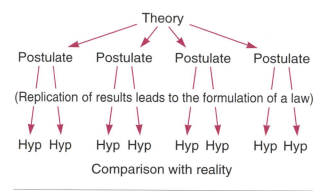

Figure 2.2   Deductive reasoning.

From *A Student Guide for Educational Research* (p. 23), by R.L. Hoenes and B.S. Chissom, 1975, Statesboro, GA: Vog Press. Copyright 1975 by Vog Press.

tive and deductive reasoning are useful. The total research setting was presented in the last chapter in Figure 1.2. Review how the deductive and inductive processes operate; that is, at the beginning of a study, the researcher deduces hypotheses from relevant theories and concepts and induces hypotheses from relevant findings in other research.

Purposes of the Literature Review

Identifying the Problem
Developing Hypotheses
Developing the Method

A major part of developing the research problem is reading what has already been published about the problem. There may already have been much research done on the problem in which you are interested. In other words, the problem has been pretty much "fished out." We hope this won't be the case when you start this phase of the research process. (In many instances, your major professor can steer you away from a saturated topic.) Whatever the topic, past research is invaluable in planning new research.

Browsing in a library confirms that information—and lots of it—exists. The dilemma lies in

---

 schema theory — Theory of motor skill learning advanced by Schmidt (1975) as an extension of Adams's closed-loop theory. The theory proposed to unify two more general explanations under one theoretical explanation.

 variability of practice — Tenet of motor skill learning advanced by Schmidt in which the practice of a variety of movement experiences facilitates transfer to a new movement when compared to practicing a single movement.

knowing how to locate the information you want and, ultimately, how to use the information once you've found it.

Reviews of literature serve several purposes. Frequently, they stimulate inductive reasoning. A scholar may seek to locate and synthesize all the relevant literature on a particular topic to develop a more general explanation or a theory to explain certain phenomena. An alternative way of analyzing the literature, mentioned in chapter 1, is meta-analysis (Glass et al., 1981), which will be discussed in detail in chapter 14.

The major problem of literature reviews is how all those studies can be related to one another in an effective way. Most frequently authors attempt to relate studies by similarities and differences in theoretical frameworks, problem statements, methodologies (subjects, instruments, treatments, designs, and statistical analyses), and findings. Results are then determined by counting votes. For example, you would write, "From the eight studies with similar characteristics, five found no significant difference between the treatments; thus, this treatment has no consistent effect."

This procedure is most easily accomplished through use of a summary sheet (see Table 2.1). This could be used to relate the frequency and intensity of exercise to the percentage of change in body fat. The conclusion from looking at these studies might be that exercising 20 minutes per day for 3 days per week for 10-14 weeks at 70% of the maximum heart rate produces moderate losses of body fat (4-5%). However, more frequent exercise bouts produce minimal increases, but less frequent or less intense

exercise is substantially less effective in eliminating body fat. Techniques of this type lend themselves to the development of the literature review around central themes or topics. Not only does this approach allow synthesis of the relevant findings, but it also makes the literature review interesting to read.

Identifying the Problem

As we have already discussed, the literature review is useful in identifying the specific problem. Of course, after locating a series of studies, the first task is to decide which studies are related to the topic area. This can frequently be accomplished by reading the abstract and, if necessary, some specific parts of the paper. Once a few key studies are identified, a careful reading will usually produce several ideas and unresolved questions. You will find it useful to discuss these questions with a professor or advanced graduate student from your area of specialization. Doing so can eliminate unproductive approaches or dead ends. After the problem is specified, an intensive library search begins.

Developing Hypotheses

Hypotheses are deduced from theory or induced from other empirical studies and real-world observations. These hypotheses are based on logical reasoning and, when predictive of the study's outcome, are labeled research hypotheses. For example, after spending a good deal of time at registration as undergraduates, graduate students, and faculty mem-

Table 2.1   Sample Form for Synthesizing Studies (Hypothetical Example)

Study	Problem statement	Subject description	Instrument	Procedure and design	Finding
Smith (1985)	Effects of exercise on body fat	30 college-age males	Underwater weighing	Exercise 3 d/wk at 70% of (220 – age) for 12 wk	4% reduction in body fat
Johnson (1978)	Effects of exercise on body fat	45 college-age males	Underwater weighing	Jog 3 d/wk at 70% or 50% of (220 – age) for 10 wk	5% for 70% gp 2% for 50% gp
Andrews (1989)	Effects of frequent and intense exercise on body fat	36 college-age males	Skinfold calipers	Jog 2, 4, 6 d/wk at 75% of (220 – age) for 12 wk	1% for 2 d 4% for 4 d 5% for 6 d
Mitchell (1980)	Effects of work load on body fat	24 high school males	Skinfold calipers	Pedaled at 30, 45, 60 rpm with 2 kp resistance for 20 min, 3 d/wk for 14 wk	1% at 30 rpm 3% at 45 rpm 4% at 60 rpm

The header spans: Characteristics of studies (over Subject description, Instrument, Procedure and design)

bers, we are able to put forth the following hypothesis for you to test: The shortest line at registration will always be the slowest. If you change lines, the one you left will speed up, and the one you enter will suddenly stop.

Developing the Method

Although considerable work is involved in identifying the problem and specifying hypotheses, one of the more creative parts of research is developing the method to test the hypotheses. If the method is planned and pilot tested appropriately, the study's outcome will allow the hypotheses to be evaluated. We believe that the researcher fails when the results of a study are blamed on methodological problems. Post hoc methodological blame results from lack of (or poor) planning and pilot work before undertaking the research.

The review of literature can be extremely helpful in identifying methods that have been successfully used to solve particular types of problems. Valuable elements from other studies may include the characteristics of the subjects, data collection instruments and testing procedures, treatments, designs, and statistical analyses. All or parts or combinations of the previously used methods are quite helpful as the researcher plans the study, but these should not limit the researcher in designing the study. Creative methodology is a key to good hypothesis testing. But neither other scholars' research nor creativity ever replaces the need to conduct thorough pilot work.

Basic Literature Search Strategies

The prospect of beginning a literature search can sometimes be frightening or depressing. How and where do you begin? What kind of sequence or strategy should you use in finding relevant literature? What services does the library offer in your search?

Authors of research texts have advanced various strategies for finding pertinent information on a topic. We know of no single "right" way of doing it. The search process depends considerably on your initial familiarity with the topic. In other words, if you have virtually no knowledge about a particular topic, your starting point and sequence will be different from that of someone already quite familiar with the literature.

 Some people are inclined to jump into the fray via a computer search. This can prove very fruitful, to be sure. However, this strategy has two weaknesses: (a) only the more recent references are available for computer searching, depending on the database, and (b) getting the necessary background and broad overview of the problem from individual studies may be difficult. For students who are not well grounded in the topic, certain preliminary sources may be helpful in locating **secondary sources** with which to become familiar with the topic at hand, and they better prepare the student to acquire and understand **primary sources**

An index, such as the *Education Index*, is a preliminary source. An index can provide the researcher with books and articles that relate to the problem. Textbooks are valuable secondary sources that can give the reader an overview of the topic and what has been done in the way of research. In fact, secondary sources such as encyclopedias and scholarly books may be the starting point for the search, by which the student becomes aware of the problem in the first place. Primary sources are ultimately the most valuable for the researcher in that the information is firsthand. Most primary sources in a literature review are journal articles. Theses and dissertations are also primary sources, but they are usually more difficult to locate if they are written at another university.

Six Steps in the Literature Search

Write the Problem Statement
Consult Secondary Sources
    Encyclopedias
    Research Reviews

---

 secondary source — Source of data in research in which an author has evaluated and summarized previous research.

primary source — Firsthand source of data in research; the original study.

Determine Descriptors
Search Preliminary Sources
    Abstracts
    Indexes
    Bibliographies
    The Library Information System
    Computer Searches
       Adjusting the Scope of the Search
       Obtaining the Primary Sources
       Personal Computers
    Other Library Services
Read and Record the Literature
Write the Literature Review

You should follow six steps when reviewing the literature. This will ensure you've been thorough and will make the search more productive.

Write the Problem Statement

We will discuss the formal writing of the problem statement in the next chapter. At this point, one is merely trying to specify what research questions are being asked. For example, a student wants to find out whether the student teaching experience influences attitude toward teaching. More specifically, the researcher wishes to examine the attitudes toward teaching before and after the student teaching experience of students in a teacher preparation program in physical education. By carefully defining the research problem, the researcher will be able to keep the literature search within reasonable limits. Write the statement as completely (but concisely) as you can at this time.

Consult Secondary Sources

This step will help you gain an overview of the topic, but it can be omitted if the researcher is knowledgeable about the topic. Secondary sources such as textbooks and encyclopedias are helpful when students have very limited knowledge about a topic and will profit from background information and a summary

of previous research. A review paper on the topic of interest is especially valuable.

Encyclopedias

Encyclopedias provide an overview of information on research topics and summarize knowledge about subject areas. General encyclopedias provide broad information about an entire field. Specialized encyclopedias pertain to much narrower topics. Examples are the *Encyclopedia of Sport Sciences and Medicine*; *Encyclopedia of Physical Fitness*; *Encyclopedia of Physical Education, Fitness and Sports*; *Encyclopedia of Educational Research*; and *Handbook of Research on Teaching*.

Because a rather lengthy period (years) often elapses from the time the authors submit their contributions until the publication date, you should be aware that the information in an encyclopedia is dated. Still, you can get important background information about a subject, become familiar with basic terms, and note references to some pertinent research journals.

Research Reviews

Reviews of research are an excellent source of information for three reasons:

- Some knowledgeable person has spent a great deal of time and effort in compiling the latest literature on the topic.
- The author has not only found the relevant literature but also critically reviewed and synthesized it into an integrated summarization of what is known about the area.
- The reviewer often suggests areas of needed research, for which the graduate student may be profoundly grateful.

Some actual review publications are the *Annual Reviews of Medicine, Annual Review of Psychology, Review of Educational Research, Physiological Reviews, Psychological Review*, and *Exercise and Sport Science Reviews*.

A number of reviews have been published by AAHPERD. One is a series called *What Research Tells the Coach*, which is about various sports including baseball, football, sprinting, distance running, swimming, tennis, and wrestling. Another AAHPERD series includes *Kinesiology Reviews I, II,*

 Three reasons why research reviews are good information sources

 Browse the review publications mentioned in the text.

and *III*. Many other research journals regularly publish reviews, to which some occasionally devote entire issues.

Determine Descriptors

Descriptors are terms that help to locate sources pertaining to a topic. For the topic of the effect of student teaching on attitude toward teaching in physical education, obvious descriptors would be attitude (toward teaching), changes in attitudes, student teaching, and physical education. Descriptors can be classified as major and minor. It is the combination of descriptors that helps the researcher pinpoint pertinent related literature. Obviously terms such as "attitude," "student teaching," and "physical education" by themselves are too broad. Various databases have their own descriptors for topics. We will discuss this further when we describe computer searching.

Search Preliminary Sources

Use preliminary (general) sources to find primary sources via computer-aided hand searches. Preliminary sources primarily consist of abstracts and indexes. Preliminary sources that are helpful to researchers in physical education, exercise science, and sport science are described below.

Abstracts

Concise summaries of research studies are valuable sources of information. Abstracts of papers presented at research meetings are available at national, district, and most state conventions. Abstracts of Research Consortium-sponsored symposia, free communications, and **poster sessions** presented at the national AAHPERD convention are published each year in the *Research Quarterly for Exercise and Sport Supplement*. *Medicine and Science in Sports and Exercise* publishes a special supplement of abstracts each year for papers to be presented at the annual meeting of the American College of Sports Medicine. *Completed Research in Health, Physical Education, Recreation and Dance*, a publication sponsored by the Research Consortium of AAHPERD, publishes hundreds of thesis and dissertation abstracts each year. It also contains a bibliographical section of research article titles from more than 160 periodicals.

Other abstract sources are *Dissertation Abstracts International*, which contains abstracts of dissertations from most colleges and universities in the United States, and the *Index and Abstracts of Foreign Physical Education Literature*, which provides abstracts from journals outside the United States. Sources of abstracts in related fields include *Biological Abstracts, Psychological Abstracts, Sociological Abstracts, Resources in Education*, and *Current Index to Journals in Education*.

Indexes

Several indexes provide references to magazine and journal articles concerning specific topics. Some general indexes commonly used in physical education, exercise science, and sport science include the *Education Index*, the *Reader's Guide to Periodical Literature*, the *New York Times Index*, the *Social Sciences Index*, and the *Physical Education Index*. Despite the title, this last source provides a comprehensive subject index to domestic and foreign periodicals in the fields of dance, health education, recreation, sports, physical therapy, and sports medicine. Researchers in the different areas within physical education, exercise science, and sport science tend to use specific indexes that pertain to their topics of interest, such as *Index Medicus, PsycINFO, ERIC*, and *Current Contents*.

• **Index Medicus**. Widely used in exercise science, the *Index Medicus* provides access to more than 2,500 biomedical journals around the world. It is published monthly, and each issue has subject and author sections and a bibliography of medical reviews. *Index Medicus* can also be searched via computer through *Medline*.

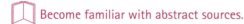
poster session — Method of presenting research at a conference in which the author places summaries of his or her research on the wall or on a poster stand and answers questions from passers-by.

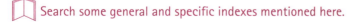
Become familiar with abstract sources.

Search some general and specific indexes mentioned here.

Specific indexes for researchers in physical activity

• **PsycINFO**. A computer search in the field of behavioral science, PsycINFO selects key words and lists appropriate titles, identifying authors and journals.

• **ERIC**. We mentioned *ERIC* with regard to abstracts. The acronym *ERIC* stands for Educational Resources Information Center. It is the world's largest source of education information. The *ERIC* system collects, sorts, classifies, and stores thousands of documents on various topics concerning education and related fields. Its basic indexes are *Resources in Education* (*RIE*) and the *Current Index to Journals in Education* (*CIJE*). Besides containing the abstracts, *RIE* provides information on how you can obtain a document: whether you can purchase it on microfilm, order an *ERIC* copy, or request the original copy from the publisher. Both *RIE* and *CIJE* provide valuable assistance in the search for information on specific topics. In addition, *ERIC* produces a thesaurus containing thousands of index terms that can be used in locating references and in conducting a computer search for information.

• **Current Contents**. This small weekly magazine, published by the Institute for Scientific Information, contains the table of contents of journals published recently within a general content area (e.g., social and behavioral sciences) and divides journals by subarea (e.g., psychology, education, rehabilitation, and special education). *Current Contents* indexes journal titles by topic and author and provides authors' addresses, so that you can obtain reprints. It also publishes a section on current books in each issue as well as weekly editions for life sciences; physical, chemical, and earth sciences; social and behavioral sciences; agriculture, biology, and environmental sciences; clinical medicine; engineering, technology, and applied sciences; and arts and humanities. *Current Contents* is now available on computer disks and CD-ROM.

Bibliographies

Bibliographies list books and articles about specific topics. They come in many forms, depending on how the information is listed. All contain the authors, titles of books or articles, journal names, and publishing information. Some bibliographies are **annotated**, meaning that a brief description of the nature and scope of the article or book is included with each reference.

The bibliography of a recent study on the topic in question is an invaluable aid to the researcher. Some authors have stated that one of the most valuable contributions of a dissertation is the review of literature and bibliography. However, you cannot simply lift the literature review from a previous study. Just because someone else has reviewed pertinent sources does not relieve you of the responsibility to read and evaluate each source yourself. Keep in mind that (a) the previous author may have been careless and cited the source or sources incorrectly, and (b) the previous author may have taken the results of a study out of context or from a point of view different from the original author's or your own.

We have found incorrect bibliographic entries on numerous occasions. A study by Stull, Christina, and Quinn (1991) revealed that of 973 citations in the 1988 and 1989 volumes of the *Research Quarterly for Exercise and Sport*, 457 contained one or more errors. This is an error rate of 47%. Such findings are by no means unique to this journal. A 50% error rate was reported for *JAMA: The Journal of the American Medical Association* (Goodrich & Roland, 1977). Stull et al. emphasized that every component in a bibliographic citation is important. Moreover, the ultimate responsibility for accuracy rests with the author. In the publishing process, mistakes can often creep in, starting with copying the source, typing the article, revising the manuscript, and checking page proofs.

A good search strategy is to look for the most recent sources of information and then work backward. You will save much time by consulting the most recent studies, and you will profit from the searches of others. Some examples of bibliographies are the *Annotated Bibliography on Movement Education*; *Completed Research in Health, Physical Education, Recreation and Dance*; *Bibliography of Research Involving Female Subjects*; *Bibliography on Perceptual Motor Development*; *Bibliography of Medical Reviews in Index Medicus*; *Annotated Bibliography in Physical Education, Recreation and Psychomotor Function of Mentally Retarded Persons*; and *Social Sciences of Sports*.

---

 annotated bibliography — List of resources that provides a brief description of the nature and scope of each article or book.

 Why you must read sources yourself

 Some good bibliographies are mentioned here.

The Library Information System

The traditional card catalog with little trays of cards containing bibliographic information by author and subject is rapidly being phased out. Most university libraries have gone to a computerized catalog system, and it seems inevitable that all libraries will adopt this method as finances permit.

Computerized catalogs abound. Usually, the searcher first selects the type of search from a menu, such as author, title, key word, or call number. When the source is found, the full display for the reference includes author, title, publication information, all the index terms, and the call number. Many libraries in colleges and universities can also be accessed by faculty and students by personal computers via modem.

Some people who have used the older system for years are nostalgically reluctant to see it disappear. They maintain that while browsing through the cards they often experienced serendipity, which is where one finds something of value when searching for something else. Nevertheless, as one becomes familiar with the computer operations, the search process becomes much faster and more productive. Remember, if you have questions about any library operations, ask a librarian. They tend to be remarkably helpful and courteous.

Computer Searches

Computer service facilities can greatly expedite the literature search. Automated searching provides more effective and efficient access to indexes and information than does manual searching. Some databases available for computer searches are listed on page 36. The computer search covers many abstracting and indexing services in the sciences, humanities, and social sciences. The search can be conducted either online or by CD-ROM. Online is directly accessing references from database tapes. Sometimes you must pay a fee for a computer search, and the more extensive the search, the more costly it is. However, the fee is usually not prohibitive, especially if the searcher is careful in selecting pertinent descriptors and limiting the number of most recent and relevant documents.

Increasingly, libraries have databases on laser-read disks called CD-ROMs (Compact Disc-Read Only Memory), which enable individuals to do the literature search from a desktop computer at no cost. It should be pointed out that in many university libraries, faculty members and students can also perform online searches at no cost. It just depends on the individual library.

Adjusting the Scope of the Search.   As we have mentioned before, in many university libraries, the individual can do the computer search from a terminal in the library, either through CD-ROM or online. The information displayed on the screen can then be printed. Remember, the key to a successful literature search is careful planning. Therefore, write down your problem statement and then formulate cogent descriptors and key indexing terms. If the database you are using has a thesaurus, by all means use it. It is also beneficial to find one or more journal articles pertaining to your topic to assist you in the search strategy.

The scope of one's search can be narrowed or broadened by using key words called "Boolean operators." The two most common operators, or connectors, are the words "and" and "or." To narrow the search, you add another term with the word "and." For example, in the proposed study on investigating changes in attitude toward teaching following the student teaching experience, there were 2,237 items listed under the descriptor "attitude change." For "attitude + teaching" there were 186 items, and for "student teacher attitudes" there were 100 items. When all were connected with the word "and" there were 44 references, which is a manageable number to examine. Figure 2.3 illustrates the Boolean logic with this example.

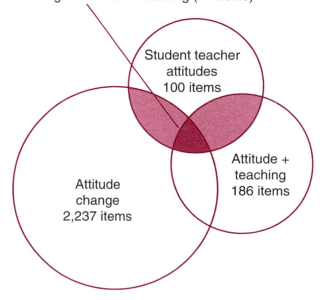

Entries dealing with changes in attitude and attitude toward teaching and student teaching (44 items)

Student teacher attitudes 100 items

Attitude + teaching 186 items

Attitude change 2,237 items

Figure 2.3   An illustration of the *AND* connector to narrow a search.

Some Databases Available for Computer Searches

ERIC (Educational Resources Information Center) (1966-   )

Descriptor Guidelines: *Thesaurus of ERIC Descriptors*

Type of Information: All topics concerning education from preschool to adult education are covered in areas of administration, curriculum, teaching, and learning. Published articles are accessed from the *Current Index to Journals in Education*, and unpublished materials can be obtained from the *Resources in Education* part of *ERIC*. These two databases can be searched simultaneously or separately. *ERIC* computer search is also available on CD-ROM.

MEDLINE (1966-   )

Descriptor Guidelines: *Medical Subject Headings*

Type of Information: The vast coverage of journal articles in biomedicine, health care, gerontology, and other areas in *Index Medicus* can be accessed through *MEDLINE*, which is available on CD-ROM.

PsycINFO (1967-   )

Descriptor Guidelines: *Thesaurus of Psychological Index Terms*

Type of Information: Journal articles, dissertations, and technical reports (book and book-chapter citations have been available since 1992) in psychology and related behavioral sciences. This database comes from *Psychological Abstracts*. *PsycLit* (1974-   ) is the CD-ROM version of *PsycINFO*.

Sociological Abstracts (1963-   )

Descriptor Guidelines: *Thesaurus of Sociological Indexing Terms.*

Type of Information: This database contains a comprehensive coverage of journal articles, conference publications, and books in social, developmental, and clinical psychology. Several database files are combined in this coverage. *Sociofile* (1974-   ) is the CD-ROM version.

Dissertation Abstracts Online (1861-   )

Descriptor Guidelines: None. Key words are listed by searcher.

Type of Information: Dissertation abstracts and master's theses (since 1962) from *Dissertation Abstracts International* and from *American Doctoral Dissertations*. It includes dissertations from nearly all American doctoral granting institutions and numerous dissertations from Canada and other countries. This service is available on CD-ROM.

UnCover (1988-   )

Descriptor Guidelines: None. Key words or names are listed by searcher.

Type of Information: Journal articles and journal tables of contents from over 15,000 journal titles with thousands of citations added daily. This is a fee-based service that offers you the opportunity to acquire a FAX of most articles usually within 24 hours.

The word "or" broadens the search. Additional related terms can be connected with "or" so that the computer will search for more than one descriptor (see Figure 2.4). For example, a researcher who seeks information about "practice teaching" (133 items) could broaden the search by using "practice teaching" (133 items) or "internship" (495 items) to get a total of 628 related terms.

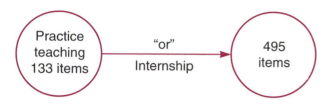

Figure 2.4 An illustration of the *OR* connector to broaden the search.

It may be that at your library you cannot conduct the computer search yourself, or you may prefer to have someone do it for you (which may be the most efficient and thorough course of action). Then you will have to consult with a librarian, and the search will have to be scheduled and carried out by library personnel. You will most likely be asked to complete a form on which the research statement, key words, and database are specified. The library personnel will be extremely helpful in selecting descriptors and in the entire literature search process. Search results can also be typed online and downloaded onto your diskette so that you can print it at your convenience. In most cases, the resulting bibliography is well worth the expense, especially in light of the comprehensiveness and the short amount of time and energy you expend.

Obtaining the Primary Sources. After you have a list of related references, you must obtain the actual studies and read them. Many references have abstracts in addition to the bibliographic information. The abstract is extremely helpful in making the decision as to whether the article is worth retrieving.

Keep in mind that a computer search does not replace the hand search. The computer is remarkably fast and effective in identifying references that may be pertinent to one's topic. However, perhaps the most valuable step in the search process is finding a recent, closely related study and reading that study's review of literature. Then, you find those studies that were cited and you read them, which leads you to other sources. Remember, as we stressed in the section on bibliographies, you are responsible for reading those studies. Don't rely on someone else's critique of the literature. Moreover, although the computer search is helpful, it is not infallible or magical. It is not unusual to have a pertinent article in your possession that is not listed on the computer search printout. This happens because somewhere in the process mistakes were made by people, not computers. It may be that the author of an article did not suggest the proper key words, or maybe the abstract did not adequately describe the study. Or perhaps someone responsible for indexing the article had a different perspective as to its subject matter. In any case, the computer search can never replace the hand search.

Your library may not have all the journals that are on the list of references (see page 38). You must consult your library's information system to see if your library carries a particular journal. If it doesn't, you will want to use interlibrary loan or possibly obtain the FAX of the article through *UnCover*.

Personal Computers. We have already mentioned that faculty and students can access library sources and conduct a literature search from personal computers in their own living quarters or office through a modem (telephone hook-up). Your library will have information about the recommended software and the Logon and Logoff procedures.

You should also be aware of the capabilities of **microcomputers** for storing bibliographic entries, abstracts, and even reprints of studies. A number of commercial programs are available for this purpose. The information can be retrieved by the use of pertinent key words, author names, or journal names. Additions, changes, and deletions are easily accomplished, and hundreds of items can be stored on a single disk. Each new entry is automatically stored in alphabetical order, and the complete bibliography is always instantly accessible. Often laboratories (e.g., exercise science and physical education) will keep files of reprints and use a software library program for a microcomputer to catalog these materials.

Other Library Services

The library services available depend mostly on the size of the institution, as larger schools generally provide more financial support for the library. However, some relatively small institutions have excellent

microcomputer — A small desktop computer.

Some Periodicals in Physical Education, Exercise Science, and Sports Science

Within the last 20 years, the number of periodicals available in our fields has increased tremendously. More specialization is one reason for this increase, as the so-called generalist is giving way to the specialist. Consequently, the vast amount of research and development of new knowledge about the special areas of interest has led to new audiences with common interests. Below is a partial list of journals that publish research in our fields.

Acta Physiological Scandinavia

Adapted Physical Activity Quarterly

American Corrective Therapy Journal

American Educational Research Journal

American Journal of Physical Anthropology

American Journal of Physical Medicine

American Journal of Physiology

American Journal of Sports Medicine

Athletic Administration

Athletic Training

Australian Journal of Sports Medicine

British Journal of Sports Medicine

Canadian Journal of the History of Sport and Physical Education

Child Development

Clinical Kinesiology

Educational and Psychological Measurement

European Journal of Applied Physiology and Occupational Physiology

Human Factors

Human Performance

International Journal of Biomechanics

International Journal of Sport Biomechanics

International Journal of Sport Psychology

International Journal of Sport Sociology

International Journal of Sports Medicine

Journal of Applied Physiology

Journal of Applied Sport Psychology

Journal of Biomechanics

Journal of Comparative and Physiological Psychology

Journal of Educational Psychology

Journal of Experimental Child Psychology

Journal of Experimental Psychology

Journal of Learning Disabilities

Journal of Motor Behavior

Journal of the Philosophy of Sport

Journal of Physical Education

Journal of Physical Education, Recreation and Dance

Journal of Physiology

Journal of Sport Behavior

Journal of Sport History

Journal of Sport Management

Journal of Sport and Exercise Psychology

Journal of Sports Medicine and Physical Fitness

Journal of Teaching in Physical Education

Medicine and Science in Sport and Exercise

The Olympian

Pediatric Exercise Science

Perceptual and Motor Skills

Physical Educator

Physical Therapy

Physician and Sportsmedicine

Physiological Reviews

Psychological Bulletin

Psychological Review

Psychology in the Schools

Quest

Research Quarterly for Exercise and Sport

Sociological Abstracts

Sociology of Sport Journal

The Sport Psychologist

library resources that provide outstanding support for the institutional and research aspects of the school.

Besides the usual services of the library information system (the computerized card catalog, reference and circulation departments, bibliographic collections, and stack areas), libraries also offer resources and services such as copy services, newspaper rooms, government document sections, telephone directories, college catalogs, and many other special features and services. One such valuable service is the interlibrary loan, which enables you to get books, theses and dissertations (occasionally), and photocopies of articles in journals that your library does not carry. An interlibrary loan usually takes 2-4 weeks from the date it is received.

 Universities typically have extensive collections of resources available on **microform**, which is a general term embracing microfilm, microfiche, microcard, and microprint. Microforms are simply miniaturized photographic reproductions of the contents of a printed page. You must use special machines called **readers** to enlarge the information so it can be read.

An obvious advantage of microforms is economy of space. In addition, they are useful for acquiring material that would otherwise not be available. Rare books and manuscripts and deteriorating materials can be preserved on microform. Some journals are on microform because it represents an economical means for the library to obtain them. Collections of government documents are often contained on microform, as are *ERIC* publications. The library will have a reader/printer that can make paper copies of microform material. Microform holdings are normally listed in the library's card catalog system and periodical listings.

Many libraries offer guided tours, short courses for orientation to the library, and self-guided tour information. Get acquainted with your library. It will be the wisest investment of time spent as a graduate student.

Read and Record the Literature

Collecting related literature is a major undertaking, but the next step is even more time-consuming. You must read, understand, and record the relevant information from the literature, keeping in mind one of the many (anonymous) Murphy's Laws: "No matter how many years you save an item, you will never need it until after you have thrown it away."

It is likely that the person originating this quote was a researcher working on a literature review. You may count on the fact that if you throw away one note from your literature search, that paper will be cited incorrectly in your text or reference list; or, if you throw away your notes on an article because you do not believe it is relevant to your research, your major professor, a committee member, or the journal to which you submit the paper will request inclusion of the article. Then, when you go back to locate the article in the library, either it will have been ripped out of the journal, the whole journal will be missing, or a professor will have checked it out and never returned it (and the librarian will not reveal the professor's name). Therefore, when you find a particular paper, take careful and complete notes, including exact citation information.

To help you understand the literature you read, try to decipher the scientific phrases on page 40. Once you understand what each phrase really means, you should have little difficulty understanding authors of research articles. Seriously, you, as researcher, should note the following information from research studies that you read:

- Statement of the problem (and maybe hypotheses)
- Characteristics of the subjects
- Instruments and tests used (including reliability and validity information if provided)
- Testing procedures
- Independent and dependent variables
- Treatments applied to subjects (if an experimental study)
- Design and statistical analyses
- Findings
- Questions raised for further study
- Citations to other relevant studies not located

When studies are particularly relevant to the proposed research, make a photocopy. Write the complete citation on the title page if the journal does not provide this. Many students (and faculty members)

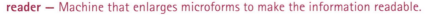

 microform — A general term that encompasses microfilm, microfiche, and any form of data storage where the pages of a book, journal, or newspaper are photographed and reduced in size.

reader — Machine that enlarges microforms to make the information readable.

What to look for as you read a research article

A Key to Understanding Scientific Research Literature

What was said	What was meant
It has long been known that . . .	I haven't bothered to look up the original reference but . . .
Of great theoretical and practical importance	Interesting to me
While it has not been possible to provide definite answers to those questions . . .	The experiment didn't work out, but I figured I could at least get a publication out of it.
The W–PO system was chosen as especially suitable to show the predicted behavior.	The researcher in the next lab had some already made up.
Three of the samples were chosen for detailed study.	The results on the others didn't make sense.
Accidentally strained during mounting	Dropped on the floor
Handled with extreme care throughout the experiment	Not dropped on the floor
Typical results are shown.	The best results are shown.
Agreement with the predicted curve is:	
excellent	fair
good	poor
satisfactory	doubtful
fair	imaginary
It is suggested that . . .	I think .
It is believed that . . .	I think.
It may be that . . .	I think.
It is clear that much additional work will be required before a complete understanding . . .	I don't understand it.
Unfortunately, a quantitative theory to account for these results has not been formulated.	Neither does anybody else
Correct with an order of magnitude . . .	Wrong
Thanks are due to Joe Glotz for assistance with the experiments and to John Doe for valuable discussion.	Glotz did the work and Doe explained what it meant.

make the mistake of simply photocopying an article without looking to see if the pages copied contain all the necessary information for a citation. Frequently, they do not, which means you have to go back to the library and try to find the journal and/or volume from which the article was taken. Also, indicate on a notecard the studies that are photocopied.

Another useful way to learn to read and understand related literature is to critique a few studies.

See the series of questions below to use when critiquing a study. Page 42 provides a sample form that we use that includes suggestions for reporting critiques. A few critiquing attempts should aid you in focusing on the important information contained in research studies.

Sometimes reviewers can go overboard in their critiques much like the critique of Schubert's Unfinished Symphony we present on page 43.

Criteria for Critiquing a Research Paper

I. **Overall impression** (most important): Is the paper a significant contribution to knowledge about the area?

II. **Introduction and review of literature**
   A. Is the research plan developed within a reasonable theoretical framework?
   B. Is current and relevant research cited and properly interpreted?
   C. Is the statement of the problem clear, concise, testable, and derived from the theory and research reviewed?

III. **Method**
   A. Are relevant subject characteristics described, and are the subjects appropriate for the research?
   B. Is the instrumentation appropriate?
   C. Are testing or treatment procedures described in sufficient detail?
   D. Are the statistical analyses and research design sufficient?

IV. **Results**
   A. Do the results evaluate the stated problem?
   B. Is the presentation of results complete?
   C. Are the tables and figures appropriate?

V. **Discussion**
   A. Are the results discussed?
   B. Are the results related back to the problem, theory, and previous findings?
   C. Is there excessive speculation?

VI. **References**
   A. Are all references in the correct format, and are they complete?
   B. Are all references cited in the text?
   C. Are all dates in the references correct, and do they match the text citations?

VII. **Abstract**
   A. Does it include a statement of the purpose; description of subjects, instrumentation, and procedures; and a report of meaningful findings?
   B. Is the abstract the proper length?

VIII. **General**
   A. Are key words provided?
   B. Are running heads provided?
   C. Does the paper provide for use of nonsexist language, protection of human subjects, and appropriate labeling of human subjects?

Form for a Critique

I. **Basic information**
   A. Name of journal
   B. Publisher of journal
   C. How many articles in this issue?
   D. Are there publication guidelines for authors? Which issue?
   E. Who is editor?
   F. Is there a yearly index? Which issue?
   G. What writing style is used (APA, *Index Medicus*, etc.)?
   H. Complete reference in APA style for article you will review

II. **Summary of the article**

III. **Critique of the article**
   A. Introduction and review
   B. Method
   C. Results
   D. Discussion
   E. References
   F. Overall

IV. **Attach one photocopy of the article.**

V. **Information about critique**
   A. It must be typed (double-spaced) in APA style.
   B. Do not put it in any type of folder; just staple the pages in upper left-hand corner.
   C. Use a cover page identifying course, purpose, and yourself.
   D. Critique may not exceed five typewritten pages exclusive of cover page.

 To summarize, the best system for recording relevant literature is probably a combination of note taking and photocopying. By using index cards (4" × 6" cards are usually large enough), the important information about most studies can be recorded and indexed by topic. Always be sure to record the complete and correct citation on the card with the appropriate citation style used by your institution (e.g., American Psychological Association [APA], *Index Medicus*).

Write the Literature Review

After you have located and read the necessary information and have recorded the appropriate bibliographic data, you are ready to begin to write the literature review. The literature review has three basic parts.

• Introduction
• Body
• Summary and conclusions

The introduction should explain the purpose of the review and the how and why of its organization. The body of the review should be organized around important topics. Finally, the review should summarize important implications and suggest directions for future research. The review's purpose is to demonstrate that your problem needs investigation and that you have considered the value of relevant past research in developing your hypotheses and methods; that is, you know and under-

 The best system for recording literature

Three parts of the literature review

Critique of Schubert's Productivity

A company CEO was given a ticket for a performance of Schubert's "Unfinished Symphony." Unable to go, he passed the invitation to the company's TQM (total quality management) coordinator. The next morning the CEO asked him how he enjoyed it. Instead of voicing a few plausible observations, he handed the CEO a memorandum which read as follows:

- For considerable periods, the oboe players had nothing to do. Their number should be reduced, and their work spread over the whole orchestra, thus avoiding peaks of inactivity.

- All twelve violins were playing identical notes. This seems unnecessary duplication, and the staff of this section should be drastically cut. If a large volume of sound is really required, this could be obtained through the use of an amplifier.

- Much effort was involved in playing the demi-semiquavers. This seems an excessive refinement, and it is recommended that all notes should be rounded up to the nearest semiquaver. If this were done, it should be possible to use trainees instead of craftsmen.

- No useful purpose is served by repeating with horns the passage that has already been handled by the strings. If all such redundant passages were eliminated, the concert could be reduced from two hours to twenty minutes.

In light of the above, one can only conclude that had Schubert given attention to these matters, he would probably have had the time to finish his symphony.

stand what other people have done and how that relates to and supports what you plan to do.

The introduction to the review (or to topical areas within the review) is very important. If these paragraphs are not well done and interesting, the reader may skip the entire section. Attempt to attract the reader's attention by identifying in a provocative way the important points to be covered.

The body of the literature review requires considerable attention. Relevant research must be organized, synthesized, and written in a clear, concise, and interesting way. There is no unwritten law dictating that literature reviews must be boring and poorly written, although we suspect that some graduate students work from that assumption. Part of the problem stems from graduate students' perceptions that they must find a way to make their scientific writing complex and circuitous as opposed to simple and straightforward. Apparently the rule is to never use a short and simple word when a longer, more complex one can be substituted. In Table 2.2, Day (1983) has provided a useful aid to potential research writers. In fact, we strongly recommend Day's book, which can easily be read in 4-6 hours. It provides many excellent and humorous examples that are valuable in writing for publication and for theses and dissertations.

In addition to removing as much jargon as possible (using Day's suggestions), you should be clear and to the point. We advocate the KISS Principle (Keep It Simple, Stupid) as a basic tenet for writing. Many grammatical errors can be avoided by use of simple declarative sentences. The list on page 46 (Day, 1983) rephrases the commandments of good writing from a 1968 Council of Biology Editors newsletter. The first 10 items are Day's, but we have included a few of our own comments as well.

Proper syntax (the way words and phrases are put together) is the secret of successful writing. Some examples of improper syntax and other unclear writing are highlighted on page 47.

As mentioned previously, the literature review should be organized around important topics. These topics serve as subheadings in the paper to direct the reader's attention. The best way to organize the topics and the information within topics is to develop an outline. The more carefully the outline is planned, the easier the writing will be. A good task is to select a review paper from a journal or from a

Day, R.D. (1983). *How to write and publish a scientific paper* (2nd ed.). Philadelphia: ISI Press.

Table 2.2   Words and Expressions to Avoid

Jargon	Preferred usage	Jargon	Preferred usage
a considerable amount of	much	in a position to	can, may
a majority of	most	in a satisfactory manner	satisfactorily
a number of	many	in a very real sense	in a sense (or leave out)
absolutely essential	essential	in case	if
accounted for by the fact	because	in close proximity	close, near
along the lines of	like	in connection with	about, concerning
an order of magnitude faster	10 times faster	in many cases	often
are of the same opinion	agree	in my opinion it is not an unjustifiable assumption that	I think
as a consequence of	because	in order to	to
as a matter of fact	in fact (or leave out)	in relation to	toward, to
as is the case	as happens	in respect to	about
as of this date	today	in some cases	sometimes
as to	about (or leave out)	in terms of	about
at an earlier date	previously	in the event that	if
at the present time	now	in the possession of	has, have
at this point in time	now	in view of the fact that	because, since
based on the fact that	because	inasmuch as	for, as
by means of	by, with	initiate	begin, start
completely full	full	is defined as	is
consensus of opinion	consensus	it has been reported by Smith	Smith reported
definitely proved	proved	it has long been known that	I haven't bothered to look up the reference
despite the fact that	although		
due to the fact that	because	it is apparent that	apparently
during the course of	during, while	it is believed that	I think
elucidate	explain	it is clear that	clearly
end result	result	it is clear that much additional work will be required before a complete understanding	I don't understand it
entirely eliminate	eliminate		
fabricate	make		
fewer in number	fewer		
finalize	end		
first of all	first	it is doubtful that	possibly
for the purpose of	for	it is evident that *a* produced *b*	*a* produced *b*
for the reason that	since, because		
from the point of view of	for	it is of interest to note that	(leave out)
give rise to	cause	it is often the case that	often
has the capability of	can	it is suggested that	I think
having regard to	about	it is worth pointing out in this context that	note that
in a number of cases	some		

(continued)

Jargon	Preferred usage	Jargon	Preferred usage
it may be that	I think	referred to as	called
it may, however, be noted that	but	relative to	about
		resultant effect	result
it should be noted that	note that (or leave out)	smaller in size	smaller
it was observed in the course of the experiments that	we observed	subsequent to	after
		sufficient	enough
lacked the ability to	couldn't	take into consideration	consider
large in size	large	terminate	end
let me make one thing perfectly clear	(a snow job is coming)	the great majority of	most
		the opinion is advanced that	I think
militate against	prohibit	the question as to whether	whether
needless to say	(leave out, and consider leaving out whatever follows it)	the reason is because	because
		there is reason to believe	I think
of great theoretical and practical importance	useful	this result would seem to indicate	this result indicates
on a daily basis	daily	through the use of	by, with
on account of	because	ultimate	last
on behalf of	for	utilize	use
on the basis of	by	was of the opinion that	believed
on the grounds that	since, because	ways and means	ways, means (not both)
on the part of	by, among, for	we have insufficient knowledge	we don't know
our attention has been called to the fact that	we belatedly discovered	we wish to thank	we thank
owing to the fact that	since, because	with a view to	to
perform	do	with reference to	about (or leave out)
pooled together	pooled	with regard to	concerning, about (or leave out)
prior to	before		
protein determinations were performed	proteins were determined	with respect to	about
quite unique	unique	with the possible exception of	except
rather interesting	interesting		
red in color	red	with the result that	so that

Reprinted from *How to Write and Publish a Scientific Paper*, 4th Edition by Robert A. Day. Used with permission of the Oryx Press, 4041 N. Central Ave., Suite 700, Phoenix, AZ, 85012. (800) 279-6799.

thesis or dissertation review of literature and reconstruct the outline the author must have used. In looking at older theses and dissertations, we find that the literature review tends to be a historical account, often presented in chronological order. We suggest that you not select one of these older studies, as this style is cumbersome and usually poorly synthesized.

To write a literature review effectively, you should write as you like to read. No one wants to read abstracts of study after study presented in chronological order. A more interesting and readable approach is to present a concept and then discuss the various findings about that concept, documenting findings by references to the various research

The Ten Commandments of Good Writing—Plus a Few Others

1. Each pronoun should agree with their antecedent.
2. Just between you and I, case is important.
3. A preposition is a poor word to end a sentence with. (Incidentally, did you hear about the streetwalker who violated a grammatical rule? She unwittingly approached a plainclothesman, and her proposition ended with a sentence.)
4. Verbs has to agree with their subjects.
5. Don't use no double negatives.
6. A writer mustn't shift your point of view.
7. When dangling, don't use participles.
8. Join clauses good, like a conjunction should.
9. Don't write a run-on sentence it is difficulty when you got to punctuate it so it makes sense when the reader reads what you wrote.
10. About sentence fragments.
11. Don't use commas, which aren't necessary.
12. Its' important to use apostrophe's right.
13. Check to see if you any words out.
14. As far as incomplete constructions, they are wrong.
15. "Last but not least, lay off cliches."

reports related to it. In this way, consensus and controversy can be identified and discussed in the literature review. More relevant and important studies can be presented in greater detail, and several studies with the same outcome can be covered in one sentence.

In a thesis or dissertation, the two important aspects of the literature review are criticism and completeness. The various studies should not simply be presented relative to a topic. The theoretical, methodological, and interpretative aspects of the research should be criticized—not necessarily on a study-by-study basis but rather across studies. This criticism demonstrates the writer's grasp of the issues and identifies problems that should be overcome in the study you are planning. Frequently, the problems identified by criticism of the literature may provide justification for your research.

Completeness (not in the sense of the length of the review but rather of reference completeness) is the other important aspect of the literature review. You should demonstrate to your committee that you have located, read, and understood all the related literature. Many studies may be redundant and only need appropriate citing, but they must be cited. The

thesis or dissertation is your passport to graduation because it demonstrates your competence; therefore, never fail to be thorough. This, however, applies only to the thesis or dissertation. Writing for publication or the use of alternate thesis or dissertation formats does not require emphasizing the completeness of the literature cited (note "cited," not "read"). Journals do not have the necessary space and usually want the introduction and literature review to be integrated and relatively short.

Summary

Identifying and formulating a researchable problem is often a difficult task, especially for the novice researcher. Some suggestions were given to help the graduate student find suitable topics. Inductive and deductive reasoning were discussed with regard to formulating research hypotheses. Inductive reasoning moves from observations to specific hypotheses to a more general theoretical model. Deductive reasoning moves from a theoretical explanation to specific hypotheses to be tested.

Examples of Unclear Writing

Sentences with improper syntax

- "The patient was referred to the hospital for repair of a hernia by a social worker."
- "As a baboon who grew up wild in the jungle, I realized that Wiki had special nutritional needs."
- "No one was injured in the blast, which was attributed to a buildup of gas by one town official."
- "Table 1 contains a summary of responses pertaining to suicide and death by means of a questionnaire." (We are aware that some questionnaires can be ambiguous, irrelevant, and trivial, but we had no idea they were fatal.)

Sentences taken from letters received by government agencies:

- I am forwarding my marriage certificate and six children. I had seven but one died which was baptized on a half sheet of paper.
- I am writing to say that my baby was born two years old. When do I get my money?
- Mrs. Jones has not had any clothes for a year and has been visited regularly by the clergy.
- I am glad to report that my husband who is missing is dead.
- This is my eighth child. What are you going to do about it?
- Please find for certain if my husband is dead. The man I am living with can't eat or do anything until he knows.
- I am very much annoyed to find that you have branded my son illiterate. This is a dirty lie as I was married a week before he was born.
- I am forwarding my marriage certificate and my three children; one of which is a mistake as you can see.
- In accordance with your instructions, I have given birth to twins in the enclosed envelope.
- I want my money as quick as I can get it. I have been in bed with a doctor for two weeks and he doesn't do me any good. If things don't improve, I will have to send for another doctor.

Sentences taken from job recommendations that are not quite clear:

- In my opinion you will be very fortunate to get this person to work for you.
- All in all, I cannot say enough good things about this candidate or recommend him too highly.
- I am pleased to say this candidate is a former colleague of mine.
- I can assure you that no person would be better for this job.

Unclear excuses for missing school:

- Please excuse Mary for being absent. She was sick and I had her shot.
- Please excuse Fred from being absent yesterday. He had diarrhea and his boots leak.
- Please excuse Mary from Jim [Gym?] yesterday. She is administrating.

A couple of others:

- This horse is an eight-year-old gelding trained by the owner who races him with his wife.
- She rode 106 miles on a bicycle with 1,400 other people.

There are no shortcuts to locating, reading, and indexing the literature and then writing the literature review. If you follow our suggestions, you can do it more effectively, but much hard work is still required. A good scholar is careful and thorough.

Do not depend on what others report, as they are often incorrect. Look it up yourself.

No one can just sit down and write a good literature review. A careful plan is necessary. First, outline what you propose to write, write it, and then write it again. When you are convinced that the review represents your best effort, have a knowledgeable graduate student or faculty member read it, then welcome their suggestions. Next, have a friend who is not as knowledgeable read it. If your friend can understand it, then your review is probably in good shape. Of course, your research methods professor will find something wrong or at least something he or she thinks should be different. Just remember that professors feel obligated to find errors in graduate students' work.

 Check Your Understanding

Throughout this chapter we have made several suggestions for exercises that will help you locate, syn-

thesize, organize, critique, and write the literature review. These suggestions are summarized below. You will need to return to various points in the chapter to read about these exercises and to refer to the necessary tables.

1. Do the library assignment in the sidebar entitled "Criteria for Critiquing a Research Paper."
2. Critique a research study in your area of interest. Use the questions in the sidebar entitled "Form for a Critique" as your model. Report the critique in the form suggested in Table 2.1.
3. Select a review paper from a journal or the literature review from a thesis or dissertation. Construct the outline the author probably used to write this paper.

CHAPTER 3

Presenting the Problem

Dear Professors of Research Methods:

I have been working on my research question and I'm having trouble narrowing the topic so that I can complete the literature review. What should I do?

Sincerely,
Ima Bookworm

Dear Bookworm:

You need to carefully study and apply "Murphy's Three Laws of the Research Question."

First Law: If you have finalized your research questions, you don't understand the literature.

Second Law: Only when you have clarified your research questions will you discover a large body of conflicting findings.

Third Law: Your study will only make sense if your research questions are hazy.

Methodologically yours,
PRM

In a thesis or dissertation, the first section or chapter serves to introduce the problem. Indeed, it is often entitled "Introduction." Its purpose is to do just that: to inform the reader about the problem being studied. Several sections in the Introduction serve to convey the significance of the problem and set forth the dimensions of the particular study. This chapter discusses each of the following sections, which are frequently required in the first part of a thesis or dissertation:

- Title
- Introduction
- Problem statement
- Hypothesis
- Definitions
- Assumptions and limitations
- Significance

Not all thesis advisors subscribe to the same thesis format, for there is no universally accepted one. Moreover, because of the nature of the research problem, there will be differences in format. For example, a historical study would not adhere to the same format as that used in an experimental study. We are merely presenting sections, each with a purpose and with specific characteristics, typically found in the Introduction.

Choosing the Title

Although discussing the title first may seem logical, it might surprise you to learn that titles are often not determined until after the study has been written. However, at the proposal meeting, you must have a title (even though it may be provisional), so we will discuss it first.

Some writers claim that there is a trend toward shortening titles (e.g., Day, 1983). However, an analysis of more than 10,000 dissertations in seven areas of education failed to demonstrate such a trend (Coorough & Nelson, in press). Many titles are, in essence, the statement of the problem (in fact, some even include the methods section). Here is an example of a too lengthy title (Note: The examples we use as representing poor practices are fictional. Frequently, they have been suggested by actual studies, but any similarity to a real study is purely coincidental.):

An Investigation of a Survey and Analysis of the Influence of PL 94-142 on the Attitudes, Teaching Methodology, and Evaluative Techniques of Randomly Selected Male and Female Physical Education Teachers in Public High Schools in Cornfield County, State of Confusion.

Simply too much information is in such a title. Day (1983) humorously responded to this problem by reporting a conversation between two students. When one asked whether the other had read a certain paper, the reply was, "Yes, I read the paper, but I haven't finished the title yet" (p. 10). A better title for the study mentioned previously would be "PL 94-142's Influence on Physical Education Teachers' Attitudes, Methodology, and Evaluations."

The purpose of the title is to convey the content, but this should be done as succinctly as possible. For example, "The Twelve-Minute Swim as a Test for Aerobic Endurance in Swimming" (Jackson, 1978) is a good title because it tells the reader exactly what the study is about. It defines the specific

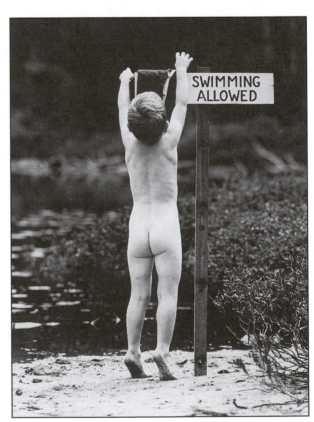

There are sometimes distinct benefits to shortening your original title.

Sections of the first part of a thesis or dissertation

purpose, which is the validation of the 12-minute swim, and it delimits the study to the assessment of aerobic endurance for swimmers.

However, do not go to the other extreme in striving for a short title. A title such as "Professional Preparation" is not very helpful. It does not include the field or the aspects of professional preparation studied. The key to the effectiveness of a short title is whether it reflects the study's contents. A title that is specific is more easily indexed and more meaningful for a potential reader who is searching for literature on a certain topic.

Avoid "waste" words and phrases such as "An Investigation of," "An Analysis of," and "A Study of." They simply increase the length of the title and contribute nothing to the description of the content. Consider this title: "A Study of Three Teaching Methods." Half the title consists of waste words: "A Study of." The rest of the title is not specific enough to be indexed effectively: teaching what? what methods?

Furthermore, always be aware of your audience. You can assume that your audience is reasonably familiar with the field, the accepted terminology, and the viable problem areas. An outsider can question the relevance and import of studies in any field. Some titles of supposedly scholarly works are downright humorous. For a rousing good time, peruse the titles of theses and dissertations completed at a university in any given year; for example, "The Phospholipid Distribution in the Testes of the House Cricket." How weird can you get? We are joking, of course. The point is that there is a tendency to criticize studies done in other disciplines simply because the critic is ignorant about the discipline. An example of this in our field could be a scholarly article by Grabe and Widule (1988) entitled "Comparative Biomechanics of the Jerk in Olympic Weight Lifting." To someone unfamiliar with the sport, this might seem to be a case study about some unpopular weight lifter in the Olympic Games.

Writing the Introduction

How to Write a Good Introduction
Examples of Good Introductions

 Hallmarks of a good introduction

The introductory portion of a thesis or research article is designed to create interest in the problem. You use the introduction to persuade readers of the problem's significance, provide background information, bring out areas of needed research, and then skillfully and logically lead to the specific purpose of the study.

How to Write a Good Introduction

A good introduction requires literary skill because it should flow smoothly yet be reasonably brief. Be careful not to overwhelm the reader with technical jargon, for the reader must be able to understand the problem to gain an interest in the solution. Therefore, an important rule is this: Do not be too technical. A forceful, simple, and direct vocabulary is more effective for purposes of communication than scientific jargon and worship of polysyllables. Day (1983) related a classic story of the pitfalls of scientific jargon:

This reminds me of the plumber who wrote the Bureau of Standards saying he had found hydrochloric acid good for cleaning out clogged drains. The Bureau wrote back, "The efficacy of hydrochloric acid is indisputable, but the corrosive residue is incompatible with metallic permanence." The plumber replied that he was glad the Bureau agreed. The Bureau tried again, writing, "We cannot assume responsibility for the production of toxic and noxious residues with hydrochloric acid and suggest that you use an alternative procedure." The plumber again said that he was glad the Bureau agreed with him. Finally, the Bureau wrote to the plumber, "Don't use hydrochloric acid. It eats the hell out of pipes." (pp. 147-148)

Audience awareness is important. Again, you can assume that the reader is reasonably informed about the topics (or he or she probably would not be reading it in the first place). However, even an informed reader needs some refresher background information to understand the nature of the problem, to be sufficiently interested, and to appreciate the author's rationale for studying the problem. You must remember that your audience has not been as completely and recently immersed in this particular area of research as you have been.

 The introductory paragraphs must create interest in the study; thus, your writing skill and knowledge of the topic are especially valuable in the introduction. The narrative should introduce the necessary background information quickly and explain the rationale behind the study. A smooth, unified, well-written introduction should lead to the problem statement with such clarity that the reader could state the study's purpose before specifically reading it.

The following introductions were selected from research journals for their brevity of presentation and for their effectiveness. This is not to say that brevity in itself is a criterion, for some topics require more comprehensive introductions than others. For example, studies developing or validating a theoretical model usually necessitate longer introductions than does an applied research topic. Furthermore, theses and dissertations (in the traditional format) almost always have longer introductions than journal articles simply because of the page-cost considerations in the latter.

Examples of Good Introductions

The following examples specify some desirable features in an introduction, including a general introduction, background information, a mention of gaps in the literature and areas of needed research, and a logical progression leading to the problem statement. After you've read them, see if you can write the purpose for each study.

Example #1   (From Sundgot-Borgen, 1994).

Reprinted by permission from *Medicine and Science in Sports and Exercise*, **26**, pp. 414-419. *Medicine and Science in Sports and Exercise* is a publication of the American College of Sports Medicine.

[General Introduction]

In recent years, there has been growing interest in eating disorders in athletes (7, 30). Studies have shown that athletes are more prone to developing eating disorders than nonathletes (4, 5, 21, 28). In addition, the highest prevalence of eating disorders is in female athletes competing in sports where leanness and/or a specific weight are considered important for either performance or appearance (4, 27, 28).

[Background Information]

There has been considerable speculation about why athletes are at increased risk for eating disorders. Predisposing personality or family interaction variables might be primary (3, 26, 32), so participation in sports favoring leanness could be a consequence

of preexisting eating problems or could be coincidental. Alternatively, participation in certain sports could be related causally to the onset of eating disorders. In all likelihood these factors interact.

[Lead-In]

One important area of inquiry, therefore, is to identify risk factors to help determine which athletes are most vulnerable, or which conditions or trigger factors elicit the pathological behavior.

Example #2   (From Dolgener, Hensley, Marsh, & Fjelstul, 1994).

Reprinted by permission from *Research Quarterly for Exercise and Sport*, **65**, pp. 152-158. *RQES* is a publication of the American Alliance for Health, Physical Education, Recreation and Dance, 1900 Association Dr., Reston, VA 22091.

[General Introduction]

Cardiorespiratory fitness is generally recognized as a major component of physical fitness. Indeed, cardiorespiratory fitness is the most significant component of physical fitness in the relationship to health. Direct measurement of maximal oxygen uptake ($\dot{V}O_2max$) is the single best measure of cardiorespiratory fitness or aerobic capacity (Astrand & Rodahl, 1986; Mitchell, Sproule, & Chapman, 1958; Taylor, Buskirk, & Henschel, 1955). However, direct measurement is time-consuming, requires extensive laboratory equipment, and does not lend itself to testing large numbers of subjects in field settings. Because of the limitations of direct measures, numerous field tests have been developed to estimate $\dot{V}O_2max$.

[Background Information]

Prediction of $\dot{V}O_2max$ from field tests requires performing at either a maximal or submaximal effort, commonly running, stepping, or bicycling. Recently, Kline, Porcari, Hintermeister et al. (1987) developed a submaximal field test for predicting $\dot{V}O_2max$ using a 1-mile walk protocol. This test, which has become known as the Rockport Fitness Walking Test (RFWT), was developed on a broad age range (30-69 years) of males and females who were heterogeneous in terms of aerobic capacity. (*Note: we are omitting some information concerning specific correlations and errors of estimate to save space*). These data indicate that the regression equations developed by Kline, Porcari, Hintermeister et al. are valid for adults between the ages of 30 and 69 years.

The RFWT has been cross-validated in samples of subjects 65 to 79 years old (Fenstermaker, Plowman, & Looney, 1992; O'Hanley et al., 1987) and 30 to 39 years old (Zwiren, Freedson, Ward, Wilke, & Rippe, 1991).

[Lead-In]

The Kline, Porcari, Hintermeister et al. (1987) equations, however, have not been validated for use with groups younger than those in the original sample.

Stating the Research Problem

Identifying the Variables
Structuring the Problem Statement

The problem statement follows the introduction. We should point out that the literature review is often included in the introductory section and thus precedes the formal statement of the problem. If this is the case, then a brief problem statement should appear fairly soon in the introductory section before the literature review.

The problem statement in example #1 from Sundgot-Borgen was to examine risk factors for eating disorders along with trigger factors that may be responsible for precipitating the onset or exacerbation of eating disorders [in elite female athletes]. The problem statement in the Dolgener et al. study was also obvious from the introduction. The purposes stated were (a) to validate the Kline, et al. 1-mile walk test in a sample of male and female college students, and (b) to develop prediction equations for $\dot{V}O_2$max on this college sample if their equations proved invalid.

Identifying the Variables

The problem statement should be succinct. However, when the study has several subpurposes, this is not always easily accomplished. The statement should identify the different variables in the study, including the independent variable, the dependent variable, and the cat-

egorical variable (if any). Usually, some **control variables** (which could possibly influence the results and are kept out of the study) can also be identified here.

The independent and dependent variables have already been mentioned in chapter 1. The independent variable is the experimental, or treatment, variable; it is the "cause." The dependent variable is what is measured to assess the effects of the independent variable; it is the "effect." A **categorical variable** is sometimes called a **moderator variable** (Tuckman, 1978). This variable is a kind of independent variable, except that it cannot be manipulated because it is categorized by, for example, age, race, and sex. It is studied to determine whether the cause-and-effect relationship of the independent and dependent variables is different in the presence of the categorical variable or variables.

The following is an actual study in which the independent, dependent, and categorical variables can be identified. Anshel and Marisi (1978) studied the effect of synchronous and asynchronous movement to music on endurance performance. One group performed an exercise in synchronization to background music; one group exercised with background music that was not synchronized to the pace of the exercise; and a third group exercised with no background music.

The independent variable was the background music condition. There were three levels of this variable: synchronous music, asynchronous music, and no music. The dependent variable was endurance performance, which was reflected by the amount of time the subject could exercise on a bicycle ergometer until exhaustion. In this study, the endurance performances of men and women under the synchronous, asynchronous, and absence-of-music conditions were compared. The authors thus sought to determine whether men responded differently than women to the exercise conditions. Gender, then, represented a categorical variable. Not all studies have categorical variables.

The researcher decides which variables to manipulate and which variables to control. One can control the possible influence of some variable by keeping it out of the study. Thus, the researcher chooses not to assess a variable's possible effect on

control variable — A factor that could possibly influence the results and that is kept out of the study.

categorical variable — A kind of independent variable that cannot be manipulated because it is categorized by age, race, sex, and so on; also called *moderator variable*.

moderator variable — See *categorical variable*.

the relationship between the independent and dependent variables, so this variable is controlled. For example, suppose a researcher is comparing stress-reduction methods on the competitive state anxiety of gymnasts before dual meets. The subjects' years of competitive experience might have a bearing on their anxiety scores. The researchers have a choice. They can include it as a categorical variable by requiring that half the subjects have had X-years of experience and that the other half have had less, or they can control the variable of experience by requiring that all subjects have similar experience.

 The decision to include or exclude some variable depends on several considerations, such as whether the variable is closely related to the theoretical model and how likely there is to be an interaction. Practical considerations include how difficult it is to make a variable a categorical variable or to control it (such as availability of subjects having a particular trait) and how much control the researcher has over the experimental situation.

In the study of the effects of synchronized music on endurance (Anshel & Marisi, 1978), the factor of fitness level was controlled by giving all the subjects a physical working capacity test. Then, on the basis of this test, each subject exercised at a work load that would cause a heart rate of 170 bpm. Thus, even though the ergometer resistance settings would be different from subject to subject, all subjects would be exercising at approximately the same relative work load; the differences in fitness were controlled in this manner. Another way of controlling fitness as a variable would be to test subjects on a fitness test and just select those subjects of a certain level of fitness.

 Extraneous variables are factors that could affect the relationship between the independent and dependent variables but are not included or controlled. The possible influence of an extraneous variable is usually brought out in the discussion section. Anshel and Marisi (1978) speculated that some differences in the performances of men and women might be due to the women's reluctance to exhibit maximum effort in the presence of a male experimenter. Consequently,

this would be an extraneous variable (all the variables are discussed in more detail in chapter 16).

Rarely are the variables labeled as such in the actual problem statement. Occasionally, the researcher will identify the independent and dependent variables, but mostly these variables are just implied.

In summary, an effectively constructed introduction leads smoothly to the study's purpose. This is expressed as the statement of the problem and should be as clear and concise as the subpurposes, or variables, allow it to be.

Structuring the Problem Statement

To achieve clarity in the statement of the problem, a final but important aspect you must consider is sentence structure, or syntax. For example, suppose a researcher conducted a study "to compare sprinters and distance runners on anaerobic power, as measured by velocity in running up a flight of stairs." Observe the difference in meaning if the researcher had worded the purpose as "to compare the anaerobic power of sprinters and distance runners while running up a flight of stairs." Apparently the researcher would have to be in good shape to make those comparisons while running up stairs. Another example of faulty syntax was the case in which the purpose of the study was "to assess gains in quadriceps strength in albino mice using electrical stimulation." Those mice had to be awfully clever to use electrical instruments.

Presenting the Research Hypothesis

 After you have stated the research problem, you must present the hypothesis. The formulation of hypotheses was discussed in chapters 1 and 2. The discussion here is on the statement of the hypotheses and the distinction between research hypotheses and the null hypothesis. Remember that **research hypotheses** are the expected results. In the study by Anshel and Marisi (1978), a

---

Considerations to help decide whether to include or exclude variables

extraneous variable — A factor that could affect the relationship between the independent and dependent variables, but that is not included or controlled.

research hypothesis — Hypothesis deduced from theory or induced from empirical studies that is based upon logical reasoning and is predictive of the outcome of the study.

research hypothesis might be that endurance performance would be enhanced by exercising to synchronized music. The introduction produces a rationale for that hypothesis. Another hypothesis might be that exercise to asynchronous music would be more effective than exercising with no background music (because of the pleasurable sensory stimuli blocking the unpleasant stimuli associated with the fatiguing exercise). As a further example, a researcher in cardiac rehabilitation might hypothesize that distance from the exercise center is more influential as a factor in exercise adherence of patients than the type of activities offered in the cardiac rehabilitation program. In the example given in chapter 1, a dance teacher hypothesized that the use of videotape in the instructional program would enhance the learning of dance skills.

In contrast, the **null hypothesis** is primarily used in the statistical test for the reliability of the results, and says that there are no differences between treatments (or no relationship between variables). For example, any observed difference or relationship is due simply to chance (see chapter 8). The null hypothesis is usually not the research hypothesis. Generally, the researcher expects one method to be better than others or anticipates a relationship between two variables. One does not embark on a study if nothing is expected to happen. On the other hand, a researcher sometimes hypothesizes that one method is just as good as another. For example, in the multitude of studies done in the 1950s and 1960s on isometric versus isotonic exercises, it was often hypothesized that the "upstart" isometric exercise was just as effective as the traditional isotonic exercise, provided there was regular specific knowledge of results. In a study on the choice of recreational activities of mentally retarded children, Matthews (1979) showed that most research in this area, which reported differences between retarded and nonretarded children, failed to consider socioeconomic status. Consequently, he hypothesized that there were no differences in frequency of participation in recreational activities between mildly mentally retarded and nonretarded children when socioeconomic status was held constant.

Furthermore, sometimes the researcher does not expect differences in some aspects of the study but does expect a difference in others. A researcher might hypothesize that children of high aptitude in learning would do better with one style of teaching, whereas children of low aptitude would fare better with another style. In a study of age differences in the strategy for recall of movement (Thomas, Thomas, Lee, Testerman, & Ashy, 1983), the authors hypothesized that because location is automatically encoded in memory, there would be no real difference between younger and older children in remembering location (where an event happened during a run). However, they hypothesized that there would be difference in remembering distance because the older child spontaneously uses a strategy for remembering and the younger child does not. The formulation of hypotheses is a very important aspect of defining and delimiting the research problem.

Operationally Defining Your Terms

Another task in the preparation of the first section of a thesis or dissertation is operationally defining certain terms so that the researcher and the reader can adequately evaluate the results. It is imperative that the dependent variable is operationally defined.

So what is an **operational definition**? It is an observable phenomenon, as opposed to a synonym definition or dictionary definition. To illustrate, a study such as Anshel and Marisi's (1978), which investigated the effects of music on forestalling fatigue, must operationally define fatigue. The author cannot use a synonym, such as *exhaustion*, because that is not concrete enough. We all might have our own ideas of what fatigue is, but if we are going to say that some independent variable affects fatigue, we must supply some observable evidence of changes in fatigue. Therefore, fatigue must be operationally defined. Anshel and Marisi did not use the term "fatigue," but from their description of procedures we can infer its operational definition as being when the subject was unable to maintain the pedaling rate of 50 revolutions per minute for 10 consecutive seconds.

---

null hypothesis — Hypothesis that is primarily used in the statistical test for the reliability of the results that says that there are no differences among treatments (or no relationship among variables).

operational definition — Observable phenomenon that enables the researcher to empirically test whether or not the predicted outcomes can be supported.

Another researcher might define fatigue as the point when a maximal heart rate was achieved; still another might define fatigue as the point of maximal oxygen consumption. In all cases, though, it must be an observable criterion.

A study dealing with dehydration must provide an operational definition such as a loss of 5% of body weight. The term "obesity" in males could be defined as having 25% body fat. A study of different teaching methods on learning must operationally define the term "learning." To use the old definition "a change in behavior" is meaningless in providing evidence of learning. Learning might be demonstrated by five successful maze traversals or some other observable performance criterion.

You may not always agree with the investigator's definitions, but at least you know how a particular term is being used. A common mistake with novice researchers is to think that every term needs to be defined. (We have seen master's students define terms not even used in their studies!) An example of an unnecessary definition would be in a study of the effects of strength training on changes in self-concept. "Self-concept" would need to be defined (probably as represented by some scale), but "strength" would not. The strength-training program used would be described in the methods section. Basically, operational definitions are directly related to the research hypotheses because, if you predict that some treatment will produce some effect, you must define how that effectiveness will be manifested.

Outlining Basic Assumptions, Delimitations, and Limitations

Assumptions
Delimitations and Limitations

Besides writing the introduction, stating the research problem and hypothesis, and operationally defining your terms, you must outline the basic assumptions and limitations under which you performed your research.

Assumptions

Every study has certain fundamental premises without which it could not proceed. In other words, you must assume that certain conditions will exist and that the particular behaviors in question can be observed and measured (along with various other basic suppositions). A study in pedagogy that compares teaching methods must assume that the teachers involved are capable of promoting learning; if this assumption is not made, the whole study is worthless. Furthermore, in a learning study the researcher must assume that the sample selection (e.g., random selection) results in a normal distribution with regard to learning capacity.

A study designed to assess an attitude toward exercise is based on the assumption that this attitude can be reliably demonstrated and measured. Furthermore, you can assume that the subjects will respond truthfully, at least for the most part. If you cannot assume those things, you should not waste your time conducting the study.

Of course, the experimenter does everything possible to increase the credibility of the premises. The researcher takes great care in selecting measuring instruments, in sampling, and in gathering data concerning such things as standardized instructions and motivating techniques. Nevertheless, the researcher still must rely on certain basic assumptions.

Consider the following studies. Johnson (1979) investigated the effects of different levels of fatigue on visual recognition of previously learned material. Among his basic assumptions were that (a) the mental capacities of the subjects were within the normal range for university students, (b) the subjects understood the directions, (c) the mental task typified the types of mental tasks encountered in athletics, and (d) the physical task demands typified the levels of exertion commonly experienced in athletes.

Lane (1983) compared skinfold profiles of black and white girls and boys and tried to determine which skinfold sites best indicated total body fatness with regard to race, sex, and age. She assumed that (a) the skinfolds caliper is a valid and reliable instrument for measuring subcutaneous fat, (b) skinfold measurements taken at the body sites are indicative of the subcutaneous fat stores in the limbs and trunk, and (c) the sum of all skinfolds represents a valid indication of body fatness.

In some physiological studies, the subjects are instructed (and agree) to fast or to refrain from smoking or drinking liquids for a specified period before testing. Obviously, unless the study is conducted in some type of prison environment, the experimenter cannot physically monitor the subjects' activities. Consequently, a basic assumption is that the subjects will follow instructions.

Delimitations and Limitations

Every study also has **limitations**. Limitations are possible shortcomings or influences that either cannot be controlled or are the results of the delimitations imposed by the investigator. Some limitations refer to the scope of the study, which is usually imposed by the researcher. These are often called **delimitations**. Kroll (1971) described delimitations as choices the experimenter makes to effect a workable research problem, such as the use of one particular personality test in the assessment of personality characteristics. Moreover, in a study dealing with individual-sport athletes, the researcher may choose to restrict the selection of subjects to just two or three sports, simply because all individual sports could not be included in one study. Thus, the researcher delimits the study. You probably notice that these delimitations resemble operational definitions. Although they are similar, they are not alike. For example, the size of the sample is a delimitation but would not be included under operational definitions.

You can also see that basic assumptions are entwined with delimitations as well as with operational definitions. The researcher must proceed on the assumption that the restrictions imposed on the study will not be so confining as to destroy the external validity (generalizability) of results.

Remember, theses or dissertations do not have one "correct" format. An examination of studies will show numerous variations in organization. You will see some studies that have delimitations and limitations described in separate sections. Some will use a combination heading, some will list only one heading but include both in the description, and so on. As with all aspects of format, much depends on how the advisor was taught. Graduate schools often allow great latitude in format as long as the study is internally consistent. You will even find considerable differences in format within the same department.

In the example Kroll (1971) used of delimiting the scope of the study to just two sports to represent individual-sport athletes, there is an automatic limitation with respect to how well these represent all individual sports. Moreover, if the researcher is studying personality traits of these athletes and delimits the measurement of personality to just one test, this results in a limitation. Furthermore, there is one (or more) limitation in all self-report instruments as to the truthfulness of the responses in which the subject responds to questions about his or her behavior, likes, or interests.

Thus, you can see that limitations also accompany the basic assumptions to the extent that the assumptions fail to be justified and, as with assumptions, the investigator tries as much as possible to reduce limitations that might stem from faulty procedures. In Johnson's 1979 study of fatigue effects on visual recognition of previously learned material, he had to have the subjects first learn the material. He established criteria for learning (operational definition) and tried to control for overlearning (i.e., differences in the level of learning). Despite his efforts, however, he recognized that a limitation was that there may have been differences in the degree of learning, which could certainly influence recognition.

In the study of skinfold profiles by Lane (1983), she had to delimit the study to a certain number of subjects in one part of Baton Rouge, Louisiana. Consequently, a limitation was that the children were from only one geographical location. She also recognized that there are changes in body fatness associated with the onset of puberty, but she was unable to obtain data on puberty or other indices of maturation, and this therefore posed a limitation. Still another limitation was the inability to control possible influences on skinfold measurement, such as dehydration and other diurnal variations. Finally, because there are no internationally recognized standard body sites for skinfold measurement, generalizability may have been limited to the body sites used in this study.

You should not be overzealous in searching for limitations, or you can apologize away the worth of the study. For example, one of our advisees who was planning to meet with his proposal committee was overly apologetic with these anticipated limitations:

- The sample size may be too small.
- The tests may not represent the parameter in question.

---

 limitation — A possible shortcoming or influence that either cannot be controlled or is the result of the delimitations imposed by the investigator.

delimitation — A limitation, imposed by the researcher, in the scope of the study; a choice the researcher makes to effect a workable research problem.

 How assumptions, delimitations, and operational definitions are related

- The training sessions may be too short.
- The investigator lacks adequate measurement experience.

As a result, the proposal was revised and the method was reassessed.

Remember, there is no perfect study. You must carefully analyze the delimitations to determine whether the resulting limitations outweigh the delimitations. In addition, careful planning and painstaking methodology will increase the validity of the results, thus greatly reducing possible deficiencies in a study.

Justifying the Significance of the Study

Basic and Applied Research Revisited

Writing the "Significance of the Study" Section

The inevitable question you face at both the proposal meeting and the final oral exams deals with the worth, or significance, of the study, which may be asked in different ways, such as, So what? or, What good is it? or, How is this of any importance to your profession? Regardless of the manner in which the question is asked, it must be answered. Perhaps because of the inevitability of the question being asked, most students are required to include a section in the first chapter entitled "Significance of the Study" or sometimes "The Need for the Study."

Basic and Applied Research Revisited

To a large extent, the worth of the research study is judged by whether it is basic or applied research. In chapter 1, we explained that basic research does not have immediate social significance; it usually deals with theoretical problems and is conducted in a very controlled laboratory setting. Applied research addresses immediate problems for improving practice. There is less control but ideally more real-world application. Consequently, basic and applied research cannot be evaluated by the same criteria.

The significance of a basic research study obviously depends on the specific purpose of the study, but usually the criteria focus on the extent to which the study contributes to the formulation or validation of some theory. The worth of applied research must be evaluated on the basis of its contribution to the solution of some immediate problems.

Writing the "Significance of the Study" Section

The significance section is often difficult to write, probably because the student thinks only in terms of the practicality of the study, for example, how the results can be immediately used to improve some aspect of the profession. Kroll (1971) emphasized the importance of maintaining continuity of the significance section with the introduction. Too often the sections are written with different frames of reference instead of a continuous flow of thought. The significance section should focus on such things as contradictory findings of previous research and gaps in knowledge in particular areas. Difficulties in measuring aspects of the phenomenon in question are sometimes emphasized. Rationale for the need to verify existing theories may be the focus of the section in some studies, whereas in others the practical application is the main concern.

Just as the length of the introduction varies, the length of the significance section varies considerably from study to study. A sample of a significance section from Lane (1983) may serve to illustrate an approach that focuses on some conflicts between previous research findings and present practice:

> Since the measurement of body composition has become an important aspect of physical fitness testing, the validity, reliability, and administrative feasibility of the measurements are of paramount concern. Adult formulas for estimating percent fat are not considered valid for children, thus skinfolds are in themselves used as measures of body composition.
>
> The AAHPERD Health Related Physical Fitness Test Manual (1980) contains two skinfold measurements: the triceps and subscapular. Norms for the total of these two

How to integrate the significance section with the introduction

measures are provided for boys and girls ages 6 to 17 years. Abbreviated norms are also given for the triceps skinfolds only. Norms were taken from HES data (Johnston et al., 1974). There is minimal evidence as to why these two body sites were selected, especially when one, the subscapular, poses some problem with regard to modesty. If the triceps and subscapular were selected as representing one from the limbs and one from the trunk, are they the most predictive of total fatness as indicated by the sum of several skinfolds from the limbs and trunk? Furthermore, if some sites are equally predictive, the ease of administration needs to be considered.

Of major significance in this study is whether the skinfolds which best represent body fatness in white children are equally suitable for black children. Authors (Cronk & Roches, 1982; Harsha et al., 1974; Johnston et al., 1974) have reported that there are differences in skinfold thicknesses between black and white children, yet the AAHPERD norms make no distinction. If norms are to be of value they must be representative of the population for which they are intended. Moreover, there may be greater differences in fatness between blacks and whites at different ages.

Similarly, it may be that a different combination of skinfolds would be more valid for girls than boys. It does not seem to be of any great administrative advantage to use the same sites for both sexes if other sites are equally valid indicators of total fatness.

A final word of warning: In being asked the inevitable question in the final orals about the significance of the study, do not reply, "It was necessary to get my degree." The stony silence will serve only to unnerve you.

The Differences Between Thesis Format and the Research Article

A mere glance at research articles in journals reveals that a number of the sections found in the traditional thesis or dissertation described in this chapter are missing. At least two reasons account for this. The first is financial: Periodicals are concerned about publishing costs, so brevity is emphasized. Second, a kind of novice-master ritual seems to be in opera-

tion. The novice is required to explicitly state the hypotheses, define terms, state assumptions, recognize limitations, and justify the worth of the study in writing. Certainly these steps are all part of defining and delimiting the research problem, and it is undoubtedly a worthwhile experience to address each step formally.

Research journal authors, on the other hand, need not explain the step-by-step procedure they used in developing the problem. Typically, a research journal has an introduction that includes a short review of literature. The length varies considerably, and some journals insist on brief introductions.

The purpose of the study is nearly always given but is usually not designated by a heading; rather, it is often the last sentence or so in the introduction. For example, in 30 articles in one volume of the *Research Quarterly for Exercise and Sport*, only 1 had a section entitled "Purpose of the Study." Twenty-four ended their introductions with sentences that began with the words "The purpose of this study was . . ." Four indicated the purpose with sentences beginning "This study was designed to . . ." or "The intent of the study was . . ." One study did not state the purpose at all. In 29 cases, the authors and editors felt that the purpose was evident from the title and introduction.

Research hypotheses are sometimes given but with little uniformity. Operational definitions, assumptions, limitations, and significance of the study are virtually never stated in research articles. Apparently, for the "master" researcher these steps were accomplished in the development of the problem and are understood, obvious, or both and need not be stated. If the article is well written, you should be able to discern the operational definitions, the assumptions and limitations, and the independent, dependent, and categorical variables even though they are not specifically stated. Moreover, the significance of the study should be implicitly obvious if the author has written a good introduction.

Summary

This chapter discussed the information that is typically presented in the first section or chapter of a thesis or dissertation (excluding the review of literature). First, we considered the length and substance of the study title. The importance of a good, short, descriptive title with respect to indexing and searching the literature is sometimes over-looked.

The introduction of a research study often proves difficult to write. It requires a great deal of thought, effort, and skill to convey to the reader the study's significance. If it is poorly done, the reader may not bother to read the rest of the study.

The problem statement and the research hypotheses commonly appear in most research studies, whether they are theses or dissertations, journal articles, or research grants. Operational definitions, assumptions, limitations and delimitations, and the significance of the study usually appear only in theses and dissertations. Their purpose is to help (or force) the researcher to succinctly define and delimit the research problem. Operational definitions specifically describe how certain terms (especially the dependent variables) are being used in a particular study. Assumptions identify the basic conditions that must be assumed to exist for the results to have credibility. Delimitations relate to the scope of the study imposed by the researcher, such as the number and characteristics of the subjects, the treatment conditions, and the specific dependent variables that are used. Limitations are possible influences on the results that are consequences of the delimitations or that cannot be completely controlled.

The significance of the study section forces the researcher to address the inevitable question of the study's worth. It should be a continuation of the introduction in terms of the contextual flow. It usually calls attention to the relationship (and differences) between this study and previous ones, controversies and gaps in the literature, and the contribution that this study might make to the practitioner, existing theoretical models, or both.

 Check Your Understanding

1. For each of the following brief descriptions of studies, write a title, the purpose or purposes, and three research hypotheses.
   The researchers assessed the following:
   a. Skill acquisition of three groups of fourth-grade boys and girls who had been taught by different teaching styles (A, B, and C).
   b. Self-concept of two groups of boys (a low-strength group and a high-strength group) before and after a strength-training program.
   c. Body composition (estimated percent fat) using the electrical impedance analysis method on subjects at normal hydration and again after they had dehydrated.
   d. Grade point averages of male and female athletes of major and minor (club) sports from large universities and small private colleges.

2. Locate five articles from research journals, and for each try to determine (a) the hypotheses, if not stated, (b) the operational definitions, (c) the limitations, and (d) the assumptions.

CHAPTER 4

Formulating the Method

Dear Professors of Research Methods:

My research hypothesis is that people who study martial arts can resist being rendered unconscious by choking significantly longer than people who have not studied martial arts. I plan to have a confederate sneak up on subjects of both groups and choke them until they are unconscious. Time from onset of choking until unconsciousness will be my dependent variable. Do you think I will have any trouble getting my topic approved by the university's Committee on the Use of Human Subjects in Research?

Sincerely,
Bruce Lee

Dear Bruce:

We don't wish to dampen your enthusiasm for research, but you may have a really big problem in getting approval for this topic (let alone finding volunteers for subjects). In other words, don't hold your breath (a little humor there). Rest assured, however. The committee will not toss your proposal lightly aside. Instead, it will likely be hurled wth great force. Find a new topic.

Methodologically yours,
PRM

The previous chapter provided an overview of the introduction in the proposal for a thesis or dissertation. As already indicated, the journal format typically includes the literature review (see chapter 2 in this book) as part of the introduction. (If the chapter format is used, the literature review may appear as a separate chapter or as part of the introduction.) Regardless, once the introduction has been completed, the researcher must describe the methodology for the research. Typically, this section is labeled "Method," and we overview the four parts of the method section here:

- Subjects
- Instruments or apparatus
- Procedures
- Design and analysis

For our purposes, let's assume that the journal format is used and the literature review is included in the introduction of your thesis or dissertation followed by the method section. Much of the remainder of this book is focused on the method: who the subjects are (this chapter), how to measure and analyze the results (Part II), and how to design the study (Part III). The purpose of the method section is to explain how to conduct the study. The standard rule is that the description should be thorough enough for a competent researcher to reproduce the study.

Science as we know it today grew out of the murky lore of the Middle Ages (e.g., sorcery and religious ritual).

> But while witches, priests, and chiefs were developing taller and taller hats, scientists worked out a method for determining the validity of their experimental results: they learned to ask, Are they reproducible?—that is, would anyone using the same materials and methods arrive at the same results? For example, it is very important to scientists that two iron balls of unequal mass dropped together from the leaning tower of Pisa hit the ground simultaneously whether dropped by Galileo in 1590 or Mr. T today. (Scherr, 1983, p. ix)

How to Present Methodological Details

Dissertations and theses differ considerably from published articles in the methodological details

provided. However, when using the journal format, the additional materials beyond what would appear in a journal article about method should be placed in the appendix. Journals try to conserve space, but space is no issue in a dissertation or thesis. Thus, where standard techniques in a journal article are referenced only to another published study (in an easily obtainable journal), a thesis or dissertation should provide considerably greater detail but in the appendix. Note that we indicated a technique could be referenced to an easily obtainable journal. When writing for publication, use common sense in this regard. Consider, for example, this citation:

> Farke, F.R., Frankenstein, C., & Frickenfrack, F. (1921). Flexion of the feet by foot fetish feet feelers. *Research Abnormal: Perception of Feet*, **22**, 1-26.

By most standards, this citation would not be considered easily obtainable. Therefore, if you are in doubt, give the details of the study or technique.

Furthermore, because theses and dissertations have appendices, much of the detail that would clutter and extend the method section should be placed there. Examples include exact instructions to subjects, samples of tests and answer sheets, diagrams and pictures of equipment, sample data-recording sheets, and informed-consent agreements.

Why Planning the Method Is Important

The purpose of this planning is to eliminate any alternative or rival hypotheses. This really means that when you design the study correctly and the results are as predicted, the only explanation is what you did in the research. Using a previous example to illustrate, our hypothesis is, "Shoe size and mathematics performance are positively related during elementary school." To test this hypothesis, we go to an elementary school, measure shoe sizes, and obtain standardized mathematics performance scores of the children in Grades 1-5. When we plot these scores, they appear as in Figure 4.1, each dot representing a single child. Moving from the dot to the x-axis shows shoe size while the

Four parts of the method section

y-axis shows math performance. "Look!" we say. "We are correct. As shoe sizes get larger, the children's mathematics performance increases. Eureka! All we need to do is buy the children bigger shoes and their mathematics performance will improve." But wait a minute! The authors have overlooked two things. First, there is a rival explanation: Both shoe size and mathematics performance are related to age. That really explains the relationship. As the kids get older, their feet get bigger and they perform better on mathematics tests. Second, just because two things are related does not mean that one causes the other. Correlation does not imply causation. Obviously, we cannot improve children's math performance by buying them bigger shoes.

In research we want to use the **MAXICON principle**: MAXimize true variance, or increase the odds that the real relationship or explanation will be discovered; minImize error vari-

ance, or reduce all the mistakes that could creep into the study to disguise the true relationship; and CONtrol extraneous variance, or make sure that rival hypotheses are not the real explanations of the relationship.

Two Principles for Planning Experiments

In an interesting paper Cohen (1990) puts forward two principles that make good sense when planning experiments. The first is **less is more**. Of course, this seldom applies to the number of subjects for a study, but it does apply to other aspects. For example, graduate students want to conduct meaningful studies that address and solve important problems. To do this they often plan complex studies with many independent and dependent variables. From one perspective, this is good: The world of physical activity is truly complex. Students often start with useful ideas to study, but the ideas become so cumbersome that the study often fails because of sheer complexity. Carefully evaluate the number of independent and dependent variables that are practically and theoretically important to your study. Don't let anyone convince you (except your major professor, of course, who can convince you of anything) to add additional variables just to see what happens. This complicates your study and causes all types of measurement and statistical problems.

This idea leads to the second principle from Cohen: **simple is better**. This statement is true from the design to the treatments, to the analysis, to displaying data, to interpreting results. Keep your study straightforward so that when you find something, you can understand and interpret what it means. Understanding your data is really an important concept. Although all the fancy statistical programs are nice and informative, there is no substitute for plotting data graphically and evaluating it carefully. Summary statistics (e.g., mean, standard deviation) are very helpful and informative, but they are no substitute for looking

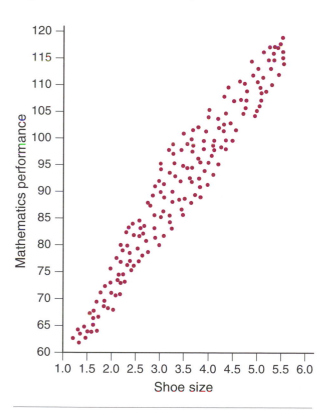

Figure 4.1 Relationship of academic performance and shoe size of children Grades 1-5.

MAXICON principle — A method of controlling any explanation for the results except the hypothesis the researcher intends to evaluate. This is done by maximizing true variance, minimizing error variance, and controlling extraneous variance.

Cohen, J. (1990). Things I have learned (so far). *American Psychologist*, **45**, 1304-1312.

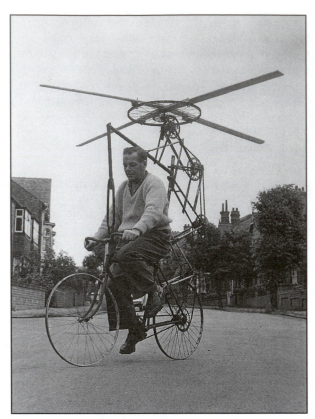

Proving the "simple is better" principle of planning experiments.

at the original data and how it is distributed. Summary statistics may not show us what we really need to know: things that become evident when we looked at a graphic display of the data.

Describing Subjects

What to Tell About the Subjects
Protecting Subjects

This section of the method of a thesis or dissertation describes how and why the subjects were selected and which of their characteristics are pertinent to the study. Issues to consider when selecting subjects revolve around these questions:

- Are subjects with special characteristics necessary for your research?
  — age (children, elderly)
  — gender
  — trained or untrained (level of training)
  — experts or novices (level of performance)
  — size (weight, fatness)
  — special types (athletes, cyclists, runners)
- Can you obtain the necessary permission and cooperation from the subjects?
- Can you find enough subjects?

Of course, you want to select subjects who will potentially respond to the treatments and measures used in the study. For example, if you want to see the results of training a group of children in overhand throwing, selecting expert 12-year-old baseball pitchers as subjects will not likely produce a change in measures of throwing outcome. It would take an intense long-term training program to have any influence on these subjects. However, selecting children who were soccer players and had never played organized baseball would offer better odds for a training program to produce changes.

In experimental research the interaction among selecting the subjects, measures, and the nature of the treatment program is essential in allowing the treatment program to have a chance to work. If you select subjects who have high levels of physical fitness, subjecting them to a moderate training program will not produce changes in fitness. Also, subjects high in physical fitness will have a small range of scores on a measure of cardiovascular endurance (e.g., $\dot{V}O_2max$). For example, you will not find a significant correlation between $\dot{V}O_2max$ and marathon performance in world-class marathon runners. This is because their range of scores in $\dot{V}O_2max$ is small as is the range of scores in marathon performance times. Because the range of scores is small in both measures, no significant correlation will be found. This does not mean that running performance and cardiovascular endurance are not related. It means you have restricted the range of subjects' performance so much that the correlation cannot be exhibited. If you had selected moderately trained runners (e.g., women who jog three times per week for 40 minutes each time), there would have been a significant corre-

Issues to consider in subject selection

lation between running performance on a 3-mile run and $\dot{V}O_2max$. (We discuss procedures for selecting sample subjects in chapter 6.)

What to Tell About the Subjects

The exact number of subjects should be given, as should any loss of subjects during the time of study. In the proposal, some of this information may not be exact. For example, the following might describe the potential subjects:

Subjects: For this study 48 males, ranging in age from 21 to 34 years, will be randomly selected from a group ($N = 147$) of well-trained distance runners ($\dot{V}O_2max = 60 \, ml \cdot kg \cdot min^{-1}$ or higher) who have been competitive runners for at least 2 years. Subjects will be randomly assigned to one of four groups ($n = 12$).

Once the study is completed, details would be available on the subjects, so now this section might read as follows:

Subjects. In this study 48 males, ranging in age from 21 to 34 years, were randomly selected from a group ($N = 147$) of well-trained runners ($\dot{V}O_2max = 60 \, ml \cdot kg \cdot min^{-1}$ or higher) who had been competitive runners for at least 2 years. The subjects had the following characteristics (standard deviations in parentheses): age, $M = 26$ years (3.3); height, $M = 172.5$ cm (7.5); weight, $M = 66.9$ kg (8.7); and $\dot{V}O_2max$, $M = 65 \, ml \cdot kg \cdot min^{-1}$ (4.2). Subjects were randomly assigned to one of four groups ($n = 12$).

The subject characteristics listed are extremely pertinent in an exercise physiology study but not at all, for example, in a study of equipment used by children on the playground. The nature of the research dictates the subject characteristics of interest to the researcher. Carefully think through the important characteristics you will report in your research. Look at related studies for ideas of important characteristics to report.

The characteristics about subjects you identify and report must be clearly specified. Note in the example that "well-trained runners" were exactly defined; that is, their $\dot{V}O_2max$ must be equal to 60 $ml \cdot kg \cdot min^{-1}$ or higher. Where subjects of different ages are to be used is another good example. It is not sufficient just to say that 7-, 9-, and 11-year-olds will be the subjects. How wide an age range is 7 years old: + 1 month, $\pm$ 6 months, or what? In the proposal, you may say that 7-, 9-, and 11-year-olds will be included in the study. At the time of testing, each age will be limited to a + 6-month age range. Then, when the thesis or dissertation is actually written, it may read as follows:

At each age level 15 children were selected for this study. The mean ages are as follows (standard deviations in parentheses): the youngest group, 7.1 years (4.4 months); 9-year-olds, 9.2 years (3.9 months); and the oldest group, 11.2 years (4.1 months).

Protecting Subjects

Most research in the study of physical activity deals with humans, often children, but it also includes animals. Therefore, the researcher must be concerned about any circumstances in the research setting or activity that could harm the humans or animals. In chapter 5, "Ethical Issues in Research and Scholarship," we provide considerable details on what the researcher must do to protect both humans and animals used in research. It is particularly important to obtain informed consent of humans and ensure the protection and care of animals. Sample forms for the use of humans and animals in research, developed at Arizona State University, are provided in Appendix D. (Such forms may be slightly different at your college or university.)

Describing Instruments

Information about the instruments, apparatus, or tests used to collect data is used to generate the dependent variables in the study. Consider the following points when selecting tests and instruments:

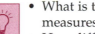

- What is the validity and reliability of the measures?
- How difficult is it to obtain the measures?
- Do you have access to the instruments, tests, or apparatus needed?
- Do you know (or can you learn) how to administer the tests or use the equipment?

 Points to consider when selecting tests and instruments

- Do you know how to evaluate subjects' test performance?
- Will the tests, instruments, or apparatus yield a reasonable range of scores for the subjects you have selected?
- Will the subjects be willing to spend whatever time is required for you to administer the tests or instruments?

For example, in a sport psychology study, you are interested in how a group of university football players will be affected by a lecture on attitudes toward steroid use. In addition, you suspect that the players' attitudes might be modified by certain personality traits. So you select three tests—a steroid knowledge test, an attitude inventory about responsible drug use, and a trait personality measure—and administer them to all subjects. The knowledge and attitude tests will probably be given before and after the lecture and the trait personality test only before the lecture (traits should not change, and this test is being used to stratify subjects in some way). In the instrument section, you should describe the three tests and probably put complete copies of each in the appendix (read the section in chapter 5 about ethical use of standardized tests). You also should describe the reliability (consistency) and validity (what the test measures) information that is available on each test with appropriate citations. Then you should explain the scoring sheets (place a sample in the appendix) and the scoring methods.

Another example might be a motor behavior study in which subjects' reaction and movement times are measured under various conditions. In this section you should describe the testing apparatus and provide a diagram or picture. If the apparatus is interfaced with a microcomputer to control the testing situation and data collection, you should describe the microcomputer (brand name and model) and how the interface was made. At least a description of how the computer program operates should be included in the appendix (if not a complete copy of the program). You should explain the dependent variables generated for reaction and movement time and give reliability estimates for these characteristics. All the necessary information could be presented by the appropriate use of both the instrument (or apparatus) part of the method section and the appendix, thus allowing the method section to flow smoothly.

Describing Procedures

In this section you should describe how the data are obtained, including all testing procedures for obtaining scores on the variables of interest. How tests are given and who gives them are important features. You should detail the setup of the testing situation and instructions given to the subjects (although you may place some of this information in the appendix). If the study is experimental, then you should describe the treatments applied to the different groups of subjects. Consider these points when planning procedures:

- **Collecting the data**
  — When? Where? How much time is required?
  — Do you have pilot data to demonstrate your skill and knowledge in using the tests and the equipment and how subjects will respond?
  — Have you developed a scheme for data acquisition, recording, and scoring (computer controlled!)?
- **Planning the treatments** (in quasi- and experimental studies)
  — How long? How intense? How often?
  — How will subjects' adherence to treatments be determined?
  — Do you have pilot data to show how subjects will respond to the treatments and that you can administer these treatments?
  — Have you selected the appropriate treatments for the type of subjects to be used?

One of our favorite summaries of the problems encountered and solutions proposed is presented on page 67. These statements are extracted from an article by Martens (1973) entitled "People Errors in People Experiments."

The procedures section contains most of the details that allow another researcher to replicate the

Points to consider when planning procedures

Errors in Experiments

Martens's method derives from the basic premise that:

> In people experiments people errors increase in disproportionate ratio to the contact people have with people.

It is obvious that the most logical deduction from this premise is:

> To reduce people errors in people experiments, reduce the number of people.

Although this solution might be preferred for its elegant simplicity, its feasibility can be questioned. Therefore, the following alternative formulation warrants consideration:

> The contact between people testers and people subjects in people experiments should be minimized, standardized, and randomized.

From "People Errors in People Experiments," by R. Martens, June 1973, *Quest*, p. 20. Copyright 1973 by the Quest Board. Reprinted with permission.

study. Tuckman (1978) outlined these details, which generally include

- the specific order in which steps were undertaken;
- the timing of the study (e.g., time for different procedures and time between different procedures);
- instructions given to subjects; and
- briefings, debriefings, and safeguards.

Avoiding Methodological Faults

Unless you carefully pilot all your procedures, "quirk theory" (p. 68) will apply to your research. *No single item in this book is more important than our advice to pilot all your procedures.* Physical education, exercise science, and sport science have produced thousands of studies in which the discussions centered on methodological faults that caused the research to lack validity. We are aware that we are repeating ourselves, but placing post hoc blame on the methodology for inadequate results is unacceptable. Every thesis or dissertation proposal should present **pilot work** that verifies that all instruments and procedures will function as specified on the type of subjects for which the research is intended. In addition, you must demonstrate that you can use these procedures and apparatuses accurately and reliably.

Don't let your procedures become so complex that you end up like Santa Claus might on Christmas Eve with more to do than it seems possible to accomplish.

According to our calculations, Santa has about 31 hours to work on Christmas (this is because of different time zones and the earth's rotation). If he travels from east to west and there are 91.8 million households to visit, Santa must make 822.6 visits per second allowing him 1/1000th of a second to park, hop out of the sleigh, jump down the chimney, fill the stockings, distribute the remaining presents under the tree, eat whatever snacks have been left, get back up the chimney, get back into the sleigh, and move on to the next house.

Importance of Pilot Work

During our years as major professors, editors, and researchers, we have seen abstracts of thousands of master's theses and doctoral dissertations. More than 75% of these research efforts are unpublishable and make no contribution to theory or practice because of major methodological flaws that could have been easily corrected with pilot work. Sadly, this reflects negatively not only on the discipline and profession but also on the graduate students who conducted the research and the faculty who directed

 Material in the procedures section

 pilot work — Verifying that you can correctly administer the tests and treatments for your study using appropriate subjects.

Law of Experiment

First Law: In any field of scientific endeavor, anything that can go wrong will go wrong.
Corollary 1: Everything goes wrong at one time.
Corollary 2: If there is a possibility of several things going wrong, the one that will go wrong is the one that will do the most damage.
Corollary 3: Left to themselves, things always go from bad to worse.
Corollary 4: Experiments must be reproducible; they should fail in the same way.
Corollary 5: Nature always sides with the hidden flaw.
Corollary 6: If everything seems to be going well, you have overlooked something.
Second Law: It is usually impractical to worry beforehand about interference; if you have none, someone will supply some for you.
Corollary 1: Information necessitating a change in design will be conveyed to the designer after, and only after, the plans are complete.
Corollary 2: In simple cases presenting one obvious right way versus one obvious wrong way, it is often wiser to choose the wrong way so as to expedite subsequent revisions.
Corollary 3: The more innocuous a modification appears to be, the further its influence will extend, and the more plans will have to be redrawn.
Third Law: In any collection of data, the figures that are obviously correct, beyond all need of checking, contain the errors.
Corollary 1: No one whom you ask for help will see the errors.
Corollary 2: Any nagging intruder who stops by with unsought advice will spot them immediately.
Fourth Law: If in any problem you find yourself doing a transfinite amount of work, the answer can be obtained by inspection.

To assist in the research suggested, the following rules have been formulated for the use of those new to this field.

Rules of Experimental Procedure

1. Build no mechanism simply if a way can be found to make it complex and wonderful.
2. A record of data is useful; it indicates that you have been busy.
3. To study a subject, first understand it thoroughly.
4. Draw your curves; then plot your data.
5. Do not believe in luck; rely on it.
6. Always leave room when writing a report to add an explanation if it doesn't work. (Rule of the way out.)
7. Use the most recent developments in the field of interpretation of experimental data.
   a. Items such as Finagle's constant and the more subtle Bougeurre factor (pronounced "Bugger") are loosely grouped, in mathematics, under constant variables or, if you prefer, variable constants.
   b. Finagle's constant, a multiplier of the zero-order term, may be characterized as changing the universe to fit the equation.
   c. The Bougeurre factor is characterized as changing the equation to fit the universe. It is also known as the "Soothing" factor; mathematically, somewhat similar to the damping factor, it has the characteristic of dropping the subject under discussion to zero importance.
   d. A combination of the two, the Diddle coefficient, is characterized as changing things so that the universe and the equation appear to fit without requiring any change in either.

it. Yet, nearly all the problems could have been corrected by increased knowledge of the topic, better research design, and pilot work on the procedures.

Graduate students frequently seek information about appropriate procedures from related literature (and they should). Procedures for intensity, frequency, and duration of experimental treatments are often readily available, as is information about testing instruments and procedures. However, it is important to remember that procedures in one area do not necessarily work well in another, as the following example illustrates.

Research Procedures May Not Generalize

Dr. I.M. Funded was a good life scientist who studied the biochemistry of exercise in a private research laboratory. He had also done several studies with a colleague in sport psychology to determine whether some biochemical responses he had found were factors in psychological responses to exercise. Thus, he had a firm grasp of some of the social science techniques as well as those of life science.

Unfortunately, Dr. Funded's funding ran out, and he lost his job. A friend of his was the superintendent of a large school district. Dr. Funded went to his friend, Dr. Elected, and said, "I am a good scientist well trained in problem-solving techniques. Surely, you must need someone like me in your administrative structure. In addition I have an undergraduate degree in physical education, so I am certified to teach, although I never have." Dr. Elected agreed to hire him as his teaching effectiveness supervisor because the school system was having difficulty identifying good teaching. Dr. Elected thought that perhaps a scientist with good problem-solving skills and the ability to make careful measurements could find a solution.

Dr. Funded decided that his first task was to identify some good teachers so he could determine the characteristics they possessed. He would use some of the techniques he had acquired from his colleague in sport psychology to identify good teachers. He had learned that questionnaires were effective in surveying large groups but that interviews were more valid. Dr. Funded drew a random sample of 6 schools from the 40 in the district. Then, he randomly selected 6 teachers in each school and interviewed them. He used a direct interview question: "Are you a good teacher?" All 36 indicated they were. So he went back to Dr. Elected, explained what he had done, and said, "You don't have a teaching problem. All of your teachers are good." (Of course, he noted there could be some sampling error, but he was certain of his results.) Dr. Elected was not very happy with Dr. Funded's procedures and results and suggested that perhaps he needed more sophisticated techniques and strategies to identify good teachers.

Dr. Funded was slightly distraught but thought to himself, I have always questioned the techniques of those psychologists anyway—I will return to my life science techniques to determine the answer. He went back to the previously selected 36 teachers with a plan to draw blood, sample urine, and do muscle biopsies (at four sites) once per week for 4 weeks. Immediately, 34 teachers said no, but 2 who were triathletes agreed to participate. Dr. Funded noted that the subject mortality rate was about normal for biopsy studies, so the data should be generalizable. He collected all the data, did the correct chemical analyses, and reported back to Dr. Elected. He indicated that effective teachers had 84% slow-twitch fiber, higher-than-average amounts of hemoglobin per deciliter of blood, and a specific profile of catecholamines (epinephrine and norepinephrine) in the urine. In addition, good teachers trained for at least 100 miles per week on the bicycle, 50 miles running, and 7,500 meters swimming. Dr. Funded sat back smugly and said, "Techniques for the life sciences can be applied to solve many problems." Dr. Elected said, "You are fired."

Describing Design and Analysis

Design is the key to controlling the outcomes from experimental and quasi-experimental research. The independent variables are manipulated in an attempt to judge their effects on the dependent variable. A well-designed study is one in which the only explanation for change in the dependent variable is how the subjects were treated (independent variable). The design and theory have enabled the researcher to eliminate all rival or alternative hypotheses. The design requires a section heading in the method for experimental and quasi-experimental research. The plans for data analysis must also be reported. In most studies some type of statistical analysis is used, but there are exceptions (e.g., historical or qualitative research).

Typically, the researcher will explain the proposed application of the statistics. In nearly all cases, descriptive statistics are provided, such as means and standard deviations for each variable. If correlational techniques (relationships among variables) are used, then the variables to be correlated and the techniques are named; for example, "The degree of relationship between two estimates of percent fat will be established by using Pearson r to correlate the sum of three skinfolds with underwater weighing." In experimental and quasi-experimental studies, descriptive statistics are provided for the dependent measures, and the statistics for establishing differences among groups are reported; for example, "A t test was used to determine whether youth league hockey players watching professional games produced more violent actions during their games than youth league players who did not watch professional hockey games."

The major problem that graduate students encounter in the description of statistical techniques is the tendency to inform everyone of their knowledge of statistics. Of course, that is not much of a problem for the new graduate student. But if your program of studies is a research-oriented one in which you take several statistics courses, your attitude may change rapidly.

Hiawatha, who at college majored in applied statistics, consequently felt entitled to instruct his fellow men on any subject whatsoever. (Kendall, 1959, p. 23)

The point of the line of poetry is for you to describe your statistical analyses but not to instruct in their theoretical underpinnings and proper use.

Establishing Cause–Effect

The establishment of cause-effect in an experimental study is much more than a statistical and design issue. The issue is one of logic. If the null hypothesis is not true, then what hypothesis is true? Of course, the scholar hopes the research hypothesis is true, but this is difficult to establish. In science the researcher seeks to explain that certain types of effects normally happen given specific circumstances or causes. For example, an effect may occur in the presence of something but not in its absence. Water boils in the presence of a high enough temperature but not in the absence of this specific temperature (given a specific air pressure).

People may (and do) differ in their opinions about what can be a cause-effect relationship or even if one can exist. For example, whether you believe in universal laws, in destiny, in free will, or in an omnipotent deity is likely to influence your view of cause and effect.

Must causes be observable? If yes, then two criteria are needed to establish cause-effect. First is the method of agreement. If an effect occurs when both A and B are present, and A and B have only C in common, then C is the likely cause (or at least part of it). Second is the method of disagreement. If the effect does not occur in E and F when C is the only common element absent, then C is the cause (or part of it). Thus, it is clear that the researcher's reasoning influences the establishment of cause and effect, because the researcher's beliefs set the stage for what may be considered a cause or even whether one can exist. This suggests that the researcher's theoretical beliefs as well as the study's design and analysis are essential factors in establishing cause-effect (for a more detailed discussion of causation, see White, 1990).

In terms of scientific progress, any statistical analysis whose purpose is not determined by theory, whose hypothesis and methods are not theoretically specified, or whose results are not related back to theory must be considered, like

White, P.A. (1990). Ideas about causation in philosophy and psychology. *Psychological Bulletin*, **108**, 3-18.

atheoretical fishing and model building, to be hobbies. (Serlin, 1987, p. 371)

Summary

This chapter has provided an overview of the method for the research study. We have identified the major parts as subjects, instruments or apparatuses, procedures, and design and analysis. The four parts of the method chapter and their major purposes are to eliminate alternative or rival hypotheses or to control any explanation for the results except the hypothesis that the researcher intends to evaluate. The MAXICON principle shows the way to accomplish this: (a) maximize the true or planned sources of variation, (b) minimize any error or unplanned sources of variation, and (c) control any extraneous sources of variation. In the following sections, we detail how to do this from the viewpoints of statistics and measurement (Part II) and of design (Part III). We will explain the final sections of the thesis or dissertation in Part IV.

 Check Your Understanding

1. Find an experimental study in *Research Quarterly for Exercise and Sport* and critique the method section. Comment on the degree to which the author provided sufficient information concerning the subjects (and informed consent), instruments, procedures, and design and analysis.
2. Locate a survey study and compare and contrast its method description with that in the study in Problem 1.

CHAPTER 5

Ethical Issues in Research and Scholarship

Dear Professors of Research Methods:

A friend of mine who is completing her thesis at another university told me about a research project a student was doing there. I am really interested in it. Can I propose the same thing to my major professor for my thesis?

Sincerely,
R.U. Ethical

Dear Ethical:

No, using another person's thesis idea would not be ethical. However, you could get some follow-up ideas from reading that student's research. Don't worry, there are plenty of ideas around.

Universities are full of knowledge

Freshmen bring a little in

Seniors take none away

So, knowledge accumulates

Methodologically yours,
PRM

As graduate students, you will encounter a number of ethical issues in research and scholarship. In this chapter we draw your attention to many of these issues and provide a framework for discussion and decision making. However, the choices will not always be clear-cut. The most important aspect of making good decisions is to have good information and obtain advice from trusted faculty. The major topics to be presented include misconduct in science, working with faculty and other graduate students, using humans as subjects in research, and using animal subjects.

Seven Areas of Scientific Dishonesty

Plagiarism
Fabrication and Falsification
Nonpublication of Data
Faulty Data-Gathering procedures
Poor Data Storage and Retention
Misleading Authorship
Sneaky Publication Practices

"When you stick a white glove in the dirt, the glove gets dirty; the dirt does not get glovy."

The Public Health Service has defined misconduct in science for us:

Misconduct or Misconduct in Science

Fabrication, falsification, plagiarism, or other practices that seriously deviate from those that are commonly accepted within the scientific community for proposing, conducting, or reporting research. . . . It does not include honest error or honest differences in interpretations or judgments of data.

(Final Regulations, Public Health Service, 42 Code, Section 50, August 8, 1989, p. 32446)

In this section we discuss issues in scientific misconduct with the notion that these concepts are generally applicable to all scholarly areas in the study of physical activity. We have also supplied a list of references on scientific misconduct as well as two "case studies" with questions for discussion.

Shore (1991) identified seven areas in which scientific dishonesty might occur; each is discussed below. The 1993 volume of *The Academy Papers* (Thomas & Gill [Eds.]) includes several thought-provoking articles on ethics in the study of physical activity. The list on pages 75-76 provides additional readings.

Plagiarism

Plagiarism means using the ideas, writings, and drawings of others as your own. Of course, this is completely unacceptable in the research process (including writing). Plagiarism carries severe penalties at all institutions. A researcher who plagiarizes work carries a stigma for life in his or her profession. No reward is worth the risk involved.

On occasion a graduate student or faculty member can inadvertently be involved in plagiarism. This generally occurs on work that is coauthored. If one author plagiarizes material, the other could be equally punished even though he or she is unaware of the plagiarism. Although there is no sure-fire means of protection (except do not work with anyone else), never allow a paper with your name on it to be submitted (or revised) unless you have seen the complete paper in its final form.

In scientific writing, originality is also important. Common practice is to circulate preprints and drafts of papers among scholars (which are often shared with graduate students) who are known to be working in a specific area. If ideas, methods, findings, and so on are borrowed from these, proper credit should always be given.

Fabrication and Falsification

There are approximately 40,000 journals that publish more than one million papers annually (Henderson, 1990). Thus, it is not surprising to learn that scientists have occasionally been caught making up or altering research data. Of course, this is completely unethical, and severe penalties are imposed on individuals who are caught. Pressures have been particularly intense in medical and health-related research because such research is often expensive, requires outside funding, and involves risk. It seems easy to make a little change here or there or to make up data because "I only

plagiarism — Using ideas, concepts, writings, and drawings of others as your own; cheating.

References on Misconduct in Science: Readings for Graduate Students

American Association of University Professors. (1981). Statement on professional ethics. *New Directions for Higher Education*, **33**, 83-85.

Association of American Medical Colleges. (1992). *Beyond the "framework": Institutional considerations in managing allegations of misconduct in research*. Author.

Anderson, A. (1988). First scientific fraud conviction. *Nature*, **335**, 389.

Bell, R. (1992). *Impure science: Fraud, compromise, and political influences in scientific research*. New York: Wiley.

Callahan, J.C. (Ed.) (1988). *Ethical issues in professional life*. New York: Oxford University Press.

Chalmers. I. (1990). Underreporting research is scientific misconduct. *Journal of the American Medical Association*, **263**, 1405-1408.

Dickersin, K. (1990). The existence of publication bias and risk factors for its occurrences. *Journal of the American Medical Association*, **263**, 1385-1389.

Engler, R.L., Covell, J.W., Friedman, P.J., Kitcher, P.S., & Peters, R.M. (1987). Misrepresentation and responsibility in medical research. *New England Journal of Medicine*, **317**, 1383-1389.

Ethics & Behavior, **3**(1), 1993 (special issue on "Whistleblowing and Scientific Misconduct").

Evans, J.T., Nadjari, H.I., & Burchell, S.A. (1990). Quotational and reference accuracy in surgical journals: A continuing peer review problem. *Journal of the American Medical Association*, **263**, 1353-1357.

Federal Register. (1991). *Federal policy for the protection of human subjects: Notices and rules*, **56**, 28001-28032.

Friedman, P.J. (1988). Research ethics, due process, and common sense. *Journal of the American Medical Association*, **260**, 1937-1938.

Friedman, P.J. (1990). Correcting the literature following fraudulent publication. *Journal of the American Medical Association*, **263**, 1416-1419.

Garfield, E., & Welljams-Dorof, A. (1990). The impact of fraudulent research on the scientific literature: The Stephen E. Breuning case. *Journal of the American Medical Association*, **263**, 1424-1426.

Goodstein, D. (1992, March 2). What do we mean when we use the term "science fraud"? *Scientist*, pp. 11-12 (Reprinted from *Windows*, fall 1991, p. 7).

Jayarama, K.S. (1990). Scientific ethics: Accusations of 'paper recycling.' *Nature*, **334**, 187.

Kimmel, A.J. (1988). *Ethics and values in applied social research*. Newbury Park, CA: Sage.

Klotz, I.M. (1986). *Diamond dealers and feather merchants: Tales from the sciences*. Boston: Birkhauser.

Kohn, A. (1988). *False prophets: Fraud and error in science and medicine*. New York: Basil Blackwell.

LaPidus, J.B., & Mishkin, B. (1991). Values and ethics in the graduate education of scientists. In W.W. May (Ed.), *Ethics and higher education* (pp. 283-298). New York: Macmillan.

Loeb, J.M., Hendee, W.R., Smith, S.J., & Schwartz, M.R. (1989). Human vs. animal rights: In defense of animal research. *Journal of the American Medical Association*, **262**, 2716-2720.

Mallon, T. (1989) *Stolen words: Forays into the origins and ravages of plagiarism*. New York: Ticknor & Fields.

(continued)

References on Misconduct in Science: Readings for Graduate Students *(continued)*

Mishkin, B. (1988). Responding to scientific misconduct: Due process and prevention. *Journal of the American Medical Association*, **260**, 1932–1936.

Mooney, C.J. (1992a). Critics question higher education's commitment and effectiveness in dealing with plagiarism. *Chronicle of Higher Education*, **38**(23), A16, A18.

Mooney, C.J. (1992b). Plagiarism charges against a scholar can divide experts, perplex scholarly societies, and raise intractable questions. *Chronicle of Higher Education*, **38**(23), A1, A14, A16.

National Academy of Sciences, National Academy of Engineering, and Institute of Medicine (1993). *Responsible science: Ensuring the integrity of the research process* (vol. 2). Washington, DC: National Academy Press.

Pfeifer, M.P., & Snodgrass, G.L. (1990). The continued use of retracted, invalid scientific literature. *Journal of the American Medical Association*, **263**, 1420–1423.

Pope, K.S., & Vetter, V.A. (1992). Ethical dilemmas encountered by members of the American Psychological Association. *American Psychologist*, **47**, 397–411.

Quest: The Academy papers, **45**(1), February 1993 (special issue, "Ethics in the Study of Physical Activity").

"Responsibilities of Awardee and Applicant Institutions for Dealing With and Reporting Possible Misconduct in Science." (1989, August 8). *Federal Register*, **54**(151), 32446–32451.

Rudolph, J., & Brackstone, D. (1990, April 11). Too many scholars ignore the basic rules of documentation. *Chronicle of Higher Education*, **36**, A56.

Schurr, G.M. (1982). Toward a code of ethics for academics. *Journal of Higher Education*, **53**, 318–334.

Taubes, G. (1993). *Bad science: The short life and weird times of cold fusion*. New York: Random House.

Wrather, J. (1987). Scientists and lawyers look at fraud in science. *Science*, **238**, 813–814.

need a few more subjects, but I am running out of time." The odds of being detected in these types of actions are high, but even if you should get away with it, you will always know you did it, and you will probably put other people at risk because of your actions.

Although graduate students and faculty may knowingly produce fraudulent research, established scholars are sometimes indirectly involved in scientific misconduct. This may occur in working with other scientists who produce fraudulent data that followed the predicted outcomes (e.g., as in a funded grant where the proposal had suggested what outcomes were probable). In these instances, the established scholar sees exactly what he or she expects to see in the data. Because this verifies the hypotheses, the data are assumed to be acceptable. For example, the case of Nobel laureate David Bal-

timore involved a paper published in *Cell* in April 1986 signed by Baltimore and coauthors Thereza Imanishi-Kari and David Weaver as principal authors. While Baltimore had checked the findings of Imanishi-Kari, he saw in the data the expected outcomes and agreed to submit the paper. The fact that the data were not accurate subsequently led to Baltimore's resignation as president of Rockefeller University. Thus, even though Baltimore was not the paper's principal author, his career was seriously damaged by being an unwilling party to scientific fraud.

Falsification can also occur with related literature. Graduate students should be careful in how they interpret what an author says. Work of other authors should not be "bent" to fit projected hypotheses. This is also a reason graduate students should read original sources instead of relying on the interpretations of others, as those interpretations may not follow the original source closely.

Nonpublication of Data

The basic idea here is that some data are not included because they do not support the desired outcome. This has sometimes been called "cooking" data. There is a very thin line between eliminating "bad" data and "cooking" data. Bad data should be caught, if possible, at the time of data acquisition. For example, if a test value seems too large or small and the researcher calibrates the instrument and finds it out of calibration, eliminating this "bad" data is good research practice. However, looking at a value when data are being examined and deciding it is inappropriate and changing it is "cooking" data.

 Another term used with unusual data is **outlier**. The term originally meant "outright liars," suggesting the data were bad. However, data now are sometimes "trimmed" if the value is extreme. Just because a score is extreme does not mean it is based on bad data. Whereas extreme scores can create problems in data analysis, trimming them *automatically* is a poor practice.

The most drastic instance in this category is the failure to publish results that do not support projected hypotheses. Journals are often accused of a "publication bias," meaning only significant results are published, but authors should publish the outcomes of solid research regardless of whether findings support projected hypotheses.

Faulty Data-Gathering Procedures

A number of unethical activities can occur at this stage of a research project. In particular, graduate students should be aware of such issues as

- continuing with data collection on subjects who are not meeting the requirement of the research (e.g., poor efforts, failure to adhere to subject agreements about diet, exercise, rest);

- malfunctioning equipment;
- inappropriate treatment of subjects (e.g., failure to follow the guidelines from the Human Subjects Committee); and
- recording data incorrectly.

For example, a doctoral student we know was collecting data on running economy in a field setting. Subjects returned several times to be videotaped while repeating a run at varying stride lengths and rates. On the third day of testing a male subject performed erratically during the run. When the experimenter questioned him, she learned he had been out drinking with his buddies very late on the previous evening and he was really hung over. Of course, she wisely discarded the data and scheduled him for another run several days later. Had she not noted the unusual nature of his performance and questioned him carefully, she would have included data that would probably have skewed her results because the subject was not adhering to previously agreed upon conditions of the study.

Poor Data Storage and Retention

Data must be stored and maintained as originally recorded and not altered. All original records should be maintained so that the original data are always available for examination.

Misleading Authorship

 A major ethical issue among researchers involves joint research projects or, more specifically, the publication and presentation of joint research efforts. Generally, the order of authorship for presentations and publications should be based on the researchers' contributions to the project. The first, or senior, author is usually the researcher who developed the idea and the plan for the research. Second and third authors are normally listed in the order of their contributions (see Fine & Kurdek, 1993, for a detailed discussion and case studies).

---

 outlier — Unrepresentative score; a score that lies outside of the normal scores.

 Unethical activities during the data-gathering process

 Fine, M.A., & Kurdek, L.A. (1993). Reflections on determining authorship credit and authorship order on faculty-student collaborations. *American Psychologist*, **48**, 1141-1147.

How to determine order of authorship

Although this sounds easy enough, the decisions are difficult at times. Sometimes researchers make equal contributions and decide to flip a coin to determine who will be listed first. In fact, the order of authorship for this book was decided in that manner. We team-taught the research methods course for several years while we were on the faculty at Louisiana State University. We contributed equally to this book. But before we began, we tossed a coin to decide who would be listed as first author (at the time Nelson was unaware of Thomas's extreme skill in games of chance; in subsequent years he has learned that lesson well). Note the phrase "before we began." This is a good procedure to follow. Decide the order of authors at the beginning of a collaborative effort. This saves hard feelings later, when everyone may not agree on whose contribution was most important.

A second issue is who should be an author (see Crase & Rosato, 1992, for a discussion of the changing nature of authorship). Studies occasionally have more authors than subjects. In fact, sometimes the authors are also the subjects. When you look at what subjects must go through in some research studies, you can see why only a major professor's graduate students would allow "that" to be done to them. Even then they insist on being an author as a reward. More seriously, these two rules should help define authorship:

- **Technicians do not necessarily become joint authors**. Graduate students sometimes feel that, because they collect the data, they should be coauthors. Only when graduate students contribute to the planning, analysis, and write-up of the research report are they entitled to be listed as coauthors. Even this rule does not apply to grants that pay graduate students for their work. A good major professor involves his or her graduate students in all aspects of his or her research program; thus, these students frequently may serve as coauthors and technicians.
- **Authorship should involve only those who contribute directly to the specific research project**. This does not necessarily include the laboratory director or a graduate student's major professor. The only thing we advocate by the chain letter on page 79 is the humor.

Sneaky Publication Practices

The final concern deals with joint publications, specifically those between the major professor and the graduate student. Major professors do (and should) immediately begin to involve graduate students in the major professors' research program (see Zelaznik, 1993, for a discussion). When this happens, the general guidelines we suggested earlier apply. However, two conflicting forces are at work. A professor's job is to foster and develop the scholarly ability of students. However, pressure is increasing on faculty to publish so they can obtain the benefits of promotions, tenure, outside funding, and merit pay. Being the first (senior) author is of benefit in these endeavors. As a result, faculty members want to be selfless and to assist students, but they feel the pressure to publish. This may not be a major issue for senior faculty, but it certainly is for untenured assistant professors. As mentioned previously, there are no hard-and-fast rules other than that everyone agrees before the research is undertaken.

The thesis or dissertation is a special case. By definition, this is how graduate students demonstrate their competence to receive the degree. Frequently, for the master's thesis, the major professor supplies the idea, design, and much of the writing and editing. In spite of this, we believe it should be regarded as the student's work. The dissertation should always be regarded as the student's work. However, second authorship for the major professor on either the thesis or the dissertation is acceptable under certain circumstances. The American Psychological Association has defined these circumstances adequately, and we recommend the use of their guidelines:

- Only second authorship is acceptable for the dissertation supervisor.
- Second authorship may be considered obligatory if the supervisor designates the

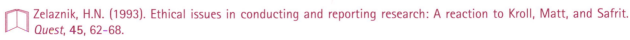
Crase, D., & Rosato, F.D. (1992). Single versus multiple authorship in professional journals. *Journal of Physical Education, Recreation and Dance*, **63**(7), 28-31.

Rules to define authorship

Zelaznik, H.N. (1993). Ethical issues in conducting and reporting research: A reaction to Kroll, Matt, and Safrit. *Quest*, **45**, 62-68.

APA guidelines for joint authorship in dissertations

Chain Letter to Increase Publications

Dear Colleague:

We are sure you are aware of the importance of publications in establishing yourself and procuring grants, awards, and well-paying academic positions or chairpersonships. We have devised a way in which your curriculum vitae can be greatly enhanced with very little effort.

   This letter contains a list of names and addresses. Include the top two names as coauthors on your next scholarly paper. Then remove the top name and place your own name at the bottom of the list. Send the revised letter to five colleagues.

   If these instructions are followed, by the time your name reaches the top of the list, you will have claim to coauthorship of 15,625 refereed publications. If you break this chain, your next 10 papers will be rejected as lacking in relevance to "real-world" behavior. Thus, you will be labeled as ecologically invalid by your peers.

Sincerely,

List as coauthors   Jerry R. Thomas, Professor
Jerry R. Thomas   Jack K. Nelson, Professor
Jack K. Nelson
I.M. Published
U.R. Tenured
C.D. Raise

primary variables or makes major interpretive contributions or provides the database.

- Second authorship is a courtesy if the supervisor designates the general area of concern, is substantially involved in the development of the design and measurement procedures, or substantially contributes to the write-up of the published report.

- Second authorship is not acceptable if the supervisor only provides encouragement, physical facilities, financial support, critiques, or editorial contributions.

- In all instances, agreement should be reviewed before the writing for publication is undertaken and at the time of the submission. If disagreements arise, they should be resolved by a third party using these guidelines.

 Authors must also be careful about **dual publication**. Sometimes this is legitimate; for example, a scientific paper published by one journal may be reprinted by another journal or in a book of readings (this should always be noted). Authors may not, however, publish the same paper in more than one copyrighted original research journal. But what constitutes "the same paper"? Can more than one paper be written from the same database? As with other concepts, the line is rather hazy. For example, Thomas (1986) indicated that

frequently, new insights may be gained by evaluating previously reported data from a different perspective. However, reports of this type are always classed as research notes whether the reanalysis is undertaken by the original author or someone else. This does not mean that reports which use data from a number of studies (e.g., meta-analyses, power analyses) are classed as research notes. (pp. iii-iv)

Generally, good scientific practice is to publish all the appropriate data in a single primary publication. For example, if both psychological and physiological data were collected as a result of a specific experiment on training, publishing these

dual publication — Occurrence of having the same scientific paper published in more than one journal or other publication; generally unethical.

separately may not be appropriate. Frequently, the main finding of interest will be in the interaction between psychological and physiological responses. But in other cases, the volume of data may be so large as to prohibit an inclusive paper. Sometimes the papers can be published as a series; at other times they may be completely separate. Another example is large-scale studies in which a tremendous amount of information is collected (e.g., exercise epidemiology or pedagogical studies). Usually, data are selected from the computer records (or videotapes) to answer a specific set of related questions for a research report. Researchers may then use a different part (or even an overlapping part) of the database to address another set of questions. This results in legitimate publications from the same database. However, authors should identify that more than one paper has been produced from this database. Researchers should follow these general types of rules, or they may be viewed as lacking scientific objectivity in their work and certainly as lacking in modesty (Day, 1983).

Most research journals require that the author include a statement that the paper has not been previously published or submitted elsewhere while the journal is considering it. Papers published in one language may not be published as an original paper in a second language.

Ethical Issues Regarding Copyright

Graduate students should be aware of copyright regulations and the concept of "fair use" as it applies to educational materials. Copyrighted material is often used in theses and dissertations, and this is acceptable if the use is fair and reasonable. Often graduate students will want to use a figure or table in their thesis or dissertation. If you use a table or figure from another source, you must seek permission from the copyright holder (for published papers usually the author, but sometimes the research journal) and cite it appropriately (e.g., used by permission of . . .).

The concept of "fair use" has four basic rules:

- **Purpose**—Is the use to be commercial or educational? More leeway is given for educational use like theses, dissertations, and published papers.

- **Nature**—Is copying expected or not? Copying a journal article for your personal use is expected and reasonable. However, copying a complete book or standardized tests is not expected and probably is a violation of the "fair use" concept.
- **Amount**—How much is to be copied? The significant issue is how important is the part copied.
- **Effect**—How does copying affect the market for the document? Making a single copy of a journal article has little effect on the market for the journal, but copying a book (or maybe a book chapter) or a standardized test reduces royalties to the author and income for the publisher. That is not "fair use."

There are no standard answers with regard to "fair use." Fair use is a flexible idea (or alternatively, a statement that can't be interpreted). Better to be safe than sorry when using material in your thesis or dissertation. If you have any doubt, seek permission. University Microfilms (produces *Dissertation Abstracts International*), the national warehouse for dissertations, reports that about 15% of dissertations require follow-up on copyright issues. A sample letter that can be used to obtain permission to use copyrighted materials appears on page 81.

Model for Considering Scientific Misconduct

Sanctions for Scientific Misconduct
Responsibilities of Graduate Students
Philosophical Positions Underlying Ethical Issues

If intention is used as the basis for differentiating between scientific misconduct and mistakes, then Drowatzky (1993) noted that the following model is often suggested:

Scientific misconduct → Sanctions
Scientific mistakes → Remedial activities

Sanctions for Scientific Misconduct

Sanctions are often imposed on individuals who are fraudulent in their scientific work. Internal sanctions

---

Four rules of fair use of copyrighted material

Sample Copyright Permission Letter

Following is a sample copyright permission letter (altered for use with a thesis or dissertation) recommended by Human Kinetics, the publisher of this textbook.

Date

Permissions Editor (or person if an individual)

Publisher (not needed if an individual)

Address

Dear _____:

I am preparing my thesis/dissertation, tentatively titled _____

I would like permission to use the following material:

title of article in journal, book, book chapter: _____

Author of article, book, or book chapter: _____

Title of journal or book (include volume and issue number of journal): _____

_____

Editor if edited book: _____

Year of publication: _____

Place of publication and name of publisher of book/journal: _____

_____

Copyright year and holder: _____

Page number(s) on which material appears: _____   ❏ to be reprinted   ❏ to be adapted

A COPY OF THE MATERIAL IS ATTACHED.

Table, figure, or page number in my thesis/dissertation:_____

I request permission for nonexclusive rights in all languages throughout the world. I will, of course, cite a standard source line, including complete bibliographical data. If you have specific credit line requirements, please make them known in the space provided below.

_____

_____

A duplicate copy of this form is for your files. Your prompt cooperation will be appreciated.

If permission is granted, please sign the release below and return to:

YOUR SIGNATURE: _____

YOUR NAME AND ADDRESS

- -

Permission granted, Signature: _____

Address: _____

_____

Date: _____

imposed by the researcher's university have included the following:

- Restriction of academic duties
- Termination of work on the project
- Reduction in professorial rank
- Fines to cover costs
- Separation from the university (either with or without loss of benefits)
- Salary freeze
- Promotion freeze
- Supervision of future grant submissions
- Verbal reprimands
- Letter of reprimand (either included or not included in the permanent record)
- Monitoring research with prior review of publications

In addition to internal university sanctions for scientific fraud, sanctions may be imposed by the agency that has funded the research, scholarly journals that published the work, and related scholarly / professional groups. In recent years external sanctions have included the following:

- Revocation of prior publications
- Letters to offended parties
- Prohibition of obtaining outside grants
- Discontinuance of service to outside agencies
- Release of information to agencies and professions
- Referral to legal system for further actions
- Fines to cover overhead costs

Responsibilities of Graduate Students

As graduate students, it is essential that you become concerned with these issues. Of course, the issues are much broader than just the science areas like exercise physiology, biomechanics, motor behavior, and sport psychology. Fraud, misrepresentation, and inaccurate interpretation of data, plagiarism, unfair authorship issues, and unethical publications practices are problems that extend to any area of scholarship (e.g., sport sociology, sport philosophy, sport history, physical education pedagogy, and exercise and wellness). Although these practices sometimes occur simply because the person is unethical, often they are caused by pressures that exist in our system of higher education:

- The need to obtain external funding for research

- Pressure to publish scholarly findings
- The need to complete graduate degree work
- The desire to obtain rewards in higher education (e.g., promotion, merit raises)

Academic units should be encouraged to develop mechanisms for discussing ethical issues in scholarship with graduate students. This might include seminars for graduate students focused on these issues. But at least some systematic means is needed to bring the issues to the forefront for discussion.

Philosophical Positions Underlying Ethical Issues

One's basic philosophical position on ethical issues drives the decision-making process in research. Drowatzky (1993) has summarized the different ethical views that underlie the decision-making process:

- The individual is precious and the individual's benefit takes precedence over the society.

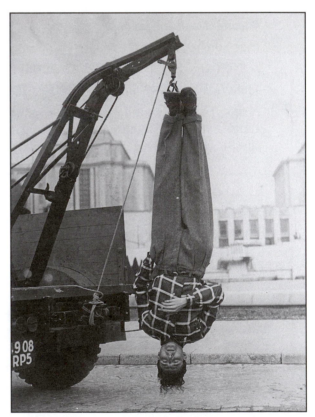

Sanctions for scientific misconduct can be severe.

 Ethical views that underlie the decision-making process

- Equality is of utmost importance and everyone must be treated equally.
- Fairness is the overriding guide to ethics and all decisions must be based on fairness.
- The welfare of society takes precedence over that of the individual and all must be done for the benefit of society.
- Truth, defined as being true, genuine, and conforming to reality, is the basis for decision making.

Of course, many statements in this list are in direct conflict with each other and will lead to substantially different decisions depending on one's view. Discussing and evaluating these statements and what they imply about decisions in scholarship should enhance graduate students' understanding of important issues.

Finally, reading some of the literature on fraud and misconduct in research is a sobering experience for anyone. A notable example is the special issue of *Ethics and Behavior* (Vol. 3, No. 1, 1993), which focused on "Whistleblowing and Scientific Misconduct." This issue gives a fascinating account of the David Baltimore and Herbert Needleman cases, including overviews and responses by the whistleblowers and those accused of scientific misconduct.

Working With Faculty

Selecting a Major Professor
Changing Your Major Professor

Ethical considerations among researchers and ethical factors in the graduate student/major professor relationship are the two topics under discussion in this section (see Roberts, 1993, for a detailed discussion). Major professors should treat graduate students as colleagues. If we want our students to be scholars when they complete their graduate work, then we should treat them like scholars from the start, for graduate students do not become scholars on receipt of a degree. By the same token, graduate students must act like responsible scholars. This means producing careful, thorough, and quality work.

Selecting a Major Professor

Students should try to select major professors who share their views in their area of interest. Master's students frequently choose an institution based on location or the promise of financial aid. Doctoral students, on the other hand, should select the institution they attend based on the program's quality and the faculty in their area of specialization (see Baxter, 1993-94, for a discussion). Do not choose your major professor hastily. If you are already at the institution, carefully evaluate the specializations available in your interest areas. Ask questions about faculty and whether they publish in these areas. Read some of these publications and determine your interest. What financial support, such as laboratories and equipment, is given to these areas? Also, talk to fellow graduate students. Finally, talk with the faculty members to determine how effectively you will be able to work with them.

We advocate a mentor model in preparing graduate students (particularly doctoral students) in physical education, exercise science, and sport science. For students to become good researchers (or good clinicians) requires a one-on-one student-faculty relationship. This means several things about graduate students and graduate faculty.

First, graduate students need to be full-time students to develop the research and clinical skills needed for success in research and teaching. They need to work with a mentor in their ongoing research program. This lends continuity to research efforts and pulls graduate students together into effective research teams. Theses and dissertation topics arise naturally from these types of settings. Additionally, more senior students become models and can offer assistance to novice graduate students. Expertise is acquired by watching experts, working with them, and then practicing the techniques acquired.

See *Ethics and Behavior* 3(1), 1993, for information on scientific fraud and misconduct.

Roberts, G.C. (1993). Ethics in professional advising and academic counseling of graduate students. *Quest*, 45, 78-87.

Baxter, N. (Winter 1993-94). Is there another degree in your future? Choosing among professional and graduate schools. *Occupational Outlook Quarterly*, pp. 19-49.

Conversely, for faculty members to be good mentors, they must have active research programs. This means that appropriate facilities and equipment must be available as well as time for faculty members to devote to research and graduate student mentoring. Potential graduate students should carefully investigate the situations into which they will place themselves, especially if they have a major interest in research (for a good description of mentors, see Newell, 1987).

However, if you are not at the institution, find out which institutions offer the specialties in which you are interested. Request information from their graduate schools and departments. Read the appropriate journals (over the past 5-10 years) and see which faculty are publishing. After you narrow your list, explore financial support and plan a visit. Speak to the graduate coordinator for the department and the faculty in your area of interest. Sometimes you can meet faculty at conventions, such as those of AAHPERD (national or district meetings), the American College of Sports Medicine, the International Society for Biomechanics, and the North American Society for Psychology of Sport and Physical Activity.

After you select a major professor, you must select a committee. Normally the master's or doctoral committee is selected in consultation with your major professor. The committee selected should be one that can contribute to the planning and evaluation of your work, not one that might be the easiest. It is preferable to wait a semester (quarter) or two (if you can) before selecting a final committee. This gives you the opportunity to have several potential committee members as teachers as well as allowing you to better evaluate your common interest.

Changing Your Major Professor

What happens, however, if you have a major professor (or committee member) who is not ideal for you? First, evaluate the reason. You need not be best friends, but it is important that you and your major professor are striving for the same goals. Sometimes students' interests change. Sometimes people just cannot get along. If handled professionally, however, this situation should not be a problem. Go to your major professor and explain the situation as you perceive it and offer him or her an opportunity to respond. Of course, the conflict may be more personal. If so, use an objective and professional approach. If you cannot, or if this does not produce satisfactory results, the best recourse may be to seek the advice of the graduate coordinator or department chairperson.

Protecting Human Subjects

What Should Research Subjects Expect? Informed Consent

Most research in the study of physical activity deals with humans, often children. Therefore, the researcher must be concerned about any circumstances in the research setting or activity that could harm the participants. Harm should be interpreted to mean to frighten, embarrass, or negatively affect the subjects (Tuckman, 1978). Of course, researchers always run the risk of creating a problem. What must be balanced is the degree of risk and the subjects' rights. The important issue is the potential value of research in contributing to knowledge, to the development of technology, and to the improvement of people's lives.

What Should Research Subjects Expect?

Tuckman (1978) has summarized the subjects' rights that experimenters must consider:

- **The right to privacy or nonparticipation.** This includes the fact that researchers should not ask for unnecessary information and should obtain direct consent from adults and consent from parents for children (as well as the consent of the children themselves where appropriate).

- **The right to remain anonymous.** The researcher should explain that the study focuses on group data and that an I.D. number (rather than the subject's name) will be used to record data.

- **The right to confidentiality.** Subjects should be told who (keep this to as few people as possible)

 Newell, K.M. (1987). On masters and apprentices in physical education. *Quest*, **39**, 88-96.

Research subjects' rights

will actually have access to original data by which the subjects might be identified.

• **The right to expect experimenter responsibility.** The experimenter should be well meaning and sensitive to human dignity. If the subject is not told the purpose of the study (or is misled), the subject must be informed immediately after the completion of testing.

Qualitative research (discussed in detail in chapter 17) lends itself to some potential ethical problems because of the close, personal interaction with subjects. The researcher often spends a great deal of time with subjects, getting to know them and asking them to share their thoughts and perceptions. Griffin and Templin (1989) raised ethical concerns as to whether to share field notes, how to protect a participant's self-esteem without compromising accuracy in the research report when the two are in conflict, and what to do if you are told about (or observe) something illegal or immoral while collecting data.

  There are no easy answers to situational ethics in **fieldwork**. Qualitative research sometimes deals with so-called deviants, such as drug addicts and unlawful motorcycle gangs. Informed consent is impossible in some circumstances. Punch (1986, p. 36) made this point when he described his research with police. The patrol car in which he was riding was directed to a fight. As the policemen jumped out and started wrestling with the combatants, Punch wondered whether he was supposed to yell "freeze," thrust his head between the entangled limbs, and, Miranda-like, chant out the rights of the participants. Similarly, when Powermaker (cited by Punch) came face to face with a lynch mob, should she have flashed her academic identity card and explained to the crowd about the nature of her presence? By these two examples we are not implying that qualitative researchers are exempt from considerations such as informed consent and deception. We are simply pointing out that certain types of qualitative research situations face special problems dealing with ethics. We invite you to read the discussion by Punch (1986) and consult some of the sources he cites concerning this issue.

Persons with disabilities are a special issue as research subjects. The fact that the subject has a disability is protected under the Right to Privacy Act.

Thus, institutions are prohibited from releasing the names of persons with disabilities as potential research subjects. The researcher must contact the institution about possible subjects. The institution will then request permission from the subject or parents to release the subject or child's name and the nature of the disability to the researcher. If the subject or parents approve, the institution allows the researcher to contact the subject or parents to seek approval for the particular research to be undertaken. Although this procedure is rather cumbersome and varies from state to state, individuals clearly have the right not to be cited in studies and labeled as "disabled" unless they so choose.

Informed Consent

Consideration must be given to the protection of human subjects. The researcher is required to protect the rights and well-being of subjects in his or her study. The regulations detailing the procedures are published by the U.S. Department of Health and Human Services (45 CFR 46.101). Most institutions regulate this protection in two ways. First, researchers are required to complete some type of form describing their research. Sample Form D.1 in Appendix D is used for conducting research with human subjects at Arizona State University.

Typically, institutions require that you include your informed-consent form with your application to conduct human-subject research. Sample Form D.2 is the model for the form used for adults at Arizona State University. If the subjects are minors, then you must obtain their parents' permission (Sample Form D.3) and the children's permission (Sample Form D.4) if they are old enough to understand. It may be useful to put this form on a microcomputer disk so that graduate students or faculty can answer the questions and print out the completed form. The researcher completes this form, attaches an abstract, and has it approved before beginning any work, including pilot work. The source of approval may vary. For example, some institutions may require that all forms be approved by a central committee. Other institutions may delegate approval for so-called standard types of research to a lower level (e.g., a college committee).

The following are basic elements of informed consent as specified by the advisory committee of

---

fieldwork — A methodology common in qualitative research in which data are gathered in natural settings.

Punch, M. (1986). *The politics and ethics of fieldwork.* Beverly Hills, CA: Sage.

the *Research Quarterly for Exercise and Sport* (Thomas, 1983, p. 221):

- A fair explanation of the procedures to be followed, including an identification of those which are experimental.
- A description of the attendant discomforts and risks.
- A description of the benefits to be expected.
- A disclosure of appropriate alternative procedures that would be advantageous for the subject.
- An offer to answer any inquiries concerning the procedures.
- An instruction that the subject is free to withdraw consent and to discontinue participation in the project or activity at any time. In addition, the agreement should contain no exculpatory language through which the subject is made to waive, or appear to waive, any legal right or to release the institution or its agents from liability or negligence.

The researcher is required to comply with any institutional guidelines both for the protection of human subjects and for informed consent. A description of this compliance should be included under the subject section in the method section of the thesis or dissertation. Most journals also require a statement with regard to this issue. The form used for informed consent is normally placed in an appendix of the thesis/dissertation.

Protecting Animal Subjects

Matt (1993) has discussed "Ethical Issues in Animal Research." As she points out, this is not a new issue, having been discussed in Europe for over 400 years and in the U.S. for over 100 years. The ground rules were established long ago when Descartes indicated it was justifiable to use animals in research because they could not reason and were therefore "lower" in the order of things than humans (Matt, 1993). However, Bentham (1970) said the issue was not whether animals could think and reason but whether they perceived pain and suffered.

As Matt (1993) argues, far fewer animals are used in research than are slaughtered for food, held in zoos, and killed as unwanted pets in animal shelters. In fact, animal studies may have more stringent criteria for approval than studies with humans. Institutional review boards typically require that investigators demonstrate that animal studies add significant knowledge to the literature and are not replications, a requirement not placed on studies using humans as subjects.

If animals are well treated, is their use in research justified? Matt (1993, pp. 46-47) says yes if the purposes of the research fall into one of five categories:

drug testing, such as the development and testing of AIDS drugs; animal models of disease, such as the development of animal models of arthritis, diabetes, iron deficiency, autoimmune dysfunction, and aging; basic research, focused on examining and elucidating mechanisms at a level of definition not possible in human models; education of undergraduate and graduate students in laboratories and lectures, with experience and information gained from the use of animal models; and development of surgical techniques, used extensively in the training of medical students and the testing of new surgical devices and procedures.

A careful consideration of these categories suggests few suitable alternatives (but see Zelaznik, 1993, for a discussion).

If animals are used as subjects for research studies in exercise science, institutions require adherence to the *Guide for the Care and Use of Laboratory Animals*, published by the U.S. Department of Health and Human Services, as detailed in the Animal Welfare Act (PL 89-544, PL 91-979, and PL 04-279). Most institutions also support the rules and procedures for recommended care of laboratory animals as outlined by the American Association for Accreditation of Laboratory Animal Care.

All these documents recognize that for advancements to be made in human and animal research, animals must be used. These animals must be well tended, and if their use results in the animals being incapacitated or sacrificed, this must be done humanely. Sample Form D.5 is the form used at

---

Basic elements of informed consent

Zelaznik, H.N. (1993). Ethical issues in conducting and reporting research: A reaction to Kroll, Matt, and Safrit. *Quest, 45*, 62–68.

Arizona State University to ensure compliance with all regulations involving the use of animals in research.

Summary

We discussed ethical issues that impact graduate students in their research and scholarly activities. We identified ethical issues and set the stage for you to think about and discuss these values as they influence your graduate and scholarly life.

Points that typically arise in scientific misconduct include plagiarism, fabrication and falsification of data, nonpublication of data, data-gathering problems, data storage and retention issues, authorship controversies, and publication practices. We discussed copyright issues in research and publication. We also suggested the model most frequently used to deal with scientific misconduct and some of the internal and external sanctions that have been imposed on individuals found guilty of scientific misconduct.

We discussed ethical and procedural issues in working relationships. How should graduate students select a mentor and committee members? Should students seek new mentors or committee members if they are unable to work effectively or amicably with their original choices?

Finally, we discussed ethics and procedures in the use of human and animal subjects. This included remembering subjects' rights, protecting human and animal subjects, and obtaining informed consent from human subjects.

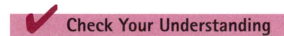

Check Your Understanding

Case Study #1

Publication of the Master's Thesis

You completed your M.S. thesis last spring in the Department of Exercise Science. You had a really good graduate experience and your major professor provided much advice and assistance with your program and research. In fact, you were supported for your master's work on your mentor's research grant from NIH.

Your thesis topic was a "spinoff" from your mentor's grant research and you were praised for the quality of the work and write-up at the thesis defense. You wrote your thesis in journal style so it could more easily be submitted for review at a scholarly journal. However, you took 40 pages to report a single experiment, and most journals prefer single experiments to be in the 20-30 page range.

After you graduated last May, you accepted a position in the fitness program of a large company and have had a very heavy workload at your new job. Yesterday, you received a letter from your mentor indicating his interest in publishing the research from your thesis. He indicated that the paper needed to be shortened to about 25 pages, which would require a substantial rewrite. In the letter he said that because your thesis was a spinoff from his research, he should serve as a second author on the paper. He was willing to continue to provide editorial assistance as you revised the paper. Alternatively, he indicated that if you wanted him to revise the paper to reduce the length, then he should be first author with you as second author.

Questions

1. What do you think of your mentor's proposal?
2. What would you do?
3. If the work was a spinoff of his work and he made major contributions to it, should he be a coauthor or first author?
4. If the situation were different and the idea had come originally from you, should he be a coauthor?
5. What if the thesis were written in chapter format and required a complete rewrite before submission?
6. What is ethical behavior in this instance—by your mentor and by you?
7. Should your mentor have discussed this process with you prior to your thesis proposal?

Case Study #2

The Problem Mentor

You came to this university to work specifically with your mentor because of her scholarly record in your area of interest within sport history. You are in your second semester and have encountered a series of problems in working with your mentor. First, she wants your courses to reflect a considerably broader interest in sport history and history than you want. In particular, there are nine credits of electives that you want to use in specific support of your research topic, but she wants six of the credits to be in two related (but not specific) courses from the history department.

You came here with considerable knowledge on the topic you are researching from your previous job in a well-known sport history museum. However, it turns out your mentor believes the interpretation given this work by the curator at the museum is incorrect. Each time you turn in a paper on the topic, your mentor wants you to consider her interpretation/perspective rather than what you had previously learned. Because you have not been willing to do this, you have received several grades that you believe are too low.

Questions

1. What are the important issues about the coursework decisions? How can a resolution be reached between the student and mentor?
2. What do you think of the mentor's/student's position on the research topic? How can/should a resolution be reached?
3. Should the student change mentors? Do mentors and students need to have the same theoretical interpretations to work together?
4. What are the problems for the student/mentor if the student decides to change mentors?

Statistical and Measurement Concepts in Research

In the following six chapters, we present some basic statistical and measurement techniques that are frequently used in physical activity research. We give more attention here to the basic statistical techniques than to the more complex methods. A general understanding of the underlying concepts of the statistical techniques has been emphasized rather than any derivation of formulas or extensive computations. Because an understanding of how the basic statistical techniques work facilitates an intuitive grasp of the more advanced procedures, we have provided the computational procedures for most of the basic statistics, as well as examples of their use. In addition, appendix C describes how basic statistical techniques may be performed on desk and mainframe computers.

Chapter 6 discusses the need for statistics. We describe different types of sampling procedures and summarize the basic statistics used in describing data, such as measures of central tendency and measures of variation. Statistics can reveal two things about data: reliability and meaningfulness. We explain the concepts of probability and significance as they relate to inference or to generalizing the results of a study. Finally, we explain power in relation to probability, sample size, and effect size.

Chapter 7 pertains to relationships among variables. We review different correlational techniques, such as the Pearson *r* for the relationship between only two variables. We explain partial correlation as a technique in which one can determine the correlation between two variables while holding the influence of a third (or more) variable constant. The use of correlation for prediction is discussed when using more than one variable to predict a criterion (multiple regression).

Chapter 8 focuses on statistical techniques for comparing treatment effects on groups, such as different training methods or different samples. The simplest comparison of differences is between two groups: the *t* test. Next, we describe analysis of variance as a means of testing the significance of the differences among two or more groups. We also discuss the use of factorial analysis of variance, in which two or more independent variables can be compared.

The approach in chapter 9 is different from the previous two. Here we deal with multivariate techniques, for which the mathematics are very complex. However, a conceptual understanding of the multivariate techniques can be gained from extending ideas from univariate procedures and the use of examples. This is what we have done. Discriminant analysis, multivariate analysis of variance, and multivariate analysis of covariance are extensions of simple analysis of variance, factorial analysis of variance, and analysis of covariance. Conceptually, these techniques represent the same idea, except a composite is formed from multiple dependent variables. From the same perspective, canonical correlation, factor analysis, and structural modeling are extensions of Pearson *r* and multiple *R*. For each technique, we present a conceptual description of the procedures and an example.

Chapter 10 provides information on nonparametric techniques for data analysis. These are procedures in which the data fail to meet one or more of the basic assumptions of parametric techniques described in chapters 6-9. Nonparametric techniques for comparisons and relationships between categories and ranked scores are discussed. Some statistical comparisons between two samples and among multiple samples are described for both independent and dependent groups. We also present simple and more complex relationships between variables expressed in nominal and ordinal forms.

Finally, chapter 11 reviews many of the measurement issues that apply when conducting research. We focus on the validity and reliability issues of the dependent variables. A short overview of measurement issues in data collected about physical performance is presented, although complete coverage of this topic is not possible. In much research in the study of physical activity, dependent variables may be affective and knowledge measures. Thus, we discuss these types of dependent variables.

After reading the six chapters in Part II, you will not be a statistician nor a measurement expert (unless you were one before you started). However, if you read and study these chapters carefully and perhaps explore some of the references further, you should be able to comprehend the statistical analysis and measurement issues of most research studies.

CHAPTER 6

Becoming Acquainted With Statistical Concepts

Dear Professors of Research Methods:

I'm not very good in math, so I'm hesitant about attempting to learn the statistical parts of research methods. What should I do?

Yours truly,
Clyde Clueless

Dear Clueless:

First, don't be like Calvin in the cartoon "Calvin and Hobbes" by Bill Watterson. Calvin says, "I already know more than I want to. . . . The fact is, I'm being educated against my will." Hobbes says, "Is it a right to remain ignorant?" Calvin says, "I don't know and I don't want to find out." Don't remain ignorant about statistics. They are simply a tool to help you make decisions!

Methodologically yours,
PRM

The concept of statistics frightens many people. If you are intimidated, you needn't be. Statistics is one of the few ways data can be reported uniformly to allow relevant, accurate conclusions and comparisons to be made. They are methodical, logical, and necessary, not random, inconsistent, or terrifying. Our approach to statistics in this book is to acquaint you with the basic concepts and give you a working knowledge; it is not our purpose to make you a statistician, especially given this well-known quotation: "There are liars, damn liars, and statisticians."

Why We Need Statistics

> Remember that throughout the process in which you conceive, plan, execute, and write up a research, it is on your informed judgment as a scientist that you must rely, and this holds as much for the statistical aspects of the work as it does for all the others. Cohen (1990, p. 1310)

Statistics is simply an objective means of interpreting a collection of observations. Various statistical techniques are necessary to allow the description of the characteristics of data, test relationships between sets of data, and test the differences among sets of data. For example, if height and a standing long jump score were measured for each person in a seventh-grade class, you could sum all the heights and then divide the sum by the number of people. The result (statistic to represent the average height) is the mean ($\Sigma\,X/N$, where Σ = sum, X = each person's height, and N = number of people; read this as "sum all Xs and divide by N"). The mean (M) describes the average height in the class; it is a single characteristic that represents the data.

An example of testing relationships between sets of data would be to measure the degree of association between height and the scores on the standing long jump. You might hypothesize that taller people can jump farther. By plotting the scores (Figure 6.1), you can see that people who are taller generally do jump farther. But note that the relationship is not perfect. If it were, the scores would begin in the lower left-hand corner of the figure and proceed diagonally in a straight line toward the upper right-hand corner. One measure of the degree of association between two variables is called **Pearson r** (or simple correlation). When two variables are unrelated, their correlation is approximately zero. In Figure 6.1, the two variables (height and standing long jump scores) have a moderately positive correlation (r is probably between .40 and .60). Relationships and correlation are discussed in greater detail in the next chapter, but for now you should see that researchers frequently want to investigate the relationship between variables.

Besides descriptive and correlational techniques, a third category of statistical techniques is used to measure differences among groups. Suppose you believe that weight training of the legs will increase the distance one can jump. You take a seventh-grade class, divide it into two groups, and have one group participate for 8 weeks in a weight-training program designed to develop leg strength. The other students continue their regular activities. You want to know whether the independent variable (weight training versus regular activity) produces a change in the dependent variable (standing long jump score). Therefore, you measure the two groups' standing long jump scores at the end of the 8 weeks (treatment period) and compare their average

Pearson r — The most commonly used method of computing correlation between two variables; also called *interclass* or *Pearson product moment coefficient of correlation.*

t **test** — A statistical technique to assess differences between two groups.

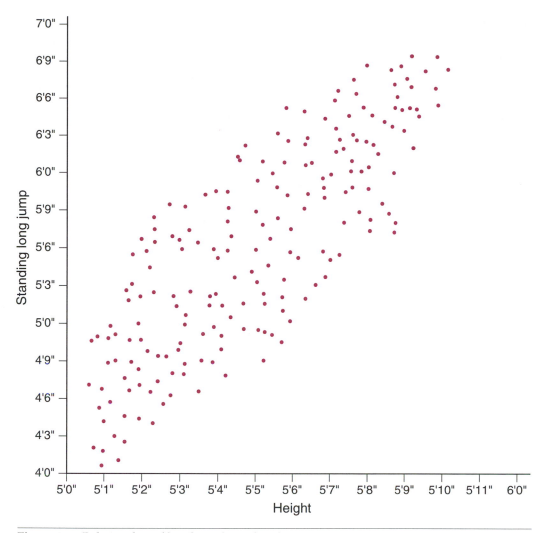

Figure 6.1   Relationship of height and standing long jump.

performances. Here, a statistical technique to assess differences between two independent groups, a *t* **test**, would be used. By calculating *t* and comparing it with a value from a *t* table, you can judge whether the two groups were significantly different on their average long jump scores. Ways for assessing differences among groups are discussed in chapter 8.

How Computers Are Used for Statistical Analysis

 Computers are very helpful in the calculation of statistics. Computers do not make the mistakes that occur in hand calculations, and they are many times faster. Two types of computers are frequently used for statistical analysis: microcomputers

 hardware — The mechanical units of a computer, such as the monitor, keyboard, disk drive, and printer.

software — The programs of instructions used to make computers function in the desired manner.

and mainframe computers. Microcomputers are frequently used in laboratories, offices, and homes for statistical calculations. Micros are small desktop computers. The computer and its attachments (disk drives, monitors, printers, hard disks, and modems) are called **hardware**, and the computer programming is called **software**. Numerous software programs have been written to calculate statistics. In Appendix C we provide a general description of software packages that integrate statistical analyses, graphic displays, and word processing for microcomputers. We are seeing more and more statistical processing being done on microcomputers because of the increased power and software available.

Three popular software packages for use on mainframe computers include the UCLA Biomedical Series (BIMED), the Statistical Package for the Social Sciences (SPSS), and the Statistical Analysis System (SAS). (These are reviewed in Appendix C.) Most colleges and universities have one or more of these packages, which can be used from a terminal or through a microcomputer (with proper hardware and software). Your computer center will have information about available equipment and services. You usually need to request an account number from the computer center. Many computer centers provide so-called user services or user consultant centers where you can get advice about the hardware and software available and instructions in how to use it.

Most institutions teach statistics courses in which these software packages are used. Statistics departments may also offer consulting services on the appropriate use of statistics for research projects. You should investigate the services your institution offers. Senior graduate students and faculty can also advise you on available services.

Description and Inference Are Not Statistical Techniques

At the beginning of this chapter we stated that statistical techniques allow the description of data characteristics, testing of relationships, and testing of differences. When we discuss description and **inference**, though, we are not discussing statistical techniques, although those two words are sometimes confused with statistical techniques. This confusion is the result of saying that correlations describe relationships and that cause-and-effect is inferred by techniques for testing differences between groups. These statements are not necessarily true. The results of any statistic describe the sample of subjects for which it was calculated. If the sample of subjects represents some larger group, then the findings can be inferred (or generalized) to the larger group. However, the statistic used has nothing to do with inference. The method of selecting the sample, procedures, and context is what does or does not allow inference.

Ways to Select a Sample

Random Selection

Stratified Random Sampling

Systematic Sampling

Random Assignment

inference — Generalization of results to some larger group.

The **sample** is the group of subjects, treatments, and situations on which the study is conducted. The key issue is how these samples are selected. In the following sections we discuss the types of sampling typically used in designing studies and using statistical analysis.

Random Selection

The sample of subjects might be randomly selected from some larger group, or a **population**. For example, if your college or university has 10,000 students, you could randomly select 200 for a study. You would assign each of the 10,000 students a number-name. The first number-name would be 0000, the second 0001, the third 0002, up through the last (the 10,000th), who would have the number-name 9999. Then a **random numbers table** (see Table A.1 in Appendix A) would be used. The numbers in this table are arranged in two-digit sets so that any combination of rows or columns is unrelated. In this instance (number-names 0000-9999), you need to select 200 four-digit numbers. Because the rows and columns are unrelated, you can choose any type of systematic strategy to go through the table. Enter the table at random (close your eyes and put your finger on the page). Suppose the place of entering the table is the sixth column of a two-digit number on row 8. The number-name here is 9953 (includes columns 6 and 7 for a four-digit number). You select the subject with that number-name (9953), then 9386, and so on until you have selected 200 subjects. Column 7 is not used because it was included with column 6 to yield a four-digit number.

The system used in the random numbers table is not the only one. You can use any systematic way of going through the table. You could read across rows rather than down columns. Of course, the purpose of all this is to select a sample of subjects randomly so that the sample represents the larger population; that is, the findings in the sample can be inferred back to the larger population. From a statistical viewpoint, this says that a characteristic, relationship, or difference found in the sample is likely also to be present in the population from which the sample was selected (inference).

Computer programs can also be used to generate a set of random numbers. These programs operate much like the procedures just described. You tell the program the population size and how many cases to randomly select.

Stratified Random Sampling

In **stratified random sampling**, the population is divided (stratified) on some characteristic before random selection of the sample. Returning to the previous example, the selection was of 200 subjects from a population of 10,000. Suppose your college is 30% freshmen, 30% sophomores, 20% juniors, and 20% seniors. You could stratify on class before random selection to make sure the sample was exact in terms of class representation. Here, you would randomly select 60 subjects from the 3,000 freshmen, 60 from the 3,000 sophomores, 40 from the 2,000 juniors, and 40 from the 2,000 seniors. This still yields a total sample of 200.

---

 sample — A group of subjects, treatments, or situations selected from a larger population.

 population — The larger group from which a sample is taken.

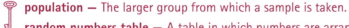 **random numbers table** — A table in which numbers are arranged in two-digit (or greater) sets so that any combination of rows or columns is unrelated.

stratified random sampling — Method of stratifying a population on some characteristic prior to random selection of the sample.

Stratified random sampling might be particularly appropriate for survey or interview research. Suppose you suspect that attitudes toward exercise participation change over the college years. You might use a stratified random sampling technique for interviewing 200 college students to test this hypothesis. Another example would be to develop normative data on a physical fitness test for grades 4-8 in a school district. Because performance would be related to age, you should stratify the population by age before randomly selecting your sample on which to collect normative data.

Systematic Sampling

If the population from which the sample is to be selected is very large, assigning a number-name to each potential subject is time-consuming. Suppose you want to sample a town with a population of 50,000 concerning the need for new sport facilities. One approach would be to use systematic sampling from the telephone book. You might decide to call a sample of 500 people. To do so, you would select every 100th name in the phone book (50,000/500 = 100). Of course, you are assuming that the telephone book represents the population or, said another way, that everyone you need to sample has a listed telephone number. This turned out to be a very bad assumption in the 1948 presidential election (Dewey vs. Truman). The pollsters had predicted Dewey to win by a substantial margin. However, the pollsters had sampled from telephone books in key areas. Unfortunately for Dewey, many people without telephones voted for Truman. His victory was called an upset, but it was an upset only because of poor sampling procedures. Systematic sampling will yield a good sample and should be equivalent to random sampling if the sample is fairly large. However, researchers generally prefer random sampling.

Random Assignment

In experimental research, groups are formed within the sample. The issue here is not how the sample is selected but how the groups are formed within the sample. Chapter 16 discusses experimental research and true experimental designs. All true designs require that the groups within the sample be randomly assigned or randomized. Although this requirement has nothing to do with selecting the sample, the procedures used for random assignment are the same. Each subject in the sample is given a number-name. If the sample has 30 subjects, the number-names range from 00 to 29. In this case, suppose three equal groups (ns = 10) are to be formed. Enter a table of random numbers; the first number-name encountered between 00 and 29 goes in Group 1, the second in Group 2, and so on until each group has 10 subjects. This process allows the researcher to assume that the groups are equivalent at the beginning of the experiment, which is one of several important features of good experimental design in which the purpose of the research is to establish cause-and-effect.

Computer programs are also available to randomize groups. You supply the sample size and the number of groups and decide whether the groups are to have an equal number of subjects. The computer program will then randomly assign subjects.

Justifying Post Hoc Explanations

Frequently, the sample for research is not randomly selected; rather, the researcher will attempt a post hoc justification that the sample represents some larger group. A typical example might include showing that the sample does not differ in average age, racial balance, or socioeconomic status from some larger group. Of course, the purpose is to allow the findings on the sample to be generalized to the larger group. A post hoc attempt at generalization may be better than nothing, but it is not the equivalent of random selection, which allows the assumption that the sample does not differ from the population on the characteristics measured (as well as any other characteristics). In a post hoc justification, only the characteristics measured can be compared. Whether those are the ones that really matter is open to speculation.

This same justification is used to compare intact groups, or groups within the sample that are not randomly formed. Except in this case, the post hoc justification is that because the groups did not differ on certain measured characteristics before the study began, they can be judged equivalent. Of course, the same point applies: Are the groups different on some unmeasured characteristic that affects the results? This question cannot be answered satisfactorily. But, as before, a good post hoc justification of equivalence does add strength to comparisons of intact groups.

Difficulty of Random Sampling and Assignment: How Good Does It Have to Be?

In many studies of physical activity, random sampling procedures are not possible. For example, when comparing experts with novice performers, typically neither group is randomly sampled, nor are group memberships (expert and novice) randomly formed. The same is true when studying well-trained versus untrained runners or cyclists. Often we are interested in comparing the responses of different age groups, ethnic groups, and genders to training in skill or exercise. Obviously, these groups are seldom randomly selected and cannot be randomly formed. In many studies sampling is not done at all; researchers are happy to have any subjects who will volunteer.

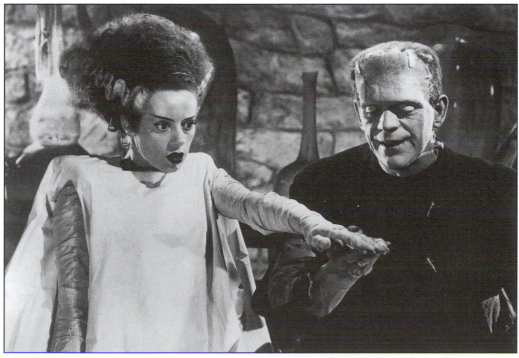

Sometimes researchers are happy to have anyone who will volunteer.

Sampling also applies to the treatments used for different groups of subjects. How are the treatments selected? Do they represent some population of potential treatments? What about the situational context under which subjects are tested or receive the experimental treatment? Are these sampled in some way? Are they representative of the potential situations?

The real answers to these questions about sampling are that we seldom sample a population at any level—subjects, treatments, or situations. Yet we hope to be able to use statistical tables based on assumptions of sampling as well as be able to infer that what we find applies to some larger group than the subjects used in the study. What is really needed is a sample that is "good enough for our purpose" (Kruskal & Mosteller, 1979, p. 259). This concept is extremely important for research in physical activity. If we cannot disregard the strict requirements of random sampling that allow study outcomes to be generalized to some similar group, we will never be able to generalize beyond the characteristics of any particular study—location, age, race, sex, time, etc. Strictly speaking, there is no basis for the findings from a sample to be similar to a population that differs in any way from the sample (even one hour after the sampling). "A good-enough principle of sampling, however, would allow generalizations to any population for which the sample is representative enough" (Serlin, 1987, p. 366).

For the sample of subjects, treatments, and situations to be "good enough" to generalize, it must be selected on some theoretical basis. For example, if the theory proposes that the cardiovascular system responds to training in a specific way in all untrained adult subjects, using volunteer untrained undergraduates in a training study may be acceptable. "It is only on the basis of theory that one decides whether the experimental results can be generalized to the responder population, to the stimulus or ecological population, or both" (Serlin, 1987, p. 367). The best likely generalization statement is to say that the findings may be "plausible" in other subjects, treatments, and situations depending on their similarity to the study characteristics.

A Review of Mathematical Concepts and Statistical Symbols

By now you should have a basic understanding of the concept of statistics: why they are necessary, how computers can be used to calculate them, why descriptions and inference aren't statistical techniques, and how good your sampling procedures need to be. It is time now to explain the "how to's" of statistics.

Before we begin discussing statistical techniques, however, a review of basic mathematical concepts may be helpful. The presentation on page 99 is rather basic, so do not hesitate to skip over it if you are proficient in the operations presented.

Statistical formulas frequently use symbols in combination with mathematical functions. The summary on page 99 also explains the symbols to be used and provides some examples of their use in connection with the mathematical functions.

Measures of Central Tendency and Variability

Central Tendency Scores

Variability Scores

Range of Scores

Mathematical Functions and Statistical Symbols

Mathematical Functions

1. + means add
2. − means subtract
3. × or · means multiply
4. ÷ or / or ‾‾ means divide
5. √‾‾ means take the square root
6. ^{2} superscript or raised number means to multiply the number by itself that many times:
   $2^2 = 2 \times 2 = 4$; $3^3 = 3 \times 3 \times 3 = 27$
7. ( ) means perform mathematical acts inside parentheses first: $3(2 + 3) = 3(5) = 15$
8. Multiply and divide before adding and subtracting unless parentheses indicate otherwise
9. Like signs are always added: $-7 - 4 = -11$

Examples

Addition of signed numbers	$+3 - 2 = 1, -3 + 1 = -2, -5 + 4 - 3 = (-5 - 3) + 4 = -8 + 4 = -4$
Subtraction of signed numbers	$-4 - 3 = -7, +4 - 3 = 1, -4 + 3 = -1, (-4) - (-3) = -4 + 3 = -1$
Multiplication of signed numbers	$(-3) \times (-4) = +12, (-3) \times 4 = -12, +5 \cdot -3 = -15, (3)(4)(-2) = -24$
Division of signed numbers	$-12/-4 = 3, -24/-3 = 8, (9/-3)(-2) = 6, 4/2 + -8/2 = -2$
Complex cases	$(3 - 4)(-5 - 2) = (-1)(-7) = 7, (3 + 5)/(-3 + 1) = 8/-2 = -4$

Statistical Symbols

1. Σ means to sum or add
2. X or Y represents a given number
3. $\bar{X}$ or M represents the mean, or average, of several numbers
4. x or y is a deviation score: $x = X - M$
5. N is the number of subjects in the sample
6. n is the number of subjects within sample subgroups
7. SD or s represents the standard deviation
8. s^2 represents the variance

Examples

1. $X_1 = 2, X_2 = 4, X_3 = 1, X_4 = 5$
   $\Sigma X = 2 + 4 + 1 + 5 = 12$

2. $Y_1 = 7, Y_2 = 3, Y_3 = 2, Y_4 = 4$
   $\Sigma Y = 7 + 3 + 2 + 4 = 16$

3. $\Sigma X^2 = 2^2 + 4^2 + 1^2 + 5^2 = 4 + 16 + 1 + 25 = 46$

4. $(\Sigma X)^2 = (2 + 4 + 1 + 5)^2 = 12^2 = 144$

Some of the more easily understood statistical and mathematical calculations are those that find **central tendency** and **variability** of scores. When you have a group of scores, one number may be used to represent the group. That number is generally the mean, median, or mode. These terms are ways of expressing central tendency. Within the group of scores, each individual score will differ to a given degree from the central tendency score. The degree of difference is the score's variability. Two terms that describe the variability of the scores are **standard deviation** and **variance**.

Central Tendency Scores

The statistic for the central tendency score with which most of you are familiar is the **mean** (*M*), or average:

$$M = \Sigma X / N \qquad (6.1)$$

Thus, if you have the numbers 4, –5, 3, 6, –2, –1, 4, –2, 3, and –3, then

$$M = [(4 + 3 + 6 + 4 + 3) + (–5 –2 –1 –2 –3)]/10$$
$$= (20 – 13)/10$$
$$= 7/10 = 0.7$$

The number 0.7 is the average and represents this series of numbers.

Sometimes the mean may not be the most representative or characteristic score. Suppose you have the numbers 4, 5, 4, 6, 3, 5, 26, 3, 4. The mean is 6.7, a number larger than all but one of the scores. It is not very representative because one score (26) made the average high. In this case, another measure of central tendency is more useful. The **median** is defined as the score in the middle; the middle score is found by the formula of $(N + 1)/2$. In our example, if you arrange the numbers from lowest to highest—3, 3, 4, 4, 4, 5, 5, 6, 26—the median [$(9 + 1)/2 = 5$; so count up 5 places from the low score] is 4, which is a much more representative score.

Most often you will be interested in the mean of a group of scores. You may occasionally be interested in the median or perhaps in another measure of central tendency, the **mode**, which is defined as the most frequently occurring score. In the previous example, the mode is also 4, as it occurs three times.

Variability Scores

Another characteristic of a group of scores is the variability. An estimate of the variability, or spread, of the scores can be calculated as the standard deviation (*s*):

---

central tendency (measure of) — A single score that best represents all of the scores.

variability — The degree of difference between each individual score and the central tendency score.

standard deviation — An estimate of the variability of the scores of a group around the mean.

variance — The square of the standard deviation.

mean — A statistical measure of central tendency that is the average score of the group.

median — A statistical measure of central tendency describing the middle score in a group.

mode — A statistical measure of central tendency that is the most frequently occurring score of the group.

$$s = \sqrt{\Sigma(X - M)^2 / (N - 1)} \qquad (6.2)$$

This formula translates as follows. Calculate the mean by Formula 6.1, subtract the mean from each subject's score $(X - M)$, square the answer, sum the squared scores, divide by the number of subjects minus one $(N - 1)$, and take the square root of the answer. Table 6.1 provides an example.

Table 6.1   Calculation of Mean and Standard Deviation

Subjects	X	$X - M$	$(X - M)^2$
1	2	−2	4
2	4	0	0
3	3	−1	1
4	5	1	1
5	6	2	4
Σ	20	0	10

$M = \Sigma X / N = 20/5 = 4$

$s = \sqrt{\Sigma(X - M)^2 / (N - 1)} = \sqrt{10/4} = \sqrt{2.5} = 1.58$

The mean and standard deviation together are good descriptions of a set of scores. If the standard deviation is large, the mean may not be a good representation. Roughly 68% of a set of scores fall between ± 1 s, about 95% of the scores fall between ± 2 s, and about 99% of the scores fall between ± 3 s. This is called a normal distribution (see next section).

Formula 6.2 was used to help you understand the meaning of the standard deviation. For use with a hand calculator, Formula 6.3 is simpler:

$$s = \sqrt{[N\Sigma X^2 - (\Sigma X)^2] / [N(N - 1)]} \qquad (6.3)$$

One final point for later consideration is that the square of the standard deviation is called the variance, or s^2.

Range of Scores

Sometimes the range of scores may also be reported, particularly when the median rather than the mean is used. The median and the mean may be used in connection with each other. For example, 15 subjects might be given 10 blocks of 10 trials (100 total trials) on a **reaction time** (RT) task. The experimenter may decide to use the median RT of a subject's 10 trials as the most representative score in each block. Thus, each subject would have 10 median scores, or 1 for each of the 10 trial blocks. Here, the range of scores from which the median was selected should be reported. Both the mean and the standard deviation would be reported for the 15 subjects' median scores at Trial Block 1, Trial Block 2, and so on. Thus, the range is reported for the selection of the median at each trial block, whereas the standard deviation is reported for the group mean at each trial block.

---

reaction time — Time elapsed from the presentation of a stimulus until the initiation of a response.

Basic Concepts of Statistical Techniques

Two Categories of Statistical Tests

What Statistical Techniques Tell About Data

Categories of Statistical Techniques

Probability

Alpha

Beta

Meaningfulness (Effect Size)

Power

Besides measures of central tendency and variability, there are other, slightly more complicated statistical techniques. Before we explain each in detail, however, you must understand some general information about statistical techniques.

Two Categories of Statistical Tests

There are two general categories of statistical tests: parametric and nonparametric. The use of the various tests depends on meeting the assumptions for those tests. The first category, **parametric statistical tests**, has three assumptions about the distribution of the data:

- The population from which the sample is drawn must be normally distributed on the variable of interest.
- The samples drawn from a population must have the same variances on the variable of interest.
- The observations are independent.

Certain parametric techniques have additional assumptions. The second category, **nonparametric statistics**, is called **distribution-free** because the previous assumptions need not be met.

Whenever the assumptions are met, parametric statistics are often said to have more **power**, although there is some debate on this issue. To have power means to increase the chances of rejecting a false null hypothesis. You frequently assume that

---

 parametric statistical test — Test based on data assumptions of normal distribution, equal variance, and independence of observation.

 Three assumptions of parametric tests

 nonparametric statistical test — Any of a number of statistical techniques used when the data do not meet the assumptions required to perform parametric tests.

distribution-free statistics — See *nonparametric statistical test.*

 power (statistical) — The degree to which the chances of rejecting a false null hypothesis are increased.

skewness — Description of the direction of the hump of the curve of distribution of data and the nature of the tails of the curve.

kurtosis — Description of the shape of the curve of the distribution of data, for example, whether the curve is more peaked or flatter than the normal curve.

the three assumptions for use of parametric statistics are met. The assumptions can be tested by using estimates of **skewness** and **kurtosis**. (Only the meaning of these tests is explained here. Any basic statistics textbook provides considerably more detail; for a helpful discussion on skewness and kurtosis, see Newell & Hancock, 1984).

To understand skewness and kurtosis, first consider the normal distribution in Figure 6.2. This is a **normal curve**, which is characterized by the mean, median, and mode being at the same point (center of the distribution). In addition, ± 1 s from the mean includes 68% of the scores, ± 2 s from the mean includes 95% of the scores, and ± 3 s includes 99% of the scores. Thus, data distributed as in Figure 6.2 would meet the three assumptions for use of parametric techniques. Skewness of the distribution describes the direction of the hump of the curve (labeled A) and the nature of the tails of the curve (labeled B and C). If the hump (A) is shifted to the left and the long tail (B) to the right (Figure 6.3a), the skewness is positive. If the shift of the hump (A) is to the right and the long tail (C) to the left (Figure 6.3b), the skewness is negative. Kurtosis describes the shape of the curve, for example, whether the curve is more or less peaked than the normal curve. Figure 6.4a shows a more peaked curve and Figure 6.4b a flatter curve.

Appendix A contains Table A.2, which is a unit normal distribution (z) for a normal curve. The column z shows the location of the mean. When the mean is in the center of the distribution, its z is equal to .00; thus, .50 (50%) of the distribution is beyond the mean, leaving .50 (50%) of the distribution as a remainder. As the mean of the distribution moves to the right in a normal curve (say to a z of + 1 s), .8413 (84%) of the distribution is to the left of the mean (remainder) and .1587 is to the right of the mean (beyond). This table allows you to determine the percentage of the normal distribution included by the mean plus any fraction of a standard deviation. Suppose you want to know

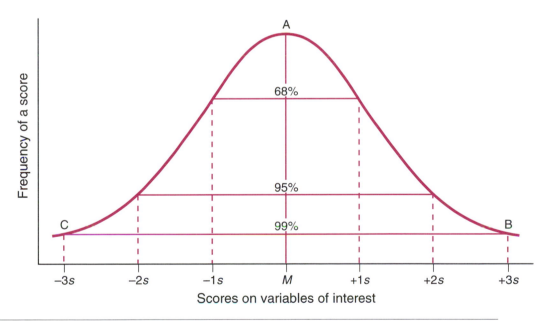

Figure 6.2   The normal curve.

Newell, K.M., & Hancock, P.A. (1984). Forgotten moments: A note on skewness and kurtosis as influential factors in inferences extrapolated from response distributions. *Journal of Motor Behavior*, **16**, 320-335.

normal curve — Distribution of data in which the mean, median, and mode are at the same point (center of the distribution) and ± 1 s from the mean includes 68% of the scores, ± 2s from the mean includes 95% of the scores, and ± 3 s includes 99% of the scores.

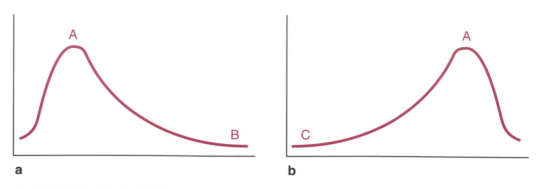

Figure 6.3   Skewed curves: a, positive skewness; b, negative skewness.

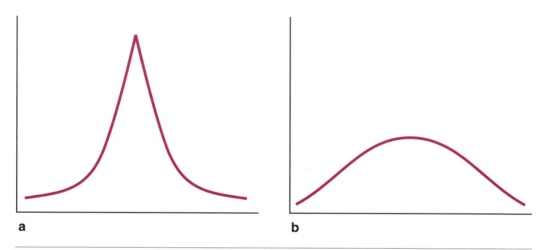

Figure 6.4   Curves with abnormal kurtosis: a, more peaked; b, more flat.

what percentage of the distribution would be included by the mean plus one half (.50) of a standard deviation. Using Table A.2 you can see that it would be .6915 (remainder), or 69%.

For chapters 7-9, consider that the three basic assumptions for parametric statistical tests have been met. This is done for three reasons. First, the assumptions are very robust to violations, meaning that the outcome of the statistical test is relatively accurate even with severe violations of the assumptions. Second, most of the research in physical activity uses parametric tests. Finally, nonparametric tests are relatively easy to understand. (Chapter 10 covers basic nonparametric techniques.)

What Statistical Techniques Tell About Data

The statistical techniques presented in the next four chapters answer the following two questions about the data to which they are applied:

- Is the effect or relationship of interest reliable? In other words, if the research is repeated, will the effect or relationship be there again (is it significant)?
- How strong (or meaningful) is the effect or relationship of interest? This refers to the magnitude, or size, of the effect or relationship.

Two facts are important about these two statements. First, Statement 1 is usually evaluated prior to Statement 2, for the strength of the relationship or effect may be of minimal

 Questions that statistical techniques answer about data

interest until it is known to be reliable (significant). Second, Statement 2 is always of interest if the effect or relationship is significant and occasionally of interest without a significant effect. Sometimes, in elating over the significance of effects and relationships, one loses sight of the need to look at the strength or meaningfulness of these relationships. This is particularly true in research in which differences among groups are compared. The experimenter frequently forgets that relatively small differences can be significant. That means only that the differences are reliable or that the same answer is likely to be obtained if the research is repeated. The experimenter then needs to look at the size of the differences to interpret whether the findings are meaningful. For each technique presented in the next four chapters, we first look at whether the relationship or effect is significant (reliable). Then we suggest ways to evaluate the strength (meaningfulness) of the relationship or effect.

Categories of Statistical Techniques

It is practical to divide statistical techniques into two categories: (a) statistical techniques used to test relationships between or among several variables in one group of subjects (regression or correlation) and (b) techniques used to test differences between or among groups of subjects (t tests and analysis of variance). This division is inaccurate because both sets of techniques are based on the general linear model and only involve different ways of entering data and manipulating variance components. However, an introduction to research methods is neither the place to reform the "world of statistics according to Thomas and Nelson" nor the place to confuse you. Thus, the techniques as two distinct groups are considered. Chapter 7 discusses relationships among variables (simple and multiple correlation), and chapter 8 discusses differences between and among groups (t tests and analysis of variance). Teaching you the simple calculations underlying the easier techniques and then building on this helps you intuitively understand the more complex ones. Chapter 9 then presents extensions of simple and multiple correlation into canonical correlation, structural modeling (LISREL), and factor analysis as well as extensions of analysis of variance into discriminant analysis and multivariate analysis of variance.

Do not panic because statistics involves manipulating numbers. You can escape from this section with a reasonable grasp of how, why, and when the various statistical techniques are used in the study of physical activity. Remember, however, that correlation between two variables does not indicate causation (recall the discussion in chapter 4). Causation is not determined from any statistic or correlation. Cause-and-effect is established by theory, logic, and the total experimental situation, of which statistics is a part. As summarized by Pedhazur (1982),

"Correlation is no proof of causation." Nor does any other index prove causation, regardless of whether the index was derived from data collected in experimental or in nonexperimental research. Covariations or correlations among variables may be suggestive of causal linkages. Nevertheless, an explanatory scheme is not arrived at on the basis of the data, but rather on the basis of knowledge, theoretical formulations and assumptions, and logical analyses. It is the explanatory scheme of the researcher that determines the type of analysis to be applied to data, and not the other way around. (p. 579)

For example, Descartes has been credited with the logical statement, "I think, therefore I am." However, the famous philosopher Edsall Murphy "recognized it as a syllogism with an unstated major premise":

 Correlation does not prove causation

Major Premise: A nonexistent object cannot think.

Minor Premise: I think.

Conclusion: Therefore, I am. (Morgenstern, 1983, p. 112)

Murphy was not satisfied with this and so tried to find deeper meaning and a better logical analysis.

Q: How can you be sure that you exist?

A: I think.

Q: How can you be sure you are thinking?

A: I can't, but I do think that I think.

Q: Does that make you sure that you exist?

A: I think so.

This should make it clear that Descartes went too far. He ought to have said:

"I think I think, therefore I am," or possibly "I think I think, therefore I think I am, I think." . . . you do not really exist unless others are aware of your existence. Murphy proclaimed, "I stink, therefore I am." (Morgenstern, 1983, p. 112)

Probability

Another concept that deals with statistical techniques is **probability**, which asks what are the odds that certain things will happen. You use probability in everyday events. What are the chances that it will rain? You hear from a weather report that probability of rain is 90%. You wonder whether that means it will rain in 90% of the places or, more likely, that the chances are 90% that it will rain where you are, especially if you are planning to play golf or tennis. The terms **subjective** or **personalistic probability** are used to describe this concept.

A second concept of probability is called **equally likely events**. For example, if you roll a die, the chances of the numbers from 1 to 6 occurring are equally likely (i.e., 1 in 6, unless you are playing craps in Las Vegas). The third approach to probability involves **relative frequency**. To illustrate, suppose you toss a coin 100 times. You would expect a head 50 times and a tail 50 times; the probability is one half, or .50. However, when you toss, you may get a head 48 times, or .48. This is the relative frequency. You might do this 10 times and never get .50, but the relative frequency would be distributed closely around .50, and you would still assume the probability as .50.

In a statistical test, you sample from a population of subjects and events. You use probability statements to describe the confidence you place in the statistical findings. Frequently, you will encounter a statistical test followed by a probability statement such as $p < .05$. This interpretation would be that a difference or relationship of this size would be expected less than 5 times in 100 as a result of chance.

---

probability — The odds that a certain event will occur.

subjective probability — Concept in probability regarding the subjective chances of occurrence of an event. Also known as *personalistic probability*.

equally likely events — A concept of probability in which the chances of one event occurring are the same as the chances of another event occurring.

relative frequency — A concept of probability concerning the comparative likelihood of two or more events occurring.

Alpha

 In research, the test statistic is compared to a probability table for that statistic, which tells you what the chance occurrence is. The experimenter may establish an acceptable level of chance occurrence (called **alpha**, α) before the study. This level of chance occurrence can vary from low to high but can never be eliminated. For any given study, the probability of the findings being due to chance always exists, or, to quote Holten's Homily, "The only time to be positive is when you are positive you are wrong."

 In behavioral research, alpha (probability of chance occurrence) is frequently set at .05 or .01 (the odds that the findings are due to chance are either 5 in 100 or 1 in 100). There is nothing magical about .05 or .01. They are used to control for a **Type I error**. In a study, the experimenter may make two types of error. A Type I error is to reject the null hypothesis when the null hypothesis is true. For example, a researcher concludes that there is a difference between two methods of training, but there really isn't. A **Type II error** is not to reject the null hypothesis when the null hypothesis is false. In the previous example, a researcher may conclude there is no difference between the two training methods, but there really is a difference. Figure 6.5 is called a **truth table**, which displays Type I and II errors. As you can see, to accept a true null hypothesis or reject a false one is the correct decision. You control for Type I errors by setting alpha. For example, if alpha is set at .05, then, if 100 experiments are conducted, a true null hypothesis of no difference or no relationship would be rejected on only 5 occasions. Although the chances for error still exist, the experimenter has specified them exactly by establishing alpha before the study.

	H_0 true	H_0 false
Accept	Correct decision	Type II error (β)
Reject	Type I error (α)	Correct decision

Figure 6.5   Truth table for null hypothesis (H_0).

 To some extent the issue is, if you had to make an error, which type of error would you be willing to make? In fact, the level of alpha reflects the type of error you are willing to make. In other words, is it more important that you avoid concluding that one training method is better than another when it really isn't (Type I), or is it more important that you avoid the conclusion that one method

---

alpha — A level of probability (of chance occurrence) set by the experimenter prior to the study; sometimes referred to as level of significance.

Type I error — A rejection of the null hypothesis when the null hypothesis is true.

Type II error — Acceptance of the null hypothesis when the null hypothesis is false.

truth table — A graphic representation of correct and incorrect decisions regarding Type I and Type II errors.

Setting the alpha to control errors

isn't any better than the other when it really is (Type II)? For example, in a study of the effect of a cancer drug, the experimenter would not want to accept the null hypothesis of no effect if there were any chance that the drug worked. Thus, the experimenter might set alpha at .30 even though the odds of making a Type I error would be inflated. The experimenter is making sure that the drug has every opportunity to show its effectiveness. On the other hand, setting alpha at .001 greatly decreases the odds of making a Type I error.

We cannot tell you where to set alpha; however, we can say that the levels .05 or .01 are widely accepted in the scientific community. If alpha is to be moved up or down, be sure to justify the reason, but consider this: "Surely God loves the .06 nearly as much as the .05" (Rosnow & Rosenthal, 1989).

Even when experimenters set alpha at a specific level (e.g., .05) before the research, they often report alpha for the specific effects of the study at the level it occurred (e.g., $p = .012$). Nothing is wrong with this procedure, as they are only demonstrating to what degree the level of probability exceeded the specified level.

It is debatable whether alpha should be specified before the research and the findings reported at the alpha that has been specified. Some argue that results are either significant at the specified alpha or they are not (not much is in between). It is like being pregnant—one either is or is not. Comparisons with alpha work the same way. It is established as a criterion, and results either meet the criterion or they do not. Although the experimenters sometimes report borderline significance (if alpha is .05), they label from .051 to .10 as borderline.

A more sound approach may be to report the exact level of probability (e.g., $p = .024$) associated with the test statistics (e.g., r, t). Then estimate the meaningfulness of the difference or relationship. Using the statistical information (significance and meaningfulness), the researcher should interpret the findings within the theory and hypotheses that have been put forward. Rather than making the decision a statistical one, this approach places the responsibility of decision making where it belongs—on the researcher who has placed the study within a theoretical model and has considered related research. Much of the criticism of statistics has revolved around the blind application of statistical techniques to data without appropriate interpretation of the outcomes. For excellent articles on the use of common sense with statistical outcomes, read Cohen (1990) and Serlin (1987).

Beta

Although the magnitude of Type I error is specified by alpha, you may also make a Type II error, the magnitude of which is determined by **beta** (β). By looking at Figure 6.6, you can see the overlap of the score distribution on the dependent variable for X (the sampling distribution if the null hypothesis is true) and Y (the sampling distribution if the null hypothesis is false). By specifying alpha, you indicate that the mean of Y (given a certain distribution) must be at a specified distance from the mean of X before the null hypothesis is rejected. However, if the mean of Y falls anywhere between the mean of X and the specified Y, you could be making a Type II error (β); that is, you do not reject the null hypothesis when, in fact, there is a true difference. As you can see, there is a relationship between alpha and beta; for example, as alpha is set increasingly smaller, beta becomes larger.

Cohen, J. (1990). Things I have learned (so far). *American Psychologist*, **45**, 1304–1312.

Serlin, R.C. (1987). Hypothesis testing, theory building, and the philosophy of science. *Journal of Counseling Psychology*, **34**, 365–371.

beta — The magnitude of committing a Type II error.

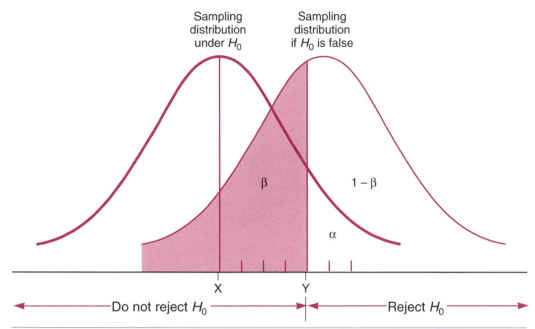

Figure 6.6   Regions under the normal curve corresponding to probabilities of making Type I and Type II errors.

From *Experimental Design: Procedures for the Behavioral Sciences*, by R.E. Kirk. Copyright © 1995, 1982, 1968 Brooks/Cole Publishing Company, a division of International Thomson Publishing Inc., Pacific Grove, CA 93950. By permission of the publisher.

Meaningfulness (Effect Size)

In addition to reporting the significance of the findings, scholars need to be concerned about the **meaningfulness** of the outcomes of their research. The meaningfulness of a difference between two means can be estimated in many ways, but the one that has gained the most attention recently is **effect size** (suggested by Cohen, 1969). You may be familiar with using effect size (ES) in meta-analysis (if not, you will be soon; see chapter 14 on research synthesis). The formula for ES is

$$ES = (M_1 - M_2)/s \tag{6.4}$$

This formula subtracts the mean of one group (M_1) from the mean of a second group (M_2) and divides the difference by the standard deviation. That places the difference between the means in the common metric called "standard deviation units," which can be compared to guidelines for behavioral research suggested by Cohen (1969): 0.2 or less is a small ES; about 0.5 is a moderate ES; and 0.8 or more is a large ES. For a more detailed discussion of the use of effect size in physical activity research, see Thomas, Salazar, and Landers (1991).

Many authors (e.g., Cohen, 1990; Serlin, 1987; Thomas, Salazar, & Landers, 1991) have indicated the need to report some estimate of meaningfulness with all tests of significance.

---

meaningfulness — The importance or practical significance of an effect or relationship.

effect size — The standardized value, the difference between the means divided by the standard deviation.

Thomas, J.R., Salazar, W., & Landers, D.M. (1991). What is missing in *p* < .05? Effect size. *Research Quarterly for Exercise and Sport*, **62**, 344-348.

Power

Power is the probability of rejecting the null hypothesis when the null hypothesis is false (e.g., detecting a real difference), or the probability of making a correct decision. Having power in the statistical analysis is important because it increases the odds of rejecting a false null hypothesis. Of course, to a degree, in behavioral research,

The null hypothesis is always false!!

What this statement reflects is that in behavioral research the means of two groups are never the same. Thus, if enough subjects are obtained (one way of obtaining power), any two means can be declared significantly different. Remember what that means. If you do it again, you will get about the same answer. The more interesting questions in behavioral research are

- How large a difference is important in theory and/or practice?
- How many subjects are needed to declare an important difference as significant?

Understanding the concept of power can answer the previous two questions. If a researcher can identify the size of an important effect through previous research or even simply estimate an effect size (e.g., 0.5 is a moderate ES, also called delta,), establish how much power is acceptable (e.g., a common estimate in the behavioral science is .8), then the size of the sample needed for a study can be estimated.

Figures 6.7 and 6.8 provide a look at the relationship among sample size, (y-axis), power (x-axis), and effect size (ES curves), when alpha is either .05 or .01. Consider the following example:

In planning a study, the investigator will have two groups that will be randomly formed but s/he does not know how many subjects are needed for each group to detect a meaningful difference between treatments. However, there are several related studies and the investigator has calculated an average ES = 0.70

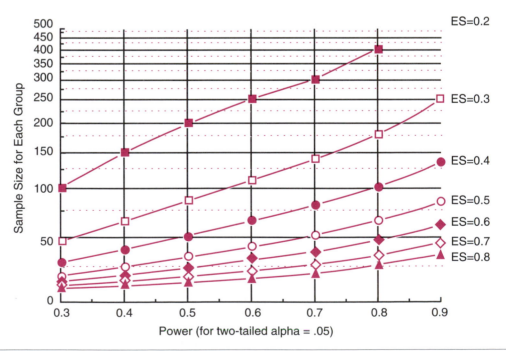

Figure 6.7   Effect size curves when alpha is .05 for a two-tailed test.

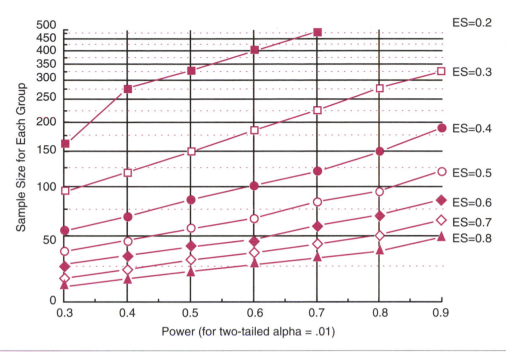

Figure 6.8   Effect size curves when alpha is .01 for a two-tailed test.

favoring the experimental group from the outcomes in these studies. The investigator decides to set alpha = .05 and wants to protect beta at 4 times the level of alpha (thus, beta = .20) because Cohen (1988) suggested that in the behavioral sciences, the seriousness of Type I to Type II error should be in a 4 to 1 ratio (.05 × 4 = .20). Since power is 1 − beta (1.0 − .2 = .8), then power is set at .8 (often recommended as appropriate power in behavioral research, Green, 1991, p. 502). When the previous information is known—alpha, ES, and power, then the number of subjects needed in each of the two groups can be estimated from Figure 6.7. Read the 0.70 ES curve to where it crosses the x-axis (power) at .8. Then, read across to the y-axis (sample size) and note that 30 subjects would be needed in each group.

Note how this relationship works: As the number of subjects in each group is reduced, power is reduced (given the same ES).

If you look at Figure 6.8 (alpha = .01), note for the same level of power (.8) and ES (0.70), the number of subjects per group increases from 30 (as in Figure 6.7, alpha = .05) to 50. So if all else stays the same but a more stringent alpha is used (e.g., .05 to .01), a greater number of subjects is required to detect a significant difference.

Of course, all the necessary information may not be available in all experiments. This is discussed further in chapter 8, although our approach is more post hoc, as it involves reporting the effect size and variance accounted for in significant findings and interpreting whether this is a meaningful effect. The procedures described previously and calculated *a priori* are more desirable but not always applicable. (For a more detailed discussion of important factors associated with establishing significance levels and determining power, see Franks & Huck, 1986.)

Finally, a summary of all this is well presented in the short poem by Rosenthal (1991, p. 221) on page 112.

Franks, B.D., & Huck, S.W. (1986). Why does everyone use the .05 significance level? *Research Quarterly for Exercise and Sport, 57,* 245-249.

Achieving Power

I. The Problem

Oh, *F* is large and *p* is small
That's why we are walking tall.

What it means we need not mull
Just so we reject the null.

Or Chi-square large and *p* near nil
Results like that, they fill the bill.

What if meaning requires a poll?
Never mind, we're on a roll!

The message we have learned too well?
Significance! That rings the bell!

II. The Implications

The moral of our little tale?
That we mortals may be frail
When we feel a *p* near zero
Makes us out to be a hero.

But tell us then is it too late?
Can we perhaps avoid our fate?
Replace that wish to null-reject
Report the *size* of the effect.

That may not insure our glory
But at least it tells a story
That is just the kind of yield
Needed to advance our field.

From "Cumulating Psychology: An Appreciation of Donald T. Campbell," by R. Rosenthal, 1991, *Psychological Science*, 2(213), p. 221. Copyright 1991. Reprinted with the permission of Cambridge University Press.

Summary

Statistics are used to describe data, to determine relationships among variables, and to test for differences among groups. In this chapter we have tried to make the point that the type of statistics used does not determine whether findings can be generalized; rather, it is sampling that permits (or limits) inference. Whenever possible, random sampling is the method of choice, but in behavioral research the more important question may be whether the sample is "good enough." In some types of research, such as surveys, stratified random sampling is desirable for the study to represent certain segments of a population. In experimental research, random assignment of subjects to groups is definitely desirable so that the researcher can assume equivalence at the beginning of the experiment.

We began our coverage of statistical techniques with basic concepts such as measures of central tendency and variability and normal distribution. It is important to remember that statistics can do two things: establish significance and assess meaningfulness. Significance means that a relationship or difference is reliable—that you could expect it to happen again if the study were repeated. Meaningfulness refers to the importance of the results.

Probability is an important component of statistics. Probability statements refer to the confidence you place in the statistical findings. The null hypothesis is used in statistical tests. It states that there is no difference (or no relationship in a study) and that any observed finding is simply a chance occurrence.

The possibility of committing statistical error always exists. A Type I error is rejecting the null hypothesis when it is true. A Type II error is accepting the null hypothesis when it is false. These two errors work in opposition: as you strive to avoid one, you increase the likelihood of committing the other. The researcher must decide what level of significance (alpha) to establish—in other words, the degree to which one is willing to be wrong.

The most important issue in statistics is using good judgment. The statistical findings must be interpreted within the context of the theory used and the results of previous work. This leads to the concept of power—estimating the characteristics needed to determine whether the outcomes of a study have merit: the combination of alpha, effect size, power, and sample size.

 ## Check Your Understanding

Two groups ($ns = 7$) of 7-year-olds are led on a 35-m jog down a 50-m string placed on the ground. The children are then asked to reproduce the distance by jogging 35 m on a second 50-m string placed at a right angle to the first string. The experimental group is told before they begin that the best way to remember the distance jogged is to count steps. The control group is told to remember as best they can. Following is the error (in meters) each subject made when asked to estimate the distance jogged.

Experimental group	Control group
2.55	7.68
3.62	6.80
3.42	5.68
2.86	3.97
2.00	7.23
1.08	5.48
1.16	6.03

1. Use Formula 6.1 to calculate the mean for each group.
2. Use Formula 6.2 to calculate the standard deviation for each group.
3. Use Formula 6.3 to calculate the standard deviations to see whether the answer is the same as that derived from Formula 6.2.
4. Make a list of 50 names. Using the table of random numbers (Table A.1 in Appendix A), randomly select 24 subjects and then randomly assign them to two groups of 12 each.

CHAPTER 7

Relationships Among Variables

Dear Professors of Research Methods:

I read about a study that reported a significant correlation between height and intelligence ($r = .11$). This being the case, basketball players should be the smartest athletes. Could one infer by this that growth hormones would make a person smarter?

Sincerely,
Pearson Arr

Dear Pearson:

As both of your authors are somewhat vertically challenged, we hasten to point out two errors in your thinking. One, the correlation between these two variables is much too small to be meaningful. Remember, statistical significance does not by itself indicate that the relationship is of any importance. Besides, we tried elevator shoes and didn't feel any smarter; in fact, many thought we looked even dumber. Secondly, just because two variables are related does not mean that one causes the other. For example, there is a strong and positive correlation between the crime rate and the number of churches. Would one conclude that churches cause crime? Or, that crime causes churches? In this situation, the obvious underlying factor that contributes both to the number of crimes and the number of churches is the size of the population.

Correlationally yours,
PRM

In chapter 6 we promised that after we had presented some basic information to help you understand statistical techniques we would begin to explain in detail some specific techniques. We begin with correlation.

Correlation is a statistical technique used to determine the relationship between two or more variables. This chapter briefly discusses several types of correlation, the reliability and meaningfulness of correlation coefficients, and the use of correlation for predictions, including partial and semipartial correlations and multiple regression equations.

What Correlational Research Investigates

Often a researcher is interested in the degree of relationship between, or correlation of, performances such as the relationship between performances on a distance run and a **step test** as measures of cardiovascular fitness. Sometimes an investigator wishes to establish the relationship between traits and behavior, such as how personality characteristics relate to participation in high-risk recreational activities. Still other correlational research problems might involve relationships between anthropometric measurements such as skinfold thicknesses and percent fat as determined by underwater weighing. Here, the researcher may wish to predict percent fat from the skinfold measurements.

Correlation may involve two variables, such as the relationship between height and weight. It may involve three or more variables, as when one investigates the relationship between a criterion (dependent variable) such as cardiovascular fitness and two or more predictor variables (independent variables) such as body weight, percent fat, speed, muscular endurance, and so on. This is multiple correlation. Another technique, canonical correlation (discussed in chapter 9), studies the relationships between two or more dependent variables and two or more independent variables.

Understanding the Nature of Correlation

Positive Correlation

Negative Correlation

Correlation and Causation

Pearson Product Moment Correlation

The **coefficient of correlation** is a quantitative value of the relationship between two or more variables. The correlation coefficient can range from 0.00 to 1.00 in either a positive or negative direction. Thus, perfect correlation is 1.00 (either + 1.00 or − 1.00), and no relationship is 0.00.

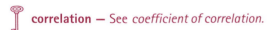

correlation — See *coefficient of correlation*.

step test — Test used to measure cardiorespiratory fitness involving the measurement of pulse rate after stepping up and down on a bench.

coefficient of correlation — A quantitative value of the relationship between two or more variables that can range from 0.00 to 1.00 in either a positive or negative direction; also called *correlation*.

Positive Correlation

 A **positive correlation** exists when a small amount of one variable is associated with a small amount of another variable and a large amount of one variable is associated with a large amount of another. Strength and body weight are positively correlated in that heavier persons are generally stronger than lighter persons. (The correlation is not perfect because some lighter people are stronger than some heavier people and weaker than some who weigh even less.)

Figure 7.1 is a graphic illustration of a perfect positive correlation. Notice that Tom's body weight is 1 s above the mean, for he weighs 110 lb, and the mean is 90. Thus, he is 20 lb heavier than the mean, which is 1 s (s = 20). His strength score is 250 lb, which is 50 lb higher than the mean of 200. Because the standard deviation is 50, he is 1 s above the mean on strength, just as he was on body weight. A second boy, Bill, is 1 s below the mean on weight and 1 s below on strength. A third boy is exactly at the mean on both variables (he weighs 90 lb and has a strength score of 200). Joe is .50 s above and Dick is .50 s below the means for weight and strength. Thus, when the scores are plotted, they form a perfectly straight diagonal line. This is perfect correlation (r = 1.00). The relative positions of the boys' pairs of scores are identical in the two distributions. In other words, each boy is the same relative distance from the mean of each set of scores. Common sense tells us that perfect correlation does not exist in human traits, abilities, and performances because of so-called people variability and other influences.

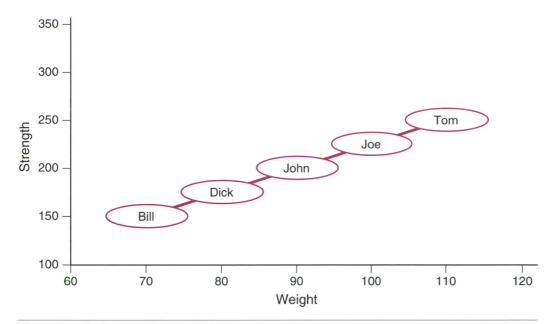

Figure 7.1   Perfect positive correlation.

Figure 7.2 illustrates a more realistic relationship between body weight and strength (r = .67). (Fictional examples have been used for purposes of presentation in this and other chapters. These examples do not represent actual data.) When these 10 sets of body weights and strength scores are plotted, they no longer constitute a straight line but do form a diagonal plot in the same lower-left-to-upper-right pattern as in Figure 7.1.

positive correlation — When a small amount of one variable is associated with a small amount of another variable, and a large amount of one variable is associated with a large amount of the other.

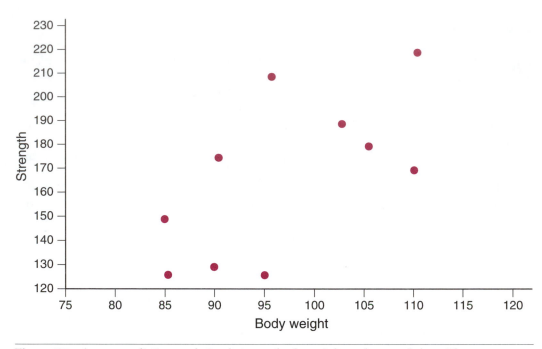

Figure 7.2   A more realistic correlation between body weight and strength (*r* = .67).

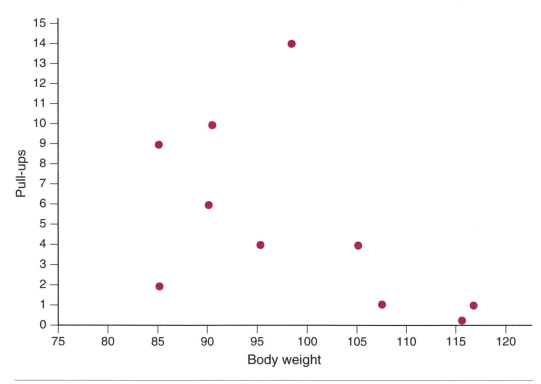

Figure 7.3   Negative correlation between body weight and pull-ups (*r* = −.54).

Negative Correlation

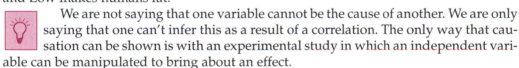

Next, in Figure 7.3, let us plot the body weights and pull-up scores for the same 10 boys. A pull-up is performed by hoisting one's body weight from a hanging position until the chin is above the bar. For this test, body weight is somewhat of a liability, often indicating that heavier persons tend to do fewer pull-ups than do lighter persons. As a result, a small number of pull-ups is associated with larger body weights and, conversely, a greater number of pull-ups with lesser body weights. This is a **negative correlation** A perfect negative correlation would be a straight diagonal line at a 45-degree angle (the upper left corner of the graph to the lower right corner). Figure 7.3 depicts a negative correlation but of a moderate degree ($r = -.54$). However, an upper-left-to-lower-right pattern is still apparent.

When virtually no relationship exists between variables, the correlation is 0.00. This denotes independence between sets of scores. The plotted scores exhibit no discernible pattern at all. The interpretation of correlations as to their reliability and meaningfulness is explained later.

Correlation and Causation

At this point we must stress again that a correlation between two variables does not mean that one variable causes the other. In chapter 4 we used an example of a research hypothesis (albeit a dumb one) that achievement in math could be improved by buying a child larger shoes. This hypothesis resulted from a correlation between math achievement scores and shoe size (with age not being controlled). This example helps to drive home the point that correlation does not mean causation.

In Ziv's 1988 study on the effectiveness of teaching and learning with humor, the experimental group subjects were told a story to illustrate the fact that correlations do not show a causal effect. In the story, aliens from another planet, who were invisible to earthlings, decided to study the differences between fat and thin people. One alien observed the coffee drinking behavior of fat and thin people at a cafeteria over an extended period. The alien then analyzed the observations statistically and decided that there was a correlation between coffee drinking behavior and body weight. Thin people tended to drink their coffee with sugar, whereas fat people mostly drank theirs with Sweet and Low. The alien concluded from this study that sugar makes humans thin, whereas Sweet and Low makes humans fat.

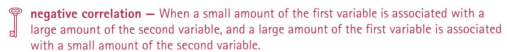

We are not saying that one variable cannot be the cause of another. We are only saying that one can't infer this as a result of a correlation. The only way that causation can be shown is with an experimental study in which an independent variable can be manipulated to bring about an effect.

Pearson Product Moment Correlation

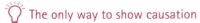

Several times in the preceding discussion we have used the symbol r. This symbol denotes the **Pearson product moment coefficient of correlation** In this type of correlation, there is one criterion (or dependent) variable and one predictor (or independent) variable. Thus, every subject has two scores, such as body weight and strength.

---

negative correlation — When a small amount of the first variable is associated with a large amount of the second variable, and a large amount of the first variable is associated with a small amount of the second variable.

The only way to show causation

Pearson product moment coefficient of correlation — The most commonly used method of computing correlation between two variables; also called *interclass* or *Pearson* r.

The computation of the correlation coefficient involves the relative distances of the scores from the two means of the distributions. The computations can be accomplished with a number of different formulas; we will present just one. This formula is sometimes called the computer method because it involves operations similar to those performed by a computer. The formula appears large and imposing but actually consists of only three operations:

1. summing each set of scores,
2. squaring and summing each set of scores, and
3. multiplying each pair of scores and obtaining the cumulative sum of these products.

The formula is

$$r = \frac{N\Sigma XY - (\Sigma X)(\Sigma Y)}{\sqrt{N\Sigma X^2 - (\Sigma X)^2} \ \sqrt{N\Sigma Y^2 - (\Sigma Y)^2}} \tag{7.1}$$

To illustrate the calculations involved, we use the body weight and pull-up scores from Figure 7.3 and designate body weight as the X variable. In a correlation problem that simply determines the relationship between two variables, it does not matter which one is X and which is Y. If the investigator wants to predict one score from the other, then Y designates the criterion (dependent) variable (that which is being predicted) and X the predictor (independent) variable. In this example, pull-up performance would be predicted from body weight, as it would not make much sense to predict body weight from pull-up scores. Prediction equations are discussed later in this section.

The computations for the correlation between body weight and pull-ups are shown in Example 7.1. Note that N refers to the number of paired scores, not the total number of scores.

Example 7.1

Known Values

Body weight X	X^2	Number of pull-ups Y	Y^2	Body weight × pull-ups XY
104	10,816	4	16	416
86	7,396	2	4	172
92	8,464	6	36	552
112	12,544	1	1	112
96	9,216	4	16	384
98	9,604	13	169	1,274
110	12,100	0	0	0
86	7,396	9	81	774
105	11,025	1	1	105
91	8,281	10	100	910

Three steps in calculating Pearson r.

Number of paired scores: $N = 10$
Sum of body weight scores: $\Sigma X = 980$
Sum of pull-up scores: $\Sigma Y = 50$
Sum of body weight scores squared: $\Sigma X^2 = 96,842$
Sum of pull-ups squared: $\Sigma Y^2 = 424$
Sum of body weight $\times$ pull-ups: $\Sigma XY = 4,699$

Working It Out
(Equation 7.1)

$$r = \frac{(10)\,4,699 - (980)\,(50)}{\sqrt{10(96,842) - (980)^2}\ \ \sqrt{10(424) - (50)^2}}$$

$$r = \frac{46,990 - 49,000}{\sqrt{968,420 - 960,400}\ \ \sqrt{4,240 - 2,500}}$$

$$r = \frac{-2,010}{\sqrt{8,020}\ \ \sqrt{1,740}}$$

$$r = \frac{-2,010}{(89.6)\,(41.7)} = \frac{-2,010}{3,736.3} = -.54$$

For the $(\Sigma X)^2$ and the $(\Sigma Y)^2$ values, the sums of the raw scores for X and Y are then squared. Notice that these values are not the same as the ΣX^2 and ΣY^2 values. The ΣXY (the sum of the cross products of the X and Y scores) determines the direction of the correlation as to whether it is positive or negative. In this example, a negative correlation was obtained because the first half of the numerator ($N\Sigma XY$) was smaller than the second half ($\Sigma X)(\Sigma Y$).

The negative correlation between body weight and pull-ups means that as body weight increased, pull-up performance decreased. Sometimes a negative correlation coefficient results when the relationship is really positive. Confusing? The following examples should clarify the meaning. Suppose we were to correlate scores on the vertical jump and the 40-yard dash. Both performances are related to explosive power. Persons who score well on the vertical jump should also do well on the 40-yard dash because the two tests are measuring much the same thing; thus, the relationship between performances is positive. However, the vertical jump is scored in inches (or centimeters), where a high score is good, and the 40-yard dash is scored in seconds, where a low number (fewer seconds) is good. Therefore, the correlation coefficient would be negative.

The correlation between the distance a person could run in 12 minutes and heart rate after exercise would also be negative. This is because a greater distance covered is good and because a lower heart rate after exercise is good. A person who has good cardiovascular endurance would have a high score on one test (the run) and a low score on the other.

What the Coefficient of Correlation Means

Interpreting Reliability of r

Interpreting Meaningfulness of r

Z Transformation of r

So far we have dealt with the nature of correlation as to direction (positive or negative) and the calculation of r. An obvious question that arises is, What does a coefficient of correlation mean in terms of being high or low, satisfactory or unsatisfactory? This seemingly simple question is not so simple to answer.

Interpreting Reliability of r

 First, there are several ways of interpreting r. One criterion is its reliability, or **significance**. Does it represent a real relationship? That is, if the study were repeated, what is the probability of getting a similar relationship? For this statistical criterion of significance, simply consult a table. In using the table, select the desired level of significance, such as the .05 level, and then enter the table in accordance with the appropriate degrees of freedom (*df*) (*df* are based on the number of subjects corrected for sample bias), which, for r, is equal to $N - 2$. Table A.3 in Appendix A contains the necessary correlation coefficients for significance at the .05 and .01 levels. Refer to the example of the correlation between body weight and pull-ups ($r = -.54$). The degrees of freedom are $N - 2 = 10 - 2 = 8$ (remember, the variable N in correlation refers to the number of pairs of scores). When entering the table at 8 *df*, we see that a correlation of .632 is necessary for significance of a two-tailed test at the .05 level (and .765 at the .01 level). Therefore, we would have to conclude that our correlation of $-.54$ is not significant. (We will explain how to know whether to find the correlation values under the column for a one-tailed or two-tailed test in the section on interpreting t in chapter 8.)

Another glance at Table A.3 reveals a couple of obvious facts. The correlation needed for significance decreases with increased numbers of subjects (*df*). In our example, we had only 10 subjects (or pairs of scores). However, if four more boys had been in the sample ($N = 14$), then there would be 12 *df*, and the correlation required for significance at the .05 level for 12 *df* would be .532. Our correlation of $-.54$ meets that test of significance. Notice, however, that very low correlation coefficients can be significant if you have a large sample of subjects. At the .05 level, a correlation of .38 is significant with 25 *df*, $r = .27$ is significant with 50 *df*, and .195 is significant with 100 *df*. In fact, with 1,000 *df*, a correlation of .08 is significant at the .01 level.

The second observation noted from the table is that a higher correlation is required for significance at the .01 level than at the .05 level. This should make sense. Remember, chapter 6 stated that the .05 level means that if 100 experiments were conducted, the null hypothesis (that there is no relationship) would be rejected incorrectly, just by chance, on 5 of the 100 occasions. At the .01 level, we would expect a relationship of this magnitude less than once in 100 experiments due to chance. Therefore, the test of significance at the .01 level is more stringent than at the .05 level, and so a higher correlation is required for significance at the .01 level.

Interpreting Meaningfulness of r

The interpretation of a correlation for statistical significance is important, but, because of the vast influence of sample size, this criterion is not always meaningful. As chapter 6 explained, statistics can answer two questions about data: Are the effects reliable? Are they meaningful?

 The most commonly used criterion for interpreting the correlation coefficient as to meaningfulness is the **coefficient of determination** (r^2). In this method, the portion of common association of the factors that influence the two variables is

 significance — The reliability of or confidence in a statistic as to its likelihood of occurring again if the study were repeated.

coefficient of determination — The squared correlation coefficient; used in interpreting meaningfulness of correlations.

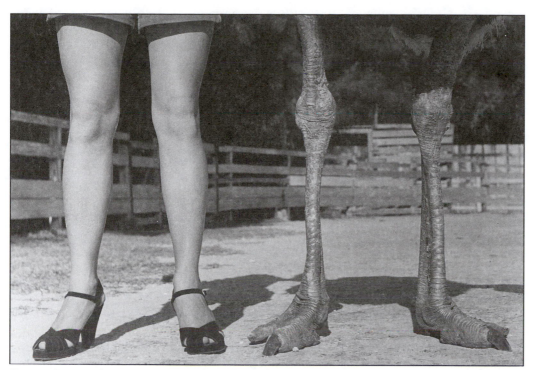

Comparison and contrast are used to determine whether groups share common traits.

determined. In other words, the coefficient of determination indicates the portion of the total variance in one measure that can be explained, or accounted for, by the variance in the other measure.

For example, the standing long jump and the vertical jump are common tests of explosive power. The tests are so commonly used that we tend to think of them as interchangeable, that is, as measuring the same thing. Yet correlations between the two tests usually range between .70 and .80. Hence, the coefficients of determination range from .49 ($.70^2$) to .64 ($.80^2$). Usually, the coefficient of determination is multiplied by 100 and then expressed as percent of variation. Thus, $.70^2 = .49 \times 100 = 49\%$ and $.80^2 = .64 \times 100 = 64\%$.

For a correlation of .70 between the standing long jump and the vertical jump, only about half (49%) of the variance (or influences) in one test is associated with the other. Both tests involve explosive force of the legs with some flexing and extending of the trunk and swinging of the arms. Both are influenced by body weight in that the subject must propel his or her body through space, both involve the ability to prepare psychologically and physiologically to generate explosive force, both involve **relative strength**, and so on. These are factors held in common in the two tests. If $r = .80$, then 64% of the performance in one test is associated with, or explained by, the factors involved in the performance of the other test.

But what about the unexplained variance ($1.0 - r^2$)? With a correlation of .70, there is 49% common (explained) variance and 51% [$(1.00 - .70^2)100$] error (unexplained) variance. What are some unique factors to each test? We cannot explain this fully, but some of the factors could be that (a) the standing long jump requires that the body be propelled forward and upward, whereas the vertical jump is only upward; (b) the scoring of the vertical jump neutralizes one's height because standing reach is subtracted from jumping reach (but in the standing long jump perhaps the taller

relative strength — The measure of the ability to exert maximum force in relation to a person's size.

person has some advantage); and (c) that perhaps more skill (coordination) is involved in the vertical jump because the person must jump and turn and then touch the wall.

The foregoing is not intended to be any sort of mechanical analysis of the two tests. These are simply suggestions of what might be some factors of common association, or explained variance, and some factors that might be unexplained or unique to each test of explosive power.

When we use the coefficient of determination to interpret correlation coefficients, it becomes apparent that a rather substantial relationship is needed to account for a great amount of common variance. It takes a correlation of .71 to account for just half the variance in the other test, and a correlation of .90 accounts for only 81%. In some of the standardized tests used to predict success, correlations are generally quite low, often around .40. You can see by the coefficient of determination that a correlation of .40 accounts for only 16% of the factors contributing to academic success; therefore, there is a great deal of unexplained variance. Still, these measures are often used very rigorously as the criterion for admission to academic programs. Of course, the use of multiple predictors can greatly improve the estimate for success. The comparative sizes of correlations by means of the coefficient of determination can also be observed. A correlation of .90 is not simply three times larger than a correlation of .30; it is nine times larger ($.30^2 = .09$, or 9%, and $.90^2 = .81$, or 81%).

Interpreting the correlation coefficient is further complicated by the fact that it depends on the purpose of the correlation with regard to whether correlation is "good" or "inadequate." For example, if we are looking at the reliability (repeatability) of a test, a much higher correlation is needed than if we are determining simply whether there is a relationship between two variables. A correlation of .60 would not be acceptable for the relationship between two similar versions of an exercise knowledge test, but a correlation of .60 between exercise knowledge and exercise behavior would be quite noteworthy.

Z Transformation of r

Occasionally, a researcher wants to determine the average of two or more correlations. It is statistically unsound to try to average the coefficients themselves because the sampling distribution of coefficients of correlation is not normally distributed. In fact, the higher the correlation, in either a positive or a negative direction, the more skewed the distribution becomes. The most satisfactory method of approximating normality of a sampling distribution of linear relationships is by transforming coefficients of correlation to Z values. This is often called the **Fisher Z transformation**. (This Z should not be confused with the z used to refer to the height of the ordinate in the area of the normal curve.)

The transformation procedure involves the use of natural logarithms. However, we need not use Fisher's formula to calculate the transformations (these conversions have been done for us in Table A.4). We simply consult the table and locate the corresponding Z value for any particular correlation coefficient.

Suppose, for example, that we obtained correlations between maximal oxygen consumption and a distance run (e.g., an 8-min run-walk) on four groups of subjects of different ages. We would like to combine these sample correlations to obtain a valid and reliable estimate of the relationship between these two measures of cardiorespiratory endurance. The data for the following steps are shown in Table 7.1.

Fisher Z transformation — Method of approximating normality of a sampling distribution of linear relationship by transforming coefficients of correlation to Z-values.

Table 7.1   Average of Correlation Coefficients by Use of the *Z* Transformation

Age-group	N	r	Z	N–3	Weighted Z
13–14	30	.69	.85	27	22.95
15–16	44	.85	1.26	41	51.66
17–18	38	.70	.87	35	30.45
19–20	35	.77	1.02	32	32.64
				135	137.70

1. First, convert each correlation to a *Z* value using Table A.4. For example, the correlation of .69 for the 13- and 14-year-olds has a corresponding *Z* value of .85, the next correlation of .85 for the 15- and 16-year-olds has a *Z* value of 1.26, and so on.

2. The *Z* values are then weighted by multiplying them by the degrees of freedom for each sample, which in this process is $N - 3$. So, in the 13- and 14-year-olds, the *Z* value of .85 is multiplied by 27 for a weighted *Z* value of 22.95. We do the same for the other three samples.

3. The weighted *Z* values are summed, and the mean weighted *Z* value is calculated by dividing by the total sample $(N - 3)$: $137.7/135 = 1.02$.

4. The mean weighted *Z* value is converted back to a mean correlation by consulting Table A.4 again. We see that the corresponding correlation for a *Z* value of 1.02 is .77.

Some authors declare that to average correlations by the Z-transformation technique you must first establish that there are no significant differences among the four correlations. A comparison for differences could be made using a chi-square test of the weighted *Z* values (chi-square is discussed in chapter 10). Other statisticians contend that averaging coefficients of correlation is permissible as long as the average correlation is not interpreted in terms of confidence intervals.

The *Z* transformation is also used for statistical tests (such as those for the significance of the correlation coefficient) and for determining the significance of the difference between two correlation coefficients. After reading chapter 8, you may wish to consult a statistics text, such as that by Mattson (1981), for further discussion on the use of the *Z* transformation for these procedures.

Using Correlation for Prediction

Working With Regression Equations
Calculating a Line of Best Fit

 Using *Z* values to compare correlations

 When to use the *Z*-transformation technique

 Mattson, D.E. (1981). *Statistics: Difficult concepts, understandable explanations.* St. Louis: C.V. Mosby.

We have stated several times that one purpose of correlation may be prediction. College entrance examinations are used to predict success. Sometimes we try to predict a criterion such as percent fat by the use of skinfold measurements or maximal oxygen consumption by a distance run. In studies of this type, the predictor variables (skinfold measurements) are less time-consuming, less expensive, and more feasible for mass testing than the criterion variable; thus, a **prediction**, or **regression**, **equation** is developed.

Prediction is based on correlation. The higher the relationship between two variables, the more accurately you can predict one from the other. If the correlation were perfect, you could predict with complete accuracy.

Working With Regression Equations

Of course, we do not encounter perfect relationships in the real world, but in introducing the concept of prediction (regression) equations, it is often advantageous to begin with a hypothetical example of a perfect relationship.

Verducci (1980) provided one of the best examples in introducing the regression equation concerning monthly salary and annual income. If there are no other sources of income, we can predict with complete accuracy the annual income of, for example, teachers simply by multiplying their monthly salaries by 12. Figure 7.4 illustrates this perfect relationship. By plotting the monthly salary (the X, or predictor,

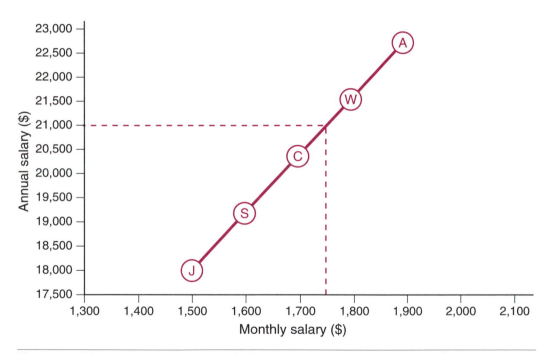

Figure 7.4   Plotting monthly and annual salaries with perfect r. *Note.* Letters refer to teachers' initials.

prediction equation — A formula to predict some criterion (e.g., some measure of performance) based on the relationship between the predictor variable(s) and the criterion; also called *regression equation.*

regression equation — See *prediction equation.*

abscissa — The horizontal, or x-, axis of a graph.

ordinate — The vertical, or y-, axis of a graph.

variable), the predicted annual income (the Y, or criterion, variable) can be obtained. Thus, if we know that another teacher (e.g., Ms. Brooks) earns a monthly salary of $1,750, we can easily plot this on the graph where $1,750 on the horizontal (x) axis (the **abscissa**) intercepts the vertical (y) axis (the **ordinate**) at $21,000. The equation for prediction ($\tilde{Y}$, predicted annual income) is thus $\tilde{Y} = 12X$. In the previous example, the teacher's monthly salary (X) is inserted in the formula: $\tilde{Y} = 12(1,750) = 21,000$.

Next, suppose that all teachers got an annual supplement of $1,000 for coaching or supervising cheerleaders or some other extracurricular activity. Now, the formula becomes $\tilde{Y} = 1,000 + 12X$. Ms. Brooks's annual income is predicted as follows: $\tilde{Y} = 1,000 + 12(1,750) = 22,000$. All teachers' annual incomes could be predicted in the same manner. This formula is the general formula for a straight line and is expressed as follows:

$$\tilde{Y} = a + bX \tag{7.2}$$

where $\tilde{Y}$ = the predicted score, or criterion; a = the intercept; b = the slope of the regression line; and X = the predictor.

In this example, the b factor was ascertained by common sense because we know that there are 12 months in a year. The slope of the line (b) signifies the amount of change in $\tilde{Y}$ that accompanies a change of 1 unit of X. Therefore, any X unit (monthly salary) is multiplied by 12 to obtain the $\tilde{Y}$ value. In actual regression problems we will not intuitively know what b is, so we must calculate it by this formula:

$$b = r(s_y/s_x) \tag{7.3}$$

where r = the correlation between X and Y, s_y = the standard deviation of Y, and s_x = the standard deviation of X.

In our previous example, application of Formula 7.3 uses these data:

$X =$	(monthly salary)	$Y =$	(annual income)
$M_x=$	1,700	$M_y=$	21,400 (1,000 added—Figure 7.4)
$s_x=$	141.42	$s_y=$	1,697.06
	$r = 1.00$		

Therefore, the computation of b is $b = 1.00(1,697.06/141.42) = 12$. The a in the regression formula indicates the intercept of the regression line on the y-axis. In other words, a is the value of $\tilde{Y}$ when X is zero. On a graph, if you extend the regression line sufficiently, you can see where the regression line intercepts $\tilde{Y}$. The a is a constant because it is added to each of the calculated bX values. Once again, in our example we know that this constant is 1,000. In other words, this is the value of $\tilde{Y}$ even if there were no monthly salary (X). But to calculate the a value, you must first calculate b. Then use the following formula:

$$a = M_y - bM_x \tag{7.4}$$

where a = the constant (or intercept), M_y = the mean of the Y scores, b = the slope of the regression line, and M_x = the mean of the X scores. In our example, $a = 21,400 - 12(1,700) = 1,000$. Then the final regression equation is $\tilde{Y} = a + bX$, or $\tilde{Y} = 1,000 + 12X$.

Next, let us use a more practical example in which the correlation is not 1.00. We can use the data from Figure 7.2, where the correlation between body weight and dynamometer strength was .67. The means and standard deviations are as follows:

X (body weight)	Y (strength)
$M_x = 98.00$	$M_y = 167.00$
$s_x = 9.44$	$s_y = 33.52$
	$r = .67$

First, we calculate b as follows from Formula 7.3:

$$b = r\left(\frac{s_y}{s_x}\right) = .67\left(\frac{33.52}{9.44}\right) = 2.38$$

Then, a is calculated as follows from Formula 7.4:

$$a = M_y - b(M_x) = 167 - 2.38(98) = -66.24$$

The regression equation (Formula 7.2) becomes

$$\tilde{Y} = a + bX$$

so

$$\tilde{Y} = -66.24 + (2.38)X$$

For any body weight, we can calculate the predicted strength score. For example, a boy weighing 100 lb (X) would have a predicted strength score ($\tilde{Y}$) of $\tilde{Y} = -66.24 + (2.38)100 = 171.8$ The main difference between this example and that of monthly and annual salaries is that there was no error of prediction in the latter because the correlation was 1.00. When we predicted strength from body weight, however, the correlation was less than 1.00, so there is an error of prediction.

Calculating a Line of Best Fit

Before presenting the formula for calculating error of prediction, let us return to the derivation of the prediction formula. Figure 7.2 shows that there was no straight line connecting the weight and strength scores as there was in the hypothetical example in Figure 7.1. Consequently, we calculate a **line of best fit** to predict $\tilde{Y}$ from the X scores. To do this, we take a high X score (body weight) such as 110 and a low body weight such as 91 and apply the prediction formula. For a body weight of 110, we predict $\tilde{Y} = -66.24 + (2.38)110 = 195.6$. For a body weight of 91, we predict $\tilde{Y} = -66.24 + (2.38)91 = 150.3$.

Then we plot these two predicted values and connect them with a straight line. This line passes through the intersection of the X and Y means. Figure 7.5 shows this line of best fit. The 10 actual body weight and strength scores are also plotted. You can readily see that the scores do not fall on the straight line as they did with perfect correlation.

In constructing this line of best fit, we selected a high body weight (110) and a low body weight (91) and predicted their $\tilde{Y}$ values. When we examine their actual $\tilde{Y}$ values, we see there is some error in prediction. The predicted strength score for the 110-lb boy was 195.6, yet the boy actually scored only 170, a difference of –25.6. The 91-lb boy was predicted to score 150.3 on the dynamometer, yet he scored 175, a difference of +24.7. These differences between predicted and actual Y scores represent the errors of prediction and are called **residual scores** . If we computed all the residual scores, the mean would be zero and the standard deviation is the **standard error of prediction** , or **standard error of estimate** $(s_{y \cdot x})$.

---

line of best fit — The calculated regression line which results in the smallest sum of squares of the vertical distances of every point from the line.

residual score — The difference between the predicted and actual scores that represents the error of prediction.

standard error of prediction — The computation of the standard deviation of all of the residual scores of a population; the amount of error expected in a prediction; also called *standard error of estimate*.

standard error of estimate — See *standard error of prediction*.

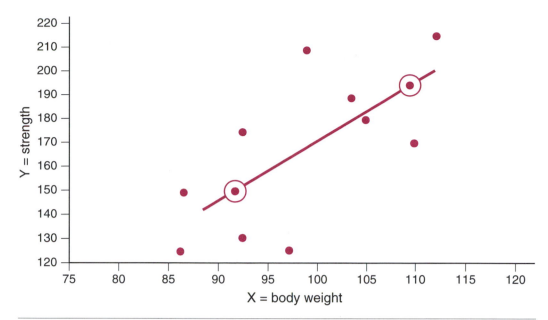

Figure 7.5   Regression line of best fit between body weight and predicted strength scores.

A simpler way of obtaining the standard error of estimate is to use the formula

$$s_{y \cdot x} = s_y \sqrt{1 - r^2}$$
$$= 33.5 \sqrt{1 - .67^2}$$
$$= 24.9 \tag{7.5}$$

The standard error of estimate is interpreted the same way as the standard deviation. In other words, the predicted value (strength) of a boy in our example, plus or minus the standard error of estimate, will occur approximately 68 times out of 100. Thus, we predict that a 104-lb boy will score 181.3 ± 24.9. To express it another way, the "prediction range" will be between 156.4 and 206.2 lb 68 times out of 100 (or the chances are 2 in 3).

The larger the correlation, the smaller the error of prediction. Also, the smaller the standard deviation of the criterion, the smaller the error. In the previous problem, if we had a correlation of .85, for example, the standard error of estimate would be only

$$s_{y \cdot x} = 33.5 \sqrt{1 - .85^2} = 17.6$$

The line of best fit is sometimes called the least squares method. This means that the calculated regression line is one about which the sum of squares of the vertical distances of every point from the line is minimal. We will not develop this point here. Sum of squares is discussed in the next chapter.

Partial Correlation

The correlation between two variables is sometimes misleading and may be difficult to interpret when there is little or no correlation between the variables other than that caused by their common dependence on a third variable.

For example, many attributes increase regularly with age from 6 to 18 years, such as height, weight, strength, mental performance, vocabulary, reading skills, and so on. Over a wide age range, the correlation between any two of these measures will almost certainly be positive and will probably be high because of the common maturity factor with which they are highly correlated. In fact, the correlation may drop to zero if the variability caused by age differences is eliminated. We can control this factor of age in one of two ways. We can select only children of the same age, or we can partial out the effects of age statistically by holding it constant.

The symbol for partial correlation is $r_{12 \cdot 3}$, which means the correlation between variables 1 and 2 with variable 3 held constant (we could partial out any number of variables, e.g., $r_{12 \cdot 345}$). The calculation of partial correlation among three variables is quite simple. Let us refer back to the correlation of shoe size and achievement in mathematics. This is a good example of **spurious correlation**, which means that the correlation between the two variables is due to the common influence of another variable (age or maturing). When the effect of the third variable (age) is removed, the correlation between shoe size and achievement in mathematics diminishes or vanishes completely. We label the three variables as follows: 1 = math achievement, 2 = shoe size, and 3 = age. Then, $r_{12 \cdot 3}$ is the partial correlation between variables 1 and 2 with 3 held constant. We can make up some correlation coefficients between the three variables: $r_{12} = .80$; $r_{13} = .90$; and $r_{23} = .88$.

The formula for $r_{12 \cdot 3}$ is

$$
\begin{aligned}
r_{12 \cdot 3} &= \frac{r_{12} - r_{13}r_{23}}{\sqrt{1 - r_{13}^2}\ \sqrt{1 - r_{23}^2}} \\[2mm]
&= \frac{.80 - (.90 \times .88)}{\sqrt{1 - .90^2}\ \sqrt{1 - .88^2}} \\[2mm]
&= \frac{.80 - .792}{\sqrt{1 - .81}\ \sqrt{1 - .77}} \\[2mm]
&= .038
\end{aligned}
\tag{7.6}
$$

Thus, we see that correlation between math achievement and shoe size drops to about zero when age is partialed out.

The primary value of partial correlation is that it is used to develop a multiple regression equation with two or more predictor variables. In the selection process, when a new variable is "stepped in," its correlation with the criterion is determined with the effects of the preceding variable partialed out. The size and the sign of a partial correlation may be different from the zero-order (two-variable) correlation between the same variables.

Uses of Semipartial Correlation

In the previous section on partial correlation, the effects of a third variable on the relationship between two other variables were partialed out. In other words, in $r_{12 \cdot 3}$, the relationship of variable 3 to the correlation of variables 1 and 2 is partialed out. In some situations, the investigator may wish to partial out a variable from only one of the variables being correlated. This is called **semipartial correlation**. The symbol is $r_{1(2 \cdot 3)}$, which indicates that the relationship between variables 1 and 2 is determined after the influence of variable 3 on variable 2 has been partialed out.

spurious correlation — Relationship in which the correlation between two variables is due primarily to the common influence of another variable.

semipartial correlation — A technique in which one variable is partialed out from just one of two variables in a correlation.

Suppose, for example, that a researcher is studying the relationship between perceived exertion (i.e., one's feelings of how hard he or she is working) and heart rate (HR) and work load (WL). Obviously, WL is going to be correlated with HR. The researcher wants to investigate the relationship between perceived exertion (PE) and HR while controlling for WL. Regular partial correlation will show this relationship. However, regular partial correlation will partial out the effects of WL on the relationship between PE and HR. But the researcher does not want to remove the effects of WL on the relationship of PE and HR; rather, he or she wants only to remove the effects of WL on HR. In other words, the main interest is in the net effect of HR on PE after the influence of WL has been removed. Thus, in semipartial correlation, WL is partialed out from HR but not from PE. The uses of semipartial correlation are discussed further in chapter 9.

Procedures for Multiple Regression

Forward Selection Multiple Regression

Backward Selection Multiple Regression

Maximum *R*-Squared Method

Stepwise Regression Procedure

Multiple Regression Prediction Equations

Some Problems Associated With Multiple Regression

Multiple regression consists of one dependent variable (usually a criterion of some sort) and two or more predictor variables (independent variables). The use of more than one predictor variable usually increases the accuracy of prediction. This should be self-evident. If you wished to predict basketball-playing ability, you would expect to get a more accurate prediction by using several basketball skills tests rather than by using only one.

The multiple correlation coefficient (R) indicates the relationship between the criterion and a weighted sum of the predictor variables. It follows then that R^2 represents the amount of the variance of the criterion that is explained or accounted for by the combined predictors. This is the same concept as coefficient of determination (r^2), which was discussed earlier with regard to the common association between two variables. Now, however, we have the amount of association between one variable (the criterion) and a weighted combination of variables.

We wish to find the best combination of variables that will give the most accurate prediction of the criterion. Therefore, we are interested in knowing how much each of the predictors contributes to the total explained variance. Another way to say this is that we want to find the variables that will best reduce the prediction errors. From a practical standpoint, in terms of time and effort involved in obtaining measures

multiple regression — Model used for predicting a criterion from two or more independent, or predictor, variables.

Cohen, J., & Cohen, P. (1983). *Applied multiple regression in behavioral research*. New York: Holt, Rinehart & Winston.

Pedhazur, E.J. (1982). *Multiple regression in behavioral research*. New York: Holt, Rinehart & Winston.

of the predictor variables, it is desirable to find the fewest number of predictors that will account for most of the variance of the criterion. There are several selection procedures used for this purpose. (For additional information on multiple regression, see Cohen & Cohen [1983], and Pedhazur [1982].)

Forward Selection Multiple Regression

In the **forward selection** method, a new predictor variable is added at each step. The first variable selected is the one that has the highest correlation with the criterion. Then, at each subsequent step, a variable is added that, with the one or more already chosen, results in the best prediction. (It is difficult to explain these methods without using terms with which you are probably not yet familiar.) The variables selected cumulatively produce the least residual sum of squares, meaning the residual sum of squares constitutes error. Recall from our discussion of linear regression with two variables that the differences between predicted and actual scores are termed residual scores.

Sometimes the researcher will set a probability level for entry, such as .05 or .01. In this way, variables are stepped in until they no longer significantly increase the prediction of the criterion. When there are a number of predictor variables, there is usually some degree of **overlap**, or redundancy. This means that predictor variables are related to each other. Some variables may be measuring the same thing, so if we have two such variables, the inclusion of both is no better than using just one.

Another important concept is that, after the first step, the selection of additional variables is determined by the combined effect, not only the additive effect. In other words, the process takes into account the interrelationship among the X variables. If there were no relationships among the X variables, prediction could be made simply in an additive fashion, but, of course, this is never the case. After each X variable is stepped in, the process identifies which one of the remaining predictor variables will account for the largest amount of the unexplained variance. Thus, in forward selection multiple regression, variables are stepped in as to their importance, and the process stops when there is no further significant contribution to the prediction.

Backward Selection Multiple Regression

In the **backward selection** procedure, the independent variables (Xs) are eliminated in respect to their lack of importance; that is, you begin with all the independent variables and drop out those variables that do not significantly contribute to the prediction of the criterion. Once again, you usually set a significance level, and those variables that do not meet this level, insofar as they are included in the linear composite of predictor variables, are dropped. In most cases (but not always), you end up with the same battery of important predictor variables with the backward selection method as you did with the forward method.

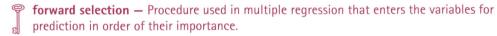

forward selection — Procedure used in multiple regression that enters the variables for prediction in order of their importance.

overlap — The use of two variables that measure the same thing, so that the inclusion of both is no more beneficial than the use of only one.

backward selection — Procedure used in multiple regression in which all the variables are entered, then those that contribute least to predicting the criterion are sequentially removed.

Maximum *R*-Squared Method

In the **maximum *R*-squared (*R*²) method**, the so-called best of all possible one-variable models is selected, as is the best two-variable model, the best three-variable model, and so on. The term "best" relates to the size of the *R*-squared value.

As explained in an earlier discussion of the coefficient of determination (r^2), squaring *r* (in this case, *R*) can estimate the degree of meaningfulness in terms of the amount of common association (or amount of variance held in common) between the dependent and the independent variables. The maximum *R*-squared method continues until the full model is included. However, the researcher usually sets some criterion as to when to stop. It may be a level of significance or a measure of meaningfulness, such as the amount of variance accounted for (see chapter 8). Usually, it is a combination of significance and meaningfulness. The researcher also may incorporate some practical criteria in the selection process, such as amount of time and effort involved in obtaining the measurements for the different-size models (as in test batteries).

Stepwise Regression Procedure

The **stepwise regression method** is a variation of the forward technique except that each time a new predictor variable is stepped in, the new relationship between the criterion and the predictor variables is reevaluated to see whether the predictor variables already selected still significantly contribute when variables are added later. It is possible, then, that a predictor entered earlier may be dropped out later when new predictors are brought into the equation. In most cases, however, the stepwise method is identical to the forward selection method.

Multiple Regression Prediction Equations

The prediction equation resulting from multiple regression is basically that of the two-variable regression model, $\tilde{Y} = a + bX$. The only difference is that there is more than one *X* variable; thus, the equation is

$$\tilde{Y} = a + b_1X_1 + b_2X_2 + ... + b_iX_i$$

We will not delve into the formula for the calculation of the *a* and the *b*s for the selected variables. As we have said before, a researcher will undoubtedly use a computer in a multiple regression problem. An example of a multiple prediction formula follows. In this equation, a man's lean body weight (LBW) is being predicted from several anthropometric measures, including skinfold thicknesses, circumferences, and diameters. The following formula, developed by Behnke and Wilmore (1974), has a correlation of .958 and a standard error of estimate of 2.358, which is interpreted just the same as in the regression equation with only one predictor variable.

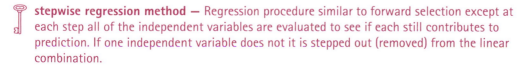

maximum R² method — A multiple regression method in which the so-called best of all possible one-variable models is selected, as is the best two-variable model, the best three-variable model, and so on until a predetermined criterion that ends the calculations is reached.

stepwise regression method — Regression procedure similar to forward selection except at each step all of the independent variables are evaluated to see if each still contributes to prediction. If one independent variable does not it is stepped out (removed) from the linear combination.

$$LBW = 10.138 + 0.9259 \text{ (wt)} - 0.1881 \text{ (thigh skinfold)} + 0.637 \text{ (bi-iliac diameter)} +$$
$$0.4888 \text{ (neck circumference)} - 0.5951 \text{ (abdominal circumference)}$$

Some Problems Associated With Multiple Regression

The basic determiner in multiple regression is the same as it is in regression with only two variables: the size of the correlation. The higher the correlation, the more accurate the prediction will be. However, some other factors should be mentioned.

 One limitation of prediction relates to generalizability. Regression equations developed with a particular sample often lose considerable accuracy when applied to others. This loss of accuracy in prediction is called **shrinkage**. The term **population specificity** also relates to this phenomenon. Shrinkage and the use of cross-validation to improve generalizability are further discussed in chapter 11. Thus, we need to recognize that the more accuracy one seeks through selection procedures (forward, backward, stepwise, maximum R-squared) that capitalize on specific characteristics of the sample, the more difficult it is to generalize to other populations. For example, a formula for predicting percent body fat from skinfold measurements that was developed with adult males would lose a great deal of accuracy if one tried to use it on adolescents. Thus, the researcher should select the sample carefully with regard to the population for which the results are to be generalized.

In prediction studies the number of subjects in the sample should be sufficiently large. Usually, the larger the sample, the more likely that the sample will represent the population from which it is drawn. However, another problem with small samples in multiple regression studies is that the correlation may be spuriously high. A direct relationship exists between the correlation and the ratio between the number of subjects and the number of variables. In fact, the degree to which the expected value of R^2 will exceed zero when it is zero in the population is dependent on two things: the size of the sample (n) and the number of variables (k). More precisely, it is the ratio of $k-1/n-1$. To illustrate, suppose you read a study in which the $R^2 = .90$. Impressive, right? However, the results would be meaningless if the study only had 40 subjects and 30 variables, because we could expect an R^2 of .74 just on the basis of chance alone ($R^2 = k-1/n-1 = 30-1/40-1 = .74$). One should be aware of this relationship between number of subjects and number of variables when reading research that uses multiple regression. In the most extreme degree you can see that with the same number of variables as subjects, $k-1/n-1$ would yield an R^2 of 1.00! A subject-to-variable ratio of 10:1 or higher is often recommended.

Methods of Association in Epidemiology Research

Epidemiology is a science that studies the frequencies and distributions of disease and health conditions among population groups. Examples of epidemiology research studies include the association between cardiovascular health and physical activity, the association between frequency and duration of running and running injuries, and the association between sedentary living and certain diseases. Comparison and contrast are used to determine whether groups of people who share a common characteristic (such as

shrinkage — Tendency for the validity to decrease when the prediction formula is used with a new sample.

population specificity — Phenomenon whereby a regression equation that was developed with a particular sample loses considerable accuracy when applied to others.

people who exercise) experience some condition (such as coronary heart disease) with the same frequency of occurrence as another group (such as sedentary people).

The rate of occurrence is the basic concept in epidemiology. The rate is the number of people with a problem divided by the population that is at risk for the problem. Two rates are commonly used: **incidence** and **prevalence**. Incidence rates refer to the number of new cases divided by the specified population during a certain period. For example, for 3 weeks researchers observed 300 people who lift weights for exercise. Nine persons were injured in the first week, 15 new injuries occurred in the second week, and 12 new injuries were reported in the third week. For simplicity, let us assume that all the weight lifters who were injured remained on the sidelines over the 3-week period. The incidence rate for the first week was 3% per week (9/300 × 100). For the second week, the denominator is 291 instead of 300 because nine people were not at risk for new injuries. So, the incidence rate for Week 2 is 5.2% (15/291 × 100). For the third week, the denominator is now 276 because 24 people (9 + 15) are not at risk for new injuries, so the incidence rate is 4.4% (12/276 × 100).

Prevalence rates are the total number of occurrences, new or old, that exist at a specified time. Prevalence and incidence are related in that Prevalence = Incidence × Duration. In this example, prevalence is directly related to the number of new injuries (incidence) and their duration. The prevalence for Week 1 is the same as the incidence (3%). At the end of Week 2, the prevalence is 8% because we include all the injured persons for the two weeks: 24/300 x 100 = 8%. Similarly, at the end of Week 3, the prevalence rate is 36 of 300 people (12%).

In epidemiological research, one must always be concerned with the size of the population being examined. To illustrate, suppose we place the 300 weight trainers into three categories based on how often they trained per month. Table 7.2 shows the number of persons injured in each category over the course of a year. If one just concentrates on the numbers of injuries, the most injuries occurred in the group that worked out the least. In fact, 50% (50/100 × 100) of all injuries came from this group, and the lowest number occurred in the group that worked out the most. However, in the third column we can see that there are considerably more people in this category (175). Now, when we look at the incidence of injuries over the year we see that the group who worked out the least had a lower incidence of injuries, 28.6% (50/175 × 100), and the group that worked out the most had the highest incidence (60%) of injuries.

As with all correlational data, one can't establish causation merely by finding association. However, experimental research studies (which can infer causation) are not feasible in most areas of concern in epidemiological research. Therefore, in the absence of experimental data, an attempt at inferring causation is made through the comparison of rates in different groups. Powell, Kohl, Caspersen, and Blair (1986) wrote an interesting paper using an epidemiological perspective.

Summary

We have explored some statistical techniques for determining relationships among variables. The simplest type of correlation is the zero-order correlation, which establishes

---

incidence — The number of new cases that occur in a particular population during a specified period of time.

prevalence — The total number of occurrences, both new and old, that exist at a particular time.

 Powell, K.E., Kohl, H.W., Caspersen, C.J., and Blair, S.N. (1986). An epidemiological perspective on the causes of running injuries. *The Physician and Sportsmedicine*, **14**(6).

Table 7.2   An Example of Epidemiological Data Showing Percentages and Incidences of Injuries to Persons Engaged in Weight Training

Workouts per month	Number of injuries	Number in category	Annual incidence of injuries
1-5	50	175	28.6
6-19	35	100	35.0
20-30	15	25	60.0
Total	100	300	33.3

the relationship between two variables. We introduced linear regression, which can be used to predict one variable from another. Correlation is interpreted for significance (reliability) and for meaningfulness (r^2), which indicates the portion of the total variance in one measure that can be explained or accounted for by the other measure.

Partial correlation is a procedure in which a correlation between two variables is obtained while the influence of one or more other variables is partialed out. Semipartial correlation partials out the influence of a third variable on only one of the two variables being correlated. Partial correlation (or semipartial correlation) is used in multiple correlation and in developing multiple regression formulas.

In multiple regression two or more predictor (independent) variables are used to predict the criterion variable. The most efficient weighted linear composite of predictor variables is determined through such techniques as forward selection, backward selection, stepwise selection, and maximum R-squared.

In epidemiological research there are methods of establishing association between the rates of occurrences of events such as disease or injuries and different population groups. The rate is the number of people with the condition divided by the population at risk for the condition. Incidence and prevalence are two kinds of rates that are frequently used.

 Check Your Understanding

1. What is the correlation (r) between fat deposits on two different body sites? Variable X is the triceps skinfold measure and variable Y the supra iliac skinfold measure.

X	Y
16	9
17	12
17	10
15	9
14	8
11	6
11	5
12	5
13	6
14	5
4	1

7	4
12	7
7	1
10	3

2. Using Table A.3, determine whether the correlation obtained in Problem 1 is significant at the .05 level. What size would the correlation need to be for significance at the .01 level if you had 30 subjects? What is the percent of common variance between the two skinfold measurements in Problem 1?

3. Compute the regression equation (Formula 7.2) for predicting maximal oxygen consumption ($\dot{V}O_2$max) from scores on the 12-min run. The information you need follows:

$$X \text{ (12-min run)} \qquad Y \text{ (}\dot{V}O_2\text{max)}$$
$$M_x = 3{,}120 \text{ yd} \qquad M_y = 52.6 \text{ ml} \bullet \text{kg} \bullet \text{min}^{-1}$$
$$s_x = 334 \text{ yd} \qquad s_y = 6.3 \text{ ml} \bullet \text{kg} \bullet \text{min}^{-1}$$
$$r = .79$$

4. Using the prediction formula developed in Problem 3, what is the predicted $\dot{V}O_2$max for a subject who ran 3,230 yd in 12 min? For a subject who ran 2,940 yd in 12 min?

5. What is the standard error of estimate (formula 7.5) for the prediction equation in Problem 3? How would you interpret the predicted $\dot{V}O_2$max for the subjects in Problem 4?

CHAPTER 8

Differences Among Groups

Dear Professors of Research Methods:

I had this really neat idea for an experiment, but when I shared it with my advisor, he said there were already several studies published on this topic. What should I do, and how can I come up with another idea?

Yours truly,
C. D. Problem

Dear Mr. Problem:

You have just encountered another version of Murphy's Law of Research.

1st Law: If you think of something new, it's been done.

2nd Law: If you think something is important, your advisor won't.

3rd Law: If you give up on an idea, someone else will publish it, obtain a grant, write a book, and appear on *Oprah*.

Almost made it twice,
PRM

Statistical techniques are used for describing and finding relationships among variables, as we discussed in chapters 6 and 7. They are also used to detect differences among groups. The latter are most frequently used for data analysis in experimental and quasi-experimental research. They enable us to evaluate the effects of an independent (cause or treatment) or categorical (gender, age, race, etc.) variable on a dependent variable (effect, outcome). Remember, however, that the techniques described in this chapter are not used in isolation to establish cause-and-effect but only to evaluate the influence of the independent variable. Cause-and-effect is not established by statistics but by theory, logic, and the total nature of the experimental situation.

How Statistics Test Differences

In experimental research, the levels of the independent variable may be established by the experimenter. For example, the experiment might involve the investigation of the effects of intensity of training on cardiorespiratory endurance. Thus, intensity of training is the independent variable (or treatment factor), whereas a measure of cardiorespiratory endurance is the dependent variable. Intensity of training could have any number of levels. If it were evaluated as a percentage of maximal oxygen consumption ($\dot{V}O_2$max), then it could be 30%, 40%, 50%, and so forth. The investigator would choose the number and the intensity of levels. In a simple experiment, the independent variable might be two levels of intensity of training, for example, 40% and 70% of $\dot{V}O_2$max. The length of each session (30 min), frequency (three times per week), and number of weeks of training (12) are controlled (equal for both groups). The dependent variable is the distance a person runs in 12 min.

 The purpose of the statistical test is to evaluate the null hypothesis at a specific level of probability (e.g., $p < .05$). In other words, do the two levels of treatment differ significantly ($p < .05$) so that these differences would not be attributable to a chance occurrence more than 5 times in 100? The statistical test is always of the null hypothesis. All that statistics can do is reject or fail to reject the null hypothesis. Statistics cannot accept the research hypothesis. Only logical reasoning, good experimental design, and appropriate theorizing can do so. Statistics can determine only whether the groups are different, not why they are different.

In using logical techniques to infer cause-and-effect after finding significant differences, you must be careful to consider all possibilities. For example, we might propose the theorem that all odd numbers are primary numbers (this example is from Ronen et al., cited in Scherr, 1983, p. 146). You know that prime numbers are those that can be divided only by 1 and by themselves. Thus, 1 is a primary number; 3 is a primary number; 5 is a primary number; 7 is a primary number, . . . Using the induction technique of reasoning, every odd number is a primary number. In Ronen et al.'s example, a very small number of levels of the independent variable (primary numbers) were sampled, and an error was made in inferring that all levels of the independent variable were the same.

When you use statistics that test differences among groups, you want to establish not only whether the groups are significantly different but also the strength of the association between the independent and dependent variables, or the size

---

 What statistical tests do

 F ratio — The ratio of true variance over error variance.

Omega squared (ω^2) — A method of interpreting the meaningfulness of the strength of the relationship between the independent and dependent variables; the proportion of total variance that is due to the treatments.

of the difference between two groups. The t and the **F ratios** are used throughout this chapter to determine whether groups are significantly different. **Omega squared (ω^2)** is used to estimate the degree of association (or percent variance accounted for) between the independent and dependent variables. To some extent, ω^2 is similar to r^2 for the correlations presented in chapter 7; both represent the same idea, which is percent variance accounted for. Another way of considering the meaningfulness of the differences is effect size (ES). Effect size (recall the discussion at the end of chapter 6) is the standardized difference between two groups and is also used as an estimate of meaningfulness.

 The uses of the t and the F distributions as presented in this chapter have four assumptions (in addition to the assumptions for parametric statistics presented in chapter 5) (Kirk, 1982, p. 74; a good book to read for more information):

- Observations are drawn from normally distributed populations.
- Observations represent random samples from populations.
- The numerator and denominator are estimates of the same population variance.
- The numerator and denominator of F (or t) ratios are independent.

Although t and F tests are robust (only slightly influenced) to violations of these assumptions, the assumptions still are not trivial. You should be sensitive to their presence and to the fact that violations affect the probability levels that may be obtained in connection with t and F ratios.

Three Types of t Tests

t Test Between a Sample and a Population Mean
Independent t Test
    Using the Independent t Test
    Checking for Homogeneity of Variance
    Estimating Meaningfulness of Treatments
        Omega Squared (ω^2)
        Effect Size
Dependent t Test

We discuss three types of t tests: t test between a sample and a population mean, t test for independent groups, and t test for dependent groups.

t Test Between a Sample and a Population Mean

First, we may want to know whether a sample of subjects differs from a larger population. For example, suppose that for a standardized knowledge test on physical fitness, the mean is 76 for a large population of college freshmen. When tested, a fitness class

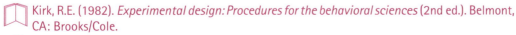

 Kirk, R.E. (1982). *Experimental design: Procedures for the behavioral sciences* (2nd ed.). Belmont, CA: Brooks/Cole.

Four assumptions for the use of t and F distributions

($n = 32$) that you are teaching has a mean of 81 and a standard deviation of 9. Does your class have significantly more knowledge about physical fitness than does the typical college freshman class?

The t test is a test of the null hypothesis, which states that there is no difference between the sample mean (M) and the population mean (μ), or $M - \mu = 0$. Formula 8.1 is the t test between a sample and a population mean:

$$t = \frac{M - \mu}{s_m / \sqrt{n}}$$

(8.1)

where s_m = the standard deviation for the sample mean and n = the number of subjects in the sample.

Example 8.1 shows this formula applied to the means and standard deviation of the example for the standardized fitness knowledge test.

Example 8.1

Known Values

Population: $N = 10,000$
Fitness class: $n = 32$
Sample mean: $M = 81$
Population mean: $\mu = 76$
Standard deviation: $s = 9$

Working It Out
(Equation 8.1)

$$t = \frac{81 - 76}{9 / \sqrt{32}} = \frac{5}{1.59} = 3.14$$

Is the value of 3.14 significant? To find out you'll need to check Table A.5 in Appendix A. To use the table, first work out the degrees of freedom (df) for the t test. Degrees of freedom are based on the number of subjects with a correction for bias:

$$df = n - 1$$

(8.2)

In our example, the degrees of freedom are $32 - 1$, or 31. Degrees of freedom are used to enter a t table to determine whether the calculated t is as large as or greater than the tabled t value. Note that across the top of Table A.5 are probability levels. We want to know if our t value is significant at $p < .05$, the level of significance that we set. Read across to the .05 level. Now read down the left side (df) to the number in the t test from Example 8.1 ($df = 31$). Read where the df row and the .05 column intersect. Is the calculated value ($t = 3.14$) larger than this value (2.04)? Yes, it is. So t is significant at $p < .05$. Thus, our sample class is reliably (significantly) different from the population average on the fitness test.

Independent t Test

The previous t test, applied to determine whether a sample differs from a population, is not used very frequently. The most frequently used t test determines whether two sample means differ reliably from each other. This is called an **independent t test**.

---

 independent t test — The most frequently used test to determine if two sample means differ reliably from each other.

Using the Independent t Test

Suppose we return to our example at the beginning of this chapter: Do two groups, training at different levels of intensity (40% or 70% of $\dot{V}O_2$max, 30 min per day, 3 days per week for 12 weeks), differ from each other on a measure of cardiorespiratory endurance (12-min run)? Let us further assume that there were 30 subjects who were randomly assigned to form the two groups of 15 each.

Formula 8.3 is the *t*-test formula for two independent samples:

$$t = \frac{M_1 - M_2}{\sqrt{s_1^2/n_1 + s_2^2/n_2}} \tag{8.3}$$

Formula 8.4 is the version of the *t*-test formula most easily performed with a calculator:

$$t = \frac{M_1 - M_2}{\sqrt{\dfrac{[\Sigma X_1^2 - (\Sigma X_1)^2/n_1 + \Sigma X_2^2 - (\Sigma X_2)^2/n_2] \cdot (1/n_1 + 1/n_2)}{n_1 + n_2 - 2}}} \tag{8.4}$$

The degrees of freedom for an independent *t* test are calculated as follows:
In our example, $df = 15 + 15 - 2 = 28$

$$df = n_1 + n_2 - 2 \tag{8.5}$$

Example 8.2 shows how these formulas would be applied to the intensity-of-training experiment.

Example 8.2

Known Values	Group 1 (70% $\dot{V}O_2$max)	Group 2 (40% $\dot{V}O_2$max)
Mean distance run:	M_1 = 3,004 m	M_2 = 2,456 m
Standard deviation:	s_1 = 114 m	s_2 = 103 m
Number of subjects:	n_1 = 15	n_2 = 15

Working It Out
(Equation 8.3)

$$t = \frac{3,004 - 2,456}{\sqrt{\dfrac{(114)^2}{15} + \dfrac{(103)^2}{15}}} = \frac{548}{39.67} = 13.81$$

$$t(28) = 13.81, p < .05$$

Thus, you can see that the 70% intensity of training allowed subjects to run reliably farther (M = 3,004 m) than did the 40% intensity of training (M = 2,456 m). If the 12-min run was a valid measure of cardiorespiratory endurance, if all other conditions were controlled, and if the theory, logic, and design of this experiment made sense, we can say that the cause of this increased level of cardiorespiratory endurance was the fact that the 70% group's training was more intense than that of the 40% group. Given that the theory and logic behind this experiment were sound, we might be able to say that the training resulted in a change in certain cardiorespiratory functions allowing more work (i.e., more distance to be covered in 12 minutes) to occur in a specific time.

Checking for Homogeneity of Variance

All comparison-between-groups techniques assume that the variances (standard deviation squared) between the groups are equivalent. Although mild violations of this assumption do not present major problems, serious violations are more likely if group sizes are not approximately equal. Formulas given here and used in most computer programs allow unequal group sizes. However, the homogeneity assumption should be checked if group sizes are very different or even when variances are very different (these techniques are not presented here but are covered in basic statistical texts).

Estimating Meaningfulness of Treatments

How meaningful is this effect? Or, stated more simply, is the increase in cardiorespiratory endurance of running an addition 548 m (3,004 – 2,456) worth the additional work of training at 70% of $\dot{V}O_2$max as compared to 40% of $\dot{V}O_2$max? Given the total variation in running performance of the two groups, what we really want to know is how much of this variation is accounted for by (associated with) the difference in the two levels of the independent variable (70% vs. 40%).

Omega Squared (ω^2).   One way to estimate this variation is to use the following formula (Tolson, 1980) to calculate omega squared (ω^2):

$$\omega^2 = \frac{t^2 - 1}{t^2 + n_1 + n_2 - 1} \tag{8.6}$$

Example 8.3 shows the application of this formula to our example.

Example 8.3

Known Values

Differences between groups: $t = 13.81$
Number of subjects in Group 1: $n_1 = 15$
Number of subjects in Group 2: $n_2 = 15$

Working It Out
(Equation 8.6)

$$\omega^2 = \frac{190.72 - 1}{190.72 + 15 + 15 - 1} = \frac{189.72}{219.72} = .86$$

We can conclude that $\omega^2 = .86$ means 86% of the total variance in the distance run scores can be accounted for by the difference in the two groups' levels of training. The remaining variance, 14% (100% – 86% = 14%), is accounted for by other factors. The question now becomes, Is this a meaningful percentage of variance? No one can answer that except you. Are you willing to increase the intensity of training 30% to produce this effect? There is no statistical answer. Only the person involved using theory, past research, and logic can answer that. The research has told you only what will happen if you increase the intensity of training from 40% to 70% of $\dot{V}O_2$max.

Effect Size.   Another way to estimate the degree to which the treatment influenced the outcome is by effect size (ES), the standardized difference between the means. Formula 8.7 is a way to estimate effect size (this concept was discussed in formula 6.4 in chapter 6 and is also used in meta-analysis, discussed in chapter 14):

$$ES = (M_1 - M_2)/s \tag{8.7}$$

where M_1 = the mean of one group or level of treatment, M_2 = the mean of a second group or level of treatment, and s = the standard deviation. The question is what standard deviation should be used. Considerable controversy exists over the answer to this question. Some statisticians think that if there is a control group, then its standard deviation should be used. If there is no control group, then the pooled standard deviation (Formula 8.8) should be used. Some advocate the use of the pooled standard deviation on all occasions. Either can be defended; however, when there is no clear control group (as in the example used here), we recommend you use the pooled standard deviation:

$$s_p = \sqrt{\frac{s_1^2(n_1 - 1) + s_2^2(n_2 - 1)}{n_1 + n_2 - 2}} \qquad (8.8)$$

where s_p = the pooled standard deviation, s_1^2 = the variance of Group 1, s_2^2 = the variance of Group 2, n_1 = the number of subjects in Group 1, and n_2 = the number of subjects in Group 2.

Effect size can be interpreted as follows: an ES of .8 or greater is large, an ES around .5 is moderate, and an ES of .2 or less is small. Thus, ES is calculated in Example 8.4:

Example 8.4

Known Values	Group 1	Group 2
Mean distance run	$M_1 = 3{,}004$ m	$M_2 = 2{,}456$ m
Standard deviation	$s_1 = 114$ m	$s_2 = 103$
Number of subjects	$n_1 = 15$	$n_2 = 15$

Working It Out
(Equations 8.7 and 8.8)

$$s_p = \sqrt{\frac{(114)^2 (15-1) + (103)^2 (15 - 1)}{15 + 15 - 2}} = 108.64$$

$$ES = \frac{3{,}004 - 2{,}456}{108.64} = 5.0$$

An ES of 5.0 is a large value and would typically be judged as a meaningful treatment effect.

Dependent t Test

We have now considered use of the t test to evaluate whether a sample differs from a population and whether two independent samples differ from each other. A third application is called a **dependent t test**. This means that the two groups of scores are related in some manner. Usually, the relationship takes one of two forms:

* two groups of subjects are matched on one or more characteristics and thus are no longer independent, or
* one group of subjects is tested twice on the same variable, and the experimenter is interested in the change between the two tests.

The formula for a dependent t test is

$$t = \frac{M_{post} - M_{pre}}{\sqrt{[(s^2_{post} + s^2_{pre}) - (2r_{pp} \cdot s_{post} \cdot s_{pre})]/(N - 1)}} \qquad (8.9)$$

Notice that the top part of this formula is the same as the independent t-test formula (8.3). In addition, the bottom (under the square-root formula) is also similar on the left

 dependent t test — A test of the significance of differences between means of two sets of scores that are related, such as when the same subjects are measured on two occasions.

 Two forms of group relationships

side (within the parentheses). However, an amount is subtracted from the bottom (error term) of the t test (formula). This series of numbers and letters is read as "two times the correlation (r) between the pre- and posttest times the standard deviation for the posttest times the standard deviation for the pretest." The independent t test (8.3) assumes that the two groups of subjects are independent. In this case, the subjects are the same people tested twice (pre and post). Thus, we adjust the error term of the t test downward (make smaller) by taking into account the relationship (r) between the pre- and posttests adjusted to their standard deviations. The degrees of freedom for the dependent t test is

$$df = N - 1 \tag{8.10}$$

where N = the number of paired observations. Formula 8.9 is cumbersome to compute because the correlation (r) between the pre- and posttest must be calculated. Thus, the raw-score formula is much easier to use:

$$t = \frac{\Sigma D}{\sqrt{[N\Sigma D^2 - (\Sigma D)^2]/(N-1)}} \tag{8.11}$$

where D = the posttest minus the pretest for each subject and N = the number of paired observations. Let's work out an example. Ten dancers are given a jump-and-reach test (difference between height they can reach and touch a wall and how high they can jump and touch), then 10 weeks of dance activity that involves leaps and jumps 3 days per week. The dancers are again given the jump-and-reach test after the 10 weeks. (This is not proposed to be a real experiment, just a simple example illustrating the statistical technique.) Our research hypothesis is that the 10 weeks of dance experience will improve jumping skills as reflected by the change in jump-and-reach scores. The null hypothesis (H_0) is that the difference between the pre- and the posttest of jumping is not significantly different from zero, $H_0 = M_{post} - M_{pre} = 0$. Example 8.5 shows how to manipulate the data.

Example 8.5

Known Values

Subject	Pretest score (cm)	Posttest score (cm)	Posttest − Pretest D	D^2
1	12	16	4	16
2	15	21	6	36
3	13	15	2	4
4	20	22	2	4
5	21	21	0	0
6	19	23	4	16
7	14	16	2	4
8	17	18	1	1
9	16	22	6	36
10	18	23	5	25

Sum of pretest scores: $\Sigma_{pre} = 165$ cm
Sum of posttest scores: $\Sigma_{post} = 197$ cm
Sum of D: $\Sigma D = 32$
Sum of D^2: $\Sigma(D^2) = 142$
Number of paired observations: $N = 10$

Posttest mean: $M_{post} = 19.7$
Pretest mean: $M_{pre} = 16.5$

Working It Out
(Equations 8.11, 8.10)

$$t = \frac{32}{\sqrt{\frac{[10\,(142) - (32)^2]}{10 - 1}}} = \frac{32}{\sqrt{\frac{1{,}420 - 1{,}024}{9}}} = \frac{32}{6.63} = 4.83$$

The results indicate that the posttest mean (19.7 cm) was significantly better than the pretest mean (16.5 cm), $t(9) = 4.83$, $p < .05$. The null hypothesis can be rejected, and if everything else has been properly controlled in the experiment, we can conclude that the dance training produced a reliable increase in the height of jumping performance of 3.2 cm.

A standard formula is not available for calculating ω^2 for a dependent t test. But we could estimate the magnitude of the effect by dividing the average gain by the pretest mean and multiplying by 100 as in Example 8.6.

Example 8.6

Known Values

Difference between post- and pretest means: $M_D = 3.2$
Mean of pretest scores: $M_{pre} = 16.5$

Working It Out
Magnitude of increase $= \dfrac{M_D}{M_{pre}} \times 100 = \dfrac{3.2}{16.5} \times 100 = 19.4\%$

The gain is 19.4% of the pretest and represents nearly a 20% improvement. Although this is a rather crude way of estimating the effect, it does suffice. On the other hand, we could estimate ES for the pretest to posttest change by subtracting the pretest M from the posttest M and dividing by the pretest standard deviation.

Interpreting t

One-Tailed Versus Two-Tailed t Tests

t Tests and Power in Research

     You have now learned to perform the calculations that determine differences among groups. What do the results mean? Are they significant? Does it matter whether they are or aren't? We answer these questions in this section by explain-

 one-tailed t test — Test that assumes that the difference between the two means lies in one direction only.

two-tailed t test — Test that assumes that the difference between the two means could favor either group.

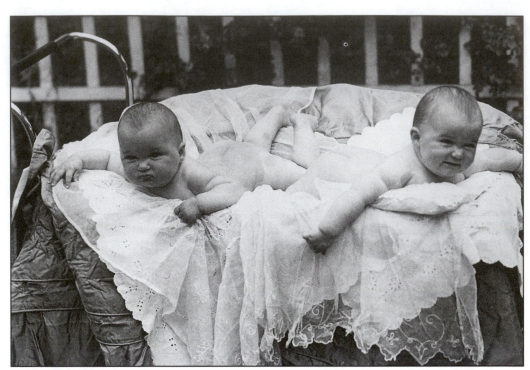

It usually becomes clear when you should use a two-tailed test.

ing the difference between **one-tailed** and **two-tailed** *t* **tests** and discussing the aspects of the *t* test that influence power in research.

One-Tailed Versus Two-Tailed *t* Tests

At this point, refer again to Table A.5 in Appendix A (the tabled values of *t* to which you compare the values calculated). Remember, you decide the probability level (we have been using .05), calculate the degrees of freedom for *t*, and read the tabled *t* value at the column (probability)-by-row (*df*) intersection. If your calculated *t* exceeds the tabled value, it is significant at the specified alpha and degrees of freedom. This table is used for a two-tailed *t* test because we assume that the difference between the two means could favor either mean. Sometimes we might hypothesize that Group 1 will be better than Group 2 or, at worst, no poorer than Group 2. In this case, the test is a one-tailed *t* test, that is, it can go only one direction. Then, when looking at Table A.5 for a one-tailed *t* test, the .05 level is .10, .025 is .05, and .01 is .02. Generally in behavioral research, however, we are not so sure of our results that we can employ the one-tailed *t* table.

t Tests and Power in Research

In chapter 6, power was mentioned as the probability of rejecting the null hypothesis when the null hypothesis is false. To obtain power in research is very desirable, as the odds of rejecting a false null hypothesis are increased. The independent *t* test is used here to explain three ways to obtain power (in addition to setting the alpha level). However, these ways apply to all types of experimental research.

Consider the formula for the independent *t* test:

$$t = \frac{M_1 - M_2}{\sqrt{\dfrac{s_1^2}{n_1} + \dfrac{s_2^2}{n_2}}}$$

1

2

3

Note that we have placed numbers (1, 2, 3) beside the three horizontal levels of this formula. These three levels represent what can be manipulated to increase or decrease power.

The first level ($M_1 - M_2$) gives power if we can increase the difference between M_1 and M_2. You should see that if the second and third levels remain the same, a larger difference between the means increases the size of the t ratio, which increases the odds of rejecting the null hypothesis and thus increases power. How can the difference between the means be increased? The logical answer is by applying stronger, more concentrated treatments. One example would be to use a 12-week treatment instead of a 6-week treatment to give the treatment a better chance to show its effect. The 12-week treatments (as compared to the 6-week) should move the means of the experimental and the control groups further apart. This results in less overlap in their distributions.

The second level is s_1^2, s_2^2, or the variances (s^2) for each of the two groups. Recall that the standard deviation represents the spread of the scores about the mean. If this spread becomes smaller (scores distributed more closely about the mean), the variance is also smaller. Because the variance term is in the denominator of the t test, if it is smaller and if the first and the third levels remain the same, the t ratio will become larger, thus increasing the odds of rejecting the null hypothesis and increasing power. How can the standard deviation and thereby the variance be made smaller? The answer is to apply the treatments more consistently. The more consistently the treatments are applied to each subject, the more the subjects will become similar in response to the dependent variable. This groups the distribution more tightly around the group means, thus reducing the standard deviation (and thereby, the variance).

Finally, the third level (n_1, n_2) is the number of subjects in each group. If n_1 and n_2 are increased and the first and second levels remain the same, the denominator will become smaller (note n is divided into s^2) and the t ratio will become larger, thus increasing the odds of rejecting the null hypothesis and obtaining power. Obviously, n_1 and n_2 can be increased by placing additional subjects in each group. Of course, power may also be influenced by varying the alpha (i.e., if alpha is set at .10 as opposed to .05, increased power is attained). But in doing this, we increase the risk of rejecting a true null hypothesis (i.e., we increase the chance of making a Type I error).

 In summary, power is desirable to obtain because it increases the odds of rejecting a false null hypothesis. Power may be obtained by using strong treatments, administering those treatments consistently, using as many subjects as feasible, or varying alpha. Remember, however, there is always a second question, even in the most powerful experiments. After the null hypothesis is rejected, the strength (meaningfulness) of the effects must be evaluated.

 The t ratio has a numerator and a denominator. From a theoretical point of view, the numerator is regarded as **true variance**, or the real difference between the means. The denominator is considered **error variance**, or variation about the mean. Thus, the t ratio is

$$t = \frac{\text{true variance}}{\text{error variance}}$$

where true variance = $M_1 - M_2$ and error variance = $\sqrt{s_1^2/n_1 + s_2^2/n_2}$. If no real differences exist between the groups, true variance = error variance, or the ratio between the two is true variance/error = 1.0. When a significant t ratio is found, we are really saying that true variance exceeds error variance to a certain degree. The amount that the t ratio

---

How to obtain power in research

true variance — The portion of the differences in scores that is (theoretically) real.

error variance — The portion of the scores that is attributed to subject variability.

must exceed 1.0 for significance is dependent on the number of subjects (df) and the alpha level established.

The estimate of the strength of the relationship (ω^2) between the independent and dependent variables is represented by the ratio of true variance to total variance.

$$\omega^2 = \frac{\text{true variance}}{\text{total variance}}$$

Thus, ω^2 represents the proportion of the total variance that is due to the treatments (true variance).

Effect size is also an estimate of the strength or meaningfulness of the group differences or treatments. ES places the difference between the means in standard deviation units, $(M_1 - M_2)/s$. Figure 8.1 shows how the normal distribution of two groups differs given two ESs, 0.5 and 1.0. In Figure 8.1a the standardized difference between the group means is an ES = 0.5; that is, the mean of Group 2 falls 0.5 standard deviations to the right

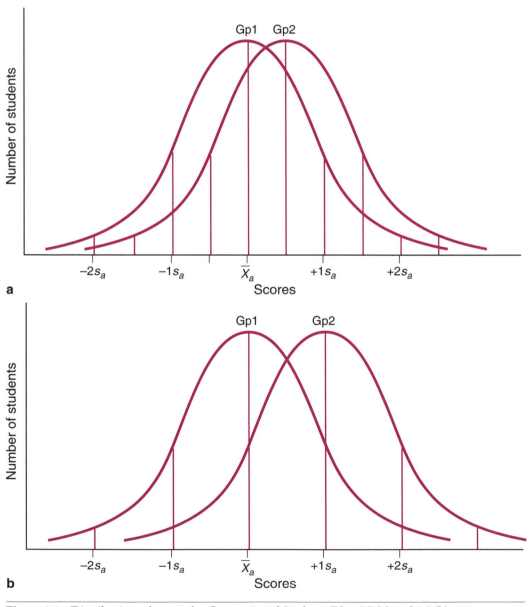

Figure 8.1   Distribution of scores for Groups 1 and 2 whom ES = 0.5 (a) and 1.0 (b).

(also, could be to the left if the ES were -0.5) of the mean of Group 1. Figure 8.1b shows the distribution when the ES $= 1.0$; that is, the mean of Group 2 is 1 standard deviation to the right (or left) of Group 1. Notice that when comparing Figure 8.1b to 8.1a, there is less overlap between the two groups' distribution of scores on the dv in 8.1b than in 8.1a. Said another way, when scores on the dv were grouped by the IV in 8.1b, the means were further apart and there was less distribution overlap than in 8.1a.

Effect size is sometimes interpreted by percentile change attributed to the treatment. For example, in Figure 8.1b, the treatment group mean was 1.0 s higher than the control group mean. If we consult Table A.2 in Appendix A, we see that a z of 1.00 (which is a distance of 1 s above the mean) shows that only .1587 (16%) of the scores are higher than 1.0. In other words, the percentile rank for such a score is 84. Consequently, in interpreting an effect size of 1.0, we can infer that the treatment improved average performance by 34 percentile points (i.e., treatment group $= 84$, control group $= 50$, $84 - 50 = 34$).

Relationship of t and r

As we mentioned previously, our separation of statistical techniques into the two categories of relationships among variables (chapter 7) and differences among groups (this chapter) is artificial because both sets of techniques are based on the general linear model. A brief demonstration with t and r should make the point. However, the idea can be extended into the more sophisticated techniques discussed in chapter 7, later in this chapter, and in chapter 9 (Understanding Multivariate Techniques). Example 8.7 provides an example of the relationship between t and r. Note that Group 1 has a set of scores (dependent variable) for five subjects as does Group 2.

Example 8.7

Known Values

Group 1		Group 2	
Subject	Dependent variable	Subject	Dependent variable
A	1	F	6
B	2	G	7
C	3	H	8
D	4	I	9
E	5	J	10

Sum of Group 1: $\Sigma_1 = 15$
Mean of Group 1: $M_1 = 3$
Standard deviation Group 1: $s_1 = 1.58$

Sum of Group 2: $\Sigma_2 = 40$
Mean of Group 2: $M_2 = 8$
Standard deviation Group 2: $s_2 = 1.58$

Working It Out

1. Conduct an independent t test (Equation 8.3) and test for significance.

$$t = \frac{3-8}{\sqrt{\dfrac{1.58^2}{5} + \dfrac{1.58^2}{5}}} = 5.0 \qquad df = (n_1 + n_2) - 2 = 8$$

$$t(8) = 5.0, p < .05$$

2. Assign each subject a dummy code that stands for his or her group.

Group 1		Group 2	
Subject	Dummy code	Subject	Dummy code
A	1	F	0
B	1	G	0
C	1	H	0
D	1	I	0
E	1	J	0

3. Apply the correlation formula (Equation 7.1, p. 120). If we treat the dummy-coded variable as X and the dependent variable as Y and ignore group membership (10 subjects with two variables), then the correlation formula used earlier can be applied to the data.

$$r = \frac{N \sum XY - (\sum X)(\sum Y)}{\sqrt{N\sum X^2 - (\sum X)^2} \ \sqrt{N\sum Y^2 - (\sum Y)^2}} =$$

$$\frac{10(15) - 5(55)}{\sqrt{10(5) - 25} \ \sqrt{10(385) - 3{,}025}} = \frac{125}{144} = .87$$

4. Apply a t test to r. In this example $t = 5.0$, the same as the t test done on the group means (within rounding error)

$$t = \sqrt{\frac{r^2}{(1 - r^2)/(N - 2)}} = \sqrt{\frac{.87^2}{(1 - .87^2)/(10 - 2)}} = \sqrt{\frac{.757}{.030}} = 5.0$$

The point is that r represents the relationship between the independent and dependent variables (in fact, r^2 is a biased estimator of ω^2) and the test of r (i.e., the t test) evaluates the reliability (significance) of the relationship.

We are not trying to confuse you. There are two sources of variance, true and error (true variance + error variance = total variance). The t test is the ratio of true variance to error variance, whereas r is the square root of the proportion of total variance accounted for by true variance. To get t from r only means manipulating the variance components in a slightly different way. This is because all parametric correlational and differences-among-groups techniques are based on the general linear model. This result can easily be shown to exist in the more advanced statistical techniques (for a thorough treatment of this topic, see Pedhazur, 1982).

You need to understand this basic concept because it is becoming increasingly common for researchers to use regression techniques to analyze what has traditionally been termed experimental data. These data have usually been analyzed by techniques discussed in this chapter. We have, however, demonstrated that what is traditional is not required. What is important is that the data have been appropriately analyzed to answer the following questions:

Pedhazur, E.J. (1982). *Multiple regression in behavioral research: Explanation and prediction* (2nd ed.). New York: Holt, Rinehart & Winston.

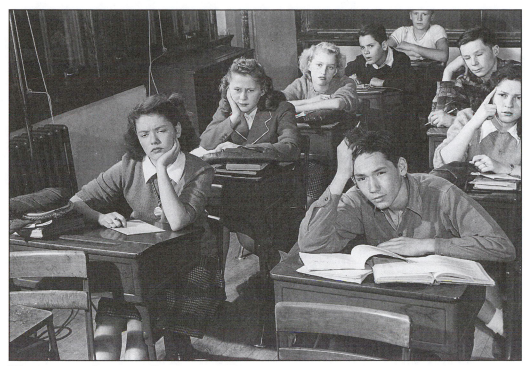

We are not trying to confuse you.

- Are the groups significantly different?
- Does the independent variable account for a meaningful proportion of the variance in the dependent variable?

Significance is always evaluated as the ratio of true variance to error variance, whereas percent variance accounted for is always the ratio of true variance to total variance.

Declaring Two Groups Equivalent

Sometimes researchers are interested in declaring groups equivalent. For example, an exercise physiologist might be interested in showing that although high-quality male cyclists ride a 30-mile race in a shorter time than high-quality female cyclists, their size and muscle mass make this possible, not differences in cardiovascular endurance as estimated by $\dot{V}O_2$max ml $\cdot$ kg $\cdot$ min^{-1}. Thus, this researcher obtains 49 male and 58 female cyclists who are excellent performers (by some definition). The males have an average $\dot{V}O_2$max of 61.4 ml $\cdot$ kg $\cdot$ min^{-1} ($s = 10.9$), and the females have an average $\dot{V}O_2$max of 59.2 ml $\cdot$ kg $\cdot$ min^{-1} ($s = 9.5$). Are these two sets of values equivalent?

Procedures have been developed to test this question. Rogers, Howard, and Vessey (1993; formulas 8.12 and 8.13 are from their paper) have given examples (based on earlier work by Westlake, 1981) of how to declare equivalency if the researcher can specify the size of a small difference that would define a range of no meaningful difference (e.g., ± 10%). In our example, we could say that high-quality male and female cyclists do not differ in their underlying cardiovascular physiological efficiency if women's $\dot{V}O_2$max when adjusted for body size (ml $\cdot$ kg $\cdot$ min^{-1}) is within 10% of men's. Thus, any difference small enough to fall within that 10% limit (in this instance 6.14 ml · kg · min⁻¹) would be declared a trivial and nonmeaningful difference.

The researcher must first define equivalency and then perform a z test to see if the groups are similar. Thus, the null hypothesis is that the groups are nonequivalent or the means are different. If the null is rejected, then the groups are declared equivalent. In the example given, we have specified a nonmeaningful difference and established alpha at .05. The first step is to find the standard error of the difference between the means (formula 8.12) because this is used as the error term in the z test.

$$s_{m_1 - m_2} = \sqrt{\left[\frac{(n_1 - 1)s_1^2 + (n_2 - 1)s_2^2}{n_1 + n_2 - 2}\right]\left[\frac{1}{n_1} + \frac{1}{n_2}\right]} \qquad (8.12)$$

Once this is known, formula 8.13 can be used to calculate the z test of the null hypothesis that the difference (X_{diff}) exceeds 6.14 (10% of the male value).

$$z = \frac{(M_1 - M_2) - (X_{diff})}{s_{m_1-m_2}} \qquad (8.13)$$

Let's work through the equations using the data from our cycling example.

Example 8.8

Known Values

Known Values	Men	Women
Mean V̇O₂max:	$M_1 =$ 61.4	$M_2 =$ 59.2
Standard deviation:	$s_1 =$ 10.9	$s_2 =$ 9.5
Number of subjects:	$n_1 =$ 49	$n_2 =$ 58

Working It Out

1. Calculate the standard error of difference between two means (Equation 8.12).

$$s_{m_1 - m_2} = \sqrt{\left[\frac{(49 - 1)(10.9)^2 + (58 - 1)(9.5)^2}{49 + 58 - 2}\right]\left[\frac{1}{49} + \frac{1}{58}\right]} = 1.96$$

2. Calculate the z test for H_o of non-equivalence (Equation 8.13).

$$z = \frac{[(61.4 - 59.2) - (6.12)]}{1.96} = -2.00$$

In Example 8.8, we see that z is 2.00. When compared with the tabled z values (two tail) in Table A.2 in the appendix, the probability of obtaining a z that large by chance is 4 times in 100 ($p = .04$). Thus, the null hypothesis of nonequivalence is rejected and the groups are declared equivalent.

Analysis of Variance

Simple Analysis of Variance
Calculating Simple ANOVA

Using t tests is a good way to determine differences between two groups. Often, though, experimenters work with more than two groups. A method of determining differences among them is needed in those cases. This section explains how analysis of variance is used to detect differences among two or more groups.

Simple Analysis of Variance

The concept of simple (sometimes called one-way but seldom considered simple by graduate students) **analysis of variance (ANOVA)** is an extension of the independent t test. In fact, t is just a special case of simple ANOVA in which there are two groups. Simple ANOVA allows the evaluation of the null hypothesis among two or more group means with the restriction that the two or more groups are levels of the same independent variable. In an earlier example, we suggested that a t test was appropriate to test between the means of two groups who trained at 40% and 70% of $\dot{V}O_2$max. This represents two levels (40% and 70%) of one independent variable (intensity of training). In fact, simple ANOVA and its test statistic, the F ratio, could just as easily have been used. But what would happen if there were more than two levels of the independent variable, for example, 40%, 60%, and 80% of $\dot{V}O_2$max? Simple ANOVA could be used in this situation to test the null hypothesis that the groups' average values on the 12-minute run were not significantly different, $H_0 = M_1 = M_2 = M_3 = 0$.

Why not do a t test between the 40% and 60% groups, a second t test between the 40% and 80% groups, and a third t test between the 60% and 80% groups? The reason is because this would violate an assumption concerning the established alpha level (let it be $p = .05$). The .05 level means 1 chance in 20 of a chance difference, assuming that the groups of subjects on which the statistical tests are made are from independent random samples. In our case, this is not true. Each group has been used in two comparisons (e.g., 40% vs. 60% and 40% vs. 80%) rather than only one. Thus, we have increased the chances of making a Type I error (i.e., alpha is no longer .05). Making this type of comparison, in which the same group's mean is used more than once, is an example of increasing the experimentwise error rate (discussed later in this chapter). Simple ANOVA allows all three group means to be compared simultaneously, thus keeping alpha at the designated level of .05.

analysis of variance (ANOVA) — Test that allows the evaluation of the null hypothesis between two or more group means.

Calculating Simple ANOVA

Table 8.1 provides the formulas for calculating simple ANOVA and the F ratio. This method, the so-called ABC method, is simple:

A $= \sum X^2$: This means to square each subject's score, sum these squared scores (regardless of which group the subject is in), and set the total equal to A.

B $= (\sum X)^2/N$: For this value, we sum each subject's score (regardless of group), square the sum, divide by the total number of subjects, and set the answer equal to B.

C $= (\sum X_1)^2/n_1 + (\sum X_2)^2/n_2 + \dots + (\sum X_i)^2/n_i$: This requires that we sum each subject's score in Group 1, square the sum, and divide by the number of subjects in Group 1; do the same for the scores in Group 2 and so on for however many groups (i) there are; then, sum all the group sums and set the answer to C.

Table 8.1   Formulas for Calculating Simple ANOVA

$$A = \sum X^2$$

$$B = \frac{(\sum X)^2}{N}$$

$$C = \frac{(\sum X_1)^2}{n_1} + \frac{(\sum X_2)^2}{n_2} + \dots + \frac{(\sum X_i)^2}{n_i}$$

Summary table for ANOVA

Source	SS	df	MS	F
Between (true)	$C - B$	$k - 1$	$(C - B)/(k - 1)$	MS_B/MS_W
Within (error)	$A - C$	$N - k$	$(A - C)/(N - k)$	
Total	$A - B$	$N - 1$		

Note. X = a subject's score, N = total number of subjects, n = number of subjects in a group, k = number of groups, SS = sum of squares, df = degrees of freedom, MS = mean square.

Next, fill in the summary table for ANOVA using A, B, and C. Thus, the between-groups (true variance) sum of squares (SS) is equal to C – B; the between-groups degrees of freedom (df) is the number of groups minus one ($k - 1$); the between-groups variance or mean square (MS_B) is the between-groups sum of squares divided by the between-groups degrees of freedom. The same follows when the source is within groups (error variance) and then for the total. The F ratio is MS_B/MS_W (i.e., true/error).

Example 8.9 shows how the formulas in Table 8.1 are used. The scores from Groups 1, 2, and 3 are the sums of two judges' skill ratings for a particular series of movements. The groups are randomly formed of 15 junior high school students. Group 1 was taught with videotape, and the teacher made individual corrections while the student viewed the videotape. Group 2 was taught with videotape, but the teacher made only general group corrections while students viewed the tape. The teacher taught Group 3 without the benefit of videotape equipment. From looking at the formulas in Table 8.1, you should be able to see how each number in this example was calculated.

The ABC method for calculating simple ANOVA

Example 8.9

Known Values	Group 1		Group 2		Group 3	
	X	X^2	X	X^2	X	X^2
	12	144	9	81	6	36
	10	100	7	49	7	49
	11	121	6	36	2	4
	7	49	9	81	3	9
	10	100	4	16	2	4
Σ	50	514	35	263	20	102
M	10	...	7	...	4	...

Working It Out

$A = \Sigma X^2 = 514 + 263 + 102 = 879$

$B = (\Sigma X)^2 / N = (50 + 35 + 20)^2 / 15 = (105)^2 / 15 = 11{,}025/15 = 735$

$C = (\Sigma X_1)^2 / n_1 + (\Sigma X_2)^2 / n_2 + (\Sigma X_3)^2 / n_3 = (50)^2 / 5 + (35)^2 / 5 + (20)^2 / 5$
$\quad = 2{,}500/5 + 1{,}225/5 + 400/5 = 825$

	Summary table for ANOVA			
Source	SS	df	MS	F
Between	90	2	45.0	10.00*
Within	54	12	4.5	...
Total	144	14	...	...

*$p < .05$.

Your main interest in Example 8.9, after you make sure you understand how the numbers were obtained, is in the F ratio of 10.00. Table A.6 in Appendix A contains tabled F values for the .05 and .01 levels of significance. Although the numbers in the table are obtained the same way as in the t table, you use the table in a slightly different way. Note in Example 8.9, that the F ratio is obtained by dividing MS_B by MS_W. The term MS_B has 2 df associated with it (numerator) and the MS_W has 12 df (denominator). Notice also that the F table (Table A.6) has degrees of freedom across the top (numerator) and down the left-hand column (denominator). For our F of 10.00, read down the 2-df column to the 12-df row; there are two numbers where the row and the column intersect. The top number (3.88) in light print is the tabled F for the .05 level, whereas the bottom number (**6.93**) in dark print is the tabled F for the .01 level. If our alpha had been established as .05, then you can see that our F value of 10.00 is larger than the tabled value of .05 (actually, it is also larger than .01). So our F is significant and could be written in the text of an article as $F(2, 12) = 10.00$, $p < .05$ (read "F with 2 and 12 degrees of freedom equals 10.00 and is significant at less than the .05 level").

Follow-up Testing

We now know that significant differences exist among the three group means (Group 1 = 10, Group 2 = 7, and Group 3 = 4). However, we do not know whether all three groups differ (e.g., whether 1 and 2 differ from 3 but not from each

Toothaker, L.E. (1991). *Multiple comparisons for researchers.* Newbury Park, CA: Sage.

other). So we next perform a follow-up test. One way to do this is to use t tests between Groups 1 and 2, 1 and 3, and 2 and 3. However, the same problem that we discussed earlier still exists with alpha (Type I error is increased). Several follow-up tests protect the experimentwise error rate (Type I error). These methods (see Toothaker, 1991, *Multiple comparisons for researchers*, for both conceptual explanations and calculations of the various techniques) include Scheffé, Tukey, Newman-Keuls, Duncan's, and several others. Each test is calculated in a slightly different way, but they all are conceptually similar to the t test in that they identify which pairs of groups differ from each other. The Scheffé method is the most conservative, followed by Tukey, which means they identify fewer significant differences. Duncan's is the most liberal, identifying more significant differences. Newman-Keuls falls between the extremes but has some other problems.

For our purpose, one example should suffice, so we explain the use of the Scheffé method of making multiple comparisons among means. Scheffé (1953) is the most widely recognized of all multiple comparison techniques (Toothaker, 1991). Because we believe one should be conservative when using behavioral data, we generally recommend the Scheffé for follow-up testing. However, other multiple comparison techniques are appropriate for various situations.

The Scheffé technique has a constant critical value for the follow-up comparison of all means when the F ratio from a simple ANOVA (or a main effect in a factorial ANOVA, discussed next) is significant. Scheffé controls Type I error (alpha inflation) for any number of appropriate comparisons. Formula 8.14 is how the critical value for t is calculated using the Scheffé technique:

$$t = \sqrt{(k-1)F^{\alpha}_{k-1,\,df,\,MS_{(W)}}} \tag{8.14}$$

where k = number of means to be compared, F^{α} = the tabled F ratio (from Table A.6) for the selected alpha (e.g., .05) given dfs of $k-1$ and $MS_{(W)}$ (degrees of freedom for the MS_{within}). Example 8.10 shows the Scheffé technique applied to the previous simple ANOVA shown in Example 8.9.

Example 8.10

Known Values

Group 1	M	Difference	Critical value
1	10	G_p 1-2 (10-7) = 3	2.24
2	7	G_p 2-3 (7-4) = 3	2.24
3	4	G_p 1-3 (10-4) = 6	4.48*

*Scheffé value, $p < .05 = 2.79$

Working It Out

1. Calculate the critical Scheffé value required for significance (Equation 8.14).

$$t = \sqrt{(k-1)\,F^{\alpha}_{k-1,\,df,\,MS_{(W)}}}$$

$$t_{.05} = \sqrt{(3-1)\,3.88} = 2.79$$

2. Calculate t for the three comparisons (Equation 8.15).

$$t = \frac{M_1 - M_2}{\sqrt{(MS_{within}/n)\,(2)}}$$

$$t_{1-2} = (10-7)/\sqrt{(4.5/5)\,(2)} = 3/1.34 = 2.24$$

$$t_{1-3} = (10 - 4)/1.34 \qquad = 4.48$$

$$t_{2-3} = (7 - 4)/1.34 \qquad = 2.24$$

3. Table calculated values of t from Step 2 as in above table and compare to Scheffé value calculated in Step 1. Any that are larger than the Scheffé value are declared significant at $p < .05$. Alpha at this level is protected from inflation due to Type I error.

You enter Table A.6 with 2 ($k - 1 = 3 - 1 = 2$) and 12 ($MS_{within} = 12$) from ANOVA in Table 8.1 dfs; the tabled F ratio is 3.88. Solving the formula 8.14 in Example 8.10, we find the Scheffé t for significance at the .05 level is 2.79. If we use the t test formula (8.15, for use when group size is equal) with the MS_{within} as the error term, we see from Example 8.10 that Group 1 is significantly different from Group 3 but not from Group 2. Also, Group 2 is not significantly different from Group 3.

$$t = \frac{M_1 - M_2}{\sqrt{(MS_w/n)(2)}} \qquad (8.15)$$

where n = number in a single group

Example 8.10 arranges the means from highest (10) to lowest (4); the means could also be arranged from lowest to highest. By following steps 1 and 2, you can see that Group 1 differs from 3 at $p < .05$. We could conclude that the techniques used in Group 1 were significantly better than those used in Group 3 but not significantly better than those used in Group 2. Also, the techniques used in Group 2 were not significantly better than those used in Group 3.

 The researcher may also use **planned comparisons** to test for differences among groups. Planned comparisons are a priori in nature; that is, they are planned (testable hypotheses developed) before the experiment. Thus, an experimenter might postulate a test between two groups before the experiment because in theory this particular comparison is important and should be significant. However, the number of planned comparisons in an experiment should be small ($k - 1$, where k = number of groups or treatment levels within an IV) relative to the total number of possible comparisons.

Determining Meaningfulness of Results

Now that we know that F is significant and have followed it up to see which groups differ, we should answer our second question: What percent variance is accounted for by our treatments, or how meaningful are our results? One way to get a quick idea is to refer to Table 8.1 and put true variance over total variance: (SS_{true}/SS_{total}) = 90/144 = .625, or 62.5% of the variance is accounted for by the treatments. Although this is sufficient for a quick estimate, it is biased. The more accurate way is to use the following formula from Tolson (1980):

$$\omega^2 = \frac{[F(k-1)] - (k-1)}{[F(k-1)] + (N-k) + 1} \qquad (8.16)$$

where F = the F ratio, k = the number of groups, and N = the total number of subjects. If we do this with the data from Example 8.9, then we have

planned comparison — Comparison among groups that are planned prior to the experiment, rather than as a follow-up of a test like ANOVA.

$$\omega^2 = \frac{[10.00(3-1)] - (3-1)}{10.00(3-1) + (15-3) + 1} = \frac{18}{33} = .545$$

Thus, ω^2 indicates that 54.5% of the total variance is accounted for by the treatments.

Putting our statistics together, we could say that the treatment was significant, $F(2, 12) = 10.00$, $p < .05$, and accounted for a meaningful proportion of the variance ($\omega^2 = 54.5\%$). In addition, a follow-up Scheffé test indicates that Group 1 had the best performance and was significantly different ($p < .05$) from Group 3. However, Group 1 was not significantly different from Group 2 nor was Group 2 significantly different from Group 3.

Summarizing Simple ANOVA

One final point to recall before leaving our discussion of simple ANOVA is that t was a special case of F when there were only two levels of the independent variable (two groups). In fact, this relationship ($t^2 = F$) is exact, within rounding error (see Example 8.11).

Example 8.11

Known Values	Experimental group			Experimental group		
	X	$(X-M)^2$	X^2	X	$(X-M)^2$	X^2
	2	.09	4	8	4	64
	4	2.89	16	7	1	49
	3	.49	9	5	1	25
	3	.49	9	4	4	16
	2	.09	4	7	1	49
	1	1.69	1	5	1	25
	1	1.69	1	6	0	36
Σ	16	7.43	44	42	12	264
M	2.3	...	...	6.0	...	...
s	1.11	...	...	1.41	...	...

Working It Out

1. Find t (Equation 8.3).

$$t = \frac{M_1 - M_2}{\sqrt{(s_1^2/n_1) + s_2^2/n_2}} = \frac{2.3 - 6}{\sqrt{(1.11^2/7) + 1.41^3/7}} = \frac{3.7}{.68} = 5.44$$

2. Compute the simple ANOVA and complete the summary table.

$A = \Sigma X^2 = 44 + 264 = 308$

$B = (\Sigma X)^2/N = (58)^2/14 = 240.29$

$C = (\Sigma X_1)^2/n_1 + (\Sigma X_2)^2/n_2 = (16)^2/7 + (42)^2/7 = 36.57 + 252 = 288.57$

Summary table for ANOVA				
Source	SS	df	MS	F
Between	48.28	1	48.28	29.80
Within	19.43	12	1.62	...
Total	67.71	13	...	...

$t^2 = F$, $(5.44)^2 = 29.6 \cong 29.8$ (within rounding error)

In other words, there is very little need for *t*, as *F* will handle two or more groups. However, *t* remains in use because it was developed first, being the simplest case of *F*.

Factorial ANOVA

Up to this point, examples of two levels (*t*) or two or more levels (simple ANOVA) of one independent variable have been discussed. In fact, what has occurred is that all other independent variables have been controlled except the single independent variable to be manipulated and its effect on a dependent variable. This is called the Law of the Independent Variable. But, in fact, we can manipulate more than one independent variable and statistically evaluate the effects on a dependent variable. This procedure is called **factorial ANOVA**, meaning that there is more than one factor or independent variable. Theoretically, a factorial ANOVA may have any number of factors (two or more) and any number of levels within a factor (two or more). However, we seldom encounter ANOVAs with more than three or four factors. This is another good place to apply the KISS principle (Keep It Simple, Stupid).

Calculating Factorial ANOVA

For our purpose we consider only a two-way factorial ANOVA, meaning the use of only two independent variables. There would be two main effects and one interaction. **Main effects** are tests of each independent variable when the other is disregarded (and controlled). Look at Table 8.2 and note that the first independent variable (IV_1) has three levels, labeled A_1, A_2, and A_3. Assume that these three levels represent the intensity of training: 40%, 60%, and 80% of VO_2max for 20 min per day for a 12-week period. The second independent variable (IV_2) represents frequency of training: 2 days per week (B_1) versus 3 days per week (B_2). We can test IV_1 by comparing the row means (M_{A1}, M_{A2}, M_{A3}) because IV_2 (B_1 and B_2) is equally represented at each level of *A*. That is, for each level of *A*, two groups (one training 2 days and one 3 days per week) are included. Thus, frequency of training is held constant to allow the test of intensity of training by the F_A ratio.

The same holds true for IV_2, frequency of training. By looking at the column means (M_{B1} and M_{B2}), you can see that the three levels of *A* (IV_1), intensity of training, are equally represented in the two levels of *B*. Therefore, the main effect of frequency of training can be tested by the F_B ratio.

In a study of this type, the main interest usually lies in the interaction. We want to know whether the effect of the levels of *A* depends on or changes across the levels of *B*, that is, whether the effect of intensity of training depends on (interacts with) the frequency of training. This effect is tested by the F_{AB} ratio, which evaluates the six cell means: M_{A1B1}, M_{A1B2}, M_{A2B1}, M_{A2B2}, M_{A3B1}, and M_{A3B2}. Unless some special circumstance exists, interest in the testing of main effects is usually limited by the presence of a significant interaction, which means that what happens in one independent variable depends on the level of the other. Thus, normally it makes little sense to evaluate main effects when the interaction is significant.

This particular factorial ANOVA is labeled as a 3 (Intensity of Training) × 2 (Frequency of Training) ANOVA (read "3-by-2 ANOVA"). As the bottom of Table 8.2 indicates, the true variance can be divided into three parts:

factorial ANOVA — Analysis of variance in which there is more than one independent variable.

main effects — Tests of each independent variable when all other independent variables are held constant.

Table 8.2   Factorial (3 × 2) ANOVA Model

IV_2

Cell means

	B_1	B_2	
A_1	$M_{A_1B_1}$	$M_{A_1B_2}$	M_{A_1}
A_2	$M_{A_2B_1}$	$M_{A_2B_2}$	M_{A_2} Row means
A_3	$M_{A_3B_1}$	$M_{A_3B_2}$	M_{A_3}

IV_1

M_{B_1} M_{B_2}

Column means

IV_1—main effect is the test of the row means by F_A.
IV_2—main effect is the test of the column means by F_B.
The interaction is the test of the six cell means by F_{AB}.

F_A = (true variance due to A)/(error variance)
F_B = (true variance due to B)/(error variance)
F_{AB} = (true variance due to $A \times B$)/(error variance)

Table 8.3   The ABC Method for Calculating a Two-Way Factorial ANOVA

$A = \sum X^2$

$B = (\sum X)^2/N$

$C \text{ (rows)} = [(\sum X_{r_1})^2 + (\sum X_{r2})^2 + \ldots + (\sum X_{r_i})^2]/n_{r_1}$

$D \text{ (columns)} = [(\sum X_{c_1})^2 + (\sum X_{c2})^2 + \ldots + (\sum X_{c_j})^2]/n_{c_1}$

$E \text{ (}r \times c\text{)} = [(\sum X_{cell_1})^2 + (\sum X_{cell_2})^2 + \ldots + (\sum X_{cell_k})^2]/n_{cell_1}$

Summary table for ANOVA

Source	SS	df	MS	F
Rows (IV$_1$)	$C - B$	$r - 1$	SS_R/df_R	MS_R/MS_E
Columns (IV$_2$)	$D - B$	$c - 1$	SS_c/df_c	MS_c/MS_E
$R \times C$	$(E - B) - (C - B)$ $- (D - B)$	$(r - 1)(c - 1)$	SS_{RC}/df_{RC}	MS_{RC}/MS_E
Error	$(A - B) - (E - B)$	$(N - 1) - [(r - 1) + (c - 1)$ $+ (r - 1)(c - 1)]$	SS_E/df_E	
Total	$A - B$	$N - 1$		

where r = number of rows or levels of IV$_1$
      c = number of columns or levels of IV$_2$

- true variance due to *A* (intensity of training),
- true variance due to *B* (frequency of training), and
- true variance due to the interaction of *A* and *B*.

Each of these true variance components is tested against (divided by) error variance to form the three *F* ratios for this ANOVA. Each of these *F*s will have its own set of degrees of freedom so that it can be checked for significance in the *F* table in Appendix A.6. Table 8.3 gives the ABC method for calculating a two-way factorial ANOVA.

Example 8.12 then uses intensity of training and frequency of training as the independent variables and distance (in meters) covered on the 12-min run as the dependent variable. Thirty subjects are randomly assigned to one of the six groups ($ns = 5$). Thus, this is a 3 x 2 ANOVA. The test for intensity is significant, $F(2, 24) = 161.57$, $p < .05$.

Example 8.12

Known Values

IV_2 (frequency of exercise)

		2 d/wk		3 d/wk		
		X	X²	X	X²	
	40%	2,940	8,643,600	2,980	8,880,400	
		3,070	9,424,900	3,160	9,985,600	
		3,100	9,610,000	3,025	9,150,625	$\sum X_{r_1} = 30,285$
		2,925	8,555,625	3,045	9,272,025	
		3,050	9,302,500	2,990	8,940,100	
		X	X²	X	X²	
IV_1		3,150	9,922,500	3,720	13,838,400	
(intensity	60%	3,020	9,120,400	3,630	13,176,900	
of exercise)		2,990	8,940,100	3,570	12,744,900	$\sum X_{c_2} = 33,510$
		3,050	9,302,500	3,690	13,616,100	
		2,980	8,880,400	3,710	13,764,100	
		X	X²	X	X²	
		3,170	10,048,900	3,920	15,366,400	
	80%	3,120	9,734,400	4,040	16,321,600	
		3,050	9,302,500	4,110	16,892,100	$\sum X_{k_3} = 35,620$
		3,110	9,672,100	4,005	16,040,025	
		3,105	9,641,025	3,990	15,920,100	

$$\sum X_{c_1} = 45,830 \qquad \sum X_{c_2} = 53,585$$

Working It Out
(Table 8.3)

$A = \sum X^2 = 8{,}643{,}600 + 9{,}424{,}900 + \ldots + 15{,}920{,}100 = 334{,}010{,}825$

$B = (\sum X)^2 / N = (2{,}940 + 3{,}070 + 3{,}100 + \ldots + 3{,}990)^2 / 30 = 329{,}444{,}741$

$C = [(\sum X_{r_1})^2 + (\sum X_{r_2})^2 + (\sum X_{r_3})^2] / n_{r_1} = [(30{,}285)^2 + (33{,}510)^2 + (35{,}620)^2] / 10 = 330{,}888{,}573$

$D = [(\sum X_{c_1})^2 + (\sum X_{c_2})^2] / n_{c_1} = [(45{,}830)^2 + (53{,}585)^2] / 15 = 331{,}449{,}408$

$E = [(\sum X_{cell_1})^2 + (\sum X_{cell_2})^2 + \ldots + (\sum X_{cell_k})^2] n_{cell_1}$

$\quad = [(15{,}085)^2 + (15{,}200)^2 + (15{,}190)^2 + (18{,}320)^2 + (15{,}555)^2 + (20{,}065)^2] / 5 = 333{,}903{,}595$

Summary table for ANOVA

Source	SS	df	MS	F
Rows (A)	1,443,832	2	721,916	161.57*
Columns (B)	2,004,667	1	2,004,667	448.68*
A × B	1,010,355	2	505,177	113.07*
Error	107,230	24	4,468	. . .
Total	4,566,084	29	. . .	. . .

*$p <.05$.

This F is then followed up with a Scheffé test (Example 8.13), and we see that the 80% group performed significantly better than both the 60% and the 40% group, whereas the 60% group was significantly better than the 40% group.

Example 8.13

Known Values

Group	M	2	3
1 40%	3,028.5	7.62*	12.61*
2 60%	3,351.0	- -	4.99*
3 80%	3,562.0	- -	- -

*$p <.05$.

Working It Out

1. Calculate the critical Scheffé value (Equation 8.14).

$$t = \sqrt{(k-1)\, F^{\alpha}_{k-1, df, MS(W)}} = \sqrt{(3-1)\, 3.40} = 2.61$$

2. Calculate the t for each comparison (Equation 8.15).

$$t_{12} = (3,028.5 - 3,351.0)/\sqrt{(4,468/5)2} = 322.5/42.3 = 7.62$$
$$t_{13} = (3,028.5 - 3,562.0)/42.3 = 12.61$$
$$t_{23} = (3,351.0 - 3,562.0)/42.3 = 4.99$$

The test for frequency of training is also significant, $F(1, 24) = 448.68, p < .05$. However, no follow-up is required for this independent variable because there are only two levels (thus, in a factorial, t^2 approximately equals F). All that is necessary is to note that the 3-day-per-week condition ($M = 3772.3$) produces significantly better performance than the 2-day-per-week condition ($M = 3055.3$).

Finally, the test for the A × B interaction is significant, $F(2, 24) = 113.07, p < .05$. Thus, what happens with intensity of training depends on the frequency of the training. Figure 8.2 is a plot of this interaction. You can see that the three intensities of training are similar in effect on the 12-min run when training is 2 days per week. However, the 80% level is clearly the best at 3 days per week, and the 60% level is better than the 40% level. The 40% level is similar to all three intensities at the 2 days per week training frequency. In looking at this interaction, we might conclude that training 2 days per week or at 40% of

$\dot{V}O_2$max is not very effective. However, if the frequency of training is at least 3 days per week and at intensities of 60% of $\dot{V}O_2$max or higher, significant cardiorespiratory benefits (as measured by the 12-min run) occur.

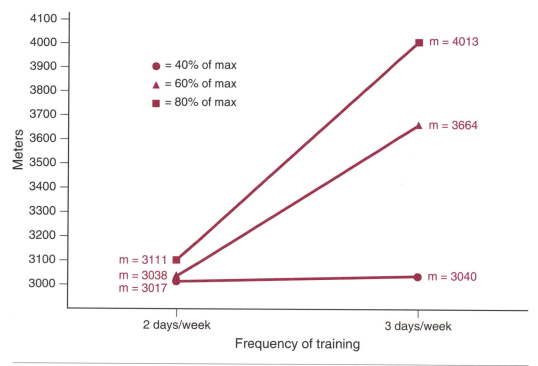

Figure 8.2   The plot of the interaction for a two-way factorial ANOVA.

As you can see, all we have done to follow up the significant interaction is to describe the plot in Figure 8.2 verbally. Considerable disagreement exists among researchers about how to follow up significant interactions. Some researchers use a multiple comparison of means test (such as Scheffé) to contrast the interaction cell means. However, these multiple comparison tests were developed for contrasting levels within an independent variable and not for cell means across two or more independent variables; thus, their use may be inappropriate. Other researchers use a follow-up called a test of simple main effects. In our example, this indicates that a multiple comparison test should be applied to the three cell means within the levels of the independent variable of *B*. That is, the three levels of intensity are tested against one another at the 2-day-per-week training and then at the 3-day-per-week training. If the interaction is to be followed up with a statistical test, simple main effects using the Scheffé procedure would be the preferred technique.

Our preference for evaluating an interaction is to do as we have done: plot the interaction and describe it. This takes into account the true nature of an interaction; that is, what happens in one independent variable depends on the other. However, you are likely to encounter all these ways of testing interactions (and probably some others) as you read the research literature. Just remember that the researcher is trying to show you how the two or more independent variables interact. Also remember that follow-ups on main effects are usually unnecessary (or at least the interpretation must be qualified) when the interaction is significant. Although we have done the follow-ups in this example to help you better understand the procedures, the follow-ups would be of limited interest in the presence of a significant and meaningful interaction.

Determining Meaningfulness of Results

We have now answered the first statistical question about a factorial ANOVA: What are the significant effects? As in previous examples, we now turn to the meaningfulness of the effects, or what percent of the variance in the dependent variable is accounted for by the independent variables and their interaction? The three formulas that follow (from Tolson, 1980) provide the (formula) test for each component of ANOVA:

$$\omega^2_A = \frac{(p-1)F_A - (p-1)}{(p-1)F_A + (q-1)F_B + (p-1)(q-1)F_{AB} + (N-pq) + 1}$$

$$\omega^2_B = \frac{(q-1)F_B - (q-1)}{(p-1)F_A + (q-1)F_B + (p-1)(q-1)F_{AB} + (N-pq) + 1} \quad (8.17)$$

$$\omega^2_{AB} = \frac{(p-1)(q-1)F_{AB} - (p-1)(q-1)}{(p-1)F_A + (q-1)F_B + (p-1)(q-1)F_{AB} + (N-pq) + 1}$$

where p = the number of levels of A, and q = the number of levels of B. These formulas involve the proportion of true variance to total variance. Note that once you calculate total variance, that value remains the same for the test of all three proportions. In Example 8.14 we have applied Formula 8.17 to the Fs calculated in Example 8.12.

Example 8.14

Known Values

$F_A = 161.57$
$F_B = 448.68$
$F_{AB} = 113.07$
Number of levels of A: $p = 3$
Number of levels of B: $q = 2$
Number of subjects: $N = 30$

Working It Out
(Equation 8.17)

$$\omega^2 = \frac{(3-1)161.57 - (3-1)}{(3-1)161.57 + (2-1)448.68 + (3-1)(2-1)113.07 + (30-6) + 1}$$

$$= \frac{2(161.57) - 2}{(2)161.57 + (1)448.68 + (2)(1)113.07 + 24 + 1}$$

$$= \frac{321.14}{323.14 + 448.68 + 226.14 + 25} = \frac{321.14}{1,022.96} = .31$$

$$\omega_B^2 = \frac{(2-1)448.00 - (2-1)}{1,022.96} = \frac{447}{1,022.96} = .44$$

$$\omega_{AB}^2 = \frac{(3-1)(2-1)113.07 - (3-1)(2-1)}{1,022.96} = \frac{226.14 - 2}{1,022.96} = \frac{224.14}{1,022.96} = .22$$

Each ω^2 represents the percent variance accounted for by that component of the ANOVA model. The ω^2s can be summed to estimate the percent of the total variance that is true variance. Thus, the independent variable of intensity accounts for 31% of the true variance; the independent variable of frequency accounts for 44% of the true variance; the interaction accounts for 22% of the true variance; and the total true variance is 97%. Of course, effect sizes can be calculated according to the previous equations (8.7 and 8.8) for any two means that you want to compare for main effects.

Summarizing Factorial ANOVA

Our discussion of simple and factorial ANOVA has dealt with studies in which the levels of the independent variables have the subjects randomly assigned. This is not always the case. Frequently, levels of the independent variable may be categorical (also called classification) in nature. For example, we could do a simple ANOVA in which the levels (or groups) of the independent variable involve novice and expert tennis players. Or, in the previously presented factorial ANOVA, we could look at the effects of intensity of training (40%, 60%, and 80% of $\dot{V}O_2$max) 3 days per week, 20 min per day for 12 weeks as one independent variable (three levels) and have the other independent be categorical (e.g., gender). That is, we would be interested in whether intensity of training affected males and females differently. The levels of the first independent variable have subjects randomly assigned, whereas subjects cannot be randomly assigned to the categorical variable (one is either male or female). Another common use of categorical variables involves age levels. A study might look at the effects of the levels of a treatment independent variable (where subjects are randomly assigned) on 6-, 9-, and 12-year-old females. Clearly, the interest in this type of factorial ANOVA is the interaction: Does the effectiveness of treatment differ according to the age of the child?

Repeated Measures ANOVA

Much of the research in the study of physical activity involves studies that measure the same dependent variable more than once. For example, a study in sport psychology might investigate whether athletes' **state anxiety** (how nervous they feel at the time) differs before and after a game. Thus, a state-anxiety inventory would be given just preceding and immediately following the game. The question of interest is, Does pregame state anxiety change significantly after the game? A dependent *t* test could be used to see whether significant changes occurred. This is the simplest case of **repeated measures ANOVA**.

Another study might have subjects measured on the dependent variable on several occasions. Suppose we wanted to know whether children (between ages 6 and 8) would increase the distance they threw a ball using an overhand throwing pattern. We decide to measure the children's distance throw every 3 months during the 2 years of the study. Thus, the children were assessed eight times on how far each could throw. We now have eight repeated measures on the same children. We would use a simple ANOVA with repeated measures on the one factor. Basically, the repeated measures is used as eight levels of the independent variable, which is time (24 months).

The most frequent use of repeated measures involves a factorial ANOVA, in which one or more of the factors (independent variables) are repeated measures. An example is an investigation of the effects of knowledge of results (KR) on skilled motor performance. There are three groups of subjects (three levels of independent variable) who receive varying types of KR (no KR, short or long of the target, and number of centimeters short or long of the target). The task is to position a handle that slides back and forth on a trackway (called a **linear slide**) as close to the target as possible. But the

---

state anxiety — An immediate emotional state of apprehension and tension in response to a specific situation.

repeated measures ANOVA — Analysis of scores on the same individuals on successive occasions such as a series of test trials; also called *split-plot ANOVA* or *subject × trials ANOVA.*

linear slide — A motor task in which a blindfolded subject attempts to move a nearfrictionless handle down a trackway to some specified location or a certain distance.

subjects are blindfolded, so they cannot see the target. They have only verbal KR to correct their estimates of where the target is located along the trackway.

In this type of study, subjects are usually given multiple trials (assume 30 trials in this example) so that the effects of the quality of KR can be judged. The score on each trial is error from the target in centimeters. This type of study is frequently analyzed as a two-way factorial ANOVA with repeated measures on the second factor. Thus, a 3 (Levels of KR) × 30 (Trials) ANOVA with error as the dependent variable is used to analyze the data. The first independent variable (levels of KR) is a true one (three groups are randomly formed). The second independent variable (30 trials) is repeated measures. Sometimes this ANOVA is called a two-way factorial ANOVA with one between-subjects factor (levels of KR) and one within-subjects factor (30 repeated trials). Although an *F* ratio is calculated for each independent variable, the major focus is usually on the interaction. For example, do the groups change at different rates across the trials?

Advantages of Repeated Measures

Repeated measures designs have three advantages (Pedhazur, 1982). First, they provide the experimenter the opportunity to control for individual differences among subjects, probably the largest source of variation in most studies. In between-subject designs (completely randomized), the variation among subjects goes into the error term. Of course, this tends to reduce the *F* ratio unless it is offset by a large number of subjects. Remember, the error term of the *F* ratio consists of dividing the variation among subjects by the degrees of freedom (based on the number of subjects). In repeated measures designs, variation from individual differences can be identified and separated from the error term, thereby reducing it and increasing power. As you can deduce from the first advantage, repeated measures designs are more economical in that fewer subjects are required. Finally, repeated measures designs allow the study of a phenomenon across time. This is particularly important in studies of change in, for example, learning, fatigue, forgetting, performance, and aging.

Problems of Repeated Measures

Several problems adversely affect repeated measures designs, including the following:

- **Carryover effects**. Treatments given earlier influence those treatments given later.
- **Practice effects**. Subjects get better at the task (dependent variables) as a result of repeated trials in addition to the treatment (also called the testing effect).
- **Fatigue**. Subjects' performance is adversely influenced by fatigue (or boredom).
- **Sensitization**. Subjects' awareness of the treatment is heightened because of repeated exposure.

Note that some problems may be the variables of interest in repeated measures designs. Carryover effects may interest the researcher of learning, whereas increased fatigue over trials may intrigue an exercise physiologist.

    The tricky part of repeated measures designs involves how to analyze the data statistically. We have already mentioned ANOVA models with repeated measures. Unfortunately, these repeated measures ANOVAs have an assumption

---

 Four issues that adversely affect repeated measures

 spherity — An assumption with regard to repeated measures to the effect that they are uncorrelated and have equal variance.

beyond the ones we have given for all techniques. This assumption is called **sphericity**: The repeated measures, "when transformed by a set of orthonormal weights, are uncorrelated with each other and have equal variances" (Schutz & Gessaroli, 1987, p. 134). If the design has a between-subjects factor, the pooled data (across all subjects) must exhibit sphericity. How well the data meet these assumptions is best estimated by a statistic called epsilon (ϵ). Epsilon ranges from 1.0 (perfect sphericity, the assumption is met) to 0.0 (complete violation). An epsilon above .75 is desirable in repeated measures experiments. Most of the widely used statistical packages (SPSS and BIMED) have repeated measures programs that provide both estimates of epsilon and tests that should be used to evaluate the F ratio for the repeated measures factors in the designs. The failure to meet this assumption results in an increase in Type I error; that is, the alpha level may be considerably larger than the researcher intended. Several statisticians (Davidson, 1972; Harris, 1985; Morrow & Frankiewicz, 1979) have suggested that multivariate techniques are the more appropriate means of analysis. However, two additional points are important (Pedhazur, 1982):

- When the assumptions are met, the ANOVA with repeated measures is more powerful than the multivariate tests.
- If the number of subjects is small, only the ANOVA repeated measures test can be used.

    If you are contemplating conducting a study that uses a repeated measures design, then an additional source of reading should be helpful to you. Schutz and Gessaroli (1987) provide a tutorial on the use of repeated measures for univariate and multivariate data that gives a sound rationale for making decisions as well as specific examples of how the data may be analyzed and evaluated.

Calculating Repeated Measures

Table 8.4 provides the formulas (ABC method) used to calculate a one-way ANOVA with repeated measures. This analysis may also be called a **subject × trials ANOVA**, within subjects ANOVA, or a two-way ANOVA with one subject per cell. Example 8.15 works out the calculations.

Table 8.4   The ABC Method for Calculating One-Way Repeated Measures ANOVA

$A = \sum X^2$

$B = (\sum X)^2/N$

$C \text{ (subjects)} = [(\sum X_{r_1})^2 + (\sum X_{r_2})^2 + \ldots + (\sum X_{r_i})^2]/n_s$

$D \text{ (trials)} = [(\sum X_{c_1})^2 + (\sum X_{c_2})^2 + \ldots + (\sum X_{c_j})^2]/n_t$

where n_t = number of trials and n_s = number of subjects

(cont.)

 Two criteria that require the use of repeated measures ANOVA

 Schutz, R.W., & Gessaroli, M.E. (1987). The analysis of repeated measures designs involving multiple dependent variables. *Research Quarterly for Exercise and Sport*, **58**, 132–149.

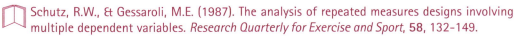 **subject × trials ANOVA** — See *repeated measures ANOVA* (page 167).

Table 8.4   (cont.)

Source	SS	Summary table for ANOVA df	MS	F
Subjects	$C - B$	$r - 1$	SS_S/df_S	MS_S/MS_R
Trials	$D - B$	$c - 1$	SS_T/df_T	MS_T/MS_R
Residual	$A - B - [(C - B) + (D - B)]$	$(r - 1)(c - 1)$	SS_R/df_R	. . .
Total	$A - B$	$N - 1$	. . .	. . .

where r = number of subjects
c = number of trials
N = number of scores (no. subjects × no. trials)

Example 8.15

Known Values

Subjects	Trial 1 X	Trial 1 X^2	Trial 2 X	Trial 2 X^2	Trial 3 X	Trial 3 X^2
1	12	144	9	81	6	36
2	10	100	7	49	7	49
3	11	121	6	36	2	4
4	7	49	9	81	3	9
5	10	100	4	16	2	4
	50	514	35	263	20	102
$\overline{M}$	10	. . .	7	. . .	4	. . .

Working It Out

$A = \sum X^2 = 514 + 263 + 102 = 879$

$B = (\sum X)^2/N = (50 + 35 + 20)^2/15 = (105)^2/15 = 11{,}025/15 = 735$

$C = (\sum X_{r_1})^2 + (\sum X_{r_2})^2 + \ldots + (\sum X_{r_i})^2/n_{r_1}$

$= [(12 + 9 + 6)^2 + (10 + 7 + 7)^2 + (11 + 6 + 2)^2 + (7 + 9 + 3)^2 + (10 + 4 + 2)^2]/3$

$= [27^2 + 24^2 + 19^2 + 19^2 + 16^2]/3 = 2{,}283/3 = 761.00$

$D = [(\sum X_{c_1})^2 + (\sum X_{c_2})^2 + \ldots + (\sum X_{c_j})^2]/n_{c_1}$

$= [50^2 + 35^2 + 20^2]/5 = 4{,}125/5 = 825.00$

Source	SS	Summary table for ANOVA df	MS	F
Subjects	26.00	4	. . .	. . .
Trials	90.00	2	45.00	12.86*
Residual	28.00	8	3.50	. . .
Total	144.00	14	. . .	. . .

Note. $\epsilon = 1.00$; no adjustment of *dfs* when $\epsilon = 1.0$.

*$p < .05$.

The example used here is the data from Example 8.9, in which Groups 1, 2, and 3 are labeled across the top. Note in Example 8.15 that the group designation has been changed to Trials 1, 2, and 3. Thus, where previously (Example 8.9) we had three groups of five subjects ($n = 15$), we now have five subjects, each measured on three trials of a task. The reason for doing this is that when Examples 8.15 and 8.9 are compared, you can see why the repeated measures design results in increased economy. Notice that the total sum of squares and degrees of freedom are the same. Also, the between effect (Example 8.9) and trials effect (Example 8.15) are the same. However, the sum of squares for the within effect (error) in Example 8.9 has been divided into two components in the repeated measures analysis (Example 8.15). The residual effect (estimating error) has a sum of squares of 28.00 with 8 *df*, and the subjects effect has a sum of squares of 26.00 with 4 *df*. This results in an *F* ratio for the repeated measures ANOVA (Example 8.15) being larger than that for the simple ANOVA (Example 8.9) despite having only one third the number of subjects. The sum of squares for subjects in Example 8.15 is not tested and simply represents the normal variation among subjects. Thus, across the three trials, the subjects' mean performance decreased significantly (Trial 1 = 10, Trial 2 = 7, and Trial 3 = 4). This analysis has all the strengths and weaknesses previously discussed.

Example 8.15 includes the epsilon estimate from this analysis, which was obtained by running a repeated measures computer program from SPSS PC. If epsilon is less than 1.00, the degrees of freedom would have been adjusted according to $df \times \epsilon = $ adjusted *df*. This is done for the degrees of freedom in both the numerator and the denominator of any *F* ratio that includes the repeated measures factor.

 A very conservative approach to this adjustment (called **Geisser/Greenhouse correction**) can also be done (Stamm & Safrit, 1975) as follows:

$$\theta = 1/(k-1) \qquad (8.18)$$

where k = the number of repeated measures. Then we multiply the degrees of freedom for trials by this value, $\theta(k-1)$, as well as the degrees of freedom for error, $\theta[(n-1)(k-1)]$. These adjusted degrees of freedom (to the nearest whole *df*) are used to look up the *F* ratio in the *F* table. If the *F* ratio is significant under the conservative test, then the effect likely is a real one. However, this procedure was advocated several years ago, and with the tests of the repeated measures designs now available, a computer program providing the epsilon estimate is more appropriate.

Analysis of Covariance

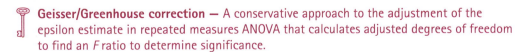

Using ANCOVA

Limitations of ANCOVA

 Analysis of covariance (ANCOVA) is a combination of regression and ANOVA. The technique is used to adjust the dependent variable for some distractor variable (called the **covariate**).

 Geisser/Greenhouse correction — A conservative approach to the adjustment of the epsilon estimate in repeated measures ANOVA that calculates adjusted degrees of freedom to find an *F* ratio to determine significance.

analysis of covariance (ANCOVA) — A combination of regression and ANOVA that statistically adjusts the dependent variable for some distractor variable called the *covariate*.

covariate — A distractor variable that is statistically controlled in ANCOVA and MANCOVA.

Using ANCOVA

Suppose we want to evaluate the effects of a training program to develop leg power on the time required to run 50 m. However, we know that reaction time (RT) will influence the 50-m dash time because those who begin more quickly after the start signal have an advantage. We form two groups, measure RT in each group, train one with our power development program while the other serves as a control group, and measure each subject's time for running 50 m. This is a study in which ANCOVA might be used to analyze the data. There is an independent variable with two levels (power training and control), a dependent variable (50-m dash time), and an important distractor variable, or covariate (RT).

Analysis of a covariance is a two-step process in which an adjustment is first made for the 50-m-dash score of each subject according to his or her RT. A correlation (r) is calculated between RT and the time in the 50-m dash. The resulting prediction equation, 50-m-dash time = $a + (b)$RT (same as formula = $a + bX$), is used to calculate each subject's predicted 50-m-dash time ($\tilde{Y}$). The difference between the actual 50-m-dash time (Y) and the predicted time ($\tilde{Y}$) is called the residual ($Y - \tilde{Y}$). A simple ANOVA is then calculated using each subject's residual score as the dependent variable* (1 df for within sums of squares is lost because of the correlation). This allows an evaluation of 50-m-dash speed with RT controlled.

Analysis of covariance can be used in factorial situations and with more than one covariate. The results are evaluated as in ANOVA except one or more distractor variables are controlled. Also, ANCOVA is frequently used in situations in which a pretest is given, some treatment applied, and then a posttest given. The pretest is used as the covariate in this type of analysis. Note that in the preceding section (Repeated Measures ANOVA) we indicated that this same situation could be analyzed by repeated measures. In addition, ANCOVA is used when comparing intact groups because the groups' performances (dependent variable) can be adjusted for distractor variables (covariates) on which they differ.

Limitations of ANCOVA

Although ANCOVA may seem to be the answer to many problems, its use does have limitations. In particular, its use to adjust final performance for initial differences can result in misleading interpretations (Lord, 1969). In addition, if the correlations between the covariate and the dependent variable are not equal across the treatment groups, standard ANCOVA (there are nonstandard ANCOVA techniques) is inappropriate.

Experimentwise Error Rate

Sometimes researchers make several comparisons on different dependent variables while using the same subjects. Usually, use of a multivariate technique (discussed in the next chapter) is the appropriate solution. However, when dependent variables are combinations of other dependent variables (e.g., cardiac output is Heart Rate x Stroke Volume), a multivariate model using all three dependent variables is

Thomas, J.R. (1977). A note concerning analysis of error scores from motor-memory research. *Journal of Motor Behavior*, **9**, 251-253.

*Actually, the procedure is slightly different, but the concept is correct.

inappropriate. (This book is not the appropriate place to explain why. For more detail, see Thomas, 1977). Thus, an ANOVA among three groups might be calculated separately for each dependent measure (i.e., three ANOVAs). The problem is that this procedure results in increasing the alpha that has been established for the experiment. One of two solutions is appropriate for adjusting alpha. The first, called the Bonferroni technique, simply divides the alpha level by the number of comparisons to be made:

$$\alpha_{EW} = \alpha/c \qquad (8.19)$$

where α_{EW} = alpha corrected for the experimentwise error rate, α = alpha, and c = the number of comparisons. In our example, if a = .05 and c = 3, then the alpha for each comparison is .05/3 or .017. This means that the F ratio would have to reach an alpha of .017 to be declared significant.

The second option is to leave the overall alpha at .05 but to calculate the upper limit that the alpha might be:

$$\alpha_{UL} = 1 - (1 - \alpha)^k \qquad (8.20)$$

where α_{UL} = alpha (upper limit) and k = the number of groups. Again, using our example, $\alpha_{UL} = 1 - (1 - .05)^3 = .14$. Thus, the hypotheses are really being tested somewhere between an alpha of .05 if the dependent variables are perfectly correlated and .14 if they are independent. In instances where researchers make multiple comparisons using the same subjects, they should either adjust alpha to the experimentwise rate or at least report the upper limit on their alpha.

Summary

This chapter has presented techniques used in situations in which differences among groups are the focus of attention. These techniques are categorized into two groups:

- A t test is used to determine how a group differs from a population, how two groups differ, how one group changes from one occasion to the next, and how several means differ (the multiple range tests).
- ANOVA shows differences among the levels of one independent variable (simple ANOVA), among the levels of two or more independent variables (factorial ANOVA), and among levels of independent variables when there is a distractor variable or covariate (ANCOVA).

Table 8.5 provides an overall look at the techniques of this chapter and chapter 7 (relationships among variables) regarding their appropriate use. Note that there are tech-

Table 8.5   Comparison of Statistical Techniques From Chapters 7 and 8

Description	Differences among groups	Relationships among variables
1 IV (2 levels) → 1 dv	Independent t test	. . .
1 predictor → 1 criterion	. . .	Pearson r
1 IV (2 or more levels) → 1 dv	Simple ANOVA	. . .
2 or more IVs → 1 dv	Factorial ANOVA	. . .
2 or more predictors → 1 criterion	. . .	Multiple regression

niques for relationships among variables that parallel each technique for differences among groups. In fact, the relationship between t and r that was demonstrated earlier in this chapter holds, as ANOVA techniques are the equivalent of multiple regression. Each technique evaluates our two basic questions: Is the effect or relationship significant? Is the effect or relationship meaningful?

Some ideas presented here are complex and may not be easily understood in one reading. We provide some suggested readings and problems in this chapter that should be helpful. If you do not feel confident in your understanding of this material, reread the chapter, do the problems, and consult some of the suggested readings. This is important because information in Parts III and IV will assume that you understand Part II.

 ## Check Your Understanding

1. Critique the statistical part of a study that uses an independent t test.
2. Calculate ω^2 for t in this study.
3. Find a study that uses a multiple range test (Newman-Keuls, Duncan's, or Scheffé) as a follow-up to ANOVA and critique the use of this test.
4. Two groups of 7-year-olds are asked to jog 35m down a string placed on the ground. Then they are asked to reproduce the distance jogged on a second string placed at a right angle to the first. One group (experimental) is cued before they begin that the best way to remember the distance is to count the number of steps. The control is just told to remember however they can. Below is the error in meters each subject made when estimating the 35m jogged on the second trial.

Experimental group		Control group	
S_1	2.55	S_8	7.68
S_2	3.62	S_9	6.80
S_3	3.42	S_{10}	5.68
S_4	2.86	S_{11}	3.97
S_5	2.00	S_{12}	7.23
S_6	1.08	S_{13}	5.48
S_7	1.16	S_{14}	6.03

   a. Are the two groups significantly different (alpha = .05)?
   b. What percent variance is accounted for by the treatment?
   c. Place the following statistics into a table: M and s for each group; t; df; ω^2
   d. Did the use of a counting strategy produce a reliable and meaningful performance difference for the experimental group when compared with the control group? Justify your answer.

5. Critique the statistical part of a study that uses simple ANOVA. Calculate ω^2 for F.
6. Critique the statistical part of a study that uses a two-way factorial ANOVA. Calculate ω^2 for each factor and the interaction.
7. Critique a repeated measures study that uses ANOVA.

CHAPTER 9

Understanding Multivariate Techniques

Dear Professors of Research Methods:

I recently went to the Statistical Advising Center on my campus to ask for help on the analysis of my master's thesis data. When I finished, the statistical consultant told me I had three independent variables, five dependent variables, and two covariates and that I needed to use MANCOVA. When I told my major professor, he just looked at me and said, "You've got to be kidding!!" What should I do?

Thanks for your advice,
I.M. Panicked

Dear Panicked:

Well, you have several options: You can take four sequenced statistics courses that will take you through MANCOVA (and two more years of study), or you can drop out of school. However, our advice is to handle it like a diagnosis from a doctor that you have doubts about—GET ANOTHER OPINION. This time we suggest you get advice from a person on this planet, or at least from our solar system.

Thinking of you graduating,
PRM

Up to this point we have discussed experimental research examples involving one or more independent variables but only one dependent variable. Multivariate cases have one or more independent variables and two or more dependent variables. For example, it seems more likely that when independent variables are manipulated, they influence more than one thing. The multivariate case allows for more than one dependent variable. To use techniques that allow only one dependent variable (called **univariate techniques**) repeatedly when there are several dependent variables increases the experimentwise error rate (sometimes called **probability pyramiding**) in the same way as doing multiple *t* tests instead of simple ANOVA when there are more than two groups. However, there are instances where using univariate techniques in a study that has multiple dependent variables is acceptable or the only choice. For example, as with all research, theory should drive decision making. You might not want to include a theoretically important dependent variable in a multivariate analysis when less theoretically important dvs could disguise its importance. Also, sometimes because the study has a small number of subjects, using multivariate techniques is just not feasible.

In evaluating relationships among variables, we have discussed having one predictor and one criterion (regression) and several predictors and one criterion (multiple regression). As with multivariate techniques for experimental data, correlational data often have several predictors and several criteria; whether variables are predictors or criteria is not always clear. In this chapter we explain various multivariate techniques frequently found in the physical education, exercise science, and sport science literature. Techniques often used in experimental studies are

- discriminant analysis,
- multivariate ANOVA (and special cases with repeated measures designs), and
- multivariate ANCOVA.

In correlational studies, techniques often used include

- canonical correlation,
- factor analysis, and
- structural modeling (often called **path analysis** or LISREL).

Remember, however, that the general linear model still underlies all the techniques, and we are still attempting to learn two things: Are we evaluating something significant (reliable)? How meaningful are significant findings?

Discriminant Analysis

Forward, Backward, and Stepwise Selection
An Example of Discriminant Analysis

 univariate technique — Statistical technique applied in the analysis of only one dependent variable.

probability pyramiding — The increasing probability of experimentwise error inherent in the application of repeated univariate tests on multiple dependent variables.

 Multivariate and correlational techniques of statistical analysis

 path analysis — Technique used to explain how certain characteristics relate to each other, with the hope of implying cause, by using correlations among all the variables to estimate the linkages among measures.

We use **discriminant analysis** when we have one independent variable (two or more levels) and two or more dependent variables. The technique combines multiple regression and simple ANOVA. In effect, discriminant analysis uses a combination of the dependent variable to predict or discriminate among the levels of the independent variable, which in this case is group membership. In the discussion of multiple regression in chapter 7, we used several predictor variables in a linear combination to predict a criterion variable. In essence, discriminant analysis does the same thing except that several dependent variables are used in a linear combination to predict which group a subject belongs to or to discriminate among two or more groups. This prediction of group membership is the equivalent of discriminating among the groups (recall how t could be calculated by r). The same methods used in multiple regression to identify the important predictors are used in discriminant analysis. These include forward, backward, and stepwise selection techniques. For greater detail as well as a useful and practical description of discriminant analysis, read Betz (1987).

Forward, Backward, and Stepwise Selection

As mentioned in chapter 7, the forward selection technique enters the dependent variables in the order of their importance; that is, the dependent variable that contributes the most to separation of the groups (discriminates among or predicts group membership the best) is entered first. By correlation techniques, the effect of the first dependent variable on all others is removed, and the dependent variable that contributes the next greatest amount to separation of the groups is entered at Step 2. This procedure continues until all dependent variables have been entered or until some criterion for stopping the process (established by the researcher) is met.

The backward selection procedure is similar except that all the dependent variables are entered and the one contributing the least to group separation is removed. This continues until the only variables remaining are those that contribute significantly to the separation of the groups.

The stepwise technique is similar to forward selection except that at each step all the dependent variables are evaluated to see whether each still contributes to group separation. If a dependent variable does not contribute, it is stepped out (removed) from the linear combination just as in multiple regression.

An Example of Discriminant Analysis

Example 9.1 shows how discriminant analysis with a forward selection technique can be used for choosing significant dependent variables.

---

discriminant analysis — A multivariate statistical technique that is used when there is one independent variable, with two or more levels, and two or more dependent variables.

Betz, N.E. (1987). Use of discriminant analysis in counseling psychology research. *Journal of Counseling Psychology*, **34**, 393-403.

Example 9.1

Original variables (df = 2, 81)

Variable	R^2	F	Probability
40-yd dash	.36	23.11	.0001
12-min run	.08	3.65	.03
Shuttle run	.21	10.48	.0001
Vertical jump	.30	17.25	.0001
Standing long jump	.27	14.85	.0001
Bench press	.39	25.90	.0001
Squat	.13	5.87	.004

Forward selection summary

Step	Variable entered	F to enter	Probability of F	Average squared canonical correlation
1	Bench press	25.90	.0001	.20
2	40-yd dash	28.22	.0001	.34
3	Vertical jump	3.21	.05	.35

$F = (6, 158) = 19.46, p < .0001$

Variables not in the equation (df = 2, 78)

Variable	R^2	F	Probability
12-min run	.03	1.19	.31
Shuttle run	.00	0.05	.95
Standing long jump	.02	0.94	.40
Squat	.06	2.42	.10

In this study (Tew & Wood, 1980), varsity football players were classified into three groups: offensive and defensive backs, offensive and defensive linemen, and linebackers and receivers. Data were collected for 28 athletes in each group (N = 84) on seven variables: 40-yd dash, 12-min run, shuttle run, vertical jump, standing long jump, bench press, and squat. Discriminant analysis was applied to determine how many of the seven dependent variables were needed to separate (predict) the three groups of football players. The top of Example 9.1 shows the seven original variables with the R^2s (estimates of percent variance accounted for) and the Fs for each variable. This F is only a simple ANOVA on this variable for the three groups. As you can see, the three groups are significantly different ($p < .05$) on all seven variables. The question not answered is, What is the relationship among these seven variables for the 84 athletes? For example, the shuttle run (which requires speed) would be expected to relate highly to the 40-yd dash.

Applying Discriminant Analysis

In applying discriminant analysis, we set two criteria for the statistical computer program, namely, to include the variable at each step with the largest F ratio and to stop when no remaining variable has an F significant at $p < .05$. By looking at the original variables in Example 9.1, you can see which one will be entered at Step 1. The bench press is entered because it has the biggest F (25.90). The program then uses a semipartial correlation procedure to remove the effects of the bench press from the remaining six dependent variables. Note that the 40-yd dash is included next at Step 2. If you looked at the computer printout (not provided here), you would see that the 40-yd dash has the largest F (28.22) at Step 2 (you should now be looking at forward selection summary in the middle of Example 9.1). At Step 3 the vertical jump is entered ($F = 3.21$, $p < .05$) because it has the largest F among the remaining five dependent variables when they are adjusted for the bench press and the 40-yd dash. At this point, none of the four remaining dependent variables had significant Fs, so the program provides the overall test of the linear composite of the dependent variables' (bench press, 40-yd dash, and vertical jump) ability to separate the three groupings of players, $F(6, 158) = 19.46$, $p < .0001$. On the right of the forward selection summary is the averaged squared canonical correlation, which is cumulative at each step. This is an estimation of the percent variance accounted for (20% with the first variable, 34% with the first and second variables, and 35% with all three). At the bottom of Example 9.1 are the dependent variables not included in the discriminant analysis equation. Note that none of the remaining four dependent variables is significant in its ability to separate the three groups when the effects of the bench press, 40-yd dash, and vertical jump are removed. This means that the characteristics underlying performance in the three dependent variables included are the same characteristics underlying performance in the four not included. Except for the 12-min run, this seems to be a reasonably good explanation. But note that it did not discriminate very effectively among the groups to begin with ($F = 3.65$, $p < .03$, 8% variance accounted for). This really addresses the issue of why the 12-min run would be expected to discriminate among football players, as their training regimens are not designed to develop cardiovascular endurance.

Following Up Discriminant Analysis

We might want to follow up the discriminant analysis with univariate techniques to determine which groups actually differed from one another on each of the three dependent variables included. There are several ways to approach this follow-up, but for simplicity, consider the fact that you could perform the Scheffé test among the three groups on the first dependent variable. Then, ANCOVA could be done among the three groups on the second dependent variable using the first dependent variable as a covariate. This would provide adjusted means (means of the second dependent variable corrected for the first) on the second dependent variable. A Scheffé test could be done among the adjusted means using the adjusted mean square for error. This procedure is continued through each dependent variable using the previously stepped-in dependent variables as covariates and is called a **stepdown F technique**. There are additional ways to follow up discriminant analysis.

Summarizing Discriminant Analysis

As you can see, we have used discriminant analysis in a situation in which the three groups were intact (i.e., not randomly formed). This is a very common application of discriminant analysis. However, discriminant analysis does not overcome the need to form the groups randomly if determination of cause and effect is the purpose of the research.

---

stepdown F technique — A procedure used as a follow-up in multivariate analysis to determine the actual differences among groups.

Discriminant analysis can also be used to place people into groups. We could write a prediction equation—$\tilde{Y} = a + $ bench press (B_1) + 40-yard dash (B_2) + vertical jump (B_3)—that could be used to classify players as backs, linemen, and linebackers and receivers. However, given that only 35% of the variance is accounted for in this model, the usefulness of this prediction equation could be questioned. Of course, football coaches would love to find a valid and reliable equation of this type because the tests could be given to high school athletes to predict those players who might be successful at the various positions on college teams.

Multivariate Analysis of Variance

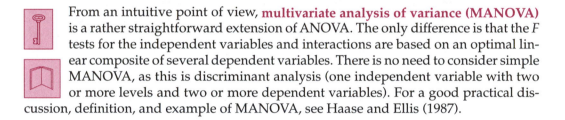

Using MANOVA

An Example of MANOVA

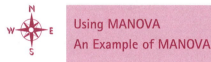 From an intuitive point of view, **multivariate analysis of variance (MANOVA)** is a rather straightforward extension of ANOVA. The only difference is that the F tests for the independent variables and interactions are based on an optimal linear composite of several dependent variables. There is no need to consider simple MANOVA, as this is discriminant analysis (one independent variable with two or more levels and two or more dependent variables). For a good practical discussion, definition, and example of MANOVA, see Haase and Ellis (1987).

Using MANOVA

The mathematics is complex for factorial MANOVA, but the idea is simple. An optimal combination (linear composite) of the dependent variables is made that will maximally account for (predict) the variance associated with the independent variables. The variance associated with each independent variable is then separated out (like in ANOVA), and a test of each of the independent variables and interactions on the optimal linear composite is done. Each test has an associated F and degrees of freedom interpreted as F for ANOVA. There are several ways to obtain this F in MANOVA: Wilks' lambda, Pillai's trace, Hotelling's trace, and Roy's greatest characteristic root. We point this out only because authors sometimes identify how the MANOVA Fs were obtained. For your purposes, these distinctions are not important: Consider only that the MANOVA F ratios are similar to ANOVA F ratios.

Once MANOVA has been used, a significant linear composite of dependent variables is identified as separating the levels of the independent variable. Then, the important question usually is, Which of the dependent variables contributes significantly to this separation? One of many ways to answer this question is to use discriminant analysis and the stepdown F procedures discussed in the previous section as follow-up techniques. This works well for the main effects but not so well for interactions. Interactions in MANOVA are most frequently handled by calculating factorial ANOVA for each de-

 multivariate analysis of variance (MANOVA) — Analysis of variance wherein a combination of dependent variables is made that will maximally separate the levels of the independent variables.

Haase, R.F., & Ellis, M.V.(1987). Multivariate analysis of variance. *Journal of Counseling Psychology*, **34**, 404–413.

pendent variable, although this procedure fails to consider the relationships among the dependent variables.

An Example of MANOVA

As an example of the use and follow-up of MANOVA, consider an experiment reported by French and Thomas (1987). One aspect of this study was to evaluate the influence of two groupings of age level (8- to 10-year-olds and 11- to 12-year-olds) and level of expertise (expert and novice players within each age level) on basketball knowledge and performance. A basketball knowledge test and two basketball skill tests (shooting and dribbling) were given to all the children. Following is French and Thomas' description of these particular results:

> A 2 × 2 (Age League × Expert/Novice) MANOVA was conducted on the scores of the knowledge test and both skill tests. The results of the MANOVA indicated significant main effects for age league, $F(3, 50) = 5.81$, $p < .01$, expert/novice, $F(3, 50) = 28.01$, $p < .01$, but no significant interaction. These main effects were followed up by a stepdown procedure using a forward selection discriminant analysis. The alpha level used as a basis for stepping in variables was set at .05. The discriminant analysis for age league revealed that knowledge was stepped in first, $F(1, 54) = 8.31$, $p < .01$. Neither skill test was entered. Older children ($M = 79.5$) possessed more knowledge than younger children ($M = 64.9$). The discriminant analysis for expert/novice revealed shooting was stepped in first, $F(1, 54) = 61.40$, $p < .01$; knowledge second, $F(1, 53) = 5.51$, $p < .05$; and dribbling was not entered. Child experts ($M = 47.2$) performed significantly better than novices ($M = 25.7$) in shooting skills. The adjusted means for knowledge showed that child experts ($M = 77.1$) possessed more basketball knowledge than novices ($M = 64.2$). (p. 22)

If more than two levels had existed within an independent variable in the MANOVA (i.e., suppose three age-league levels had been used), then following the discriminant analysis, there would have been three means (one for each age-league level) to test among for significance. It would be appropriate to use a Scheffé test for this follow-up just as we did for ANOVA.

Multivariate Analysis of Covariance

Conceptually, **multivariate analysis of covariance (MANCOVA)** represents the same extension of ANCOVA that MANOVA did for ANOVA. In MANCOVA there are one or more independent variables, two or more dependent variables, and one or more covariates. Recall how ANCOVA was done (chapter 8). A variable was used to adjust the dependent variable by correlation, and then ANOVA was calculated on the adjusted dependent variable. In MANCOVA each dependent variable is adjusted for one or more covariates, then an optimal linear composite is

multivariate analysis of covariance (MANCOVA) — An extension of MANOVA in which there are two or more independent variables, two or more dependent variables, and one or more covariates.

Porter, A.C., & Raudenbush, S.W. (1987). Analysis of covariance: Its model and use in psychological research. *Journal of Counseling Psychology*, **34**, 383–392.

formed from the adjusted dependent variables that best discriminates among the independent variables, just as in MANOVA. Follow-up procedures are the same as in MANOVA except that the linear composite of adjusted dependent variables is used. This technique is seldom used and typically used incorrectly. Normally, there is no reason to adjust a dependent variable for a linear composite of covariates. We have purposely not provided an example of MANCOVA use from the physical activity literature. MANCOVA is a fine technique if you understand what it does and you specifically want to test for that. However, many researchers misunderstand MANCOVA and do not use it properly. Of course, we indicated the same was true of ANCOVA; for a good discussion of the issues, see Porter and Raudenbush (1987).

Repeated Measures With Multiple Dependent Variables

Sometimes experiments have multiple dependent variables that are measured more than once (over time). For example, in an exercise adherence study, both physiological and psychological variables might be measured once a week for a 15-week training program. If there were two training groups (different levels of training) and a control group (each with 15 subjects), all of which were measured every week (i.e., 15 times) on two psychological and three physiological measures, we would have a design that is three levels of exercise × 15 trials (3 × 15) for five dependent variables. This design offers several options for analysis.

We could do five 3 × 15 ANOVAs with repeated measures on the second factor. Here, we would follow the repeated measures procedures described in chapter 8. However, we would be inflating the alpha by doing multiple analyses on the same subjects. Of course, the alpha could be adjusted by the Bonferroni technique ($\alpha = .05/5 = .01$), but this fails to take into account the relationships among the dependent variables, which might be substantial and of considerable interest. An excellent tutorial on how to handle this problem is provided by Schutz and Gessaroli (1987). The following brief discussion is taken from their study, but if you are using this design and analysis, you should read their complete study and example.

There are two options for this analysis: multivariate mixed model (MMM) analysis and doubly multivariate (DM) analysis. Which is used depends on the assumptions that your data meet. Using the study previously described (three levels of exercise × 15 trials for five dependent variables), the MMM analysis treats the independent variable (levels of exercise) as a true multivariate case by forming a linear composite of the five dependent variables to discriminate among the levels of the independent variable. If this composite is significant, it can be followed up by the stepdown F procedures (for an alternative procedure, see Schutz and Gessaroli, 1987). For the repeated measures factor (and interaction), a linear composite is formed for each trial, and the linear composite at each trial is treated as a regular repeated measures analysis. This means that the sphericity assumption must be met as previously described and the epsilon can be used to test this assumption with the same standards described in chapter 8. The interpretation of the resulting F ratio for main effects for groups, trials, and the Group × Trial interaction are the same as in other designs. The question usually posed here is, Do the groups change at different rates across the trials on the linear composite of dependent variables? This is the preferred analysis if the sphericity assumption can be met because most authors believe it offers more power. However, this is a difficult assumption to meet, especially if

Schutz, R.W. & Gessaroli, M.E. (1987). The analysis of repeated measures designs involving multiple dependent variables. *Research Quarterly for Exercise and Sport*, **58**, 132-149.

there are more than two or three dependent variables measured on more than three to five trials.

The DM analysis does not require that the sphericity assumption be met. The analysis is the same for the independent variable of exercise. In the repeated measures part of the analysis, however, a linear composite is formed not only of the dependent variables at each trial but also of the 15 trials (which themselves become a linear composite), thus the name DM. The interpretations of the Fs for the two main effects and interaction remain essentially the same, but follow-ups become more complex.

Canonical Correlation

In chapter 7, we discussed correlation in which there was one dependent (or criterion) variable and one independent (or predictor) variable (zero-order correlation, r) and in which there was one dependent variable and two or more independent variables (multiple regression, R). There is also a correlational technique that can determine the relationship in which there are two or more dependent variables (criteria) and two or more independent variables (predictors). This technique is called **canonical correlation** (R_c).

In essence, there are two optimal linear combinations: one of Y variables and one of X variables. These composites are weighted so that the maximum correlation is achieved. This is the canonical correlation (R_c), and R_c^2 is the estimated amount of common association (shared variance) between the two linear composites of these variables. This is similar to multiple regression, in which the X variables were weighted in terms of their linear combination effects.

Canonical correlation is sometimes used in an exploratory manner to discover which variables might best be manipulated for use as the independent variables and which will best show results as dependent variables. For example, suppose we have several physical characteristics for a group of athletes, such as height, weight, percent fat, and several performance measures of power, speed, endurance, and aerobic capacity. We may wish to learn which among the physical characteristics are the best predictors of performance. Canonical correlation will identify the best solution, and multiple regression is often used to follow up for interpretation and prediction purposes. For a more detailed but understandable explanation of canonical correlation, read Thompson (1991).

For example, McPherson and Thomas (1989) studied expert and novice tennis players at two age levels (10-11 and 12-13). They measured tennis knowledge and tennis skill (serve and ground strokes) in these children, then videotaped them as they played six games. The videotapes were coded for three qualities of game performance (control, decisions, and execution). McPherson and Thomas were interested in the relationship between tennis knowledge and skill (predictor variables) and several aspects of game performance (criterion variables) and used canonical correlation to evaluate this relationship. Following is a description of their results:

The canonical correlation to examine the relation of knowledge and groundstroke skill and the components of tennis play following the serve . . . revealed one signifi-

---

canonical correlation — A correlational technique that can determine the relationship when there are two or more criterion variables and two or more predictor variables.

 Thompson, B. (1991). Methods, plainly speaking: A primer on the logic and use of canonical correlation analysis. *Measurement and Evaluation in Counseling and Development, 24,* 80-95.

cant function, $R_c = .79$, $F(6, 70) = 7.58$, $p < .01$. The standardized canonical coefficients indicated that both knowledge (0.42) and groundstrokes (0.69) were important in the relation to decisions (0.65) and execution (0.41). (p. 198)

McPherson and Thomas used canonical correlation to establish the general nature of the relationships between knowledge, skill, and game performance before they analyzed in more detail how expert and novice players organize tennis knowledge differently at this age.

Factor Analysis

Using Factor Analysis

An Example of Factor Analysis

Additional Types of Factor Analysis

Many performance variables and characteristics are used to describe human behavior. Often it is useful to reduce a large set of performance and characteristic measures to a more manageable structure. We have already discussed the likelihood that two performance measures might to some extent assess the same underlying characteristic. This represents the degree to which they are correlated. **Factor analysis** is an approach to reducing a set of correlated measures to a smaller number of latent or hidden variables (Tinsley & Tinsley, 1987). There are numerous procedures grouped under the general topic of factor analysis. We do not discuss in detail the various techniques, but we do provide a general explanation that allows you to read and understand studies that use factor analysis. For a good explanation and example of factor analysis, read Tinsley and Tinsley (1987).

Using Factor Analysis

Factor analysis is performed on a group of individuals on whom a series of measures have been taken. The researcher usually wants to describe a reduced number of underlying constructs and possibly select the one or two best measures of each construct. Factor analysis begins by calculating an intercorrelation matrix of all the measures used (correlation between all possible pairs of variables; thus, if eight measures were made, the correlation would be determined between variables 1 and 2, 1 and 3, and so on for a total of 28 correlations). The goal of factor analysis is to discover the factors (underlying or hidden constructs) that best explain a group of measures and describe the relation of each measure to the factor or underlying construct. Thus, the computer program first provides a choice about how many factors to use. The more tests that have high loadings (correlations) on a factor, the more important the factor is in accounting for the total variance of the tests (the more important the factor, the bigger the eigenvalue). In addition, measures that have high loadings on a factor are more closely related (correlated) to that factor.

---

 factor analysis — A statistical technique used to reduce a set of data by grouping similar variables into basic components (factors).

Tinsley, H.E., & Tinsley, D.J. (1987). Uses of factor analysis in counseling psychology research. *Journal of Counseling Psychology*, **34**, 414-424.

There are rules of thumb about how many factors to use, the best of which is probably the **scree curve**. Figure 9.1 shows a scree curve for a factor analysis. The y-axis is called **eigenvalues** (the correlation of each test with that factor squared and summed). The x-axis is the number of factors (and is equal initially to the number of variables). You decide to keep the number of factors before the elbow of the scree curve (note the scree curve has the greatest bend at the fourth factor with the remaining factors forming a line parallel to the x-axis). So, in this example three factors would be rotated. These factors are then rotated according to a criterion to maximize the tests' loadings and to minimize the relation among factors (having the factors uncorrelated is called **orthogonal rotation**). Or the researcher may decide to allow the factors to correlate with one another (called **oblique rotation**). The researcher then decides what represents a significant loading (correlation of a test or item with a factor): .4 is often used as an arbitrary number, but there are other ways of deciding.

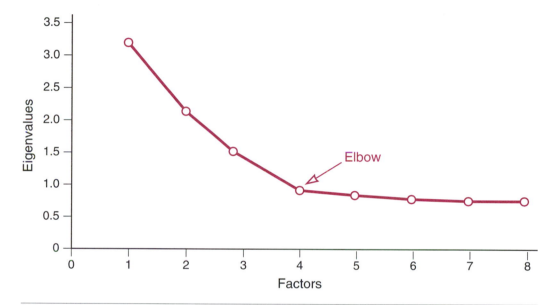

Figure 9.1   Scree curve for factor analysis.

An Example of Factor Analysis

Example 9.2 shows a factor analysis of a sports orientation questionnaire (Gill & Deeter, 1988) that was administered to a group of subjects. Gill and Deeter did both orthogonal and oblique rotations (columns under each of three factors of Competitiveness, Goal, and Win). The numbers in each column represent the correlation

scree curve — A method used in factor analysis to determine the number of important factors.

eigenvalues — The squared and summed correlations of each variable, or test, for a factor; the y-axis on a scree curve.

orthogonal rotation — Technique in factor analysis designed to maximize the loadings of the tests, or variables, and minimize the relation among factors; also called *varimax rotation.*

oblique rotation — A method in factor analysis in which the factors are redefined (and allowed to correlate) in order to make sharper distinctions in the meanings of the factors.

simple structure — Research design in which the investigator wants each item to correlate highly on the one factor that item was designed to measure and load to a low degree on the other factors.

(called loadings) of each item with the hypothesized factor. Ideally, the authors wanted each item to load heavily (correlate highly) on the one factor that the item was designed to measure and to load to a low degree on the other two factors. Such a solution is called **simple structure**

Example 9.2

Item	Competitiveness Varimax	Competitiveness Oblique	Goal Varimax	Goal Oblique	Win Varimax	Win Oblique
Competitiveness						
I am a competitive person	.71	.74	.05	.18	.21	.34
I try my hardest to win	.75	.78	.10	.24	.21	.34
I am a determined competitor	.77	.79	.12	.26	.09	.22
I want to be the best every time I compete	.54	.62	.24	.33	.27	.34
I look forward to competing	.82	.83	.10	.25	.11	.25
I thrive on competition	.74	.80	.12	.26	.31	.42
My goal is to be the best athlete possible	.68	.74	.23	.36	.22	.32
I enjoy competing against others	.79	.80	.07	.22	.17	.30
I want to be successful in sports	.71	.75	.17	.30	.18	.29
I work hard to be successful in sports	.73	.78	.28	.41	.10	.20
The best test of my ability is competing against others	.69	.72	.06	.19	.23	.35
I look forward to the opportunity to test my skills in competition	.79	.80	.16	.30	.08	−.21
I perform my best when I am competing against an opponent	.64	.70	.12	.24	.34	.44
Goal						
I set goals for myself when I compete	.35	.46	.58	.64	.04	.04
I am most competitive when I try to achieve personal goals	.01	.11	.50	.50	−.04	−.09
I try hardest when I have a specific goal	.01	.15	.64	.63	.01	−.07
Reaching personal performance goals is very important to me	.08	.24	.77	.77	.04	−.04
The best way to determine my ability is to set a goal and try to reach it	.03	.15	.61	.60	.01	−.07

Item	Factors					
	Competitiveness		Goal		Win	
	Varimax	Oblique	Varimax	Oblique	Varimax	Oblique
Performing to the best of my ability is very important to me	.27	.37	.57	.61	−.03	−.05
Win						
Winning is important	.50	.62	.16	.26	.57	.63
Scoring more points than my opponent is very important to me	.38	.50	.10	.18	.59	.63
I hate to lose	.27	.43	.19	.24	.69	.70
The only time I am satisfied is when I win	.17	.28	−.09	−.04	.70	.73
Losing upsets me	.20	.33	.02	.07	.72	.74
I have the most fun when I win	.44	.52	.06	.14	.47	.54
Percent variance	33.5		10.8		5.3	
Cumulative percent variance	33.5		44.3		49.6	

From *Research Quarterly for Exercise and Sport*, **59**(3), p. 196. Reproduced with permission from the American Alliance for Health, Physical Education, Recreation and Dance.

As you can see, the structure is fairly simple for the Competitiveness and Goal factors, but the loadings are not so clear-cut for the Win factors. Gill and Deeter reported a clear bend in the scree curve at the fourth factor (thus, they rotated the three factors before the bend, presented in Example 9.2). You can see that the first factor accounts for 33.5% of the total variance, the second factor for 10.8%, and the third factor for 5.3%. The total variance accounted for in this solution is 49.6%.

Additional Types of Factor Analysis

There are other types of factor analysis. The one previously discussed is often called **exploratory factor analysis**. Once a pattern is identified, the researcher may want to see whether the structure fits a new data set from a different sample. Solutions such as the previous one can sometimes be very sample specific, especially if a unique group (e.g., athletes) is used. Thus, Gill and Deeter took the

exploratory factor analysis — Factor analysis performed for the purpose of identifying basic constructs, or factors, that underlie a set of measures.

confirmatory factor analysis — A type of factor analysis that tests hypotheses about the structuring of variables with regard to the expected number of significant factors.

goodness of fit — Term used to describe how well a factor structure fits the hypothesized structure.

solution and applied it to two new samples in a **confirmatory factor analysis**. In this approach, an important element is how well the proposed solution fits the new sample. Several ways of determining this are available, and Gill and Deeter report most of them (coefficient of determination, chi-square/*df* ratio, **goodness of fit**, and root mean square residuals). All the statistics supported that the three-factor model was a good one.

Numerous other approaches to factor analysis exist, but the previous example should enable you to follow what the researchers are doing. They should provide you with a good description of the following:

- Whether the factor analysis is exploratory or confirmatory
- The type of solution selected
- How the number of factors selected to be rotated was determined
- How the rotation was done
- What was considered a significant loading

It is also important to have a large number of subjects for factor analysis (some suggest at least 10 per variable). Remember also that solutions tend to be very specific to the sample on which they were determined. So a battery established by factor analysis on one sample may not prove useful on a different sample (e.g., sample of general college students to sample of college athletes, adults to children, etc.)

Structural Modeling

Path Analysis
Linear Structural Relations

Path analysis and **linear structural relations (LISREL)** are structural, or causal, modeling techniques that are used to explain the way certain characteristics relate to one another and attempt to imply cause. You should remember from the discussion in chapters 4 and 8 that cause-and-effect is not a statistical result but a logical one. That is, if the experimenter can argue theoretically that changing a certain characteristic should result in a specific change in behavior, and if the actual experiments (and statistical analysis) support this hypothesis, then cause is often inferred for a particular independent variable on a dependent variable. Of course, this is true only if all other possible influences have been controlled.

The way variables influence one another is not always clear; for example, $X \rightarrow Y \rightarrow Z$, or $X \leftarrow Y \rightarrow Z$. In the first case, X influences Y, which in turn influences Z; however, in the second case, Y influences both X and Z. This is a very simple explanation. Path analysis and LISREL allow a more complex modeling of the way variables influence one another. But all you can say about these models is that they are either consistent or inconsistent with the data and hypotheses. Whether this infers

What a report using factor analysis should describe

linear structural relations (LISREL) — A statistical approach used to establish relationships and examine the structural equations model.

Fassinger, R.E. (1987). Use of structural equation modeling in counseling psychology research. *Journal of Counseling Psychology*, **34**, 425-436.

cause-and-effect depends on other things (e.g., control of all other variables, careful treatments, logical hypotheses, valid theories). For a nice overview and practical explanation of structural modeling, read Fassinger (1987).

Path Analysis

 Path analysis uses correlations among all the variables (much like multiple regression) to estimate the linkages among measures where the experimenter has a rationale for how these measures should influence one another. Path analysis labels two types of variables: **exogenous**, whose variance is explained by factors outside the model, and **endogenous**, whose variance is explained by exogenous variables, other variables within the model, or both. Researchers often assume that the flow of cause to effect is in one direction, and arrows are used to depict this flow (see Figure 9.2). Path analysis has rarely been used since the evolution of LISREL.

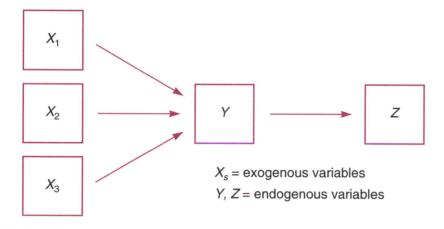

X_s = exogenous variables
Y, Z = endogenous variables

Figure 9.2   Example of a structural model with the flow of influence in one direction.

Linear Structural Relations

Linear structural relations, or LISREL, is an approach to structural modeling that has gained widespread use, particularly among social scientists. It is much like path analysis, except path analysis assumes that all variables are measured without error. Of course, this is a very weak assumption, as we know all types of errors creep into real data (measurement error, coding errors, testing errors, etc.). A good way for you to gain a basic understanding of LISREL is through an example (Greenockle, Lee, & Lomax, 1990) from the physical education literature. These researchers were interested in describing the relationship between student characteristics and exercise behavior. Figure 9.3 shows how they found this relationship to be in a sample of 10 intact high school physical education classes in which the teacher had agreed to teach a specific physical

---

exogenous variable — A characteristic in path analysis whose variance is explained by factors outside the model.

endogenous variable — A characteristic in path analysis whose variance is explained by exogenous variables, other variables within the model, or both.

Greenockle, K.M., Lee, A.M., & Lomax, R. (1990). The relation between selected student characteristics and activity patterns in required high school physical education class. *Research Quarterly for Exercise and Sport*, **61**, 59–69.

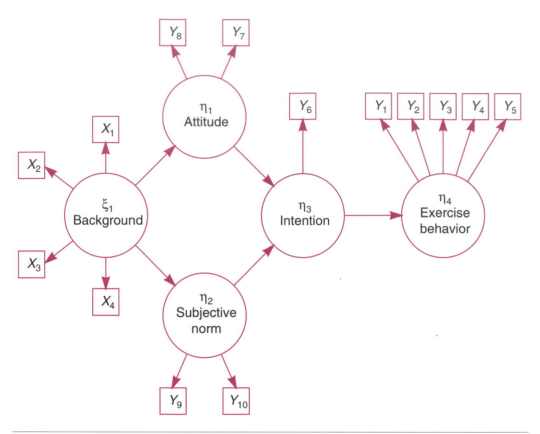

Figure 9.3   LISREL Model.

From *Research Quarterly for Exercise and Sport*, **61**, March 1990, pp. 59-69. Reproduced with permission from the American Alliance for Health, Physical Education, Recreation and Dance.

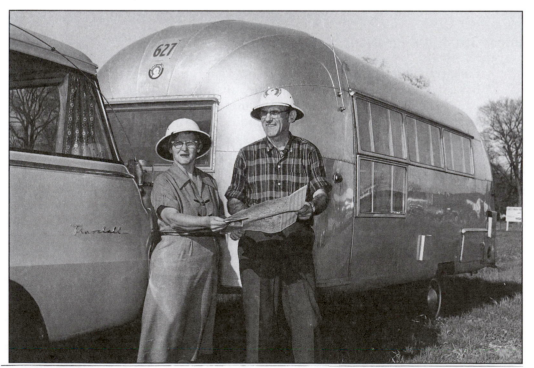

Path analysis.

fitness unit. They measured four background variables on the students: past activity level, perception of father's activity level, perception of mother's activity level, and knowledge of physical fitness. Two measures of attitude toward exercise were taken from a valid and reliable questionnaire. Two subjective norm measures were obtained from the same questionnaire, which indicated subjects' perceptions concerning how others felt about the subjects' exercise behavior. One measure of intention to exercise was obtained. Five exercise behaviors were measured: jogging, fitness test score, percent participation, heart rate, and perceived exertion.

The technique of LISREL was used because it allows related measures to be grouped (as in factor analysis) into components (e.g., exercise behavior) and it shows the relationship among the components in terms of magnitude and direction. The estimates of each component are grouped together in a linear equation (using their factor loadings). Then a series of general linear equations (as in multiple regression) shows the relationships among the components. "The general intent of the analysis is to reconstruct the observed correlation matrix as well as possible by imposing a theoretical structure on the data" (Greenockle et al., 1990, p. 63). Model fitting indexes are used to assess the nature of the fit. These are similar to those discussed previously for confirmatory factor analysis: chi-square and goodness of fit. The results of the study by Greenockle et al. indicated "the prediction of exercise behavior by attitude and subjective norm to be significantly mediated by intention" (p. 59). You can see, then, that structural modeling techniques provide a way to evaluate the complex relationships that exist in real-world data. By establishing the directions that certain relationships go, stronger inferences can be made about which characteristics are likely to cause other characteristics.

Summary

The multivariate techniques discussed here are mathematically complex. However, we think you can gain enough understanding from the explanations offered to read a research study using one of these techniques and to follow what happens. The techniques were grouped as experimental (discriminant analysis, MANOVA, MANCOVA, and repeated measures) and correlational (canonical, factor analysis, and structural modeling). However, as we have noted several times, whether cause-and-effect exists depends very little on statistics but mostly on logical, theoretical, and design rationale.

Check Your Understanding

1. Locate a study that used discriminant analysis and briefly describe how it was used to address the purpose of the study. Identify any follow-up procedures used.
2. Locate a study that used MANOVA in its data analysis. Identify the independent and the dependent variables.
3. Locate a study that used canonical correlation in its data analysis. Identify the dependent variables (criteria) and the independent variables (predictors).

Nonparametric Techniques

Dear Professors of Research Methods:

I am using a nonparametric test in the statistical analysis for my thesis because of the skewness of the scores. My friend says this is too bad because parametric statistics are more scientific and I won't be able to get my study published. I say that the use of nonparametric statistics does not make a study less worthy, nor constitute grounds for rejecting a paper for publication. Instead, it would be wrong to use a parametric test when the data do not meet the assumptions. Is my argument right or wrong?

Sincerely,
Normal I.R. Knott

Dear Normal:

As the song says, "You got the right one, baby! Uh huh!" Nonparametric tests should not be viewed as a substitute for the "preferred" parametric tests. The ultimate question is whether the statistical test that one chooses does the job more effectively than other procedures. In other words, if the shoe fits, wear it (assuming one can find the other one).

Methodologically yours,
PRM

In the preceding chapters, various parametric statistics have been described. As you recall, parametric statistics make assumptions about the distribution with regard to normality and homogeneity of variance. Another category of statistics is called nonparametric statistics. This category is also referred to as distribution-free statistics because no assumptions are made about the distribution of scores.

Nonparametric statistics are versatile in that they can deal with ranked scores and categories. This can be a definite advantage when the investigator is dealing with variables that do not lend themselves to precise, interval-type data (that are more likely to meet parametric assumptions), such as categories of responses on questionnaires and various affective behavior rating instruments. Data from qualitative research are often numerical counts of events that can be effectively analyzed with nonparametric statistics.

The main drawback to nonparametric statistics that has often been voiced is that they are less powerful than parametric statistics. As you recall, power refers to the ability of a statistical test to reject a null hypothesis that is false. It should be pointed out that there is not unanimous agreement regarding the supposed power advantage of parametric tests (Harwell, 1990). Another drawback in the use of nonparametric tests has been the lack of available statistical software in computer programs for the more complex statistical tests, such as multivariate cases.

 Nevertheless, there are numerous occasions when a researcher's data do not meet the assumptions of normality. Micceri (1989), for example, maintains that much of the data in education and psychology are moderately or largely nonnormal, and thus nonparametric tests should be considered. Moreover, sometimes the only scores available are frequencies of occurrence or ranks (which often are not normally distributed), and the researcher should use nonparametric tests. Several nonparametric methods are available. In this chapter, we describe a few of the more common ones. You may also find enlightening information about nonparametric statistical tests in Conover (1971).

Chi-Square: Testing the Observed Versus the Expected

The Contingency Table
Restrictions in Using Chi-Square

Data are often sorted into categories, such as gender, age, grade level, treatment groups, or some other **nominal** (categorical) **measure**. A researcher is sometimes interested in evaluating whether the number of cases in each category is different from what would be expected on the basis of chance, some known source of information (such as census data), or some other rational hypothesis about the distribution of cases in the population. **Chi-square** is a technique that provides a statistical test as to the significance of the discrepancy between the observed and the expected results.

 Conover, W.J. (1971). Practical nonparametric statistics. New York: Wiley.

 nominal measure — Method of classifying data into categories, such as gender, age, grade level, or treatment groups.

chi-square — Technique that provides a statistical test as to the significance of the discrepancy between the observed and the expected results.

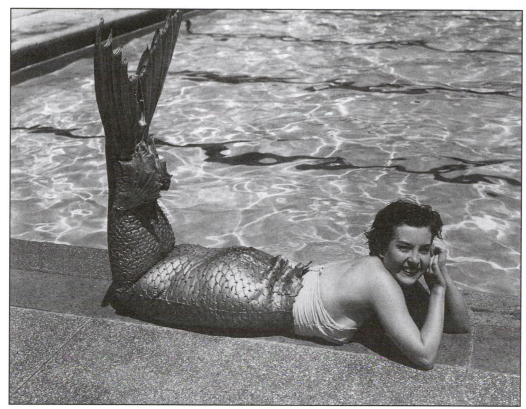

There are numerous occasions when a researcher's data do not meet the assumptions of normality.

The formula for chi-square is

$$\chi^2 = \sum[(O - E)^2 / E] \qquad (10.1)$$

where O = the observed frequency and E = the expected frequency. Thus, the expected frequency in each cell is subtracted from the observed (or obtained) frequency. This difference is then squared (which means all differences will be positive), and these values are divided by the expected frequency for their respective cells and are then summed.

For example, tennis coach Roger Rabbitfoot believes in jinxes. He believes that one court at his university is definitely unlucky for his team. He has kept records of matches on four courts over the years and is convinced that his team has lost significantly more matches on court number 4 than on any other. Roger has set out to prove his point by comparing the number of losses on each of the four courts. The same number of matches has been played on each court, and his team has lost a total of 120 individual matches on these courts during this period. Theoretically, it would be expected that each court would have one fourth, or 30, of the losses. The observed frequencies and the expected frequencies are shown in Example 10.1.

Example 10.1

Known Values		Court number				
		1	2	3	4	Total
Observed number of losses:	$O =$	24	34	22	40	120
Expected number of losses:	$E =$	30	30	30	30	120

Working It Out
(Equation 10.1)

	Court number			
	1	2	3	4
$(O - E)$	−6	+4	−8	+10
$(O - E)^2$	36	16	64	100
$(O - E)^2/E$	1.20	.53	2.13	3.33
$\Sigma(O - E)^2/E = 7.19 = \chi^2$				

The resulting chi-square is then interpreted for significance by consulting Table A.8 in Appendix A. Because there are four courts (or cells), the number of degrees of freedom (df) is $c - 1 = 3$. The researcher finds the critical value for 3 df, which is 7.82 for the .05 probability level. Roger's calculated value of 7.19 is less than this, so the null hypothesis that there were no differences among the four courts in the number of losses is not rejected. The observed differences could be attributed to sample error. Roger probably still believes in his heart that he is right (called cardiac research).

In some cases, the expected frequencies for classifications can be obtained from existing sources of information, such as in the following example. A new assistant professor, Nancy Niceperson, is assigned to teach the large sections of an introductory physical education course. After a few semesters, the department chairperson hears rumors that Dr. Niceperson is too lenient in her grading practices, so he uses chi-square to compare the grades of the 240 students with the department's prescribed normal curve grade distribution: 3.5% As and Fs, 24% Bs and Ds, and 45% Cs. If Dr. Niceperson were adhering to this normal curve distribution, she would be expected to have given 8 As and 8 Fs, (3.5% × 240), 58 Bs and 58 Ds (24% × 240), and 108 Cs (45% × 240). The observed frequencies (Nancy's grades) and the expected frequencies (the department's mandated distribution) are worked out in Example 10.2.

Example 10.2

Known Values

		Grade					
		A (3.5%)	B (24%)	C (45%)	D (24%)	F (3.5%)	Total
Observed number of grades given:	$O =$	21	75	114	28	2	240
Expected number of grades given:	$E =$	8	58	108	58	8	240

Working It Out
(Equation 10.1)

	Grade				
	A	B	C	D	F
$(O - E)$	13	17	6	−30	−6
$(O - E)^2$	69	289	36	900	36
$(O - E)^2/E$	21.13	4.98	0.33	15.52	4.50
$\Sigma(O - E)^2/E = 46.46 = \chi^2$					

The chairperson, who is always fair, does not want to make a bad decision, so he decides to use the .01 level of probability. Table A.8 shows that for 4 df (there are five grades, or cells), a chi-square of 13.28 is needed for significance at the .01 level. The obtained chi-square of 46.46 exceeds the value, indicating a significant deviation from the expected grade distribution. Clearly, Nancy's grades show too many As and Bs and too few Ds and Fs. The chairperson does the only fair thing by firing her on the spot.

The Contingency Table

Often a problem involves two or more categories of occurrences and two or more groups (a two-way classification). A common example is in the analysis of the results of questionnaires or attitude inventories in which there are several categories of responses (e.g., agree, no opinion, disagree) and two or more groups of respondents (e.g., exercise adherents and nonadherents). This type of two-way classification is called a **contingency table**.

To illustrate, suppose a group of athletes and a group of nonathletes respond to the following statement on a sportsmanship inventory: "A baseball player who traps a fly ball between the ground and his glove should tell the umpire that he did not catch it." In the previous examples of one-way classification, the expected frequencies were determined by some type of rational hypothesis or source of information. In a contingency table, the expected values are computed from the marginal totals. Example 10.3 shows the subjects' responses.

Example 10.3

Known Values

Observed responses	Agree	No opinion	Disagree	Total
Athletes	30	46	124	200
Nonathletes	114	80	56	250
Total	144	126	180	450

Working It Out

1. Find the expected values (Column total × row total)/N

Expected responses	Agree	No opinion	Disagree	Total
Athletes	$144 \times 200/450$ = 64	$126 \times 200/450$ = 56	$180 \times 200/450$ = 80	200
Nonathletes	$144 \times 250/450$ = 80	$126 \times 250/450$ = 70	$180 \times 250/450$ = 100	250
Total	144	126	180	450

2. Compute χ^2 (Equation 10.1)

	$O - E$	$(O - E)^2$	$(O - E)^2/E$
Athletes agree	–34	1,156	18.06
Nonathletes agree	34	1,156	14.45
Athletes no opinion	–10	100	1.79
Nonathletes no opinion	10	100	1.43
Athletes disagree	44	1,936	24.20
Nonathletes disagree	–44	1,936	19.36
			$\chi^2 = 79.29$

---

contingency table — A two-way classification of categories of occurrences and two or more groups that is used for computing the significance of the differences between observed and expected scores.

A total of 144 respondents agreed with the statement. Because there are 450 people in all, then 144/450, or 32% of the total group, agreed with the statement. Thus, if there were no difference between athletes and nonathletes on sportsmanship (the null hypothesis) as reflected by this statement, then 32% of the athletes ($.32 \times 200 = 64$) and 32% of the nonathletes ($.32 \times 250 = 80$) would be the expected frequencies for these two cells.

A much faster method of calculating these expected frequencies is simply to multiply the column total by the row total for each cell and divide by the total number (N), as we've worked out in Step 1 of Example 10.3. Chi-square is computed in the same manner as in the examples of one-way classification.

The degrees of freedom for a contingency table is $(r-1)(c-1)$, where r stands for rows and c for columns. Here, we have two rows and three columns, so $df = (2-1)(3-1) = 2$. As before, the investigator then looks up the tabled value for significance (in this study, the investigator had decided on the .01 level) and sees that a chi-square of 9.21 is needed. The obtained chi-square of 79.29 is clearly significant. This tells us that the null hypothesis is rejected: There is a significant difference between athletes and nonathletes in their responses to the statement. After inspecting the table, we could conclude that a significantly greater proportion of nonathletes agreed that the player should tell the umpire he had trapped the ball and, conversely, that a higher proportion of athletes felt he should not.

Restrictions in Using Chi-Square

Although we indicated that nonparametric statistics do not require the same assumptions concerning the population as do parametric statistics, some restrictions apply in using this technique. The observations must be independent and the categories mutually exclusive. By this we mean that an observation in any category should not be related to or dependent on other observations in other categories. You could, for example, ask 50 people about their activity preferences. If each gave three preferences, you would not be justified in using a total (N) of 150 because the preferences of any subject would likely be related and the chi-square inflated. Moreover, an observation can be placed in only one category. The observed frequencies are exactly that—numbers of occurrences. Ratios and percentages are not appropriate. Another related point is that the total of the expected frequencies and the total of the observed frequencies for any classification must be the same. In Example 10.3, for example, notice that the total of the expected frequencies for athletes is the same as the total of the observed frequencies. The same is also seen for nonathletes and for the column totals.

Chi-square is usually not applicable for small samples. The expected frequency for any cell should not be less than 1.0. Furthermore, some statisticians claim that no more than 20% of the cells can have expected values of less than 5. Opinions vary on this, however. Some say no cell should have less than 5, whereas other statisticians would allow as many as 40%. A common tactic in cases with several cells with expected frequencies less than 5 is to combine adjacent categories, therefore increasing the expected values.

 Researchers generally agree that a 2 × 2 contingency table should have a so-called correction for continuity. This correction, usually referred to as **Yates' correction for continuity**, is to subtract 0.5 from the difference between the observed and the expected frequencies for each cell before it is squared:

$$\text{Corrected } \chi^2 = \Sigma[(O - E - .5)^2/E] \qquad (10.2)$$

Another limitation imposed on the 2 × 2 contingency table is that the total number (N) should be at least 20.

Yates' correction for continuity — Method of correcting a 2 × 2 contingency table by subtracting 0.5 from the difference between the observed and expected frequencies for each cell before it is squared.

Finally, the expected distribution should be logical and established before the data are collected. In other words, the hypothesis (probability, equal occurrence, census data, etc.) precedes the analysis. Researchers are not allowed to look over the distribution and then conjure up an expected distribution that will fit their hypothesis.

Mann–Whitney *U* Test

The Mann-Whitney *U* test is analogous to the parametric independent *t* test. The *U* test is one of the more powerful of the nonparametric tests. It can be used with very small or fairly large groups and requires only ordinal (rank) measurement. We can use this test when we have two independent groups and one dependent variable.

There is more than one way to compute the Mann-Whitney *U* test. We demonstrate only the ranking method recommended for larger groups because the counting procedure for small groups is too time-consuming if you have, say, 20 or more scores.

Suppose a researcher wishes to test the hypothesis that experienced teachers require less time (duration of eye fixation) than novice teachers while observing skill performance. A group of golf teachers with more than 10 years of experience are compared with a group of novice golf teachers. Both groups observe the same individuals performing a golf drive. An eye movement recorder is used to measure the duration of eye fixation in milliseconds (ms). The scores for the 11 experienced and 12 novice teachers are shown in Example 10.4. The median time for experienced golf teachers is 117 ms and 128 ms for novice teachers.

Example 10.4

Known Values

Group 1 (experienced) raw score: 111, 114, 120, 101, 118, 128, 125, 117, 106, 120, 110.

Group 1 rank: 4, 5.5, 10, 1, 8, 17, 14, 7, 2, 10, 3

Group 2 (inexperienced) raw score: 130, 123, 124, 138, 142, 120, 127, 140, 136, 129, 127, 114

Group 2 rank: 19, 12, 13, 21, 23, 10, 15.5, 22, 20, 18, 15.5, 5.5

Sum of ranks of group 1: $\Sigma R_1 = 81.5$

Sum of ranks of group 2: $\Sigma R_2 = 194.5$

Working It Out

1. **Rank the scores for both groups (all 23 teachers).** We ranked the shortest time as 1 and the longest as 23. Of course, we must maintain group identities in the ranking process. When you have ties in ranks, you give each score the average of the ranks they occupy. For example, two people have scores of 114, which occupy the 5th and the 6th ranks. So, we give each person the average of those two ranks (5.5), and the next rank is now 7. Three teachers had scores of 120, which occupy the 9th, 10th, and 11th ranks. Therefore, all three are given the middle rank (10), and the next rank is 12.

2. **Sum the ranks for each group.** You can check your accuracy in ranking by using the formula $N(N + 1)/2$, where N is the total number of scores in all groups combined. In this example, it would be $23(23 + 1)/2 = 276$,

which agrees with the sum of the ranks of Group 1 (81.5) plus the sum of Group 2 (194.5), or 276.

3. **Calculate U.** The difference between the groups will be maximum when there is little overlap between samples. In other words, if there is no overlap, then all measurements for one sample would be greater than the other. On the other hand, if the null hypothesis is true, scores from the two groups will be mixed, in which case the ranks of one sample will be greater than the other sample about half the time and the same for the other sample. Thus, U would be near $(n_1)(n_2)/2$ if there is no difference between groups. Conversely, a real difference between groups will show a high U for one group and a low U for the other. The formula for calculating U for Group 1 follows:

$$U = n_1 n_2 + [n_1(n_1 + 1)/2] - \Sigma R_1 \tag{10.3}$$

where n_1 = the number of subjects in Group 1, n_2 = the number of subjects in Group 2, and R_1 = the sum of ranks for Group 1.

In our example, U for Group 1 is

$$U = (11)(12) + [11(11 + 1)/2] - 81.5 = 116.5$$

The formula for U for Group 2 is

$$U = n_1 n_2 + [n_2(n_2 + 1)/2] - \Sigma R_2 \tag{10.4}$$

In our example, U for Group 2 is

$$U = (11)(12) + [12(12 + 1)/2] - 194.5 = 15.5$$

4. **Determine probability.** This can be accomplished either by consulting a table of U values (for the smaller of the two Us) or by calculating z and consulting a table of areas of the standard normal probability curve (Table A.2). The U tables are used with small samples. If samples are of moderate size (say 10 or more in each sample), the sampling distribution of U will be approximately normal, and the calculation of z is appropriate. Most statistics textbooks contain U tables if you want to use the Mann-Whitney U test with very small samples.

The calculation of z is as follows:

$$z = \frac{U - (n_1)(n_2)/2}{\sqrt{n_1 n_2 (n_1 + n_2 + 1)/12}} \tag{10.5}$$

Substituting the values from our example, we calculate z using the U for Group 1:

$$z = \frac{116.5 - (11)(12)/2}{\sqrt{(11 \times 12)(11 + 12 + 1)/12}}$$

$$= \frac{116.5 - 66}{\sqrt{(132)(24)/12}}$$

$$= \frac{50.5}{\sqrt{264}}$$

$$= 50.5/16.25 = 3.11$$

It does not matter which U is used. If we had used the U for Group 2, the resulting z would be -3.11. So the absolute value of z is the same (only the sign is different).

Consult Table A.2 and find the z for 3.11. We see that the probability that a difference this large would occur by chance is less than 1%. Thus, there appears to be a real difference between the two groups of teachers on duration of eye fixation, with novice golf teachers watching significantly longer than experienced teachers.

Wilcoxon Matched–Pairs Signed–Ranks Test

You recall from chapter 8 that there are studies in which one has matched groups, or the same group of people is tested twice on a dependent measure, and the investigator wants to know whether the difference between the matched groups (or the change in scores for the same subjects) is significant. In such situations, the independent t test is not appropriate, and the researcher must use a dependent t test (or repeated measures ANOVA). The same principle applies in nonparametric statistics. The researcher would not be correct in using a test such as the Mann-Whitney U test with dependent (paired) groups.

The Wilcoxon matched-pair signed-ranks test is a powerful nonparametric test for comparing related samples. In the Wilcoxon test, the size of the difference between scores (such as between pre- and posttest scores) is determined and ranked. An example illustrates the steps and the interpretation of this test. A researcher, Dr. Marlo Perkins, believes that adventure programs are conducive to raising one's self-concept. She gathers scores on a self-concept scale for a group of boys before and after an adventure activity program. (They are listed in Example 10.5.) She wishes to assess whether they gained in self-concept. So, in this case, she is using a one-tailed test because she is hypothesizing a positive change and is not interested in any changes that might occur in the opposite direction. (Note: This example is to illustrate the Wilcoxon statistical test and is not intended as a model for experimental design.) In such a case, other influences certainly could explain changes in self-concept other than the adventure program. A control group would definitely add validity to such a study. Unfortunately, Dr. Perkins never read this book.

Example 10.5

Known Values

Subject	Self-concept scores before program	Self-concept scores after program	Posttest – Pretest (D)	Rank of differences	Signed rank	Fewest
A	33	36	+3	6.5	+6.5	. . .
B	30	31	+1	2	+2	. . .
C	40	37	−3	6.5	−6.5	−6.5
D	27	36	+9	13	+13	. . .
E	18	24	+6	10	+10	. . .

Subject	Self-concept scores before program	Self-concept scores after program	Posttest – Pretest (D)	Rank of differences	Signed rank	Fewest
F	26	25	–1	2	–2	–2
G	35	35	0	. . .	. . .	. . .
H	20	16	–4	8	–8	–8
I	38	33	–5	9	–9	–9
J	16	24	+8	12	+12	. . .
K	26	28	+2	4.5	+4.5	. . .
L	21	20	–1	2	–2	–2
M	18	20	+2	4.5	+4.5	. . .
N	24	24	0	. . .	. . .	. . .
O	11	18	+7	11	+11	. . .

$$T = 27.5$$

Working It Out

1. **Determine the differences (column 4) by subtracting the pretest scores from the posttest scores**. Of course, some differences are positive and some negative. In two cases, no score changes occurred. Therefore, these two are dropped from further analysis because they would have no influence.

2. **Rank the differences *without* regard to sign (column 5)**. We started with the lowest difference, and we see that three people have a difference of one (+1, –1, –1). As before, because they occupy the first three ranks, each is given the average rank of 2.

3. **Place the appropriate sign in front of the ranks (column 6)**.

4. **Determine if there are more plus or minus ranks and enter the values for the smaller number in column 7**. Here, there are eight plus ranks and five minus ranks, so we enter all the minus ranks in column 7. These ranks are summed, which is designated as T.

5. **Test the T statistic for significance**. Dr. Perkins had specified in advance that she would be using a one-tailed test with significance at .01. With a sample size of greater than 10, we compute z and consult Table A.2 for the critical value. (With N less than 10, special tables provided in textbooks for nonparametric statistics should be consulted.)

6. **With a sample size of greater than 25, compute z and consult Table A.2 for the critical value**. We use the data in Example 10.5 to demonstrate the calculation of z:

$$z = \frac{T - N(N + 1)/4}{\sqrt{N(N + 1)[2(N + 1)]/24}} \tag{10.6}$$

$$= \frac{27.5 - 13(13 + 1)/4}{\sqrt{13(13 + 1)[2(13 + 1)]/24}}$$

$$= \frac{-18}{14.57}$$

$$= -1.24$$

The sign of the z does not matter. Table A.2 shows a probability of 0.11 for the one-tailed test (not significant). Dr. Perkins sadly concludes that no significant gains in self concept followed participation in the adventure program.

Kruskal–Wallis ANOVA by Ranks

The Kruskal-Wallis test is a nonparametric test of group differences when there are more than two independent groups. This is comparable to one-way ANOVA in parametric statistics. The data are converted to ranks for the analysis.

To illustrate this technique, we use the example at the beginning of chapter 1 concerning the effectiveness of aerobic dance and jogging on loss of fat as measured by the sum of skinfolds. A control group was also used in which the subjects did not engage in any exercise program but were measured before and after the 10-week period. For this analysis we use small numbers of subjects in each group and assume that our data were skewed, thus prompting the use of a nonparametric test. Example 10.6 shows the scores for the three groups. The scores represent the loss of fat; thus, negative numbers are "good," and positive numbers represent gains in fatness and are "bad."

Example 10.6

Known Values

Aerobic		Jogging		Control	
Score	Rank	Score	Rank	Score	Rank
−10	10	−25	15.5	+10	3
−29	19	−31	20	−5	7
−8	8	−19	12	+20	1
−32	21	0	6	−10	10
−22	14	−28	18	+9	4
−25	15.5	−27	17	+13	2
+2	5	−10	10		
−20	13				

Sum of aerobic ranks: $\Sigma R_A = 105.5$
Sum of jogging ranks: $\Sigma R_J = 98.5$
Sum of control ranks: $\Sigma R_C = 27$

Average aerobic rank: $\bar{R}_A = 13.2$
Average jogging rank: $\bar{R}_J = 14.1$
Average control rank: $\bar{R}_C = 4.5$

Working It Out

1. **Combine all scores and rank them.** The poorest score (a gain of fatness of 20 mm in skinfold thickness) is given a rank of 1 and the best score (a loss of 32 mm) the highest rank of 21. As in previous examples, ties are given the average ranking.

2. **Place the overall ranking for individuals next to their raw scores and sum the rankings for each group.** It should be obvious by now that if the null hypothesis were true, the average rank for each group would be the same. In other words, any differences in scores would be attributable to sampling error. We see that the average ranks for the three groups are as follows: aerobic dance (13.2), jogging (14.1), and control (4.5).

3. **Test for the significance of the differences among the groups by the Kruskal-Wallis test (H):**

$$H = [12/N(N + 1)] \times \Sigma[(\Sigma R_i)^2/n_i] - 3(N + 1) \qquad (10.7)$$

   where N = the total number of scores, ΣR^2 = the sum of the squared sum of ranks for the three groups, and n = the number of scores in a group.

4. **Do the simple computations.** For each group we need to square the sum of ranks and divide by the number of scores in that group; we then sum R_i^2/n for all three groups:

$$\frac{(105.5)^2}{8} + \frac{(98.5)^2}{7} + \frac{(27)^2}{6} = 2,898.8$$

   This sum is multiplied by $12/N(N + 1)$:

$$[12/21(21 + 1)] \times 2,898.8 = .026 \times 2,898.8 = 75.37$$

   from which we subtract $3(N + 1)$:

$$75.37 - 3(21 + 1) = 75.37 - 66 = 9.37$$

5. **When there are at least five subjects in each group, test H by chi-square with $df = k - 1$ (where k is number of groups). If there are five or fewer subjects in each group, use a special table.** If there are many tied ranks (e.g., over 25%), a correction for H should be calculated (Siegel, 1956). Because we have sufficient numbers in each group, we consult Table A.8 and see that the tabled chi-square value at the .05 level for 2 df is 5.99. As our value of 9.37 surpasses that, we can conclude that there are significant differences among the groups.

When we described one-way ANOVA in chapter 8, you will remember that when F is significant, a follow-up procedure (e.g., Scheffé) is used to find where the differences are. A similar procedure can be performed to test the differences between the average ranks. This procedure allows the investigator to make all possible pairwise comparisons while holding the overall alpha level at a specified value. In our Example 10.6, suppose we wish to make all possible comparisons while holding the overall alpha level to .05 or less. With three groups, three comparisons are possible, i.e., $k(k - 1)/2$. We set the confidence level for each comparison. First, we can use the Bonferroni technique and divide the alpha level (.05) by the number of comparisons (3), which results in .017. Consulting Table A.2, we find the z value that corresponds to this percentage of area in the tails of the distribution and find the z value of 2.39. This will be multiplied by the standard error of difference (SE) between any two samples:

$$SE_{\bar{R}_1 - \bar{R}_2} = \sqrt{[N(N+1)/12] \times (1/n_1 + 1/n_2)} \qquad (10.8)$$

where N = the total sample size and n = the size of the groups being compared.

For our three comparisons, the standard error of differences are as follows:

aerobic dance (A) versus jogging (J):

$$SE_{\bar{R}_A - \bar{R}_J} = \sqrt{[[21(21+1)/12](1/8 + 1/7)} = 3.21$$

aerobic dance (A) versus control (C):

$$SE_{\bar{R}_A - \bar{R}_C} = \sqrt{[21(21+1)/12](1/8 + 1/6)} = 3.35$$

jogging (J) versus control (C):

$$SE_{\bar{R}_J - \bar{R}_C} = \sqrt{[21(21+1)/12](1/7 + 1/6)} = 3.45$$

The confidence interval can now be established for each comparison. The confidence interval equals the observed difference between groups plus or minus z for .017, or 2.39 $(SE_{\bar{R}_1 - \bar{R}_2})$:

aerobic dance versus jogging:

$$\bar{R}_A(13.2) - \bar{R}_J(14.1) \pm (2.39)(3.21) = 0.9 \pm 7.67 = -6.77 \text{ to } 8.57$$

aerobic dance versus control:

$$\bar{R}_A(13.2) - \bar{R}_C(4.5) \pm (2.39)(3.35) = 8.7 \pm 8.01 = 0.69 \text{ to } 16.71$$

jogging versus control:

$$\bar{R}_J(14.1) - \bar{R}_C(4.5) \pm (2.39)(3.45) = 9.6 \pm 8.25 = 1.35 \text{ to } 17.85$$

A comparison is considered statistically significant when the confidence interval does not include zero. In the previous comparisons, the significant differences appear in the two comparisons involving the control group with the exercise groups. Here too we conclude that both the aerobic dance and the jogging groups result in significant reductions in fatness and that there is no difference between the two types of exercise in this regard.

Friedman Two-Way ANOVA by Ranks

The Friedman test is analogous to repeated measures ANOVA in parametric statistics. The scores are ranked, and chi-square is used as the test of significance. An example will explain the steps in the analysis.

Twelve people have been measured for percent fat by three different methods: (a) hydrostatic weighing, (b) total body water, and (c) potassium-40. The investigator wishes to discover whether there is any difference among the three methods. The values for Methods a, b, and c for the 12 subjects are shown in Example 10.7.

Example 10.7

Known Values

Subject	Method a	Method b	Method c	R(a)	R(b)	R(c)
1	16.0	15.7	15.2	3	2	1
2	11.6	10.9	11.5	3	1	2
3	18.1	18.0	17.6	3	2	1
4	16.3	16.8	17.0	1	2	3
5	12.0	13.1	12.8	1	3	2
6	12.5	12.2	12.3	3	1	2
7	9.3	8.8	9.0	3	1	2
8	18.8	17.5	18.0	3	1	2
9	19.2	19.7	19.7	1	2.5	2.5
10	22.3	22.8	21.6	2	3	1
11	20.7	20.3	19.6	3	2	1
12	24.1	23.7	24.4	2	1	3
			Sums of ranks =	28	21.5	22.5

Working It Out

1. **Convert the three scores for each individual to ranks from 1 to 3.**
   Subject 1, for example, has percent fat values of 16.0, 15.7, and 15.2 for
   Methods a, b, and c, respectively. Method c yields the lowest percent fat,
   so it is ranked 1, the next lowest (b) is ranked 2, and Method a is ranked
   3. This procedure is followed for the rest of the subjects (ranks are also
   shown in the table). The familiar procedure of averaging tied ranks is
   followed.

2. **Sum the ranks for each column.** Under the null hypothesis, these sums
   should be about the same because the ranks should be evenly distributed
   over all three methods. On the other hand, if one method shows consistently low percent fat values, for example, it would have more ranks of 1,
   and the result would be a lower sum of ranks.

3. **Compute the chi-square.** The Friedman two-way ANOVA by ranks
   yields a chi-square with $df = k - 1$. The formula is as follows:

$$\chi^2 = [12/Nk(k + 1)] [\Sigma(\Sigma R)^2] - 3N(k + 1)] \qquad (10.9)$$

where N = the total subjects (number of rows), k = the number of columns,
and $\Sigma(\Sigma R)^2$ = the sum of the squared column totals.
   The computations for our example are as follows:

$$\chi^2 = [12/12(3)(3 + 1)][(28)^2 + (21.5)^2 + (22.5)^2] - 3(12)(3+1)$$

$$= (12/144)(784 + 462.25 + 506.25) - 144$$

$$= .083(1,752.5) - 144 = 1.46$$

From Table A.8, with $df = k - 1 = 2$, the chi-square needed for significance at
the .05 level is 5.99. Therefore, we conclude that there are no significant differences among the three methods of estimating percent fat.

A special table (Siegel, 1956) of critical values of chi-square is needed if one uses very small samples (e.g., $k = 3$ and $N < 10$ or $k = 4$ and $N < 5$).

Spearman Rank–Difference Correlation

There are times when an investigator wishes to determine the relationships between variables when the assumptions of parametric statistics cannot be met or perhaps when precise measurements are not available. If the data can be converted to ranks, the Spearman rank-difference method can be used to find the correlation between two sets of ranks. It is a quick and simple process:

$$r_s = 1 - 6\Sigma D^2/[N(N^2 - 1)] \qquad (10.10)$$

where ΣD^2 = the sum of the squared differences between ranks and N = the number of pairs of ranks.

To demonstrate the method, suppose an English teacher ranked 10 boys on social behavior in class. The basketball coach ranked the same 10 boys on his perception of their social behavior in sport participation. The research question is, Are social behaviors of boys perceived similarly across various contexts (e.g., English class and basketball practice)? Example 10.8 contains the data for the rank-difference method.

Example 10.8

Known Values

	A	B	C	D	E	F	G	H	I	J
					Student					
Score from classroom teacher:	4	6	8	1	7	3	9	5	2	10
Score from basketball coach:	1	9	8	6	2	4	3	10	5	7
Classroom score – coach score: $D =$	3	–3	0	–5	5	–1	6	–5	–3	3
Differences squared: $D^2 =$	9	9	0	25	25	1	36	25	9	9

Sum of differences squared: $\Sigma D^2 = 148$

Working It Out
(Equation 10.10)

$r_s = 1 - 6\,(148)/10\,(100 - 1)$
$\quad = 1 - 888/990$
$\quad = 1 - .897$
$\quad = .10$

Table A.9 contains the values of r_s that are necessary for significance at the .05 and .01 levels. We enter the table with our N of 10 and find the tabled values for r_s at the .05 level to be .65. Because our r_s is much lower than that, we are forced to conclude that our coefficient is not significantly different from zero, and social behavior appears to be specific to the setting rather than a general trait.

The Spearman r_s can be computed on variables in which one or both of the values are interval measurements. The measurements simply must be converted to ranks. Of course,

Siegel, S. (1956). *Nonparametric statistics for the behavioral sciences.* New York: McGraw-Hill.

tied ranks are averaged. In a negative correlation, D_2 is very large, so the fraction to be subtracted from 1 is greater than 1, which results in a negative r_s.

The Spearman r_s and the Pearson r will not necessarily yield the same coefficient for the same data, especially if there are a number of tied ranks. Also, because r_s is based on ranks that are not continuous or normally distributed, the coefficient may differ from Pearson r. However, the Spearman r_s is a valuable tool for special cases in which r cannot or should not be used.

Other Indexes of Association

Contingency Coefficient

Multivariate Contingency Tables: The Loglinear Model

The Puri and Sen L Statistic

Several correlational techniques can be used in situations in which data are discrete (i.e., not continuous).

Contingency Coefficient

You can compute the relationship between dichotomous variables such as gender and race by using a **contingency coefficient** The test of significance is the chi-square. You recall that we described the contingency table in this chapter for use in detecting differences between groups or sets of data. The contingency table can also be used to determine relationships. You can have any number of rows and columns in a contingency table. After the chi-square is computed, the contingency coefficient can be computed:

$$C = \sqrt{\chi^2/N + \chi^2} \tag{10.11}$$

If χ^2 is significant, C is also significant. The direction of the relationship is established by examining the data. There are several limitations concerning the ability of the contingency coefficient to estimate correlation. In general, one needs several categories and many observations to obtain a reasonable estimate.

Multivariate Contingency Tables: The Loglinear Model

Categorical data can be analyzed in combination with other variables. In other words, contingency tables can be studied in more than two dimensions. One can therefore identify associations among many variables, for example, the interrelationships among age, gender, skill level, and teaching method. This would be similar to parametric multivariate analysis except that in continuous quantitative data, variables are expressed as linear composites. However, with categorical variables, the researcher deals with contributions to the expected frequencies within each cell of the multivariate contingency table. Any given cell represents the intersection of many marginal proportions.

 contingency coefficient — Method of computing the relationship between dichotomous variables such as gender and race.

Loglinear models are used to analyze multivariate contingency tables. Relative frequencies are transformed to logarithms, which are additive and similar to sum of squares in analysis of variance. Main effects and interactions can be tested for significance. The probability of membership in a particular category can be predicted as a function of membership in other categories using a logistic regression equation and is based on the log odds of membership (called a **logit**).

The loglinear model has considerable potential application in qualitative research (Schutz, 1989). The type of analysis is attracting much attention from researchers and theoreticians. The loglinear analysis provides a means for sophisticated study of the interrelationships among categorical variables. Readers who are interested in pursuing this topic are directed to the text by Kennedy (1983).

The Puri and Sen *L* Statistic

The *L* statistic was developed by Puri and Sen (1969, 1985). This general linear model-based nonparametric test allows the testing of any of the hypotheses encompassed by the canonical correlation model. The hypotheses can be tested using existing computer programs.

 Harwell (1990) provides an interesting and informative illustration of how the Puri and Sen model can be used with simple and multiple regression, ANOVA, ANCOVA, MANOVA, and canonical correlation. The statistical tests by the Puri and Sen model require that the measures are sampled from a common distribution and are independent across subjects. Also, the sample size must be large enough to justify the validity of the chi-square approximation. The method involves ranking the values and then using the appropriate statistical package. From the results, the *L* statistic is calculated and subjected to a chi-square test in order to reject or retain the null hypothesis.

As an illustration, we will use the data in Example 10.6 that were used to explain the Kruskal-Wallis comparison method. The ranks are treated as scores in a simple ANOVA, as described in chapter 8. The *L* technique consists of multiplying r^2 times $N - 1$. For ANOVA, r^2 is *SS* (between groups)/*SS* (total). For the data in Example 10.6, *SS* (between) = 357.8, *SS* (total) = 767.5, and $r^2 = .466$. Then *L* is $(21 - 1)(.466) = 9.32$, which is the same (with rounding error) as was obtained with the Kruskal-Wallis method. A table of critical values of chi-square (Table A.8) is consulted using $df = 2(k - 1)$, where *k* = number of groups. At the .05 level, 5.99 is needed for significance; we therefore reject the null hypothesis.

Harwell presents a strong argument for the flexibility and ease of use of the Puri and Sen model. He recommends consideration of this method especially for multivariate tests because of the difficulty of evaluating the normality assumption with such tests.

Summary

In this chapter we have presented some nonparametric tests that can be used as alternatives to corresponding parametric tests. Researchers sometimes consider the use of non-

---

 loglinear model — A system that analyzes multivariate contingency tables by transforming relative frequencies into logarithms.

logit — Probability of membership in a particular category occurring as a function of membership in other categories in multivariate contingency tables.

Kennedy, J.J. (1983). *Analyzing qualitative data: Introductory loglinear analysis for behavioral research.* New York: Praeger.

Harwell, M.R. (1990). A general approach to hypothesis testing for nonparametric tests. *Journal of Experimental Education*, **58**, 143-156.

parametric statistics as inferior to or less scientific than parametric tests. They are often almost apologetic. Remember that just because a nonparametric test is easy to compute does not mean that something more has to be done before it can be considered fit to be reported.

Whether nonparametric tests are less powerful than the corresponding parametric test seems debatable. Marascuilo and McSweeney (1977), for example, argue that nonparametric tests are strong competitors of parametric tests regarding power efficiency. Moreover, nonparametric procedures are as **robust** as, or more robust than, parametric procedures to distribution differences and the lack of homogeneity of variance. This is especially pertinent in studies in the behavioral sciences because of the small samples that are often used. The conclusion is that if one's data do not meet the assumptions of parametric tests, then nonparametric tests should be employed. The lack of software programs for the more sophisticated tests such as multivariate tests appears to be resolved by the Puri and Sen model.

Table 10.1 summarizes the nonparametric statistics described in this chapter and their application with regard to the type of data (ordinal or nominal), the nature of the sample (independent or dependent), and the number of groups and correlational techniques.

Table 10.1   Summary of Nonparametric Tests

Comparisons of nominal (category) data

Type design	Non-parametric test
One classification:	Chi-square
Two or more classifications:	Contingency tables

Comparisons with ordinal (ranked) data*

Type design	Independent groups	Dependent groups
Two groups:	Mann-Whitney *U* test	Wilcoxon matched pair
More than two groups:	Kruskal-Wallis ANOVA	Friedman ANOVA

Correlations

Type design	Dependent groups
Ordinal (rank) data:	Spearman rank difference
Nominal (category) data (two classifications):	Contingency coefficient
Nominal (category) data (more than two classifications):	Loglinear analysis

*The Puri and Sen *L* statistic can be used with all ranked data analyses.

✔ Check Your Understanding

1. Compute chi-square for the following contingency table of activity preferences of men (*n* = 110) and women (*n* = 90). Determine the significance of the chi-square at

 robust — Characteristic of a statistical test when it is relatively accurate even with fairly severe violations of the assumptions.

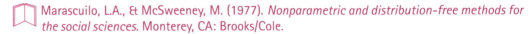 Marascuilo, L.A., & McSweeney, M. (1977). *Nonparametric and distribution-free methods for the social sciences.* Monterey, CA: Brooks/Cole.

the .01 level using Table A.8. When calculating the expected values, round off to whole numbers of expected frequencies.

   a. Write a brief interpretation of your results.
   b. What would be the critical value for significance at the .05 level if you had five rows and four columns?

	Racquetball	Weight training	Aerobic dance
Men	35	45	30
Women	28	13	49

2. Critique the statistical part of a study that uses chi-square in the analysis.
3. Find whether there is a significant difference among the following four groups using the Kruskal-Wallis ANOVA method. First convert the scores to ranks (smallest score = 1), then determine the significance at the .05 level.

Group 1	Group 2	Group 3	Group 4
52	36	32	51
42	37	44	54
51	40	32	46
44	49	45	43
60	50	38	58
39	32	. . .	41
. . .	30	. . .	35

CHAPTER 11

Measuring Research Variables

Dear Professors of Research Methods:

To obtain the measurements I need in my thesis research requires that I both directly observe and videotape during the experimental treatment of the subjects. Do you think that will matter in the way subjects perform?

Carefully collecting data,
Valery Validity

Dear Valery:

Two verses from a 1991 poem by Schuyler W. Huck (*Journal of Experimental Education*, **59**, 193-196) answer your question.

The subjects may be told or know
Observers are watching . . . and so
They'll work with great skill
But only until
The watchers stop watching and go

Or what if the subjects perceive
What you hope and want to believe
Unconscious or not
Like robots they trot . . .
And data you want you'll receive.

Sincerely,
PRM

A basic step in the scientific method of problem solving is the collection of data; therefore, an understanding of basic measurement theory is necessary. (We should point out that although measurement is discussed here as a research tool, measurement itself is an area of research.) In this chapter, we discuss fundamental criteria for judging the quality of measures used in collecting research data: validity and reliability. We explain different types of validity and different ways by which evidence of validity and reliability may be established. The validity and reliability of qualitative research are also a topic. We conclude with some issues concerning the measurement of movement and the measurement of written responses used in paper and pencil-type instruments.

Four Basic Types of Measurement Validity

Logical Validity

Content Validity

Two Contexts of Criterion Validity

    Concurrent Validity

    Predictive Validity

Construct Validity

 In gathering the data on which the results are based, we are also greatly concerned with the validity of the measurements we are using. If, for example, a study seeks to compare training methods for producing strength gains, the researcher must have a valid measure of strength to evaluate the effects of the training methods. **Validity** of measurement, then, indicates the degree to which the test, or instrument, measures what it is supposed to measure. Thus, validity refers to the soundness of the interpretation of a test, the most important consideration in measurement.

There are different purposes for using certain measures. Consequently, there are different kinds of validity. According to the American Psychological Association (APA) and the American Educational Research Association (AERA), the four basic types of validity are *logical*, *content*, *criterion*, and *construct*.

You will notice that logical validity was listed as a separate type of validity; however, the APA and the AERA consider logical validity to be a special case of content validity. Because our main concern in this book is measurement for research purposes, logical, content, criterion, and construct validity are discussed only briefly. A more comprehensive discussion would be necessary if we were discussing the evaluation of educational objectives.

Logical Validity

 Logical validity is sometimes referred to as **face validity**, although measurement experts dislike that term. Logical validity is claimed when the measure obviously involves the performance being measured. In other words, it means that the test is

 validity — Degree to which a test or instrument measures what it purports to measure; can be categorized as *logical*, *content*, *criterion*, and *construct*.

logical validity — Condition that is claimed when the measure obviously involves the performance being measured; also known as *face validity*.

face validity — See *logical validity*.

static balance — The ability to hold a stationary position.

valid by definition. A **static balance** test that consists of balancing on one foot has logical validity. A speed-of-movement test, in which the person is timed in running a specified distance, must be considered to have logical validity. Occasionally, logical validity is used in research studies, but a researcher would prefer to have more objective evidence as to the validity of measurement.

Content Validity

 Content validity pertains almost exclusively to learning in educational settings. A test has content validity if it adequately samples what was covered in the course. As with logical validity, no statistical evidence can be supplied for content validity. The teacher should prepare a table of specifications (sometimes called a test blueprint) before making out the test. The topics and course objectives, as well as the relative degree of emphasis accorded each, can then be keyed to a corresponding number of questions pertaining to each area.

Two Contexts of Criterion Validity

Measurements used in research studies are frequently validated against some criterion. **Criterion validity** is used in two main contexts: concurrent validity and predictive validity.

Concurrent Validity

Concurrent validity involves a measuring instrument being correlated with some criterion that is administered at about the same time (i.e., concurrently). Many physical performance measures are validated in this manner. Popular criterion measures include an already validated or accepted measure, judges' ratings and tournament results, and some other observable performance criterion. Concurrent validity is usually employed when the researcher wishes to substitute a shorter, more easily administered test for a criterion that is more difficult to measure.

To illustrate: Maximal oxygen consumption is regarded as the most valid measure of cardiorespiratory fitness. However, it requires a laboratory, expensive equipment, and considerable time for testing; furthermore, only one person can be tested at a time. Let us assume that a researcher, Douglas Bag, wishes to screen subjects as to their fitness levels before assigning them to experimental treatments. Rather than using such an elaborate test as maximal oxygen consumption, Douglas determines it would be advantageous to use a stair-walking test he has devised. To determine whether it is a valid measure of cardiorespiratory fitness, he could administer both the maximal oxygen consumption test and the stair-walking test to a group of subjects (from the same population as will be used in the study) and correlate the results of the two tests. If a satisfactory relationship exists, Doug can conclude that his stair-walking test is valid.

Written tests may also be validated in this way. For example, a researcher might wish to use a group intelligence test rather than one such as the lengthy Stanford-Binet, which must be administered individually.

 content validity — Condition that is claimed (usually in educational settings) when a test adequately samples what was covered in the course.

 criterion validity — The degree to which scores on a test are related to some recognized standard, or criterion.

 concurrent validity — Type of criterion validity in which a measuring instrument is correlated with some criterion that is administered at about the same time, or concurrently.

Judges' ratings serve as criterion measures for some tests (sport skills are sometimes validated this way). A great amount of time and effort is required to secure competent judges, teach them to use the rating scale, test for agreement among judges, arrange for a sufficient number of trials, and so on. Consequently, judges' rating cannot be used routinely to evaluate performances. The use of some skills tests would be more economical. Furthermore, the skills tests usually provide knowledge of results and measures of progress for the students. The skills tests could be initially validated, however, by giving the test and having judges rate the subjects on those skills. A validity coefficient can be obtained by correlating the scores on the skills tests with the judges' ratings.

Choosing the criterion is critical in the concurrent validity method. All the correlation can tell you is the degree of relationship between a measure and the criterion. If the criterion is inadequate, then the concurrent validity coefficient is of little consequence.

Predictive Validity

Predictive validity involves the use of a criterion to be predicted. Often the criterion is some later behavior, e.g., entrance examinations used to predict later success. Suppose that a physical education instructor wished to develop a test that could be given in beginning gymnastics classes to predict success in advanced classes. Students would take this test while they were in the beginner course. At the end of the advanced course, those test results would be correlated with the criterion of success (grades, ratings, etc.). In trying to predict a certain behavior, one should try to ascertain whether there is a known "base rate" for that behavior. For example, someone might attempt to construct a test that would predict women students who might develop bulimia at a university. Suppose that the incidence of bulimia is 10% of the female population at that school. Knowing this, one could be correct 90% of the time in predicting that no one in the sample will be bulimic. If the base rate is very low or very high, a predictive measure may have little practical value because the increase in predictability will be negligible.

Chapters 7 and 15 discuss aspects of prediction in correlational research. Multiple regression is often used because several predictors are likely to have a greater validity coefficient than the correlation between any one test and the criterion. Previously, we used the example of the prediction of percent fat from skinfold measurements. The criterion—percent fat—is measured by the underwater (hydrostatic) weighing technique. Several skinfold measures are taken, and multiple regression is used to determine the best prediction equation. The researcher hopes to use the skinfold measures in the future if the prediction formula demonstrates an acceptable validity coefficient.

One limitation of such studies is that the validity tends to decrease when the prediction formula is used with a new sample. This tendency is called shrinkage. Common sense suggests that shrinkage is more likely when a small sample is used in the original study and particularly when the number of predictors is large. In fact, if enough predictor variables (equal to the number of subjects) are added to the multiple regression equation, one can achieve perfect prediction. The problem is that the correlations are unique to the sample, and when the results are applied to another sample (even similar to the first one), the relationship does not hold. Consequently, the validity coefficient decreases substantially (i.e., shrinkage occurs).

A technique recommended to help estimate shrinkage is **cross-validation**. In this technique, the same tests are given to a new sample from the same population to check whether the formula is accurate. For example, a researcher might administer the criterion measure and predictor tests to a sample of 200 subjects. Then, using

---

predictive validity — Degree to which scores of predictor variables can accurately predict criterion scores.

cross-validation — Technique to assess the accuracy of a prediction formula in which the formula is applied to a sample not used when the formula was developed.

100 subjects, he or she would employ multiple regression to develop a prediction formula. This formula is then applied to the other 100 subjects to see how accurately it predicts the criterion for them. Because the researcher has the actual criterion measures on these subjects, the amount of shrinkage can be ascertained by correlating (Pearson r) the predicted scores with the actual scores. A comparison of the R^2 from the multiple prediction with the r^2 between the actual and the predicted criteria yields an estimate of shrinkage.

Construct Validity

 Many human characteristics are not directly observable. Rather, they are hypothetical constructs that carry a number of associated meanings concerning how a person who possesses the trait(s) to a high degree would behave differently from someone who possesses a low degree of the trait(s). Anxiety, intelligence, sportsmanship, creativity, and attitude are a few such hypothetical constructs. Because these traits are not directly observable, measurement poses a problem. **Construct validity** is the degree to which a test measures a hypothetical construct and is usually established by relating the test results to some behavior. For example, a number of behaviors are expected of someone with a high degree of sportsmanship. This person might be expected to compliment the opponent on shots made during a tennis match. As an indication of construct validity, a test maker could compare the number of times the person scoring high on a test of sportsmanship complimented the opponent with the number of times a person scoring lower on the test did so.

 The **known group difference method** is sometimes used in establishing construct validity. For example, construct validity of a test of anaerobic power could be demonstrated by comparing test scores of sprinters and jumpers with distance runners. Sprinting and jumping require greater anaerobic power than distance running. Therefore, the tester could determine whether the test differentiates between the two kinds of track performers. If the sprinters and jumpers score significantly better than the distance runners, this would provide some evidence that the test measures anaerobic power.

An experimental approach is occasionally used in demonstrating construct validity. For example, a test of cardiovascular fitness might be assumed to have construct validity if it reflected gains in fitness following a conditioning program. Similarly, the originator of a motor skills test could demonstrate construct validity with regard to its sensitivity in differentiating between groups of instructed and noninstructed children.

Correlation can also be used in establishing construct validity. Hypothesized structures or dimensions of the trait being tested are sometimes formulated and verified with factor analysis. The tester also uses correlation to examine relationships between constructs, for example, when it is hypothesized that someone with high scores on the test being developed (e.g., cardiovascular fitness) should also do well on some total physical fitness scale. Conversely, individuals with low scores on the cardiovascular test would do poorly on the fitness test.

Validity Generalization

In the discussion on criterion validity, we mentioned the problem of population (or situation) specificity, whereby the prediction is most accurate for the sample used in

construct validity — Degree to which a test measures a hypothetical construct; usually established by relating the test results to some behavior.

known group difference method — Method used in establishing construct validity in which the test scores of groups that should differ on a trait or ability are compared.

developing the formula. For example, a researcher produces a formula for predicting percent body fat from skinfold measures for young adult females. If you look at the literature on this topic you will see that many researchers have done this particular study and that various correlation coefficients have been obtained between skinfold measurements and a criterion of percent fat (such as derived from underwater weighing).

A pertinent question is, Just how generalizable is the prediction of percent body fat from skinfold measurements? How valid is the prediction when you wish to look at other ages, such as older or younger women? What about using athletic and nonathletic women? What about predicting for men? Certainly, a person does not want to have to compute a new criterion-predictor formula every time he or she wants to predict percent fat. Validity generalization is a statistical model designed to address this problem.

 Validity generalization was developed by Schmidt, Hunter, and Urry (1976). The method uses the ideas of meta-analysis (see chapter 14) for generalizing the results of many studies employing the same criterion-predictor combinations. Patterson (1989) has provided a clear and readable summary and application of the method in exercise science.

As with any innovative idea, validity generalization and its assumptions provoke controversy. One drawback is that one needs a very large number of studies (samples) to achieve adequate power. Nevertheless, it is a potentially valuable tool for estimating generalizability and has widespread applications for certain tests.

Establishing Validity in Criterion-Referenced Tests

The methods discussed so far relate to norm-referenced measurement. Research studies also use criterion-referenced measurement, in which a test purports to establish that subjects have achieved certain levels of proficiency or development. For example, a developmental study may wish to establish that the subjects have reached mature behavior in some motor task such as throwing or jumping.

• **Domain-Referenced Validity.**   A test is used that contains the essential components (or objectives) of that task weighted as to their importance. This is **domain-referenced validity**. It is usually validated by using a pool of judges and measurement specialists to assess the representativeness of items and item bias (Safrit, 1989). Written tests may also be validated in this manner, for example, when a researcher wishes to establish that the subjects possessed suitable knowledge about a topic. Safrit (1989) listed the steps for demonstrating domain-referenced validity in written tests.

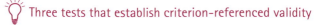

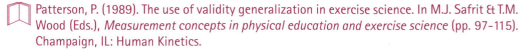
Patterson, P. (1989). The use of validity generalization in exercise science. In M.J. Safrit & T.M. Wood (Eds.), *Measurement concepts in physical education and exercise science* (pp. 97-115). Champaign, IL: Human Kinetics.

Three tests that establish criterion-referenced validity

domain-referenced validity — The degree to which a test measures essential components or objectives of a domain.

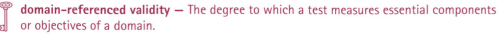
Safrit, M.J. (1989). Criterion-referenced measurement: Validity. In M.J. Safrit & T.M. Wood (Eds.), *Measurement concepts in physical education and exercise science* (pp. 119-135). Champaign, IL: Human Kinetics.

• **Decision Accuracy**. Another approach to validity of criterion-referenced tests (besides domain-referenced ones) is **decision accuracy**. This approach involves decisions of mastery-nonmastery classifications. Contingency tables are generally used in this procedure. An example of a study in exercise science that dealt with decision accuracy is that by Washburn and Safrit (cited in Safrit, 1989). This study assessed the validity of an aerobic capacity cutoff score for U.S. Forest Service firefighters. The study involved three analytical procedures to test the cutoff decision score: the calculation of the outcome probabilities in a contingency table, calculation of the phi coefficient, and a utility analysis to determine relative weighing. Cross-validation was performed.

• **Adaptive Testing**. In this type of testing, researchers use a computer to constantly adapt the administration of questions to the student's performance. If the student is having difficulty, the computer adapts by giving easier questions. Conversely, if the student is having no difficulty, harder questions are given. Thus, little time is wasted with items that are too hard or too easy, and testing time is greatly reduced. Item response theory is used in adaptive testing to match the student with the test so as to yield the most precise information about the individual's mastery of material (see Spray, 1987, 1989). Item response theory is discussed further later in this chapter.

Validity of Observations in Qualitative Research

Chapter 17 discusses internal and external validity of qualitative research. Here we are concerned with the validity of the observations or of data collection. The qualitative researcher does not usually attempt to provide numerical evidence of the validity of the observations. "The issue of validity is not a matter of methodological hair splitting about the fifth decimal point, but a question of whether the researcher sees what he or she thinks he or she sees" (Kirk & Miller, 1986, p. 21).

The qualitative researcher is constantly doing something comparable to hypothesis testing. The researcher's perceptions are continuously checked against possible alternatives or sources of error. When the hypothesis is incorrect, the researcher will usually find out about it (Kirk & Miller, 1986).

Reliability does not assure validity in qualitative research any more than in quantitative research. You can get the same answers to the same questions consistently, but the answers may not be correct. Whereas the criticism often levied at qualitative research is the lack of supporting numerical data, the qualitative researcher counters that the quantitative researcher tends to simply accept results without question and tests them for significance. The qualitative researcher, on the other hand, will suspect faulty data and then search for the error.

In chapter 17 we define Type III error as that of asking the wrong questions. This is probably the cause of most validity problems in qualitative research. However, through multiple sources of data and simultaneous analysis with the data collection, the qualitative researcher contends that his or her interpretations of the data are valid. In fact, the

---

decision accuracy — Approach used to validate criterion-referenced tests that assesses the accuracy of classifications of individuals to mastery and nonmastery categories.

Spray, J.A. (1989). New approaches to solving measurement problems. In M.J. Safrit & T.M. Wood (Eds.), *Measurement concepts in physical education and exercise science* (pp. 229-248). Champaign, IL: Human Kinetics.

intensive firsthand presence of the researcher is the strongest support for validity in the data-gathering process in qualitative research.

An Overview of Measurement Reliability

Sources of Measurement Error

Expressing Reliability Through Correlation

Interclass Correlation

Three Methods of Testing Intraclass Correlation

Calculating F

Discarding Trials

Ignoring Trial-to-Trial Variance

An integral part of validity is reliability, which pertains to the consistency, or repeatability, of a measure. A test cannot be considered valid if it is not reliable. In other words, if the test is not consistent—if you cannot depend on successive trials to yield the same results—then the test cannot be trusted. Of course, a test could be reliable yet not valid, but it could never be valid if it were not reliable. For example, weighing oneself repeatedly on a broken scale would give reliable results but not valid ones. Test reliability is sometimes discussed in terms of observed score, true score, and error score.

A test score obtained on an individual is the **observed score.** It is not known whether this is a true assessment of this person's ability or performance. There may well be measurement error involved pertaining to the test directions, the instrumentation, the scoring, or the emotional-physical state of the subject. Thus, an observed score theoretically consists of the person's **true score** and **error score.** Expressed in terms of score variance, the observed score variance consists of true score variance plus error variance. The goal of the tester is to remove error to yield the true score. The coefficient of reliability is the ratio of true score variance to observed score variance. Because true score variance is never known, it is estimated by subtracting error variance from observed score variance. Thus, the reliability coefficient reflects the degree to which the measurement is free of error variance.

Sources of Measurement Error

Measurement error can come from four sources: the subject, the testing, the scoring, and the instrumentation. Measurement error associated with the subject includes many factors, including mood, motivation, fatigue, health, fluctuations in memory (and performance), previous practice, specific knowledge, and familiarity with the test items.

 Three components of test reliability

 observed score — In classical test theory, an obtained score which is comprised of a person's true score and error score.

true score — In classical test theory, the part of the observed score that represents the individual's real score and does not contain measurement error.

error score — In classical test theory, the part of an observed score that is attributed to measurement error.

Errors in testing are those that can arise due to the lack of clarity or completeness in the directions, to whether the instructions are rigidly followed, to whether supplementary directions or motivation is applied, and so forth. Errors in scoring relate to the competence, experience, and dedication of the scorers as well as to the nature of the scoring itself. The extent to which the scorer is familiar with the behavior being tested and the test items can greatly affect scoring accuracy. Carelessness and inattention to detail produce measurement error. Measurement error due to instrumentation includes such obvious causes as inaccuracy and lack of calibration of mechanical and electronic equipment. It also refers to the inadequacy of tests in discriminating between abilities and to the difficulty of scoring some tests.

Expressing Reliability Through Correlation

The degree of reliability is expressed by a correlation coefficient, ranging from 0.00 to 1.00. The closer the coefficient is to 1.00, the less error variance it reflects and the more the true score is assessed. Reliability is established several ways, which are summarized in the next section. The type of correlation technique used in computing the reliability coefficient differs from that used in establishing validity. Pearson r is often called **interclass correlation**. This is used in correlating two different variables (bivariate statistic), such as in determining validity where judges' ratings are correlated with scores on a skill test. However, interclass correlation is not appropriate in establishing reliability because the same variable is being correlated. When a test is given twice, the scores on the first test are correlated with the scores on the second test to determine the degree of consistency. Here, the two test scores are for the same variable, so interclass correlation should not be used. Rather, **intraclass correlation** is the appropriate statistical technique. This method uses ANOVA to obtain the reliability coefficient.

Interclass Correlation

There are three main weaknesses of Pearson r (interclass correlation) for reliability determination. The first is that, as mentioned previously, the Pearson r is a bivariate statistic, whereas reliability involves univariate measures. Second, in Pearson r, the computations are limited to only two scores, X and Y. Often, however, more than two trials are given, and the tester is concerned with the reliability of multiple trials. For example, if a test specifies three trials, the researcher must either give three more trials and use the average or best score of each set of trials for the correlations or perhaps correlate the first trial with the second, the first with the third, and the second with the third. In the first case, extra trials must be given only for reliability; in the second case, multiple correlations often lose meaningfulness. Finally, the interclass correlation does not provide a thorough examination of different sources of variability on multiple trials. For example, changes in means and standard deviations from trial to trial cannot be assessed in the Pearson r method but can be analyzed with intraclass correlation.

Three Methods of Testing Intraclass Correlation

Intraclass correlation provides estimates of systematic and error variance. For example, systematic differences among trials can be examined. The last trials may differ significantly from the first trials because of a learning phenomenon or fatigue effect (or both). If the tester

interclass correlation — The most commonly used method of computing correlation between two variables; also called Pearson r or *Pearson product moment coefficient of correlation*.

intraclass correlation — An ANOVA technique used in estimating reliability of a measure.

Three weaknesses of interclass correlation for determining reliability

recognizes this, then perhaps initial (or final) trials can be excluded or the point at which performance levels off can be used as the score. In other words, through ANOVA the tester can truly examine test performance from trial to trial and then select the most reliable testing schedule.

Example 11.1 shows how to determine intraclass correlation (R). The example consists of three trials. The procedures leading to the calculation of R are the same as those of the simple ANOVA with repeated measures presented in chapter 8.

Example 11.1

Known Values

Student	Trial 1	Trial 2	Trial 3
A	3	3	4
B	4	6	6
C	2	3	4
D	1	3	4
E	2	4	2
M	2.4	3.8	4.0

Working It Out
(See Example 8.15)

Summary of ANOVA

Source	SS	df	MS	F
Subjects	14.9	4	3.73	. . .
Trials	7.6	2	3.80	5.94*
Residual	5.1	8	.64	. . .

*$p < .05$.

By using the formulas in Example 8.15 we can calculate the necessary sums of squares (SS) and mean squares (MS). We find the total sum of squares to be 27.6. The sum of squares for subjects is 14.9 and that for trials 7.6. We can then calculate the residual sum of squares by subtraction and get 5.1. Next, we compute the mean squares (MS) for subjects, trials, and residual by the formulas in the example.

Calculating F. You can determine any significant differences among the three trials by calculating the F for trials as in Example 8.15. Then enter Table A.6 in Appendix A and read down the 2-df column to the 8-df row. Our F of 5.94 is found to be greater than the tabled F of 4.46 for the .05 level of probability. Thus, there are significant differences among trials. At this point we need to recognize that there are different opinions as to what should be done with trial differences (Baumgartner & Jackson, 1991; Johnson & Nelson, 1986; Safrit, 1976). Some test authorities argue that the test performance should be consistent from one trial to the next and that any trial-to-trial variance should be attributed simply to measurement error. If we decide to do this, the formula for R is

$$R = (MS_S - MS_E) / MS_S \tag{11.1}$$

in which MS_S = the mean squares for subjects (from Example 11.1) and MS_E = the mean squares for error, which is computed as follows:

Baumgartner, T.A., & Jackson, A.S. (1991). *Measurement for evaluation in physical education* (4th ed.). Dubuque, IA: Wm. C. Brown.

Johnson, B.L., & Nelson, J.K. (1986). *Practical measurements for evaluation in physical education* (4th ed.). Minneapolis: Burgess.

Safrit, M.J. (1976). *Reliability theory.* Washington, DC: American Alliance for Health, Physical Education, and Recreation.

$$\frac{SS \text{ for trials} + SS \text{ for residual}}{df \text{ for trials} + df \text{ for residual}}$$

$$= \frac{7.6 + 5.1}{2 + 8}$$

$$= 1.27$$

The R is thus calculated: $R = (3.73 - 1.27)/3.73 = .66$

Discarding Trials.   Another way of dealing with significant trial differences is to discard the trials that are noticeably different from the others (Baumgartner & Jackson, 1991). Then a second ANOVA is conducted on the remaining trials, and another F test is computed. If F is nonsignificant, R is calculated using Formula 11.1, in which trial variance is considered measurement error. If F is still significant, additional trials are discarded, and another ANOVA is conducted. The purpose of this method is to find a measurement schedule that is free of trial differences (nonsignificant F that yields the largest possible criterion score) and that is most reliable. This method is especially appealing when there is an apparent trend in trial differences, as when a learning phenomenon (or release of inhibitions) is evident in the initial trial or trials. For example, if five trials on a performance test yielded mean scores of 15, 18, 23, 25, and 24, one might discard the first two trials and compute another analysis on the last three trials. Similarly, a fatigue effect may be evidenced by a decrease in scores on the final trials in some types of tests.

In Example 11.1, note that Trial 1 is considerably lower than Trials 2 and 3. So, we discard the first trial and compute another ANOVA on Trials 2 and 3 (results are shown in Table 11.1). The F for trials in the table is nonsignificant, so we compute R with Formula 11.1: $R = (2.85 - .7)/2.85 = .75$.

Table 11.1   Summary of ANOVA for Reliability Estimation (2 Trials)

Source	SS	df	MS	F
Subjects	11.4	4	2.85	...
Trials	.1	1	.10	.11
Residual	3.4	4	.85	...

Note that we computed MS_E (.7) by combining the sum of squares for trials and residual and dividing by their respective degrees of freedom: $(.1 + 3.4)/(1 + 4) = .7$. We see that R is considerably higher when we discarded the first trial.

Ignoring Trial-to-Trial Variance.   A third approach is simply to not consider trial-to-trial variance as measurement error and to compute R as follows:

$$R = (MS_S - MS_{res}) / MS_S \tag{11.2}$$

Using the data in Example 11.1, we calculate R as follows: $R = (3.73 - .64)/3.73 = .83$. In this approach, trial-to-trial variance is not considered as true score variance or error score variance. Consequently, R is notably higher than it was in the previous approaches because all trial-to-trial variance is removed. Although some measurement authorities advocate this approach, it does not seem to follow the theory that observed score variance equals true score variance plus error score variance. Other measurement specialists argue that every source of variance not attributable to subjects should be considered error score variance (Safrit, 1976). Although we do not intend to enter into the argument, we do believe it should be of interest to the researcher (tester) to ascertain whether there are trial-to-trial differences. Consequently, if significant differences are found, the tester can decide whether to eliminate some trials (as with a learning trend) or simply to consider trial-to-trial differences as measurement error.

 Intertester reliability is determined the same way. Thus, the objectivity of judges or different testers is analyzed by intraclass R, and judge-to-judge variance is calculated in the same way as trial-to-trial variance. Of course, more complex ANOVA designs can be used in which trial-to-trial, day-to-day, and judge-to-judge sources of variance all can be identified. Baumgartner (1989) and Safrit (1976) discuss some models that can be used for establishing reliability.

Three Methods of Establishing Reliability

Determining Stability
Constructing Alternate Forms
Obtaining Internal Consistency
   Same-Day Test-Retest
   Split-Half Technique
   Kuder-Richardson Method
   Coefficient Alpha

It is easier to establish reliability than validity. We first look at three types of coefficients of reliability: stability, alternate forms, and internal consistency.

Determining Stability

The coefficient of **stability** is determined by the test-retest method on separate days. This method is used frequently with fitness and motor performance measures but less often with pencil-and-paper tests. This is one of the most severe tests of consistency because the errors associated with measurement are likely to be more pronounced when the two test administrations are separated by a day or more.

In the **test-retest method**, the test is given one day and then repeated a day or so later. The interval may be governed to some extent by how strenuous the test is and whether more than a day's rest is needed. Of course, the interval cannot be so long that actual changes in ability, maturation, or learning occur between the two test administrations.

Intraclass correlation is used to compute the coefficient of stability of the scores on the two tests. Through ANOVA procedures, the tester can determine the amount of variance

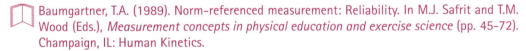

Baumgartner, T.A. (1989). Norm-referenced measurement: Reliability. In M.J. Safrit and T.M. Wood (Eds.), *Measurement concepts in physical education and exercise science* (pp. 45-72). Champaign, IL: Human Kinetics.

Safrit, M.J. (1976). *Reliability Theory*. Washington, DC: American Alliance for Health, Physical Education and Recreation.

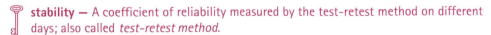

stability — A coefficient of reliability measured by the test-retest method on different days; also called *test-retest method*.

test-retest method — Method of determining reliability in which a test is given one day and then administered exactly as before a day or so later; also called *stability*.

accounted for by the separate days of testing as well as test trial differences, subject differences, and error variance.

Constructing Alternate Forms

 The **alternate-forms method** of establishing reliability involves the construction of two tests that supposedly sample the same material. This method is sometimes referred to as the **parallel-form method** or the **equivalence method**. The two tests are given to the same subjects. Ordinarily, some time elapses between the two administrations. The scores on the two tests are then correlated to obtain a reliability coefficient. The alternate-forms method is a widely used technique with standardized tests, such as those of achievement and scholastic aptitude. The method is rarely used with physical performance tests, probably because it is more difficult to construct two different sets of good physical test items than it is to write two sets of questions.

Some test experts maintain that, theoretically, the alternate-forms method is the preferred method. Any test is only a sample of test items from a universe of possible test items. Thus, the degree of relationship between two such samples should yield the best estimate of reliability.

Obtaining Internal Consistency

 An **internal consistency** reliability coefficient can be obtained by several methods. Some common methods are the same-day test-retest, the split-half method, the Kuder-Richardson method of rational equivalence, and the coefficient alpha technique.

Same-Day Test-Retest

 The **same-day test-retest method** is used almost exclusively with physical performance tests , as practice effects and recall tend to produce spuriously high correlations when this technique is used with written tests. The test-retest on the same day results in a higher reliability coefficient than does a test-retest on separate days. One would certainly expect more consistency of performance within the same day than on different days. Intraclass correlation is used to analyze trial-to-trial (internal) consistency.

Split-Half Technique

 The **split-half technique** has been widely used to determine internal consistency. This method has been used for written tests and occasionally in performance tests that require numerous trials. The test is divided in two, and the two halves are

---

alternate-forms method — Method of establishing reliability involving the construction of two tests, both that supposedly sample the same material; also called *parallel-form method* or the *equivalence method*.
parallel-form method — See *alternate-form method*.

equivalence method — See *alternate-form method*.

internal consistency — An estimate of the reliability that represents the consistency of scores within a test.

same-day test-retest method — Method of establishing reliability in which a test is given twice to the same subjects on the same day.

split-half technique — Method of testing reliability in which the test is divided in two and the two halves are correlated, usually by making the odd numbers one part and the even numbers the other part.

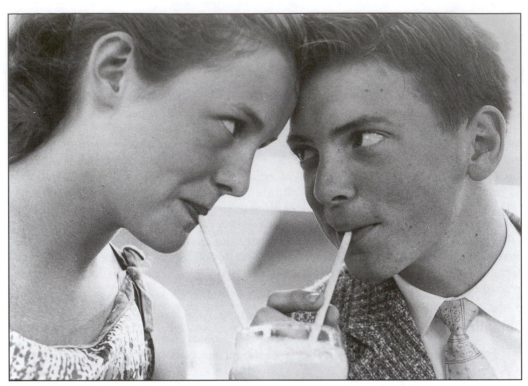

The split–half technique: a good way to test reliability.

then correlated. A test could be divided into first and second halves, but this is usually not deemed satisfactory. Sometimes a person tires near the end of the test, and sometimes easier questions are placed in the first half. Usually, the odd-numbered questions are compared with the even-numbered ones. That is, the number of odd-numbered questions a person got correct is correlated with the number of correct answers on the even-numbered questions.

 Because the correlation is between the two halves of the test, the reliability co-efficient represents only half the size of the total test; that is, behavior is sampled only half as thoroughly. Thus, a step-up procedure, the **Spearman-Brown proph-ecy formula**, is used to estimate the reliability for the entire test because the total test is based on twice the sample of behavior (twice the number of items). The formula is

$$\text{corrected reliability coefficient} = \frac{2 \times \text{reliability for 1/2 test}}{1.00 + \text{reliability for 1/2 test}}$$

If, for example, the correlation between the even-numbered items and the odd-numbered items was .85, the corrected reliability coefficient would be

$$\frac{2 \times .85}{1.00 + .85} = \frac{1.70}{1.85} = .92$$

 Another split-half method is the **Flanagan method**, which analyzes the vari-ances of the halves of the test in relation to the total variance. No correlation or Spearman-Brown step-up procedure is involved.

Spearman–Brown prophecy formula — Equation developed to estimate the reliability for the entire test when the split-half technique is used to test reliability.

Flanagan method — A process for estimating reliability of a test in which the test is split into two halves, and the variances of the halves of the test are analyzed in relation to the total variance of the test.

Kuder–Richardson Method

 The **Kuder–Richardson (K-R) method of rational equivalence** can be used for items scored dichotomously (e.g., right or wrong). Only one test administration is required, and no correlation is calculated. Two formulas, known as KR-20 and KR-21, are the most widely used. The resulting coefficient represents an average of all possible split-half reliability coefficients.

Highly regarded by many test experts, the KR-20 involves the proportions of students who answered each item correctly and incorrectly in relation to the total score variance. The KR-21 is a simplified, less accurate version of the KR-20. Quickly and easily computed, KR-21 is applicable to the teacher (or researcher) for "homemade" tests. The KR-21 formula is

$$KR\text{-}21 = 1.00 - \frac{M(n - M)}{n(s^2)}$$

where M = the mean score for the test, n = the number of test items, and s^2 (standard deviation squared) = the test variance. The KR-21 formula always results in a lower reliability coefficient than the KR-20. One can assume, then, that the coefficient represents a minimum reliability estimate.

Coefficient Alpha

 Coefficient alpha is sometimes referred to as the **Cronbach alpha coefficient** (see Cronbach, 1951). It is a generalized reliability coefficient that is more versatile than other methods. One particularly desirable feature of coefficient alpha is that it can be used with items that have various point values such as essay tests and attitude scales that have "strongly agree," "agree," etc. The method involves calculating variances of the "parts" of a test. The parts can be items, test halves, trials, or a series of tests such as quizzes. When the items are dichotomous (i.e., either right or wrong), the alpha coefficient will result in the same reliability estimate as KR-20 (in fact, KR-20 is just a special case of coefficient alpha). When the parts are halves of the test, the results will be the same as the Flanagan split-halves method, and when the parts are trials or tests, the results will be the same as intraclass correlation. Coefficient alpha is probably the most commonly used method of estimating reliability in standardized tests.

Ensuring Intertester Reliability (Objectivity)

 A form of reliability that pertains to the testers is called **intertester (interrater) reliability**, or often **objectivity**. This facet of reliability is the degree to which different testers can achieve the same scores on the same subjects.

Overall, most teachers and students prefer objective over subjective measures because so much depends on how valid and reliable the measures are. Objective measures are not automatically better than subjective ones, but they do yield quantitative scores that

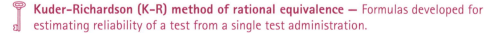

Kuder–Richardson (K–R) method of rational equivalence — Formulas developed for estimating reliability of a test from a single test administration.

coefficient alpha — A technique used in estimating reliability of multiple trial tests; also called *Cronbach alpha coefficient.*

Cronbach alpha coefficient — See *coefficient alpha.*

intertester (interrater) reliability — The degree to which different testers can obtain the same scores on the same subjects; also called *objectivity.*

objectivity — See *intertester reliability.*

are more "visible" and that, statistically, can be handled more easily. In most research techniques, objective measurements are essential.

The degree of objectivity (intertester reliability) can be established by having more than one tester gather data; then the scores are analyzed with intraclass correlation techniques to obtain an intertester reliability coefficient. It is possible to assess a number of sources of variance in one analysis, such as variance caused by testers, trials, days, subjects, and error (for discussion of the calculations involved, see Safrit, 1976).

Some forms of research in physical activity involve the observation of certain behaviors in real-world settings, such as during physical education classes or sport participation. This involves the use or development of some sort of coding instrument. Most frequently, the instrument has a series of categories into which the various motor behaviors may be coded. The behaviors are observed using techniques described in chapter 15 such as event recording, time sampling, and duration recording.

 In these types of scales, as with any measure, validity and reliability are important. However, it is usually much more difficult to obtain consistency in recording children's activities in a physical education class or sport than in recording error measurements from a laboratory task such as the linear slide. Consequently, observational researchers are concerned about coder consistency. Typically, coders are trained to a criterion level of reliability, and reliability is checked regularly throughout the project. A common way of estimating reliability among coders is called **interobserver agreement (IOA)**, which uses the following formula:

$$IOA = \frac{agreements}{(agreements + disagreements)}$$

Agreements are commonly coded behaviors, whereas disagreements are behaviors coded differently. IOA is typically reported as the percent of agreement.

Generalizability Theory

Earlier we said that intertester reliability is determined the same way as intraclass reliability. An extension of intraclass reliability is **generalizability theory (G-theory)**. This model enables the researcher to identify sources of error in estimating reliability of test scores. To illustrate, in the measurement of strength, we can think of many variables that affect the reliability of the scores. Among these are the subjects and their ages, gender, and levels of experience; the tester; the types of instruments used; the types of contraction; and the muscle groups being studied.

The G-theory employs two approaches, the G study and the D study. The **G study** uses repeated measures ANOVA to help identify the relative importance of different sources of variance that contribute to measurement error. In the **D study**,

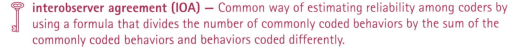

interobserver agreement (IOA) — Common way of estimating reliability among coders by using a formula that divides the number of commonly coded behaviors by the sum of the commonly coded behaviors and behaviors coded differently.

generalizability theory (G–theory) — An extension of intraclass reliability that enables the researcher to identify sources of error in estimating reliability of scores on a test.

G study — An approach employed in generalizability theory that uses repeated measures ANOVA to help identify the relative importance of different sources of variance that contribute to measurement error.

D study — An approach employed in generalizability theory in which the researcher calculates generalizability coefficients for the various facets in the study.

the researcher calculates generalizability coefficients for the study's various components. The combined results of the G and the D studies provide the researcher with an optimal measurement format for collecting the data. Morrow (1989) has provided an excellent description and tutorial for G theory, and Wood and Safrit (1987) compared different multivariate models in estimating reliability of a test battery. Generalizability theory should play an increasingly important role in estimating test reliability in the future.

Reliability in Criterion-Referenced Measurements

In criterion-referenced measurements, the tests are not designed to discriminate among subjects' abilities; instead, they are often used for screening and measuring competencies (Safrit, 1986). The statistical methods used to establish reliability with criterion-referenced measurements are different than those used with norm-referenced tests. Both are concerned with consistency, but criterion-referenced tests try to consistently replicate a person's domain (or true) score independently of other persons' performances (Looney, 1989).

Hambleton and Novick (1973) first suggested the **proportion of agreement index** to assess the consistency of correct decisions. The index is now usually corrected for chance. Looney (1989) described and discussed the various procedures involved as well as estimates for single-test administration.

Two Ways of Examining Reliability in Qualitative Research

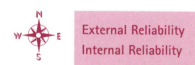
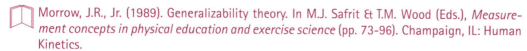

External Reliability
Internal Reliability

In qualitative research, one cannot very well replicate the data-gathering process simply for the purpose of establishing reliability. The subjects would probably think the researcher was suffering from senility if he or she tried to interview the same people with the same questions twice on the same day. However, qualitative researchers sometimes do ask the same questions of different (but similar) subjects and occasionally interview the same subjects over time as evidence of consistency, or agreement.

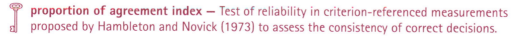

Morrow, J.R., Jr. (1989). Generalizability theory. In M.J. Safrit & T.M. Wood (Eds.), *Measurement concepts in physical education and exercise science* (pp. 73-96). Champaign, IL: Human Kinetics.

Wood, T.M., & Safrit, M.J. (1987). A comparison of three multivariate models for estimating test battery reliability. *Research Quarterly for Exercise and Sport*, 58, 150-159.

proportion of agreement index — Test of reliability in criterion-referenced measurements proposed by Hambleton and Novick (1973) to assess the consistency of correct decisions.

Hambleton, R.K., & Novick, M.R. (1973). Toward an integration of theory and method for criterion-referenced tests. *Journal of Educational Measurement*, 10, 159-170.

We repeat that repeatability is not validity because repeatable results may be repeatedly wrong. Furthermore, a large number of people saying the same thing does not guarantee that what is said is real. Merriam (1988, p. 171) offered a good example: An audience's account of a magician was not as reliable as that of one stagehand who watched the show from behind the curtain.

The researcher can become more reliable through practice. Triangulation (described in chapter 17) can also work to increase reliability. The reliability of the data can be enhanced by using various techniques and sources.

Goetz and LeCompte (1984) interpreted reliability as the extent to which studies can be replicated. That is, can a researcher using the same methods obtain the same results as those obtained in a prior study? They pointed out that the difficulties of replication in qualitative research stem from the fact that a study takes place in natural settings and is often undertaken for the purpose of recording processes of change. Reliability in qualitative research can be examined from the standpoint of external reliability and internal reliability.

External Reliability

External reliability refers to the content of the data. Goetz and LeCompte (1984) discussed five major problems associated with external reliability: researcher status, choice of subjects, social situations and conditions, analytic constructs and premises, and methods of data collection and analysis.

Researcher status relates to the role of the researcher in the group. Is the researcher a participant observer or a nonparticipant observer? Is the researcher considered a friend or some sort of evaluator? Margaret Mead's data on adolescent sexual behavior in Samoan society were challenged by Daniel Freeman, who studied Samoan society many years later (Agar, 1986). The discrepancy in their findings may result from the researcher's status position. Mead was a young woman at the time she talked with the Samoan adolescent girls. Freeman's status was more that of a distinguished visitor when he conducted much of his study with male parents. Clearly, the researcher's role and status within the group should be described.

Choice of subjects is closely related to the role of the researcher. The nature of the data will be greatly influenced by the source. In the previous discussion concerning Mead and Freeman, one can easily understand how there could be discrepancies when Mead's subjects were largely adolescent females and Freeman's subjects were male parents. The researcher needs to carefully describe both the characteristics of the subjects and the rationale for their selection (Kirk & Miller, 1986).

Social situations and conditions can have a significant bearing on what information the subjects are willing to reveal. A subject may speak freely under some conditions yet be quite guarded when asked the same questions in another context. The presence of others is obviously a factor that can affect what people say. The researcher's description of the social situations and conditions is an important aspect of external reliability.

Analytic constructs and premises refer to the manner in which the researcher defines and categorizes the data. Some concepts and operational definitions are constant from the inception of the proposal, whereas others change as the data unfold.

Methods of data collection and analysis must be carefully described if the content of the data is to be assessed. Delineate all details as to how observations were gathered and recorded, how interviews were conducted, and how multiple sources of data were integrated into the study. You must also specify and discuss general strategies employed in analyzing the data. The credibility of the data is closely tied to the clarity and thorough-

external reliability — The content of the data in qualitative research that determines the degree to which a study can be repeated.

ness of the accounts of how the data were examined and synthesized (Goetz & LeCompte, 1984).

Internal Reliability

Internal reliability concerns interobserver agreement. In other words, what is the extent of agreement among different observers concerning the description of events? According to Goetz and LeCompte (1984), qualitative researchers use any of the following strategies to reduce threats to internal reliability: low-inference descriptors, peer examination, and mechanically recorded data.

"Low-inference descriptors" relates to the method of rich, thick description used in data collection. Verbatim accounts of conversations and complete field notes provide reviewers with the means for judging the researcher's findings.

Multiple researchers are involved in a team effort. This sometimes occurs when researchers in different geographical areas collaborate on a study. In such studies that have more than one researcher, it is imperative that all team members are extensively trained in the methods of observation and descriptive techniques. Participant researchers are local observers who confirm what has been seen and recorded. This is not done to any great extent in our field.

Peer examination involves having colleagues corroborate a researcher's findings. This may be informally done by asking people to evaluate one's study, and it is a standard practice when an article is submitted for publication. The manuscript is reviewed by qualified researchers in that area.

Mechanically recorded data offer an effective means of assessing internal reliability in a qualitative study. Tape recorders, photographs, and videotapes are used frequently, and other qualified researchers can be asked to examine the data. In this process it is essential that all observers are carefully trained and that they follow the same coding procedures. Interobserver reliability can be established in some qualitative research studies by having other competent people evaluate or code the behavior of the same subjects. Videotapes are advantageous because more judges can be used and the evaluations done at any time and as many times as desired. A percent of agreement (IOA) can be computed by dividing the number of agreements between raters by the total number of coded behaviors. Observer "drift" is often tested by checking interobserver values at the beginning, middle, and end of data collection. If desired, intraobserver reliability can be established by having the researcher evaluate the same videotapes on another occasion. However, this is usually done as a training procedure before the study begins.

Finally, some qualitative research experts maintain that reliability evidence is unnecessary if internal validity can be demonstrated. Guba and Lincoln (1981) used the logic that it is impossible to have internal validity without reliability. Therefore, reliability is simultaneously demonstrated.

Using Standard Error of Measurement to Interpret Results

Previous chapters have touched on the idea of standard error several times with regard to t and F tests and in interpreting significance levels. Chapter 7 also discussed standard error of prediction in correlational research. The standard error of measurement is an important concept in interpreting the results of measurement. Sometimes

internal reliability — The extent of agreement among different observers concerning the description of events.

we get too carried away with the aura of scientific data collection and fail to realize that the possibility of measurement error always exists. For example, maximal oxygen consumption ($\dot{V}O_2$max) has been mentioned several times in this book as the most valid measure of cardiorespiratory fitness. Field tests are frequently validated through correlation with $\dot{V}O_2$max. We must be careful, however, not to consider $\dot{V}O_2$max as a perfect test that is error free. Every test yields only observed scores; we can obtain only estimates of a person's true score. It is much better to think of test scores as falling within a range that contains the true score. The formula for the standard error of measurement ($S_{y \cdot x}$) is

$$S_{y \cdot x} = s \sqrt{1.00 - r} \tag{11.5}$$

where s = the standard deviation of the scores and r = the reliability coefficient for the test. In the measurement of percent body fat for female adults, assume that the standard deviation is 5.6% and the test-retest correlation is .83. The standard error of measurement would be

$$S_{y \cdot x} = 5.6 \sqrt{1.00 - .83} = 2.3\%$$

Assume further that a particular woman's measured percent fat is 22.4%. We can use the standard error of measurement to estimate a range within which her true percent fat probably falls.

Standard errors are assumed to be normally distributed and are interpreted in the same way as standard deviations. About two thirds (68.26%) of all test scores will fall within plus or minus one standard error of measurement of their true scores. In other words, there is a 68% chance that a person's true score will be found within a range of the obtained score plus or minus the standard error of measurement. In the example of the woman who had an obtained score of 22.4% fat, chances are 2 in 3 that her true percent fat is 22.4% ± 2.3% (standard error of measurement) or somewhere between 20.1% and 24.7%.

We can be more confident if we multiply the standard error of measurement by 2 because about 95% (95.44%) of the time the true score can be found within a range of the observed score plus or minus two times the standard error of measurement. Thus, in the present example, we can be about 95% sure that the woman's true percent fat will be 22.4% ± 4.6% (± 2.3% × 2), that is, between 17.8% and 27.0%.

From the formula we see that the standard error of measurement is governed by the variability of the test scores and the reliability of the test. If we had a higher reliability coefficient, the error of measurement would obviously decrease. In the present example, if the reliability coefficient was .95, the standard error of measurement would be only 1.3%. With the same reliability (.83) but with a smaller standard deviation, such as 4%, the standard error of measurement would be 1.7%.

Remember the idea of standard error of measurement when you are interpreting test scores. As indicated earlier, people sometimes have absolutely blind faith in some measurements, particularly if the measurements seem scientific. With percent fat estimation from skinfold thicknesses, for example, we need to keep in mind that error is connected not only with the skinfold measurements but also with the criterion that these measurements are predicting, that is, the density obtained from underwater weighing and the determination of percent fat from the body density values. Yet we have observed people accepting as gospel that they have a certain amount of fat because someone measured a few skinfolds. Newspapers have reported that some athletes have only 1% fat. This would be impossible from a physiological standpoint. Moreover, obtaining a predicted negative percent fat from regression equations is possible. Please do not misunderstand. We are not condemning skinfold measurements. We are simply trying to emphasize that all measurements are susceptible to errors and that common sense, coupled with knowledge of the concept of standard error of measurement, can help us better understand and interpret the results of measurements.

Four Types of Measurement Scales

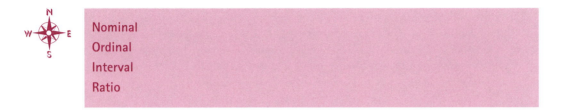

Nominal

Ordinal

Interval

Ratio

Interval scale measures and ordinal data have been mentioned several times in the discussion of statistics and measurement. There are four types of scales: nominal, ordinal, interval, and ratio.

Nominal

When scores are grouped into categories, or classes, the result is a **nominal scale**, or a classification by name. Scores of boys and girls can be assigned to two mutually exclusive groups, which means that no score can fall in more than one classification. Because the nominal scale classification is for identification only, there is no differentiation as to order of magnitude of differences between groups. Examples of nominal scales include such categories as gender and race.

Sometimes a researcher creates groups based on some measurement criterion. For example, subjects might be categorized as high or low anxious on the basis of an anxiety measure. High-, average-, and low-fitness groupings and highly skilled and poorly skilled classifications are other examples. In these cases, the classifications are not strictly nominal because there is some kind of distinction regarding order. Such scales could be considered somewhere between nominal and ordinal.

Ordinal

Ordinal scales are ranks. They provide more information than do nominal data. The highest ordinal number is better than the next highest, which in turn is better than the third highest. With an ordinal scale, we do not know how much better one score is than another. Therefore, we must use caution in making comparisons. For example, John is 6 inches taller than Joe, and Joe is a half-inch taller than Bob. Yet, by merely ranking them, we have John first, Joe second, and Bob third, and the ordinal difference between the first and second ranks is the same as that between the second and third. We cannot assume equal intervals between ranks in terms of their actual raw scores.

Percentiles are ordinal numbers; thus, a teacher should not try to average percentiles or interpolate between two percentile ranks. A score falling between the

 nominal scale — Scale of measurement in which the scores are classified by name.

 ordinal scale — Scale of measurement in which scores are classified by ranks.

60th and the 65th percentiles should not be assigned a value of 62.5, because it cannot be assumed that the scores are evenly distributed between those two percentile ranks.

Interval

 Interval scales provide not only the order between scores but also the magnitude of the distance between them. A score of 35 sit-ups is not only higher than a score of 25; it is 10 sit-ups higher. Similarly, a difference between 35 and 25 sit-ups is the same absolute difference as that between 25 and 15. Interval scoring enables us to interpret performances with standard scores (discussed later in this chapter).

Ratio

Ratio scales have all the properties of the other three scales plus a true zero value, which represents a complete absence of the characteristic. An interval measure does not have a true zero. A common example frequently used to distinguish between the interval and the ratio scales is the IQ scale, the scores of which are interval because there is no "zero intelligence." We cannot say that an IQ of 160 is twice as high as an IQ of 80 because zero on the IQ scale is an arbitrary point. We can say only that a score of 160 is 80 points higher than a score of 80.

On the other hand, measures of force, time, and distance are ratio scales because they have true zero points. A force of 50 lb is twice as high as one of 25 lb. A jump of 20 ft is twice as far as one of 10 ft. Actually, although many of the measures used in physical education, exercise science, and sport science are ratio scales, they are treated the same as interval scores. For example, even though distance is a ratio scale, the relative differences between performances may not be equal. The 2-in. difference between high jumps of 7 ft 2 in. and 7 ft is probably more significant than the 2-in. difference between jumps of 5 ft 2 in. and 5 ft.

Using Standard Scores to Compare Performance

	z Scores
	T Scales

Direct comparisons of scores are not possible without having some point of reference. Is a score of 46 cm on the vertical jump as good as a score of 25 push-ups? How can you compare centimeters and repetitions? If we know that the class mean for the vertical jump is 40 cm and that 20 is the mean for push-ups, we know that the performances of 46 cm and 25 push-ups are better than average, but how much better? Is one performance better than the other?

 interval scale — Scale of measurement that provides not only the order between scores, but also the magnitude of the distance between them.

 ratio scale — Scale of measurement that has all of the properties of nominal, ordinal, and interval measures, plus a true zero value that represents a complete absence of the characteristic.

One way to compare the performances is to convert each score to a standard score. A standard score is a score expressed in terms of standard deviations from the mean. Standard scores are interval scores because the standard deviation is a constant interval unit throughout the scale. We now discuss how to determine standard scores by using z scores and T scales.

z Scores

The basic standard score is the **z score**. The z scale converts raw scores to a mean of zero and to a standard deviation of 1.0. The formula is

$$z = (X - M) / s \tag{11.6}$$

Suppose that the mean and standard deviation for vertical jump scores are 40 and 6 cm, respectively, and for push-ups 20 and 5, respectively. Thus, a score of 46 cm for the vertical jump is a z score of + 1.00: $z = (46 - 40) / 6 = 6 / 6 = 1.00$. A score of 25 push-ups is also a z score of + 1.00: $z = (25 - 20) / 5 = 5 / 5 = 1.00$.

We see that the person performed exactly the same on the two tests. Both performances were 1 s above the mean. Similarly, scores of different students can be compared on the same test by z scores. A person jumping 37 cm has a z score of – 0.5, a student who jumps 44 cm has a z score of 0.67, and so on. All standard scores are based on the z score. However, because z scores are expressed in decimals and have positive and negative numbers, they are not as easy to work with as are some other scales.

T Scales

The **T scale**, for example, sets the mean at 50 and the standard deviation at 10. Hence, the formula is $T = 50 + 10z$. This removes the decimal and makes all the scores positive. A score 1 s above the mean ($z = 1.0$) is a T score of 60. A score 1 s below the mean ($z = -1.0$) is a T score of 40. Because more than 99% (99.73%) of the scores fall between ± 3 s, it is rare to have T scores below 20 ($z = -3.0$) and above 80 ($z = +3.0$). Some standardized tests that use different transformations of means and standard deviations using the z-score distribution are shown in Table 11.2.

The decision as to which standard score to use depends on the nature of the research study and the extent of interpretation required for the test takers. In essence, then, it is a matter of choice in light of the use of the measures.

Table 11.2   Standardized Means and Standard Deviations of Well–Known Tests

Scale	M	s
Graduate Record Examination	500	100_z
Stanford–Binet IQ	100	16_z
College Entrance Examination	500	100_z
National Teachers Examination	500	100_z
Wechsler IQ	100	15_z

z score — The basic standard score that converts raw scores to a mean of 0 with a standard deviation of 1.0.

T scale — Type of standard score that sets the mean at 50 and standard deviation at 10 to remove the decimal found in z-scores and to make all scores positive.

Measuring Movement

Much of the research in physical activity obviously involves movement. The measurement of physical fitness has fascinated exercise physiologists and physical educators for years. The concept of health-related physical fitness is widely accepted as being represented by the components of cardiorespiratory endurance, muscular strength, **muscular endurance**, **flexibility**, and body composition. In addition, many research studies have pertained to other fitness parameters that are needed primarily for skilled performances, such as in athletics and dance. These components include power, speed, reaction time, **agility**, balance, kinesthetic perception, and coordination. Research in motor behavior generally deals with the acquisition and control of motor skills. Types of measurements include tests of basic movement patterns, sport skills, and controlled (often novel) laboratory tasks.

Research in **biomechanics** involve such measurements as **high-speed cinematography**, **force transducers**, and **electromyography**. Research in pedagogy typically involves observations of behavior in real-world settings, such as during physical education classes or sport participation. Videotaped observations are often used to allow for more precise analyses.

All forms of measuring movement must be defended by the researchers with regard to their validity and reliability. In some respects, measuring movement is simpler and more straightforward than measuring cognitive or affective behaviors. For example, the amount of force a person can apply in a given movement can be accurately and directly measured. The distance a person can jump can be assessed by a measuring tape, and everyone accepts that as a valid and reliable measure. On the other hand, cognitive and affective behaviors must usually be inferred from marks made on a sheet of paper. Nevertheless, the measurement of movement is rarely a simple manner of measuring distance jumped. It is usually complex and often difficult to standardize. Each type of measurement has its own methodological difficulties, which pose problems for the researcher with regard to validity and reliability. We do not attempt a more thorough description of measuring movement because much of this is specific to your area of specialization (e.g., motor behavior, exercise, and wellness). The focus of your graduate program will be on many of these issues.

Measuring Written Responses

The measurement of written (and oral) responses is part of the methodology of numerous research studies in physical education and exercise science. Research questions fre-

---

 muscular endurance — The ability to persevere in working against a submaximal resistance.

flexibility — The range of movement about a joint.

agility — The accuracy and speed of changing direction while moving.

 biomechanics — The application of the physical laws of motion to the study of biological systems.

high-speed cinematography — Most widely used measure in biomechanics in which a camera or cameras allow motion to be studied.

force transducer — Device in biomechanical research that measures the forces exerted during motor performance, including the reactions between a runner's or jumper's feet and the ground as well as the forces exerted against equipment.

electromyography (EMG) — Technique that uses skin or muscle electrodes to pick up electrical activity caused by muscle contraction during movement.

quently deal with affective behavior, which includes attitudes, interests, emotional states, and personality and psychological traits.

Measuring Affective Behavior

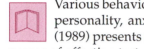 Attitude Inventories

Personality Research

Various behaviors fall into the category of affective behavior, including attitudes, personality, anxiety, self-concept, social behavior, and sportsmanship. Nelson (1989) presents an extensive discussion of the construction, strengths, and weaknesses of affective tests, as well as scaling.

Attitude Inventories

A large number of attitude inventories have been developed. Undoubtedly, many test developers see a direct link between attitude and behavior. For example, if a person has a favorable attitude toward physical activities, that person will participate in such activities. Research, however, has seldom substantiated this link between attitude and behavior, although such a link seems logical.

Researchers usually try to locate an instrument that has already been validated and that is an accepted measure of attitude rather than having to construct one. Finding a published test that closely pertains to the research topic is a problem. Another problem is that often the researcher wants to determine whether some treatment will bring about an attitude change. A source of invalidity discussed in chapter 16 is the reactive effects of testing. The pretest sensitizes the subject to the attitudes in question, and this may promote a change rather than the treatment.

Another problem (mentioned in chapter 15) inherent in any self-report inventory is whether the person is truthful. It is usually evident what a given response to an item in an attitude inventory indicates. For example, a person is asked to show his or her degree of agreement or disagreement to the statement "Regular exercise is an important part of our daily lives." The individual may perceive that the socially desirable response is to agree with this statement regardless of his or her true feelings. Some respondents deliberately distort their answers to appear "good" (or "bad"). Tests sometimes use so-called filler items to make the true purpose of the instrument less visible. For example, a test designer might include several unrelated items, like "Going to the opera is a desirable social activity," to disguise the fact that the instrument is designed to measure attitude toward exercise. This is especially important when social desirability considerations may be biasing factors.

When a researcher seeks an attitude instrument to use in a study, validity and reliability must, of course, be primary considerations. Unfortunately, published attitude scales have not always been constructed scientifically, and limited information is provided about validity and reliability. Reliability can be established easily regarding methodology. (We are not saying that attitude scales are easily made reliable.) Validity is usually the prob-

Nelson, J.K. (1989). Measurement methodology for affective tests. In M.J. Safrit & T.M. Wood (Eds.), *Measurement concepts in physical education and exercise science* (pp. 229-248). Champaign, IL: Human Kinetics.

lem because of the failure to develop a satisfactory theoretical model for the attitude construct.

Personality Research

Many research studies in physical education and sports have attempted to explore the relationship between personality traits and various aspects of athletic performance. Interest in this topic can be attributed to several factors, including the great deal of public attention focused on athletics. Athletes are obviously "special" people with regard to physical characteristics. Beyond that, however, is the hypothesis that athletes have certain personality traits that distinguish them from nonathletes.

 One area of investigation has been to identify personality traits that might be uniquely characteristic of athletes in different sports. For example, do persons who gravitate toward vigorous contact sports differ in personality from those individuals who prefer noncontact sports? That is, is there a "football type" or a "bowler type"? Are superior athletes different from average athletes in certain personality traits? Can participation in competitive sport modify one's personality structure? Moreover, do athletes within a sport differ on some traits that, if known, could point to different coaching strategies or perhaps be used to screen and predict those athletes who will be "hard" to coach or who will lack certain qualities associated with success?

Persons with a strong interest in sports, such as former coaches and players, have been greatly attracted to the study of personality and athletics. However, having a strong interest in athletics does not compensate for a lack of preparation and experience in psychological evaluation. Unfortunately, there have been cases in which personality measuring instruments have been misused. Recently, sport psychologists have recognized the value of sport-specific measures of various behaviors and perceptions. Much of the impetus for this approach can be traced to Martens's *Sport Competition Anxiety Test* (Martens, 1977).

Some sport-specific measures relate to group cohesiveness (Carron, Widmeyer, & Brawley, 1985), intrinsic and extrinsic motivation (Weiss, Bredemeier, & Shewchuck, 1985), confidence (Vealey, 1986), and sport achievement orientation (Gill & Deeter, 1988). The rationale for the sport-specific approach is that general measures of achievement, anxiety, motivation, self-concept, social behavior, and fair play do not have high validity for sport situations. Recent studies in test development indicate a commitment by sport psychologists to develop measures of affective behavior that are multidimensional and specific to the competitive environment.

Scales for Measuring Affective Behavior

The Likert Scale

The Semantic Differential

Thurstone-Type Scales

Rating Scales

　Types of Rating Scales

　Rating Errors

 Areas of investigation of athletes' personality traits

 Some sport-specific affective measures

In measuring affective behavior, a variety of scales are used to quantify the responses. Three of the most commonly used are the **Likert scale**, the **semantic differential scale**, and the **Thurstone-type scales**

The Likert Scale

The Likert Scale is referred to in chapter 15 in connection with survey research techniques. It is usually a 5- or 7-point scale with assumed equal intervals between points. The Likert scale is used to assess the degree of agreement or disagreement with statements and is widely used in attitude inventories. An example of a Likert scale item follows:

I prefer quiet recreational activities such as chess, cards, or checkers rather than activities such as running, tennis, or basketball.

Strongly Agree   Agree   Undecided   Disagree   Strongly Disagree

A principal advantage of scaled responses such as the Likert is that it permits a wider choice of expression than items such as "always," "never," "yes," or "no." The five, seven, or more intervals help increase the reliability of the instrument (for more comprehensive information concerning the Likert, semantic differential, and other scales, see Edwards, 1957, or Nunnaly, 1978).

The Semantic Differential

The semantic differential scale employs bipolar adjectives at each end of a 7-point scale. The respondent is asked to make judgments about certain concepts. The scale is based on the importance of language in reflecting a person's feelings. A sample of a semantic differential item follows:

The Coach

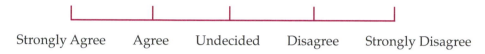

1. creative | | | | | | | unoriginal
2. supportive | | | | | | | critical
3. fair | | | | | | | unfair

The 1-7 scale between adjectives is scored with 7 being the most positive judgment. Factor analysis studies have consistently identified the same three dimensions being

---

 Likert scale — Type of closed question that requires the subject to respond by choosing one of several scaled items with the assumption that there are equal intervals between items.

semantic differential scale — Scale used to measure affective behavior in which the respondent is asked to make judgments about certain concepts by choosing one of seven intervals between bipolar adjectives.

Thurstone–type scale — Scale used to measure affective behavior in which the respondent expresses agreement or disagreement with each item, which has been rated by a panel of judges and scaled with a numerical value to reflect the most positive attitude.

Edwards, A.L. (1957). *Techniques of attitude and scale construction.* New York: Appleton-Century-Crofts.

Nunnaly, J.C. (1978). *Psychometric theory* (2nd ed.). New York: McGraw-Hill.

assessed by the semantic differential technique: evaluation (e.g., fair-unfair), potency (e.g., powerful-feeble), and activity (e.g., dynamic-static).

Thurstone–Type Scales

The Thurstone-type scales were the first to use judges to determine comparative weightings for psychological stimuli. The respondent expresses agreement or disagreement with a series of statements. In developing Thurstone scales, each item is first scaled by a panel of judges. Judges rate each statement with a numerical value from 1 to 11, with 11 reflecting the most positive attitude. Their median score for each item is then used to weight the statements for use in scoring.

An example of a statement as it would appear on the tester's manual follows:

    1. Physical education should be required in the elementary school.   (9.1)

The final score (9.1) is the sum of all the weighted scores divided by the number of "agree" items. The Thurstone-type scales are more difficult to construct than the Likert and semantic differential scales because of the judges' involvement.

Rating Scales

Rating scales are sometimes used in research to evaluate performance. For example, in a study that compares different strategies in teaching diving, the dependent variable (diving skill) would most likely be derived from expert ratings because diving does not lend itself to objective skill tests. Thus, after the experimental treatments have been applied, persons knowledgeable in diving rate all the subjects on their diving skills. To do this in a systematic and structured manner, the raters need to have some kind of scale with which to assess skill levels in different parts or phases of the performance.

A self-rating scale concerning an individual's perceived efforts during exercise that has been widely used in research is the **Ratings of Perceived Exertion (RPE)** scale by Borg (1962). The underlying rationale for the scale is that the many physiological indicators of exertion are combined and integrated into a whole, or gestalt, of subjective feeling of physical effort. This feeling of perceived exertion was quantified by Borg into a scale with numbers ranging from 6 to 20, reflecting a range of exertion from "very, very light" to "very, very hard."

Types of Rating Scales

There are different kinds of rating scales. Some scales use numerical ratings, some use checklists, some have verbal cues associated with numerical ratings, some require forced choices, and still others use rankings. Some scales are simple, whereas others are rather complex. Whatever the degree of complexity, however, practice in using the scale is imperative.

When more than one judge is asked to rate performances, some common standards must be set. Training sessions with videotaped performances of persons of different levels of ability are helpful in establishing standard frames of reference before judging the subjects' actual performances. Intertester agreement and reliability were discussed earlier in this chapter.

 rating scale — A measure of behavior that involves a subjective evaluation based on a checklist of criteria.

 Rating of Perceived Exertion (RPE) — Self-rating scale developed by Borg (1962) to measure an individual's perceived effort during exercise.

Rating Errors

 Despite efforts to make ratings as objective as possible, there are inherent pitfalls in the process. Recognized errors in rating include leniency, central tendency, the halo effect, proximity, observer bias, and observer expectation.

 Leniency is the tendency for observers to be overly generous in their ratings. This error is less likely to occur in research than in evaluating peers (e.g., co-workers). Thorough training of raters is the best means of reducing leniency. **Central tendency errors** result from the inclination of the rater to give an inordinate number of ratings in the middle of the scale, avoiding the extremes of the scale. Several reasons are attributed to this. Sometimes it may be due in part to ego needs or status. For example, the judge is acting in the role of an expert and, perhaps unconsciously, may grade good performers as average to suggest that he or she is accustomed to seeing better performances. Sometimes, errors of central tendency are due to the observer's wanting to "leave room" for better future performances. A common complaint in large gymnastics, diving, and skating competitions is that the performers scheduled early in the meet are scored lower for comparable performances than athletes scheduled later in the competition.

Another central tendency error is the inclination to avoid assigning very low scores and is likely due to a judge's reluctance to be too harsh (wanting to "give the poor devil a break"). It is, of course, a form of leniency.

The **halo effect** is the commonly observed tendency for a rater to allow previous impressions or knowledge about a certain individual to influence ratings on all that individual's behaviors. For example, knowing that an individual excels in one or more activities, a judge may rate that person highly on all other activities. The halo effect perhaps is not the most appropriate term because negative impressions of a person tend to lead to lower ratings in subsequent performances.

Proximity errors are often the result of overly detailed rating scales, the lack of sufficient familiarity with the rating criteria, or both. Proximity errors are manifested when the rater tends to rate behaviors that are listed close together as more nearly the same than when the behaviors are separated on the scale. For example, if the qualities "active" and "friendly" were listed side by side on the scale, proximity errors would result if raters evaluated performers as more similar on those characteristics than if the two qualities were listed several lines apart on the rating scale. Of course, if the rater does not have adequate knowledge about all facets of the behavior, he or she may not be able to distinguish between different behaviors that logically should be placed close together on the scale. Thus, the different phases of behavior are rated the same.

Observer bias errors vary with the judge's own characteristic and prejudices. For example, a person who has a low regard for movement education may also tend to rate students from such a program too low. Racial, sexual, and philosophi-

 Recognized errors in rating scales

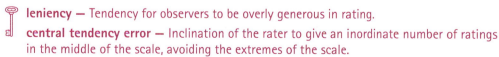 **leniency** — Tendency for observers to be overly generous in rating.

central tendency error — Inclination of the rater to give an inordinate number of ratings in the middle of the scale, avoiding the extremes of the scale.

halo effect — A threat to internal validity wherein raters allow previous impressions or knowledge about a certain individual to influence ratings on all of that individual's behaviors.

proximity error — Occurs when a rater considers behaviors to be more nearly the same when they are listed close together on a scale than when they are separated by some distance.

observer bias error — Inclination of a rater to be influenced by his or her own characteristics and prejudices.

cal biases are potential sources of rating errors. Observer bias errors are directional in that they produce errors that are consistently too high or too low.

Observer expectation errors can operate in various ways, often stemming from other sources of errors such as the halo effect and observer bias. Observer expectations can contaminate the ratings in that a person who expects certain behaviors will be inclined to see evidence of those behaviors and interpret observations in the "expected" direction.

Research has demonstrated the powerful phenomenon of expectation in classroom situations in which teachers are told that some children are gifted or slow learners. The teachers tend to treat the pupils accordingly, giving more attention and patience to the "gifted" and less time and attention to the "slow learners."

In the research setting, potential observer expectation errors are likely when the observer knows what the experimental hypotheses are and is thus inclined to watch for these outcomes more closely than if the observer were unaware of the expected outcomes. The double-blind experimental technique described in chapter 16 is useful in controlling for expectation errors. In the double-blind method, the observers do not know which subjects received which treatments. They also should not know which performances they are shown are the pretest and which are the posttest.

In summary, rating errors are always potentially present. The researcher must recognize and strive to eliminate or reduce them. One way to minimize rating errors is to define the behavior to be rated as objectively as possible. In other words, avoid having the observer make many value judgments. Another suggestion is to keep observers "ignorant" of the hypotheses and which subjects received what treatment. Bias and expectation can be reduced if the observer is given no information about the subjects' achievements, intelligence, social status, and other characteristics. The most important precaution the researcher can take is to train the observers adequately to achieve high levels of accuracy and interrater reliability.

Measuring Knowledge

Analyzing Test Items
   Item Difficulty
   Item Discrimination
Types of Knowledge Test Items

Obviously, the measurement of knowledge is a fundamental part of the educational thrusts in physical education, exercise science, and sport science. However, the construction of knowledge tests is relevant for research purposes as well. Most pencil-and-paper measuring instruments used in research involve similar procedures in establishing validity and reliability. However, we must also determine whether the individual items are functioning in the desired manner as to their difficulty and their ability to discriminate between levels of ability, i.e., item analysis (for

---

observer expectation error — Inclination of a rater to see evidence of certain behaviors and interpret observations in the expected direction.

 Mood, D.P. (1989). Measurement methodology for knowledge tests. In M.J. Safrit & T.M. Wood (Eds.), *Measurement concepts in physical education and exercise science* (pp. 251-270). Champaign, IL: Human Kinetics.

a more thorough discussion of measurement methodology for knowledge tests, see Mood, 1989).

Analyzing Test Items

The purpose of **item analysis** is to determine which items are suitable and which need to be rewritten or discarded. Two important facets of item analysis are the difficulty of the test items and the power to discriminate between different levels of achievement.

Item Difficulty

Analysis of **item difficulty** is usually accomplished easily. One simply divides the number of persons who correctly answered the item by the total number of people who responded to the item. For example, if 80 people answered an item, and 60 answered it correctly, the item would have a difficulty index of .75 (60/80). A "hard" item has a low difficulty index. For example, if only 8 of 80 answered an item correctly, the index is 8/80, or .10. Most test authorities recommend that questions with difficulty indices below .10 or above .90 should be eliminated. The best questions are those that have difficulty indices around .50. Occasionally, a test maker may wish to set a specific difficulty index for screening purposes. For example, if only the top 30% of a group of applicants are to be chosen, this could be accomplished by using questions with difficulty indices of .30. Questions that everyone answers correctly or that everyone misses provide no information about people differences in norm-referenced measurement scales.

Item Discrimination

Item discrimination, or the degree to which test items discriminate between persons who did well on the entire test and those who did poorly, is an important consideration in analyzing norm referenced test items. There are many ways to compute an **index of discrimination**. The simplest way is to divide the completed tests into a high group and a low group on the basis of scores and then use the following formula:

$$\text{Index of Discrimination} = (n\text{H} - n\text{L})/n$$

where $n\text{H}$ = number of high scorers who answered the item correctly, $n\text{L}$ = the number of low scorers who answered the item correctly, and n = the number in either the

---

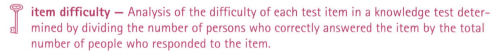

 Two facets of item analysis

 item analysis — Process in analyzing knowledge tests in which items are evaluated as to their suitability with regard to difficulty and discrimination.

item difficulty — Analysis of the difficulty of each test item in a knowledge test determined by dividing the number of persons who correctly answered the item by the total number of people who responded to the item.

item discrimination — The degree to which a test item discriminates between persons who did well on the entire test and those who did poorly; also called *index of discrimination*.

index of discrimination — See *item discrimination*.

high or the low group. To illustrate, if we have 30 in the high group and 30 in the low group, and 20 of the high scorers answered an item correctly and 10 of the low scorers answered it correctly, the index of discrimination would be .33: $(20 − 10)/30 = 10/30 = .33$

Various percentages of high and low scorers are used in determining discrimination indices, such as the upper and lower 25%, 30%, or 33%. The Flanagan method uses the upper and the lower 27%. The proportion of each group answering each item correctly is calculated; then a table of normalized biserial coefficients is consulted to obtain the item reliability coefficient. Thus, item reliability is the relationship between responses to each item and total performance on the test.

If approximately the same proportion of high scorers answer an item correctly as did the low scorers, the item is not discriminating. Most test makers strive for an index of discrimination of .20 or higher for each item. Obviously, a negative index of discrimination would be unacceptable. In fact, when this happens, the question needs to be examined closely to see whether something in the wording is throwing off the high scorers.

Types of Knowledge Test Items

The most common types of test items are completion, essay, matching, multiple choice, and alternate choice (true-false). Each type of question has its strengths and weaknesses (these are discussed in detail in measurement and evaluation textbooks). Knowledge tests have been used in research studies concerning facts and fallacies about diet and exercise, game rules and strategies, and basic information. Knowledge testing in such research studies invariably uses objective items, such as multiple choice or alternate choice. Matching test items are objective, but they are time-consuming and limited as to the effective number of items that can be presented.

Multiple-choice items are considered by testing authorities as the most reliable of the test items. Good multiple-choice items are difficult to write. The stem should be presented clearly and concisely, and the alternatives must be meaningful and attractive. Poor alternatives simply limit the choices and can reduce multiple-choice items to alternate-choice items. The number of alternatives influences reliability. The more choices, the greater the reliability because the likelihood of getting the correct answer by chance is reduced. However, as you increase the number of alternatives, practical considerations (e.g., time required for testing) negate the advantage. Between three and five choices are recommended.

Alternate-choice items, such as true-false, are used occasionally in research studies. This type of item has been criticized for various reasons, but often the weaknesses cited can be minimized by careful test construction. Alternate-choice items are less reliable than multiple-choice tests of the same length. However, more alternate-choice items can be given in a set period, and this can increase the test reliability. The items are easier to write than those of multiple choice, but considerable skill is required to write good test questions. With care, alternate-choice tests can be employed to assess knowledge effectively.

Making a Case for Item Response Theory

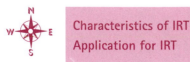

Characteristics of IRT

Application for IRT

Most of the information concerning the validity, reliability, and item analysis thus far pertains to what is called **classical test theory (CTT)**. There have been some radical changes recently in the study of the measurement of cognitive and affective behaviors. The advance that has received the most attention in the educational and psychological literature is **item response theory (IRT)**

Characteristics of IRT

Whereas in the CTT, inferences are made about items and student abilities from *total* test score information, IRT, as the name implies, attempts to estimate an examinee's ability on the basis of his or her responses on test *items*. Classical test theory requires only a few assumptions with regard to the observed scores and the true scores of individuals on a test. Group statistics pertaining to the total score on a particular test for the total group being examined are used to make generalizations to an equivalent test and population. The estimate of error is assumed to be the same for all individuals.

Item response theory is based on stronger assumptions than CTT. The two major assumptions are unidimensionality and local independence. Unidimensionality means that a single ability or trait is being measured. This ability is not directly measurable, so IRT is sometimes referred to as **latent trait theory** (for an introduction to IRT and some of its applications, see Spray, 1989). According to Spray, the real advantage of IRT is that the measurement of an examinee's ability from responses to test items is not limited to a particular test. Rather, it can be measured by any collection of test items that are considered to be measuring the same trait.

In traditional CTT, item difficulty is measured as a function of the total group. In IRT, item difficulty is fixed and can be assessed relative to an examinee's ability level. Thus, the probability of an examinee with a particular ability level making a correct response to an item can be mathematically described by an **item characteristic curve (ICC)**. The ICC is a nonlinear regression for any item that increases from left to right, indicating an increase in the probability of a correct response with increased ability, or latent trait. The item difficulty remains constant regardless of the group of examinees (**parameter invariance**). The item's discriminating power is indicated by the steepness of the curve. The ICC can be analyzed in relation to the difficulty of the item, the discriminating power of the item, and a so-called guessing parameter.

Application for IRT

Space limitations (and lack of knowledge by the authors) prohibit a detailed description and discussion of IRT. It is not a simple concept, and complex computer programs are

---

classical test theory (CTT) — A measurement theory built on the concept of observed scores being composed of a true score and an error score.

item response theory (IRT) — A theory that focuses on the characteristics of the test item and the examinee's response to the item as a means of determining the examinee's ability; also called *latent trait theory*.

latent trait theory — See *item response theory*.

item characteristic curve (ICC) — Nonlinear regression curve for any item that increases from left to right, indicating an increase in the probability of a correct response with increased ability, or latent trait.

parameter invariance — A postulate in item response theory that the item difficulty remains constant regardless of different populations of examinees and that examinees' abilities should not change when a different set of test items is administered.

required. Large sample sizes are needed for item calibration and ability estimates. The IRT model has been the subject of intense research in psychology and education for several years. It definitely has potential application for assessment problems in physical education, exercise science, and sport science.

 Spray (1989) has described several ways IRT can be used: item banking, adaptive testing, mastery testing, attitude assessment, and psychomotor assessment. **Item banking** is the creation of large pools of test items that can be used for constructing tests that have certain characteristics concerning the precision of estimating latent ability. **Adaptive testing**, sometimes called **tailored testing**, refers to selecting items that will best fit (items neither too difficult nor too easy) the ability level of each individual. This function must be done on a computer by using items drawn from an item bank.

In criterion-referenced measurement, tests are constructed that use a cutoff score to show the proportion of items that should be answered correctly to represent mastery of the subject matter. Item response theory can be used to select the optimal number of items that will yield the most precise indication of mastery for an examinee. In other words, subjects of different ability levels would require different numbers of items.

Item response theory has considerable potential application for assessing attitudes and other affective behaviors. Models of IRT have been proposed that will estimate the attitude or trait parameter of each respondent on an interval scale regardless of the ordinal nature of the scale. A score for each trait level is available for each category of each item. Changes in attitude or other traits over time can also be assessed with IRT models. To date, few affective measuring instruments have been constructed using IRT procedures. In our field, Tew (1988) used IRT methods in the construction of a sport-specific test of mental imagery.

The potential use of IRT for psychomotor assessment has been postulated (Spray, 1987) but has not yet been proved to any extent. The nature of motor performance tests is different from written tests in terms of the numbers of items and trials. Also, some assumptions (particularly local independence) of IRT are not easily accommodated in psychomotor testing. Preliminary research on the application of IRT to motor performance has been conducted by Safrit, Cohen, and Costa (1989). More research will undoubtedly be done on the application of IRT models to our field.

Summary

In this chapter we discussed the concepts of validity and reliability of measurements and how they apply to research. Criterion validity (which includes both concurrent and predictive validity) and construct validity are two of the most popular methods of validating measures used in research studies. One problem often identified regarding predictive measures is population or situation specificity. A current area of interest among

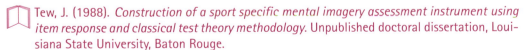

item banking — The creation of large pools of test items that can be used for constructing tests that have certain characteristics with regard to the precision of estimating latent ability.

adaptive testing — Practice of selecting test items that will best fit the ability level of each individual; also called *tailored testing*.

tailored testing — See *adaptive testing*.

Tew, J. (1988). *Construction of a sport specific mental imagery assessment instrument using item response and classical test theory methodology*. Unpublished doctoral dissertation, Louisiana State University, Baton Rouge.

measurement specialists is validity generalization, which attempts to estimate the generalizability of the results of different studies on the same topic.

The methods used in validating norm-referenced measurements are not applicable to criterion-referenced measurements. We identified methods used to establish domain-referenced validity and decision accuracy.

Qualitative research has special problems regarding validity. We discussed some of the issues raised concerning data collection in qualitative research studies and some of the arguments and approaches used to address the problems.

The topic of test reliability has prompted hundreds of studies and innumerable discussions among test theorists and researchers. The reason for this interest is that a measure that does not yield consistent results cannot be valid. Classical test theory views reliability in terms of observed scores, true scores, and error scores, and the coefficient of reliability reflects the degree to which the measure is free of error variance. The rationale for using intraclass R instead of r for reliability was presented, as well as the computational procedures for intraclass R. Various methods of estimating reliability were mentioned such as stability, alternate forms, and internal consistency. Generalizability theory (G-theory) is an extension of intraclass reliability that enables the researcher to identify sources of error in estimating reliability of scores on a test. Reliability techniques used in criterion-references measurements were summarized, and reliability in qualitative research was addressed.

An understanding of the concept of standard error of measurement is vital. Any test score should be viewed as only an estimate of an individual's true score that probably falls within a range of scores.

There are four types of scales of measurement: nominal, ordinal, interval, and ratio. Standard scores allow direct comparisons of scores of different tests and types of scoring. The basic standard score is the z score, which interprets any score in terms of standard deviations from the mean.

Research studies in physical activity frequently use instruments involving written responses to measure knowledge as well as affective attributes like attitudes, interests, emotional states, and psychological characteristics. Many general measures of these constructs have been used over the years (e.g., **Cattell 16 Personality Factor (PF) Questionnaire**, Spielberger State-Trait Anxiety Inventory). More recently, specific sport and exercise tests have been developed for affective measures.

Responses to items on these scales often use the Likert-scale (a 5-point scale ranging from strongly agree to strongly disagree) and the semantic differential scale (a 7-point scale anchored at the extremes by bipolar adjectives). When using scales like these, researchers must be aware of specific problems like rating errors, leniency, central tendency, halo effects, proximity, observer bias, and observer expectation.

Knowledge testing requires that the researcher use item analysis techniques for objective responses. The difficulty and discrimination must be established for each test item to determine the quality of the knowledge test.

Item response theory (IRT, also called latent trait theory) differs from classical test theory. It allows item difficulty to be fixed so that the subject's ability level can be determined. Item response theory is useful in tailoring tests for adaptive testing, mastery testing, attitude assessment, and psychomotor assessment.

Cattell 16 Personality Factor (PF) Questionnaire — Instrument that has frequently been used in research studies to assess personality traits.

Check Your Understanding

1. Briefly describe two ways that evidence of construct validity could be shown for either a motor performance test (such as throwing), a test of power, or a test of manipulative skill. How could criterion validity be shown in your example?

2. In a research journal find a study that used a written test (for example, an attitude inventory). Describe how the author reported the reliability of the instrument. What is another technique that could have been used to establish reliability?

3. A girl received a score of 78 on a test for which the reliability is .85 and the standard deviation is 8. Interpret her score in terms of the range in which her true score would be expected to fall (with 95% confidence).

III
PART

Types of Research

 esearch may be divided into five basic categories: analytical, descriptive, experimental, qualitative, and creative (the last category includes art and dance but is not presented in this book). Chapter 12 discusses historical research, which is a type of analytical research that answers questions through the use of past knowledge and events. Substantial changes have occurred in recent years in the reporting of historical research, particularly regarding the integration of the events of interest with other related events. In this chapter, Nancy Struna provides an excellent overview of historical research methods. Note that this chapter is written in University of Chicago style because that is the style most commonly used in reporting historical research.

Chapter 13 describes another type of analytical research that can be applied to physical activity—philosophic methods. Scott Kretchmar does a fine job of explaining and grouping philosophic research methods, and uses various examples to identify the strengths and weaknesses of these methods. Chapter 14 presents research synthesis (specifically meta-analysis), another type of analytical research that focuses on the short-comings of the typical literature analysis. Meta-analysis is a more useful solution in analyzing a large body of literature. Although several other types of research are considered analytical, historical, philosophic, and meta-analysis are the most common and useful in the study of physical activity.

Chapter 15 discusses descriptive research and focuses on the present, showing the relationship among people, events, and performances as they now exist. Included as descriptive research are surveys, case studies, correlational studies, developmental studies, and observational studies.

Chapter 16 introduces experimental research, which deals with future events or the establishment of cause-and-effect. Which independent variables can be manipulated to create change in the future in a certain dependent variable? After reviewing how difficult cause-and-effect is to establish, we divide the chapter according to the strengths of various designs: preexperimental, true experimental, and quasi-experimental. Our purpose is to demonstrate which designs and principles are best suited for controlling the various sources of invalidity that threaten experimental research.

Finally, chapter 17 presents qualitative research techniques, which are increasingly used in the study of physical activity. The assumptions underlying qualitative research differ from types of research that adhere to the traditional scientific method. That does not mean qualitative research is not science (i.e., systematic inquiry); however, the techniques for acquiring and analyzing knowledge differ from the typical steps in the scientific method. This chapter discusses differences in the quantitative and qualitative paradigms, procedures used in qualitative research, and interpretation and theory construction.

If you are either a producer or a consumer of research in physical education, exercise science, and sport science, you understand accepted techniques for solving problems systematically. The following six chapters attempt to provide the basic underpinnings of research planning. Many research types reported here are closely associated with the appropriate statistical analyses previously presented. We refer to the appropriate statistics as we discuss the many types of research. Use the knowledge gained from the previous section to understand this application. You should learn about the relationship between the correct type of design and the appropriate statistical analysis as soon as possible.

CHAPTER 12

Historical Research in Physical Activity

Nancy L. Struna

Dear Professors of Research Methods:

I am writing a thesis using the historical method, and my advisor wants to make sure that I apply both internal and external criticism to my sources. I have a hard time explaining to my roommate the difference between the two types of criticism. He claims that internal criticism is done indoors and external criticism is done outdoors. Any suggestions?

Sincerely,
Albert S. Authentic

Dear Albert:

Ascertain that he really did say that (external criticism) and then point out how stupid it is (internal criticism). You might ask him if he thinks that gross ignorance is 144 times worse than the ordinary kind.

Methodologically yours,
PRM

The ways of the historian often mystify the scientist. For one thing, historians study the past rather than the present, and the reality of the past is often elusive. Further, historians can rarely be as certain about past relationships, causes, or consequences as can scientists, for they just cannot isolate variables as concisely and independently. Finally, historians do not write like scientists. A historical report has no distinct *purpose, methods, results,* and *conclusions* sections, and the "storytelling" format of the historical study can mask the systematic, rational procedures that produced it.

The historian's work need not be so mysterious, however, for history, if not exactly a science, is certainly "sciencelike." Historians, who attempt to describe and explain change and continuity in human experience in the past, undertake many of the tasks that characterize scientific research. They carefully derive questions from the literature, thoroughly gather and translate evidence (data), and test inferences. Like scientists, historians work to disprove rather than to prove findings, and this requires that their minds be "trained in a discipline of attentive disbelief."[1]

The similarities between historical and scientific research are many, and these will become clearer as this chapter proceeds. One significant difference requires some comment, however. This is about the role of law and theory. In traditional science, laws and theories are generalizations about natural phenomena. Laws describe what some "thing" is, and the relationships among the components are often expressed mathematically. A theory builds upon such a description, but it also proposes to explain a phenomenon. Moreover, if a scientific theory is adequate, it will also be predictive: It will account for future or further occurrences.

Many historians do not view social phenomena—or, consequently, laws and theories about them—as scientists do natural phenomena. One of the prevailing assumptions in historical scholarship is that humans, who are rational beings, make and give meaning to social phenomena. Their thoughts and actions, as well as the individual character of experience and meaning, are neither predetermined nor predictable. This human agency thus diminishes the probability of covering laws, as well as the predictive function of theory.[2] So the role of theory in history is limited to account-

ing for—meaning to both describe and explain—particular events and processes. One such social theory that historians of sport and leisure have employed is that of modernization.[3] This maintains that "progressive increases in per capita productivity set in motion" a whole series of changes common to a range of human institutions and activity.[4] Modernization thus describes and, to some extent, explains how a society became what it did. However, it also works only in particular societies. Consequently, a social theory like modernization does not predict events and processes as scientific theories do.[5]

As do good scientists, however, good historians do expect to construct meaningful generalizations from the historical evidence, or data. Generalizations are "large," synthetic statements that offer the historian's "sense" of multiple pieces of evidence or data. They present one's interpretation of the data, usually from a time or a set of humans' experiences. Many historical generalizations also draw on, or are informed by, social science theories and they can be tested on data from other periods or sets of experiences. In effect then, few historians proceed to or from the evidence of the past (the data) without some attention to theory and without some regard for theoretical generalizations. If a study of the past did not produce such generalizations, it would not be a history.[6]

The Historian Begins

Defining Research Paradigms
Exploring Lines of Inquiry and Topics
Investigating Secondary Sources
Developing Good Questions

The possibilities and limits of theory in history are probably not the first issues that graduate students would ponder as they begin to study **historical research**. The discussion of social theory does, however, serve two purposes. First, it helps students to understand why history is "sciencelike" and not science. Second, it intro-

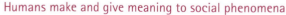

 Humans make and give meaning to social phenomena

historical research — Type of research that deals with events that have already occurred.

duces students to the kinds of issues that face working historians. There are many such issues, and how one resolves them affects how and what one sees in the past. Three other issues are particularly crucial to one's conception of the past. First, what is historical evidence? When one has a piece of data from the past, what is it that one really has? Second, how does social change proceed? Is change in humans' activities and institutions gradual, progressive, and cumulative—in a word, "evolutionary"? Or is the process not linear, in part because at any given time both change and continuity are in evidence? Finally, when one is investigating past sports, or exercise programs, or leisure practices, what is one really studying?[7]

Defining Research Paradigms

The answers to questions about such things as the nature of evidence, historical change, and the subject are a part of what Thomas Kuhn in *The Structure of Scientific Revolutions* has called the researcher's **paradigm**. Research **perspective**, **tradition**, or, in the historian's ordinary language, **approach** are synonyms. They say the same thing, however. A paradigm encompasses beliefs about every part of the researcher's work, including the role of theory, interpretive tools and rules, the nature of evidence, and what significant questions are asked. All researchers, scientists and historians alike, have such a body of beliefs, beliefs resulting from the things one has thought about in the course of research. Researchers also have a responsibility for grasping and explaining their beliefs, because every research methodology is also an ideology.[8]

Beginning students of history will probably not be able to define an integrated and logically consistent paradigm. Most historians readily admit that it takes them a long time to do so, and this is one reason why they maintain that they become good historians only late in their careers. So I introduce the notion of paradigms to help students contemplate the things that historians think about and the beliefs that bear on the doing of history.

Exploring Lines of Inquiry and Topics

About the only limit on possible topics for historical research today is one's imagination! Within the past decade, the field that we call the history of sport has broadened dramatically. One has only to look at the major journal in the field on this continent, the *Journal of Sport History*, published by the North American Society for Sport History, to see that historians are pursuing many lines of inquiry, not all of which are suggested by Americans' use of the term *sport*. Articles about the history of health, sports medicine, the body, and leisure are now nearly as common as articles about sport leagues, teams, and institutions. Books published by academic and popular presses also make the point that the field is broader than its name could

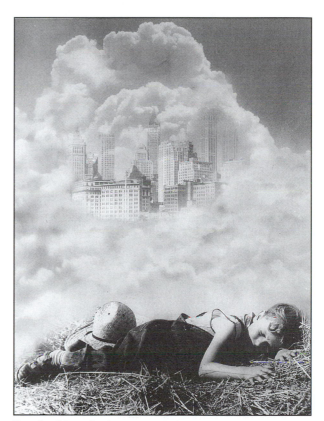

For the historical researcher, imagination is the only limit on possible research topics.

---

paradigm — A scientific model and the approaches used to test that model; also called *perspective*, *tradition*, and *approach* in historical research.

perspective — See *paradigm*.

tradition — See *paradigm*.

approach — See *paradigm*.

Kuhn, T.S. (1970). *The structure of scientific revolutions* (2nd ed.). Chicago: University of Chicago Press.

imply. In part this topical expansion reflects the awareness of historians in the United States and Canada that sports as organized physical contests are part of their broad physical cultures. But it also reflects the impact of other fields of history and of scholars from other countries around the world. Sport history is a global enterprise, which is expanding in subject matter and depth of understanding even as you read this.

 Historians of sport in the United States have taken great strides recently in exploring various topics, but we have only really "broken the surface." The particular history of baseball, for example, has an extensive literature, but many dimensions of historic baseball experiences remain un- or underexplored. These include local community programs, the experiences of women and minorities, struggles between professional players and owners, and the international transmission and adaptation of the game. Other organized sports like professional football, basketball, and hockey remain to be fully examined, as do the many sports about which few histories have been written: rodeo, water and winter sports, and more recent forms like rollerblading. There are also volumes yet to be written about collegiate athletics beyond the Ivy League, industrial recreation programs, a broad range of sport business enterprises, and sport policies in both the public and the private sectors.

Research is also needed on such broad topics as health, leisure, and public recreation. We have only just begun to reconstruct the histories of sports medicine, the use of drugs to enhance human physical performance, and health programs. Indeed, little is known about health programs beyond the nineteenth century. Sport historians have also begun to turn, or return, to historical studies of leisure experiences and to examine the experiences, both in and out of sports activities, that people who have not received adequate attention—women, European ethnic groups, African Americans, Asian Americans, and Native Americans—have found meaningful. Histories of the relationships between the media and sports organizations, between government agencies and sports groups, sports spectatorship, gender relations and the gendering of sports, and health interests and programs, among other things, are also waiting for interested and well-prepared students of history. For

graduate students looking for historical topics, any of these lines of inquiry, and many others, would provide solid topics and loads of fun! [9]

Investigating Secondary Sources

Where does a student go to find out whether anyone has investigated any of these topics or what historians think they know about a given topic? To the secondary sources, or the existing literature, which is the history student's real beginning point, as they are for all researchers. The secondary literature includes the existing body of books, articles, and other media that are histories, in contrast to the primary or firsthand sources that are the actual evidence. In the literature, a student will actually become more aware of the nature and effect of researchers' paradigms. One may read about the "evolution" of a club, conflicting accounts of a given event or person's life, or a different view of history than the one presented in this chapter. Each book or article is shaped by the historian's assumptions, beliefs, and cultural influences—his or her unstated paradigm. But students will also take information from the secondary sources.

 Today historians of sport and leisure, **kinesiology**, physical education, and exercise science have a vast array of secondary literature upon which to draw. In fact, we have several literatures. First, of course, is the direct literature, which consists of monographs, anthologies, journal articles, films about the history of sport, health, and so on.[10] There is also an ever-widening body of ancillary literature. This literature derives both from traditional disciplines—history, anthropology, sociology, political science, and economics, among others—and from interdisciplinary fields such as American studies, women's studies, African American studies, public policy, and management. Individual topics may also require a student to examine the literatures in medicine, law, and other fields.

Students will often not know precisely what their exact secondary literatures are until they have begun to search for background reading on their topic. Most students generally start their study of history with a general interest area, some thing or person or era about which or whom they wish to know more—the amorphous topic. One's advisor will undoubtedly suggest some books and articles for

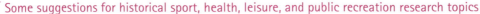

Some suggestions for historical sport, health, leisure, and public recreation research topics

kinesiology — The study of human movement.

the student to read and understand in order to begin to realize what is already known about this topic. But graduate advisors will invariably encourage the student to do precisely what they do to locate the literatures: Use the computer searches to proceed systematically through various literature banks. Not too many years ago, students searched for secondary literature through the various published indexes, such as *America: History and Life*, *Education Index*, or *Social Science Abstracts*. Today students can define a string of key words and search online databases such as Online Computer Library Center Union Catalog (OCLC) and Research Libraries Information Network (RLIN), which register the catalog records of many contributing libraries.[11] A student may also converse via electronic mail with working historians about topics they have investigated and secondary sources they find important.

What does one take from this secondary literature? The simple answer is as much as possible. At one level, a student reads as much as possible on a topic so that she or he knows what other scholars do and do not know about that topic. At another level, a student reads the literature to understand both the broader society that affected the subject and the conceptual frameworks and social theories that will bear on any interpretations and conclusions. Finally, the student reads the literature to uncover sources of evidence. In historical research, evidence is discussed in the text, but the actual identification and location of that evidence usually appear in the notes and appendices. For this reason, historians often study the notes as long and hard as they do the body of an article or book.

The history student's eventual success or failure often hinges on how thoroughly she or he is grounded in the literature. This literature will assist the student in shaping the approach or framework (or paradigm) that directs the research. It will direct the student to the data and the many ways of interrogating the evidence. And perhaps most important, at least as one begins to investigate the past, the literature will help the student to refine and transform the original amorphous topic into a researchable question.

Developing Good Questions

All research is about answering questions, and on this point history is exactly like science. Still, one

issue critical to the life of the historian may raise the stake of the question in historical research: the issue of objectivity. Not too many years ago, historians would find themselves on one of two sides in a debate about objectivity. Either they were objective, or they were not. The nots were known as subjectivists or relativists.[12] Today, however, most working historians admit that they will be more or less objective, or relatively objective. Beginning with questions helps the historian to operate with more rather than less objectivity—or, in simple terms, as an open-minded detective. Questions about what one will find encourage this open-mindedness, as propositions about what one wants or expects to find do not.

How does a student develop a good beginning question, and what criteria can one apply to distinguish a good question from another kind? On the general matter of questions, the French historian Henri-Irenee Marrou offered some sage advice: "There is an unlimited number of different questions to which the documents can provide answers." However, he cautioned, one must ask each question "properly."[13] And that proper questioning of the past begins with the secondary sources. A good question, at the very least, is one that is grounded in and derived from the literature. The unknown it focuses upon is thus clear, as is the significance of the question. But a good question is something more: It is also answerable.[14]

Let us work through two examples, which move us from the vague topic to the good beginning question(s). The first example, for which there is a good deal of secondary literature, involves the topic of baseball in the late nineteenth century. The student comes to this topic in the usual way, from personal interest and/or some knowledge of the literature. In the beginning the advisor will probably tell the student to narrow the topic, so that it can be accomplished in the span of the graduate experience. The student, in turn, focuses on a particular period and on a given city or town, where he or she has access to records and will not spend a fortune traveling. At this point, or perhaps up to this point, the student will read the histories of baseball, the histories of the particular city or region, and the more general histories of the period. From all this, the student will conclude that his or her town did have a baseball club by 1865; that the town—say, Cleveland, Ohio—did have a rapidly

 What to look for in secondary literature

 A good question is one that is grounded in the literature, has a clear unknown, and is answerable

expanding population and industrial base by the same date; and that baseball was still controlled by players in loosely linked clubs. The student can now delimit the topic with a set of questions that are significant and answerable and most of which test the conclusions offered in the literature. Who were the earliest members of the Cleveland baseball club? Was baseball the middle-class, upper-class, or working-class sport? Where did they play, and what rules did they use? Was baseball a refuge from their industrial work, or did it replicate the players' work life?

The second topic presents a bit more of a challenge because there is less secondary literature to help in framing the questions. The topic is the women's high school athletic association in a state, in this case Louisiana. In the beginning the student knows only that the organization first appeared about 1925. Still, he or she begins in the literature. The topic itself suggests the background reading, for every word in that topic has a literature: social histories of the 1920s (and subsequent decades), women's and gender histories, organized athletics, histories of schools and education, and Louisiana history. From all this, the student learns nothing about the particular athletic federation but much about the issues concerning competition for girls and women; about occupational and social expectations and roles for women; about other organizations that women formed; and about the changing curriculum, population, and context of high schools in Louisiana. The logical transformation of topic to questions can now occur. Who were the organizers, and what goals did they have? What activities and what kinds of competitive format did they incorporate? When did they introduce different or additional sports? What were the relationships of athletic competitions to other physical education, health, and recreational programs? What was the structure of the association, and what were the relationships of the association to other governing structures within the school and community? Questions such as these will be precursors to some bigger questions. How did the association change over time? What social factors affected the organization? How did the association affect the student body and school life, especially in gender relations? Why did it come into being?

Designing the Research

| Descriptive History |
| Analytic History |

Once students have replaced the vague topic with specific beginning questions, they can begin to construct a research design. This is not a phrase working historians frequently use, and the apparent lack of discussion about constructing the study's design may be one of the things that mystifies scientists about the work of their colleagues in history. But good historians do design their research, even if such designs lack the formulaic precision found in experimental designs. A design in historical research is precisely what it is in scientific research: a systematic, even hierarchical, layout of the questions and a plan for answering them. In science there are three broad categories of designs:

- Description, which produces a statement of what something is and from which variables are identified
- Correlation, which examines relationships among variables
- Experimentation, which examines one set of relationships, cause and effect

 Most historians reduce this list to two designs, on the grounds of the questions asked: description ("what happened") and analysis ("how" and/or "why" something happened).[15] The first broad historical design category is virtually the same as descriptive scientific research. The second plan parallels the correlational and cause-effect research in science, minus the experimentation.[16]

 How does a student decide which design, descriptive or analytic, to undertake? The critical factors should be the existing litera-

 Two broad categories of historical research designs

 descriptive history — A method of constructing a "map" of past experience that locates in time and place a person, a trend, an event, or an organization by providing answers to particular questions.

chronicle — A listing of the happenings in time; used in historical research.

antiquarianism — Collecting of old things; appropriate for historical research.

ture and the questions one wishes to answer. If virtually nothing is known about a particular event or person or program, then a good **descriptive history** is in order. Good descriptive history, which is distinct from **chronicle** (the listing of happenings in time) or **antiquarianism** (the collecting of old things), is also an appropriate goal for students who are just learning to ask historical questions and to work with evidence. As is the case in science, however, descriptive research in history has its limits. Students who wish to explore beyond the "what" to the "how" and "why" of a historical person or process will develop analytic designs, even if this means doing some descriptive work as well. Doctoral students especially, who can expect to publish their dissertations, should look to the existing literature for models of analytic histories. Such recently published models include monographs like Ann Fabian's *Card Sharps, Dream Books, and Bucket Shops: Gambling in 19th-Century America* and Bruce Kuklick's *To Every Thing a Season: Shibe Park and Urban Philadelphia, 1909-1976.*[17] Good historians aim to write such analytic histories.

Descriptive History

The world's oceans present us with a useful analogy for understanding descriptive history. Today, scientists know much about these huge bodies of water—their depths, their total sizes, the plants and animals that live in them, even the courses that ships need to travel across them. Not too many centuries ago, however, the oceans were truly "uncharted seas," a situation that made captains and navigators double as map makers. Today, much of the history of sport, exercise, education, athletics, health, and leisure is like those uncharted seas of old; and like earlier ocean travelers, one who makes that journey to the past becomes a mapmaker. In short, the goal of a descriptive history is a map of past experience.

A good map locates roads and landmarks, and this is precisely what good descriptive history does. It locates in time and place a person, a trend, an event, or an organization in the past by providing answers to particular questions. Such questions are many, but they include "where" something took place or someone lived, "when" an event happened or a person lived, "who" a person was, and "what" an organization or program was. In effect, descriptive history identifies as fully as possible a set of experiences in the past.

Identifying the appropriate questions is the first step in designing a descriptive study, as the earlier discussion of questions suggested. A student begins with a broad topic, say, the "history of intercollegiate athletics at Arizona State University." Then he or she digests the secondary literature on intercollegiate athletics, higher education, the state, and the university. This literature reveals that nobody really knows anything about ASU athletics, so questions are needed to formulate a "map" of the experiences. When did competition emerge, in what sports did the competitors participate, and where did the matches occur? Who were the competitors, in terms of gender, race, and social class? Who were the officials and spectators, and what were their roles? How were athletics gendered? What did the larger university community have to say about these contests, and what values and meanings did its members assign to intercollegiate athletics? The results will contribute to a detailed map of athletic experiences. This map will "locate" the people and the program, as well as the place of athletics in the context of university life.

However, because this is a historical study, our ASU athletics map will also contain a particular set of markers—the periods or time phases that contain events within time and indicate change over time.[18] To produce these patterns in time, the student will have to ask a second set of questions, drawing directly from the secondary literature. When were different sports and opponents added to the athletic program? At what point did administrators or faculty attempt to govern the program? When did the program incorporate women's and minority experiences?

The secondary literature suggests more than just another set of questions to be asked about the ASU experience, however. Because it also offers answers to these questions in the form of conclusions about the patterns of athletic experience at other institutions, it sets up the student with hypotheses to test. Logically deduced, just as are scientific hypotheses, these broad statements of probability about intercollegiate athletics may look something like this:

Initially, the students created, funded, and organized athletics. As athletics began to com-

Fabian, Ann. (1990). *Card sharps, dream books, and bucket shops: Gambling in 19th-century America.* Ithaca: Cornell University Press.

Kuklick, Bruce. (1991). *To every thing a season: Shibe Park in urban Philadelphia, 1909-1976.* Princeton: Princeton University Press.

pete with students' academic responsibilities and to draw support from alumni, faculty and administrators sought to become actors on the athletic stage. Even later, departments of athletics became embroiled in racial and gender controversies. One effect of the expanding athletic program, then, was to reproduce and reinforce divisions among the university's constituents rather than to erase them.

All these statements need to be tested against the evidence about the ASU program before students can achieve their goal of writing an adequate descriptive history.

Analytic History

In effect, what the student has done to "design" this descriptive study is to develop two sets of questions about ASU athletics. The first set includes the ones that result in the student's knowing what happened at ASU. The second set enables the student to make sense of the ASU experiences, both in terms of patterns within and over time and in terms of the existing literature. What the student has not done, however, is to pose questions about the relationships among experiences and the factors, or variables, that affected them. Such questions are the domain of our second type of history, **analytic history**, which focuses on "how" something occurred and even "why" someone did something. The analytic historian, in other words, begins with the map (or description) of experiences, breaks apart and relates the constituents of those experiences, and ends with "making sense" of the entire scene.

If we continue with the example of intercollegiate athletics at Arizona State University, we can design an analytic investigation. Assume for the moment that one of the simple conclusions of the previous description is that by about 1920 the types of sports included in the athletic program had changed. The earliest forms, football and basketball for men, now existed alongside rodeo, riflery, swimming, a distinctive women's version of basketball, track, and swimming, among other things. The questions thus become, How did this situation come to be and why did the athletic program diversify?

Finding the answers is not simple. A simple sounding "how" question, which asks about the process of the experience, is one of the most diffi-

cult to answer in historical research. A "why" question, which focuses on the cause, is even more difficult to resolve. Before one can even begin to answer the "how" questions, a student needs to identify clearly all the variables, the agents and social factors and structures, that operated in the process of change. In the case of the ASU athletic program, as the prior descriptive history established, the variables include three main groups of actors (students, alumni, and faculty and administrators); the beliefs and interests and the material conditions of each group; and the social setting and structures in which they existed. It is the relationships among these three sets of variables that the student needs to analyze before answering the "how" question.

Hence, our initial "how this situation came to be" needs to be restated as a series of answerable subquestions about relationships and changes in relationships within and across time. Such questions might include the following: What were the relationships between the changing ethnic and gender composition of the student body and the emergence of new forms of sport? How did students react to (or act upon) faculty efforts to monitor the times and funding of competition? What were the relationships between alumni and students or between administrators and alumni? What were the relationships between the university's teams and the broader community and government officials?

At this point the biophysical science student would probably be able to identify the predictor variable and proceed to test for cause-effect in the laboratory via a controlled experiment. The science student would then be able to answer "what caused" a given phenomenon, which is our "why" question: Why did the ASU athletic program change? Students of history, however, will find the trip from determining relationships among variables in a given set of past experiences to determining cause much more difficult, even in a quantitative study.[19] In fact, looking for a single cause may be an impossible task for several reasons. A major reason is theoretical: Historical experiences and events are "massive clusters" of behavior and thought, only some of which may even have been "known" to the historical actors.[20] Put another way, unlike some natural science phenomena, social phenomena are complexes of human action, thoughts and beliefs, social factors, and conse-

---

analytic history — Type of historical research that focuses on how something occurred and why someone did something.

quences (both intended and unintended). The final form of any given event or experience is something more, and perhaps even something other than its components. A second reason is a methodological one: Historians cannot be certain that they have uncovered all the evidence about a given event or person. Consequently, descriptions and explanations will fall short of absolute truth, no matter how well refined and valid are the interpretive schemes and techniques.

So we are left expecting the answer to our "why" question to be complex and perhaps inexact. Why did the ASU athletic program broaden about 1920? The probable cause(s) will lie in three areas, or dimensions of experience. One source of cause is the material conditions and ideological interests of the participants themselves. A second dimension is the material conditions and ideological interests of the university administration, alumni, and faculty. The third area is the political relationships among students, faculty, alumni, and other supporters of the university. Unfortunately perhaps, the historian cannot "control" for student "effect," nor can one isolate the alumni as a group and apply different "treatments" to them. We also do not have the means to separate out and then recombine in an experimental fashion all the variables that affect human experience in the past: class, gender, motive or interest, received traditions, social structures, and so on. Consequently, the student must logically weigh the changes in all these areas. For example, what was happening to the student population? To what pressures was the university responding? Had students or alumni gained some political leverage? Then one must logically assess the relative power of any or all of these and other factors. In effect, the student analyst will produce a complex explanation or even a complex of explanations that take the shape of a true logical inference which is theoretically informed and methodologically driven.

Working With the Evidence

Locating Primary Sources
Criticizing the Sources

 Historical evidence is "everything made or recalled"

 Where to find historical sources

Reading the Evidence
Considering the Context

The preceding discussion may have left the impression that historical research depends almost entirely on the kinds of questions one asks. In the real world of the historian, however, nothing could be further from the truth. A student will, of course, use questions to structure her or his study. But questions require answers, and answers require evidence or, in the scientist's terms, data. Moreover, the evidence that one identifies and uses will affect the increasingly specific questions that one will ask. Located in primary sources, or firsthand accounts, historical evidence is a major determinant in the research process.[21]

What is historical evidence, or data? In *Truth in History*, Oscar Handlin offered a simple and clear definition: Evidence is "everything made or recalled."[22] Each "thing" is a piece of the past, and such pieces come in many forms—artifacts such as equipment and clothes; photographs; oral tales and reminiscences; numerical evidence such as prize money and census accounts; and literary materials such as letters, laws, and written stories. The evidence that a student will use depends, of course, on the questions that he or she is asking. The questions also determine whether a student uses qualitative or quantitative, or both, forms of evidence.[23] However, about one thing there is no "depending": There can be no answers to questions without evidence.

Just as a physiologist must have raw data about heart rate to answer questions about cardiovascular condition or the psychologist must have records of brain activity to study hemispheric dominance, the historian must have information created and constructed by his or her subjects in the past.

Locating Primary Sources

Before a student can actually begin to work with evidence, he or she needs to identify the sources that may contain the evidence. To locate where historical sources exist—usually in distinct kinds of laboratories such as archives, libraries, or private collections—the student can proceed in a number of ways. If one is working on a particular sport, recreational facility, curricular program, or any other project that is locale-specific, she or he may go directly to the catalogs or indexes to the holdings of the local historical society (state or town), to the college or university archives, to a hall of fame, or to an organization's archives and library. Some of these are identified in Appendix 1 at the end of this chapter. A student may also draw upon the online databases noted earlier and published catalogs, like the *National Union Catalog of Manuscripts,* found in most university libraries. Students will discover that many newspapers, censuses, and government records have indexes that aid in locating potential information. There are also many published topical bibliographies of sources.

Particularly for students who are interested in recent history, another form of historical evidence consists of oral sources. Unlike many of us, some historians have the luxury of working with people who are very much alive and well. These are people who have lived through experiences and processes that are of historic value and who can provide "firsthand" accounts. Many of the suggestions this chapter makes about doing history are applicable to oral history projects, but there are also a number of issues that are particular to oral history research. This chapter will not address those issues, but there are many books and articles that can help students through the process of doing oral history. Most university libraries will have oral history research methods books, so interested students should search them out.

Criticizing the Sources

 Once a student has located existing primary sources, even though the identification of all the sources will probably not yet be complete, he or she begins to criticize the sources. This is an evaluative process that has two steps: **external criticism** and **internal criticism**.

The first step, external criticism, determines the form of the material. In this step we ask whether a given artifact or document is really a source of evidence about the past. This phase of the evaluation establishes the authenticity of the source. A student has only to think about Watergate or the Iran-Contra affair to realize why the historian must establish a source as an authentic witness to the past. For any number of reasons, people in the past—who were the makers of historical evidence—could, and have been known to, forge documents. More common than outright forgeries, however, are the unintended errors that resulted when time or another person intervened between the actual occurrence of an event and the period when a record of the event or person was made. So historians must either know how to establish that a piece of evidence is really a record of what it purports to be—through a technique like Carbon-14 dating for very old artifacts or through textual and stylistic analysis for documents—or they must rely on experts to perform these tests. The simple point, of course, is that a piece of evidence must be the genuine article![24]

Internal criticism deals with the nature of the source. It asks specifically whether a now-determined genuine artifact or document is credible. Internal criticism thus involves matters of consistency and accuracy, and at one level it is comparable to the scientist's efforts to establish validity.[25] Just as the scientist must establish the adequacy and accuracy of a test, instrument, or construct, so the historian must determine both whether an observation or some other form of record is believable and what the context and perspective of the record are. Historians who use quantitative data and sampling techniques will actually use the same techniques to establish validity as biophysical scientists do. Investigators who rely on more traditional historical data sources, especially literary documents, cannot approach the mathematical precision of validity coefficients, but they do ask appropriate questions systematically. In fact, there are three rules for a student to apply in the process of internally criticizing a document:

 • The **rule of context**. This rule maintains that a word must be understood in relation to the words that precede and follow it—and not in the historian's own contemporary usage.

---

 external criticism — Phase of historical research process that establishes the authenticity of the source.

 internal criticism — Phase of historical research process that establishes the credibility of a genuine artifact or document.

rule of context — A rule of internal criticism in historical research that maintains that a word must be understood in relation to the words that precede and follow it and not in the historian's own contemporary usage.

Reading sentences and paragraphs requires the same sequence and connotation guidelines.

 • The **rule of perspective**. The second guideline encourages the student to ask who (or what agency or group) left the record, what a source's relationship to an event or group was, and even how the source collected the information.

• The **rule of omission** or **free editing**. This rule holds that most historical sources—whether official records, newspaper accounts, diaries, or formal agreements—are not accounts of complete scenes. The minutes of an NCAA meeting, a photograph of a home run, a day's diary entry by someone like Albert Spalding or Senda Berenson, and even a census or map will record some things and leave out others. Diarists may omit things that happened or words that were spoken in the course of a day, whereas the editing of a meeting or newspaper report may use different words, leave out entire sections of a report, or even purposefully misrepresent conversations and actions.[26] Thus, because sources may leave information out, whether intentionally or not, the historian needs to use more than one source to view any event or program or person in the past—in much the same way as a biomechanist may use several cameras to view one movement from different angles.

Reading the Evidence

The location and criticism of historical sources are important tasks that all historians perform, over and over again. They are not, however, ends in themselves. A newspaper, for example, is a source of information about the past, just as an EMG record is a source of information about muscle contractions. And like the EMG firing pattern, the newspaper text or picture requires a "reading." In short, a student needs to know what information the newspaper, or any historical source, contains.

To accomplish this, the student will ask a relatively simple question of each piece of information:

"What is this evidence evidence of?" Consider a practical example—a health and physical education curriculum from, say, 1950. Most students in our fields are familiar with curricula; they lay out goals, activities, and learning outcomes. But about what or whom can a curriculum really inform us? Is it evidence of what went on in a classroom or gymnasium? Is it evidence of all the thoughts about health and physical education that the writers may have held? Is it evidence of the state of health and physical education in the country? The answer, of course, is "none of the above." Insofar as it was written in behavioral terms, the health and physical education curriculum is nothing more, or less, than evidence of a set of expected behaviors. Moreover, a curriculum is evidence of behaviors expected by the writers rather than of those for whom the curriculum was written.

Students will see that all historical sources provide us with evidence that is narrow in scope, once they ask "what the evidence is evidence of." Typical newspaper accounts of a ball game, for example, provide us with a portion of the reporter's observations, rather than a comprehensive picture of all that occurred in the contest. The same is true of diaries and letters. Rule books provide information about what behaviors should and/or should not occur, but they do not tell us about what behaviors actually did or did not occur. Likewise, numerical evidence can inform us of only certain things. A salary figure, for instance, informs us only of dollars paid to a player, not of the athlete's value. The number of fans at an event tells us how many people were present, rather than whether the event was popular.[27]

 This process of determining what the evidence "is evidence of" thus really has two goals. The more obvious of the two is knowing what information we *can* obtain or read from any given piece. Less obvious but no less important is knowing what information we *cannot* read from a source. A student must come to grips with both sides of the coin if she or he is to determine whether the evidence is or is not adequate and ap-

---

 rule of perspective — A rule of internal criticism in historical research that requires the researcher to determine who left the record, relationship of a source to an event or group, and how the source collected the information.

 rule of omission — A rule of internal criticism in historical research that maintains that most historical sources are not accounts of complete scenes. Also called *free editing.*

free editing — See *rule of omission.*

 Three rules to apply in internal criticism

 Two goals for determining what the evidence proves

propriate. If someone finds that the evidence meets both criteria, then she or he can proceed to answer the research questions. If it does not, however, the student has a "big" problem, and he or she cannot proceed with the questions as originally asked. This situation might have occurred with our health education curriculum—had we expected it to be evidence of behaviors in the classroom. It is also a situation that can, and does, occur when historians ask questions about beliefs, attitudes, values, processes, and conditions. Most of our common forms of evidence, whether literary or numerical evidence, provide data about what people did or said rather than about what they believed. Consequently, unless an historian makes some hard-to-establish assumptions about the relationships between what one saw or did and what one believed, he or she will find that most historical sources do not provide the "right" information about an individual's or a society's beliefs and attitudes.

There are several ways of resolving this dilemma of having the wrong (or inadequate) evidence for the questions one wants to ask. First, a student can change the questions. Second, he or she can retain the question and search for other appropriate sources of evidence. Finally, the student can translate what is evidence of one thing, usually behavior, into evidence of another thing, such as beliefs or other concepts. This is an inferential process that requires the careful construction of indicators and the testing of relationships between the "thing" we cannot observe or find direct evidence of and the "thing" we think will indicate or implicate it. It is also a process about which historians can learn much from their peers in science, who frequently investigate what they cannot directly observe. Physiologists, for example, examine cardiovascular fitness, a condition that cannot be directly observed or measured. So they have developed and validated an inferred indicator: expired air. In studying aggression, psychologists have proceeded similarly. They cannot observe and measure aggression directly, but they can observe and measure an inferred indicator: violent acts.

Constructs and inferential relationships are important to historians when they wish to examine concepts, values, or attitudes that cannot be directly observed. Social class is such a concept. It is also a complex of behaviors and attitudes about which no one piece of evidence is direct evidence. Historical sources do, however, provide numerous and appropriate indicators—occupation, income, goods purchased and used, club membership, and so on—which altogether may be inferred as evidence of class. Indicators and inferences are also essential to the study of beliefs and values, as in the case of research on the beliefs of health club members. A student may suspect that particular beliefs—in good health, fitness, even beauty—may have even motivated people to join a given club. The hypothesis is not directly testable, however, because of the nature of the evidence. All the records of the clubs and even the members—daily logs, accounts, equipment used and purchased, exercise regimens, diaries—are readable only as evidence of what the members did and not what they believed. Again, the student must infer a relationship between the observed and the unobservable and, of course, test it.

In part because of the critical role of inferences in historical description and explanation, other information about a person, an event, or a process becomes essential to the historian. This other information will often be in sources that may, at first, seem tangential to a student's major sources. In the previous example of the research about beliefs of health club members, one might not think that evidence about members' occupations, the other activities and groups in which they participated, their eating habits and medical histories, and their neighborhoods, among other things, would be particularly important. All these are, of course. Only with this large body of evidence can a student test the inferences about beliefs that he or she has produced from the health club behavior data. If the student projected a belief in fitness as one of the factors, perhaps even a "motive" for a subject's membership in the health club, he or she must "test" that belief in other behavioral situations, the evidence for which lies in this other information. If no such evidence is forthcoming, or if there is even counterevidence—if the subject drank heavily, ate high-cholesterol food, or did not regularly see a doctor—the student will have to look for a "new" belief within the health club behaviors. In effect, this seemingly tangential evidence did not bear out the inferred relationship between behavior and belief.[28]

Considering the Context

 This seemingly tangential evidence is important in historical research for another reason, as well. It is a part of the **context** in which a

---

 context — In historical research, the total network of data (information) about a person, event, or period.

historical subject lived or a historical process occurred and in which sport, recreation, or health experiences and processes they need to be placed, if they are to be understood. Context refers to the "ensemble" of data about a person, event, or period. Rather than background material, in other words, context means the network of facts and meanings in which a given piece of historical evidence existed. The term is so important in historical research that one scholar has defined the field with the term: History is the "discipline of context."[29]

Context figures in many tasks that the historian performs. Students may recall the "rule of context" discussed in the section on internal criticism. They may also recognize the allusions to context in the paragraphs on indicators and inference. But it is in the reading of evidence that the importance of context becomes most obvious, as one extended example should reveal. The source here is a typical literary document, the *American Turf Register and Sporting Magazine*, which was an urban journal published in the 1820s and 1830s. The particular article, "The Great Foot Race" (reprinted in Appendix 2), is an account of a pedestrian race held at the Union Race Track on Long Island in June 1835. Beyond the kind of race and its site, the piece contains information about the distance covered (10 miles), the numbers of competitors (nine), some descriptive information about the runners (name, age, weight, occupation, dress), the order in which they ran, the prize money ($1,300), and the times for each mile achieved by the winner.[30]

From this evidence, we can construct a description of the event. Nine men, ranging in age from twenty-two to thirty-three and of various manual occupations, competed against one another on a Friday in June 1835 over a distance of 10 miles on what was normally a horse track. The winner, Henry Stannard, covered the distance in the prescribed time (just under an hour) and won the purse of $1,300 in the presence of a crowd estimated at between 16,000 and 20,000. With any certainty, this is all the information we can "read" in this account.

The rest of the information in the article is in bits and pieces and generally in the form of judgments and suggestions by the reporter. For example, the first sentence of the piece introduced the event as the "great trial of human capabilities." We cannot accept this statement at face value; the phrase may have been a literary device employed by the writer to interest readers. The report also mentions that a tenth runner, a Francis Smith, had appeared but did not run because he had not entered his name "by a

certain day." Such a "reason" may or may not be true; the runner was a black man, who may have been excluded on the grounds of race. The report also indicates that another man, John Cox Stevens, was particularly active in the race; he even rode around the track with Stannard. But Stevens's exact role remains unclear. Finally, we cannot be certain that the purse represented the sum total of Stannard's winnings or that he was the only one who "won" money. The reporter also noted that betting, even by the runners, was a part of the scene.

So beyond the earlier "barebones" and not very telling description of this event, we cannot proceed from this piece. As a consequence, many fairly simple questions must go unanswered. Was pedestrianism common? Was the $1,300 purse typical or "a lot"? Was this really a "Great Race"? Was Smith prevented from running because of his late entry or his race? Was the crowd large? Answers to these questions hinge on a student's willingness to read the evidence in relation to, or in conjunction with, other pieces of evidence. The first question, for example, requires data on other races—in fact, a counting of them and a numerical comparison to other sport and public events in this period. The second question can only be answered by a comparison of this purse to other purses and to the annual incomes of similar working men. The last question, concerning the size of the crowd, requires a major shift in the evidential base, from qualitative to quantitative evidence. Descriptive statistics from both sport and nonsport crowds are essential; inferential statistics would be more informative. The remaining questions demand additional data on other sports, events, and social practices of the times.

The significance of this practice of reading the evidence in its full and appropriate context should not be underestimated. Divorced from the network of facts and meanings in which any given piece of evidence about a sport, a health practice, or a recreational program originally existed, the evidence becomes drab and lifeless. To picture such a situation, consider a ball. Unless a student places a ball in the context of a game, played by real people who hit and threw and caught it, it exists only as a round object. Taken out of its context, a ball becomes just another bit of rubber, or cloth packing, or even an animal bladder. Considering your own life as a graduate student might even make the point a bit more dramatically. Taken out of the context of graduate school, in a particular place at a particular time in your life, much of what you do (like reading this chapter) would make absolutely no sense to anyone, even to you! So like you, if historians are to achieve their goal of making sense of the past, they must place their subjects in context.

Some Final Thoughts

We now have some of the components for the making of a good history. From the secondary literature, we have derived our research questions: significant ones, telling ones, answerable ones. We have laid out the questions in a logical, hierarchical order and identified the evidence needed to answer them. We have located and criticized the sources, and we have spent hours reading the evidence and putting it into context. We have, in effect, been both scientist and detective. So, are we finished?

Not quite! The historian is not finished until he or she makes sense of whatever piece of the past one has investigated. This is clearly a matter of constructing a case, a theme, or, perhaps more pointedly, an argument. With everything done so far—the questions raised, the evidence read and interrogated—the historian now assumes the guise of both architect and prosecuting attorney.

The construction of a history demands an answer to one final question: So what happened here? Another way of asking this is "so what does all this mean?" Regardless of how one poses it, however, this question needs an answer before a student can begin to write. Like the architect who would not presume to build a house before he or she knew what the house should look like, the historian would not presume to write the story before he or she was certain of its content and meaning.

How does one answer the question, So what does all this mean? I do not believe that there is any single or simple answer, nor is there any intellectual formula. An analogy of the prosecuting attorney may be helpful, however, for like the attorney, the historian is committed to making a case (or interpretation). This goal, in turn, requires laying out the evidence and the interpretations of various pieces of evidence in a logical fashion, which leads to the climax, the "point." When we talk about laying out the evidence, historians usually mean discussing and analyzing the primary material (even in descriptive studies) and pointing out and discussing the patterns of experiences about which particular

sources are revealing. We also lay out the evidence, and our interpretations of its meanings, in a sequence that leads through and to the "end" of the story. No prosecuting attorney would take his or her case to court until the sequence of events was clear and until he or she knew which evidence to produce when. So it is with the historian's story, or case. Good historians never "list" sentences within paragraphs or paragraphs within an article or chapter. Each sentence and each paragraph has a logical "fit" in a sequence of sentences and paragraphs.

What determines this sequence? The historian's mind, of course, and the "big" story or argument that he or she wishes to offer, which in turn is the answer to the question one asked. And this "story," in turn, moves us to the task of writing, which many people, working scholars and students alike, view as the hardest task of doing history. When I hear my students, or my colleagues, complain about how hard writing is, I usually respond with a short and cryptic "nuts!" It's not the writing that is hard. It's the thinking that is difficult. And too often, many of us try to write before we have labored through all the thinking that "good" history requires. And that thinking must include the answer to "so what happened here?" In other words, a student needs to know precisely what her or his storyline, interpretation, or argument is before he or she sits down to write. One must work out in one's head precisely what the story is that one is going to write and in what sequence the evidence and conclusions from it should be presented so that they lead the reader through the argument and to the "big" conclusion.

There are undoubtedly as many ways to work through the "end of the story" and determine the best sequencing of evidence and subarguments as there are historians. A couple of suggestions, however, may be in order. Some people work well with topical outlines, in part because each part of such an outline is really a code for a more extensive thought that they retain in memory. For other people, however, topical outlines are insufficient to prevent the "problem" they have with writing. Single words or phrases are often vague; they fall short of the complete answers that historical questions require. Students in history may find themselves in this second category, and they would be better off spending their time drafting complete sentences or even paragraphs that answer specific questions. In effect, one may find the writing of a history easier after she or he has already done a lot

The final question that must be answered

of thinking (and writing) and can honestly say, "This is how the story ends" or "This is the point," as well as saying, "This is how I am going to develop it."

The writing of history deserves a more extended treatment than this. It is a skill that, like most others, takes practice, and it actually warrants several volumes of material. But that is not in the purview of this book or this chapter. There are many chapters and books that students can consult about the writing of history.[31] There is not, however, such an extensive literature on historical research, especially oriented to graduate students in sport studies, exercise science, and physical education. I hope this chapter provides that orientation. Perhaps only time—and good history—will tell.

Summary

History is the systematic study of change and continuity in past human affairs. The historian carefully derives questions, gathers and interrogates evidence (data), and frames and tests inferences. He or she also incorporates and tests social theories and operates within distinctive research paradigms or conceptual frameworks. Questions important to the historian include the following:

- How does social change proceed?
- How did people in the past use sport and exercise practices to construct categories such as gender and class?
- Why did particular forms of sport and exercise emerge at particular times, and what cultural meanings did they have?
- How and why did sport forms, structures, and meaning change over time (or fail to change)?
- In what ways did sport, health, and exercise affect the social structures and economic and political systems?

Secondary sources—the written accounts of others—provide the beginning point for historians to develop questions and the design of the research. The construction of viable answers, however, requires primary evidence, which one subjects to both internal and external criticism, and context. This matter of reading the evidence in its full and appropriate context is essential to historical research. Finally, the historian must make sense of his or her conclusions by answering the question, So what happened here?

Check Your Understanding

1. Select a historical article from the *Journal of Sport History*. Summarize the arguments that the author made, identify the evidence that he or she used, and analyze how the author used the evidence to make the arguments.

2. Locate one of the serials identified in Appendix 1. Read one article in it about sport, health, or exercise. What kind of evidence does this article contain, and about what questions does this evidence provide information? What can this evidence not tell us anything about?

Endnotes

[These endnotes represent the substance and style of notes as they would appear in a research manuscript according to *The Chicago Manual of Style* (14th ed.). Direct quotations are cited immediately, whereas the citations for information and ideas borrowed and adapted from one or more sources, either secondary or primary, occur at the end of a sentence or paragraph.]

 Some additional discursive material may also appear in an endnote. Consult these sources for additional information about the topics discussed in this chapter.

1. E. P. Thompson, *The Poverty of Theory and Other Essays* (New York: Monthly Review Press, 1978), 28-29.

2. For readily available and readable discussions of theoretical differences between natural and social phenomena, see R. Gerald Glassford, "Methodological Reconsiderations: The Shifting Paradigm," *Quest* **39** (Fall 1987): 295-312; and Roberta J. Park, "Hermeneutics, Semiotics, and the Nineteenth-Century Quest for a Corporeal Self," *Quest* **38** (Spring 1986): 33-49. About social theory, human agency, and other issues related to theory, see Pauline M. Rosenau, *Post-Modernism and the Social Sciences: Insights, Inroads, and Intrusions* (Princeton: Princeton University Press, 1992); Alex Callinicos, *Making History* (Ithaca: Cornell University Press, 1988); Anthony Giddens, *The Constitution of Society* (Berkeley: University of California, 1984); Alfred Schmidt, *History and Structure*, trans. Jeffrey

Herf (Cambridge: Harvard University Press, 1981); Gordon S. Wood, "Intellectual History and the Social Sciences," in *New Directions in American Intellectual History*, ed. John Higham and Paul Conkin (Baltimore: Johns Hopkins University Press, 1979); Peter Burke, *Sociology and History* (London, 1980); Eric Monkkonen, "The Challenge of Quantitative History," *Historical Methods* 17 (Summer 1984): 89-90; Carey B. Joynt and Nicholas Rescher, "The Problem of Uniqueness in History," *History and Theory* 2 (1961): 150-62.

3 See, for example, Allen Guttmann, *From Ritual to Record: The Nature of Modern Sport* (New York: Columbia University Press, 1978); Melvin Adelman, *A Sporting Time: New York City and the Rise of Modern Athletics, 1820-1870* (Urbana: University of Illinois Press, 1986).

4 Joyce Appleby, "Modernization Theory and the Formation of Modern Social Theories in England and America," *Comparative Studies in Society and History* 20 (1978): 261.

5 One of the earliest discussions remains appropriate: Peter N. Stearns, "Modernization and Social History: Some Suggestions and a Muted Cheer," *Journal of Social History* 14 (Winter 1980): 189-210.

6 Maurice Mandelbaum, *The Anatomy of Historical Knowledge* (Baltimore: Johns Hopkins University Press, 1977).

7 On the dilemmas associated with thinking about the evidence, see Stephen R. Humphrey, "The Historian, His Documents, and Elementary Modes of Historical Thought," *History and Theory* 19 (1980): 1-20. Students may find that reading some histories will help them to see how and why these questions and the answers to them do affect a historian's writing. So, for what is a fine history and an example of both history as an evolutionary process and evidence "speaking" for itself, see Ronald A. Smith, *Sports and Freedom: The Rise of Big-Time College Athletics* (New York: Oxford University Press, 1988). An alternative model of historical experience, one that incorporates change and persistence, or continuity, informs Elliott Gorn, *The Manly Art: Bare-Knuckle Prize Fighting in America* (Ithaca: Cornell University Press, 1986). The polar position, to Smith's, on the evidence—that it will not reveal anything until something has been asked of it—is evident in Nancy L. Struna, "Sport and Society in Early America," *International Journal of the History of Sport* 5 (December 1988): 292-311;

and Patricia Vertinsky, *The Eternally Wounded Woman: Women, Exercise, and Doctors in the Late Nineteenth Century* (Manchester: Manchester University Press, 1990).

8 Thomas Kuhn, *The Structure of Scientific Revolutions* (Chicago: University of Chicago Press, 1962). About the implications of Kuhn's work for history and the social sciences, see Barry Barnes, *T. S. Kuhn and Social Science* (New York: Columbia University Press, 1982); David Hollinger, "T. S. Kuhn's Theory of Science and Its Implications for History," *American Historical Review* 78 (April 1973): 370-93.

9 A student may find exemplary articles in the *Journal of Sport History* and in the *International Journal of the History of Sport*, as well as in many other historical journals that do not focus on sport. A few books that highlight important recent, nontraditional research directions include Jack W. Berryman and Roberta J. Park, eds., *Sport and Exercise Science: Essays in the History of Sports Medicine* (Urbana: University of Illinois Press, 1992); Richard Butsch, ed., *For Fun and Profit: The Transformation of Leisure into Consumption* (Philadelphia: Temple University Press, 1990); Matt Cartmell, *A View to a Death in the Morning: Hunting and Nature Through History* (Cambridge: Harvard University Press, 1993); J. A. Mangan and James Walvin, eds., *Manliness and Morality: Middle-Class Masculinity in Britain and America, 1800-1940* (New York: St. Martin's Press, 1987); Kathryn Grover, ed., *Fitness in American Culture: Images of Health, Sport, and the Body, 1830-1940* (Amherst: University of Massachusetts Press, 1989).

10 Reviews of the literature on the history of sport, leisure, and health can be very helpful to students and working historians alike. Some earlier reviews include Melvin L. Adelman, "Academicians and American Athletics: A Decade of Progress," *Journal of Sport History* 10 (Spring 1983): 80-106; Stephen Hardy and Alan Ingham, "Games, Structures, and Agency: Historians on the American Play Movement," *Journal of Social History* 17 (Winter 1983): 285-301; Roberta J. Park, "Research and Scholarship in the History of Physical Education and Sport," *Research Quarterly for Exercise and Sport* 54 (June 1983): 93-103; Nancy L. Struna, "In 'Glorious Disarray': The Literature of American Sport History," *Research Quarterly for Exercise and Sport* 56 (June 1985): 151-60. Recently, and in fact still to come, the *Journal of Sport History* is publishing another series of litera-

ture reviews and assessments. See the numbers for 1994 for discussions of women's experiences and gender; health, the body, and sports medicine; social class and other subtopics. For a history of sport history, see Nancy L. Struna, "Sport History," in *History of Exercise and Sport Science*, ed. John Massengale and Richard Swanson (Champaign: Human Kinetics, in press).

[11] Joyce Duncan Falk, "OCLC and RLIN: Research Libraries at the Scholar's Fingertips," American Historical Association Newsletter *Perspectives* **27** (May/June 1989): 1, 11-13, 17. See also Robert L. Oakman, *Computer Methods for Literary Research* (Athens: University of Georgia Press, 1984).

[12] This debate really commenced over a century ago with the introduction of "scientific history" by the German scholar Leopold Von Ranke. He maintained that objective history, "written as it really happened," was both possible and necessary. Wilhelm Dilthey just as clearly stated the opposing position, the subjectivist or interpretivist position, which was predicated on his view that the "historical world was a text to be deciphered." Later relativists raised the level of the debate by establishing a clear role for the present; the past had meanings for the present and could be used to solve current problems. This objective vs. subjective issue has some bearing on questions about theory in history and on the nature of evidence; see note 2 above. See also John R. Hall, "Temporality, Social Action, and the Problem of Quantification in Historical Analysis," *Historical Methods* **17** (fall 1984): 206-18. See also Joyce Appleby, Lynn Hunt, and Margaret Jacob, *Telling the Truth about History* (New York: W.W. Norton, 1994).

[13] Henri-Irenee Marrou, *The Meaning of History*, trans. Robert J. Olsen (Baltimore: Helicon, 1967), 76-77.

[14] For a more extended discussion of the question-deriving process, see Nancy L. Struna, "E. P. Thompson's Notion of 'Context' and the Writing of Physical Education and Sport History," *Quest* **38** (Spring 1986): 24-27.

[15] Description and analysis are the common categories of historical research presented in methodology books, such as Robert Shafer, *A Guide to Historical Method*, 3rd ed. (Homewood, Ill.: Dorsey Press, 1980); Jacques Barzun and Henry F. Graff, *The Modern Researcher*, 3rd ed. (New York, 1977). Two other terms, however,

often make their way into such discussions, narration and explanation, and can confound students' understandings of historical designs. Narration, or narrative history, does not mean the same thing as does description. Narration refers to a mode of historical thought, specifically the "recounting" of something in the past. Narration will then take place in the creation of a descriptive history. But so may explanation, if the word is used in the general sense of "making clear." Both the narrative and explanatory modes of thought may appear in analytic histories. See Robert F. Atkinson, *Knowledge and Explanation in History* (Ithaca: Cornell University Press, 1978); Mandelbaum, *Anatomy of Historical Knowledge*; and Dale H. Porter, *The Emergence of the Past: A Theory of Historical Explanation* (Chicago: University of Chicago Press, 1981); Allan Megill, "Recounting the Past: 'Description,' Explanation, and Narrative in Historiography," *American Historical Review* **94** (June 1989): 627-53.

[16] Some historians also describe a third design, synthetic history, that builds primarily on existing histories (secondary sources) to produce overarching generalizations. See Thomas Bender, "Wholes and Parts: The Need for Synthesis in American History," *Journal of American History* **73** (June 1986): 120-36.

[17] Ann Fabian, *Card Sharps, Dream Books, and Bucket Shops: Gambling in Nineteenth-Century America* (Ithaca: Cornell University Press, 1990); Bruce Kuklick, *To Every Thing a Season: Shibe Park and Urban Philadelphia, 1909-1976* (Princeton: Princeton University Press, 1991).

[18] Fernand Braudel, *On History*, trans. Sarah Matthews (Chicago: University of Chicago Press, 1980), 25-54; Humphrey, "The Historian, His Documents"; Hall, "Temporality, Social Action."

[19] Carole Shammas, "Dealing with Dichotomous Dependent Variables," *Historical Methods* **14** (Winter 1981): 47-51; Michael D. Ornstein, "Discrete Multivariate Analysis: An Example from the 1871 Canadian Census," *Historical Methods* **16** (Summer 1983): 101-8; David P. Gagan, Peter J. George, and Ernest H. Oksanen, "On Regression Models with Observation-specific Dummy Variables," *Historical Methods* **19** (Winter 1986): 5-8. See also note 23 below.

[20] Dale H. Porter, "History as Process," *History and Theory* **14** (1975): 297-313.

[21] Thompson, *Poverty of Theory*, 27-28. In Thompson's exact words: "A historian is entitled . . . to make a provisional assumption . . . : that the evidence which he handles has a 'real' (determinant) existence independent of its existence within the forms of thought, that this evidence is witness to a real historical process, and that this process (or some approximate understanding of it) is the object of historical knowledge." However, he continued, "The historical evidence is there . . . not to disclose its own meaning but to be interrogated" (pp. 28-29).

[22] Oscar Handlin, *Truth in History* (Cambridge: Harvard University Press, 1979), 120.

[23] Quantitative evidence, numerical evidence, is slowly but surely finding its way into historical research in HPER. Much more needs to be used, particularly in cases where historians want to establish conditions, extent of change, and social class. The most helpful journal about quantitative techniques in history is *Historical Methods*, cited several times in this chapter. The most adequate "methods text" belongs to Konrad H. Jarausch and Kenneth A. Hardy, *Quantitative Methods for Historians: A Guide to Research, Data, and Statistics* (Chapel Hill: University of North Carolina Press, 1991).

[24] One classic case of a document of questionable authenticity that had a longstanding impact on the history of a sport was a diagram of a baseball field, presumably authored by Abner Doubleday when he was a schoolboy in 1839. Abner Graves, who claimed to have been a classmate and eyewitness, included the diagram in a letter to the Mills Commission, which had been set up to establish the "origin" of baseball in 1907. The commission accepted the diagram and Graves's testimony as "proof" that Doubleday had "invented" the game.

Shafer, *Historical Method*, 127-47; Handlin, *Truth in History*, 111-24. For a marvelous and humorous discussion of a suspect document and the problems it created, see John D. Milligan, "The Treatment of an Historical Source," *History and Theory* **18** (1979): 177-96.

[25] Shafer, *Historical Method*, 149-70; Handlin, *Truth in History*, 124-44.

[26] Shafer, *Historical Method*, 150-58.

[27] Handlin, *Truth in History*, 165-226.

[28] Adrian Wilson, "Inferring Attitudes from Behavior," *Historical Methods* **14** (Summer 1981): 143-44.

[29] E. P. Thompson, "Anthropology and the Discipline of Historical Context," *Midland History* **3** (Spring 1972): 41-55.

[30] Anon., "The Great Foot Race," *American Turf Register and Sporting Magazine* **6** (June 1835): 518-20.

[31] Savoie Lottinville, *The Rhetoric of History* (Norman: University of Oklahoma Press, 1976); Henry W. Fowler and F. G. Fowler, *The King's English* (Oxford: Oxford University Press, 1954).

APPENDIX 1

Selected Historical Sources*

Collections

Source	*Location*
AAHPERD Archives Extensive material on physical education, exercise, sport programs, etc.	Reston, VA
AIAW Archives Extensive material about the Association for Intercollegiate Athletics for Women during the 1970s and early 1980s	University of Maryland College Park
Avery Brundage Collection Some 310 boxes, 100+ scrapbooks; Brichford Guide to the collection.	University of Illinois, Champaign
YMCA Library	St. Paul, MN
International Sports and Games Research Collection	University of Notre Dame
National Baseball Library Individual files for all players, many topics; runs of personal papers.	Cooperstown, NY
Albert Spalding Collection Henry Chadwick Scrapbooks, Harry Wright Notebooks; runs of Spalding Guides and instruction books.	New York Public Library
Sporting Books Collection	Princeton University, Firestone Library
Basketball Hall of Fame	Springfield, MA
National Track Hall of Fame Historical Library 15,000 items including programs, rule books, statistical guides.	Butler University, Indianapolis, Irwin Library Rare Book Room
Pro Football Hall of Fame Archives	Canton, OH

*These sources are provided courtesy of Prof. Stephen Hardy, University of New Hampshire. Hardy collected the sources from various scholars around the country, developed the bibliography, and presented it at the AAHPERD national convention, April 1989.

Source	Location
Strong Museum and Library Extensive collection of 19th- and early-20th-century papers, artifacts, books, etc., relating to exercise and health movements.	Rochester, NY
College and University Archives Often rich in material about sport, exercise, athletics.	Individual institution archives
City, County, or Town Historical Societies Contain records, artifacts, diaries, papers of all kinds relating to exercise, sport, recreation.	Individual state, county, or city archives

Governmental or Organization Documents

Source	*Location*
NCAA Proceedings, 1906-date Official records and debates.	NCAA headquarters and university libraries.
Records of Governing Bodies AAU, NCAA, Big 10, NHL, NFL, or any governing body from which one may request information.	Organization headquarters and archives
Public Statutes and Legislative Records For any historical period, these are published and usually indexed.	State and local archives
State and Federal Tax Lists and Censuses Typically published and indexed; contain economic and demographic data.	State archives and libraries
Probate Records Estate inventories, court cases, wills, land records for demographic and economic analyses.	Individual state, county, or city archives
Court Records Occasionally indexed; contain legal data as well as information about sport/exercise practices and attitudes	Individual state and county archives

Manuscripts

Source	*Location*
Walter Byers Papers Now being processed; about 40 boxes.	NCAA Headquarters, Mission, KS

Source	*Location*
Amos Alonzo Stagg Papers Runs for years ca. 1892-1933.	University of Chicago Archives
Walter Camp Papers Covers collegiate and amateur sports; includes 100 pp. index, 1876-1925.	Yale University Archives *Available on microfilm*
E.M. Hartwell Papers One of founders of profession of Physical Education.	Johns Hopkins University, Eisenhower Library, Special Collection
Edward Hitchcock, Jr., Room Correspondence, papers, early books and journals in physical education.	Amherst College, Frost Library
Lou Henry Hoover Papers Leader in the organization and promotion of sport for girls and women.	Herbert Hoover Library
Arthur H. Steinhaus Papers One of founders of American College of Sports Medicine, 40 boxes.	University of Tennessee Library
Senda Berenson Papers	Smith College Archives
Joe Louis Scrapbooks	University of Michigan Archives
Branch Rickey Papers Cover all aspects of Rickey's life in baseball, especially the business side.	Library of Congress
Papers of U. S. Presidents For example, T. Roosevelt on football issue, D. Eisenhower on Jesse Owens, G. Ford on amateur sports. Often there are some real gems.	Presidential Libraries
Papers of University Presidents Typically contain material on athletics and physical education.	Individual institutional archives

Serials

Source	*Location*
The Afro-American (1982+) Reports on black sports, especially in the East.	Enoch Pratt Library, Baltimore, MD *Available on microfilm*
American Turf Register and Sporting Magazine Early-19th-century magazine focusing on outdoor field sports and racing.	American Periodical Series microfilm; National Agricultural Library, Beltsville, MD, *originals*

Source	*Location*
Boston Medical and Surgical Journal Early history of exercise, fitness, health issues in 19th century.	National Library of Medicine, Bethesda, MD; University of Chicago, Crerar Library
Clipper (New York, 1853-1924) Sporting newspaper from mid-19th century on; later became *Variety*. Henry Chadwick wrote extensively for it.	New York Public Library *Available on microfilm*
Country Life (1901-1917) Covers elite sports, clubs, resorts.	Various libraries
Foreign Language Press Survey WPA project, translations include aspects of social life related to sport.	University of Chicago, Chicago Public Library
Frank Leslie's Illustrated (1854-1904)	Various libraries
Journal of Health (1829-1833)	American Periodical Series microfilm
Journal of HPE (HPERD, PER, etc.)	AAHPERD Archives, various libraries
Local Newspapers At any level; often contain important details of everyday life and practices.	Local public libraries and/or historical societies
New York Times (1851+) Increasing coverage of all sports over time; indexed; tends toward bourgeois practices.	*Available on microfilm*
Outing Magazine (1888-1923)	Various libraries
The Playground (1907+) Professional journal covers play and recreation issues; became *Recreation*.	Various libraries
Spirit of the Times (1831-1903) Excellent coverage of a range of sports across social classes.	*Available on microfilm*
Sporting Life (1883-1922)	*Available on microfilm*
Sporting News (1886+)	*Available on microfilm*
Sports Illustrated (1954+)	Various libraries
The Sportswoman (1924-1936) Published by U.S. Field Hockey Assoc; also considered lacrosse and some general issues about sport for women.	Scattered in college libraries, including Vassar, Penn, Bryn Mawr, and Smith

APPENDIX **2**

The Great Foot Race

The great trial of human capabilities, in going ten miles within the hour, for $1,000, to which $300 was added, took place on Friday, on the Union Course, Long Island; and we are pleased to state, that the feat was accomplished twelve seconds within the time, by a native born and bred American farmer, Henry Stannard, of Killingworth, Connecticut. Two others went the ten miles—one a Prussian, in a half a minute over; the other an Irishman, in one minute and three quarters over the time.

As early as nine o'clock, many hundreds had crossed the river to witness the race, and from that time until near two, the road between Brooklyn and the course presented a continuous line, (and in many places a double line) of carriages of all descriptions, from the humble sand cart to the splendid barouche and four; and by two o'clock, it is computed that there were at least from sixteen to twenty thousand persons on the course. The day, though fine, being windy, delayed the start until nineteen minutes before two, when nine candidates appeared in front of the stand, dressed in various colors, and started at the sound of a drum.

The following are the names, &c. of the competitors, in the order in which they entered themselves:

Henry Stannard, a farmer, aged twenty-four years, born in Killingworth, Connecticut. He is six feet one inch in height, and weighed one hundred and sixty-five pounds. He was dressed in black silk pantaloons, white shirt, no jacket, vest, or cap, black leather belt and flesh colored slippers.

Charles R. Wall, a brewer, aged eighteen years, born in Brooklyn. His height was five feet ten and a half inches, and he weighted one hundred and forty-nine pounds.

Henry Sutton, a house painter, aged twenty-three years, born in Rahway, New Jersey. Height five feet seven inches; weight one hundred and thirty-three pounds. He wore a yellow shirt and cap, buff breeches, white stockings and red slippers.

George W. Glauer, rope-maker, aged twenty-seven, born in Elberfeldt, Prussia. Height five feet six and a half inches; weight one hundred and forty-five pounds. He had on an elegant dress of white silk, with a pink stripe and cap to match; pink slippers and red belt.

Isaac S. Downes, a basket-maker, aged twenty-seven, born at Brookhaven, Suffolk county. Height five feet five and a half inches; weight one hundred and fifty pounds. He was dressed in a white shirt, white pantaloons, blue stripe, blue belt, no shoes or stockings.

John Mallard, a farmer, aged thirty-three, born at Exeter, Otsego Co., New York. Height five feet seven and a half inches; weight one hundred and thirty pounds. Dress, blue calico, no cap, shoes or stockings.

William Vermilyea, shoemaker, aged twenty-two years, born in New York. Height five feet ten and a half inches; weight one hundred and fifty pounds. Dressed in green calico, with black belt; no shoes or stockings.

Patrick Mahony, a porter, aged thirty-three, born in Kenmar county, Kerry, Ireland. Height five feet six inches. Weight one hundred and thirty pounds. Dress, a green gauze shirt, blue stripe calico breeches, blue belt, white stockings, and black slippers.

John M'Gargy, a butcher, aged twenty-six, born at Harlaem. Height five feet ten inches. Weight one hundred and sixty pounds. Dressed in shirt, pink stripe calico trowsers, no shoes or stockings.

There was a tenth candidate, a black man, named Francis Smith, aged twenty-five, born in Manchester, Virginia. Mr. Stevens was willing that this man should run; but as he had not complied with the regulation requiring his name to be entered by a certain day, he was excluded from contesting the race.

The men all started well, and kept together for the first mile, except Mahony, who headed the others several yards, and Mallard, who fell behind after the first half mile. At the end of the second mile, one gave in; at the end of the fourth mile, two more gave up; in the fifth, a fourth man fell; at the end of the fifth mile, a fifth man gave in; during the eighth mile, Downes, one of the fastest, and decidedly the handsomest runner, hurt his foot, and gave in at the termination of that mile, leaving but three competitors, who all held out the distance.

The following is the order in which each man came up to the judges' stand at the close of each mile.

American Turf Register and Sporting Magazine 6 (June 1835): 518-20.

					Miles					
	1st.	2d.	3d.	4th.	5th.	6th.	7th.	8th.	9th.	10th.
Stannard	3	4	3	3	3	2	2	1	1	1
Glauer	2	2	1	1	2	3	3	3	2	2
Mahony	1	1	5	5	5	4	4	4	3	3
Downes	5	3	2	2	1	1	1	2	gave in.	
McGargy	6	7	7	7	4	gave in.				
Wall	4	5	4	4	gave in.					
Sutton	8	8	6	6	gave in.					
Mallard	9	9	8	8	fell and gave in.					
Vermilyea	7	6	gave in.							

The following is the time in which each mile was performed by Stannard, the winner. Mahony, the Irishman, did the first mile in five minutes twenty-four seconds.

	Min.	Sec.
1st mile	5	36
2d "	5	45
3d "	5	58
4th "	6	25
5th "	6	2
6th "	6	3
7th "	6	1
8th "	6	3
9th "	5	57
10th "	5	54
	59	44

The betting on the ground both before and after starting, was pretty even, and large sums were staked both for and against time. Downes was undoubtedly the general favorite; and was well known in the neighborhood; he did the eight miles in forty-eight and a half minutes; he had been well trained under his father, who in his thirty-ninth year, performed seventeen miles in one hour and forty-five minutes; accomplishing the first twelve and a half miles in one hour and fifteen minutes.

Mallard was known to be an excellent runner; he had performed sixteen miles in one hour and forty-nine minutes, stopping during the time to change his shoes. He was not sober when he started, and he fell in the fifth mile.

The German had performed the distance between New York and Harlaem, and returned thence (twelve miles) in seventy minutes; his friends were very sanguine of his success. He betted nearly $300 that he would win the prize. He was within the time until the sixth mile, and he performed the ten miles in one hour and twenty-seven seconds. He was four seconds behind time in the eighth mile. Part of the distance he carried a pocket handkerchief in his mouth.

Mahony, the Irishman, had undergone no training whatever; he left his porter's cart in Water street, went over to the course, ran the first mile in less than five and a half minutes; at the end of the sixth mile he was one minute and a quarter behind; at the end of the eighth mile two minutes behind; at the ninth he was three minutes behind, and he performed the ten miles in sixty-one and three quarter minutes. On the 25th of last month, this man ran eight miles in forty-one minutes fifty-six seconds. M'Gargy was out of condition; but he did the five miles in thirty-two and a half minutes. Vermilyea was very thin and in a wreched state of health; he travelled thirty-eight miles on foot, on Tuesday last, to be here in time to enter, and the next day performed eight miles in forty-six minutes; he is an excellent runner, but gave in at the end of the second mile from a pain in the side; he was also thrown down by a man crossing the course in the first mile. Wall and Sutton ran remarkably well, but gave in at the end of the fourth mile for want of training.

Stannard, the winner, we understand, has been in good training for a month. He is a powerful stalwart young man, and did not seem at all fatigued at the termination of the race. He was greatly indebted to Mr. Stevens, for his success; Mr. S. rode round the course with him the whole distance, and kept cheering him on, and cautioning him against over-exertion in the early part of the race; at the end of the sixth mile, he made him stop and take a little brandy and water, after which his foot was on the mile mark just as the thirty-six minutes were expired; and as the trumpet sounded he jumped forward gracefully, and cheerfully exclaimed "Here am I to time;" and he was within the time every mile. After the race was over, he mounted a horse and rode round the course in search of Mr. Richard Jackson, who held his overcoat. He was called up to the stand and his success (and the reward of $1,300) was announced to him, and he was invited to dine with the Club; in which he replied in a short speech thanking Mr. Stevens, and the gentlemen of the Club for the attention shewn to the runners generally throughout the task. After this, it was announced by Mr. King, the President of the Jockey Club, that the German and the Irishman, who had both performed the ten miles, though not within the time, would receive $200 each.

We are happy to state that none of the men seemed to feel any inconvenience from their exertions; every thing went off remarkably satisfactory, nor did we hear of the slightest accident the whole day. After the foot race was over, a purse of $300, two mile heats, for all ages, was run for by the following horses, and decided as under:

	1st.	2d.
Tarquin	1	1
Post Boy	2	3
Columbia Taylor	3	dist.
Rival	4	2
Ajax	5	dist.
Sir Alfred	6	d'rn.

The first heat was performed in three minutes forty-seven seconds—the second in three minutes fifty seconds.

During the running of this match, a written paper was handed to Mr. King, stating that two native Americans were willing to attempt to walk five hundred miles without eating or drinking, as soon as a purse of $500 should be made up.

The day was remarkably fine, but the wind blew very strongly on the course, and considering the vast amount of money (in bets, &c.) at stake, Mr. Stevens felt uncertain at first how to act, and decided to postpone the race; but the general opinion and desire seem to be against any postponement, and he yielded to this. The result on this account was most fortunate. The race was won handsomely; although when it wanted but twenty eight seconds to the hour, bets at five to three were offered, and taken, that the task would not be accomplished. It is certain that if the wind had not been so high, Stannard would have performed the ten miles in fifty-seven minutes.

CHAPTER 13

Philosophic Research in Physical Activity

R. Scott Kretchmar

Dear Professors of Research Methods:

I know there is a vast difference between philosophical research and merely stating opinions, so I try to be reflective, to clearly define the problem, and to analyze it in a sound manner. However, I find that I spend a great deal of time just trying to organize my thoughts before I get anything down on paper. Does this ever happen to you?

Sincerely,
Paralysis by Analysis Phil

Dear Phil:

We are pleased that you recognize the difference between a philosophy and a bumper sticker. Many do not. We are also empathetic with your writer's block. Anyone who has written to any extent has a hard time explaining to others, such as one's spouse, that they are working when they are staring out a window.

Philosophically yours,
PRM

Philosophic research for many in our field is neither well understood nor highly valued. This is due partly to the rise of empirical science and the onset of related doubts about the validity of reflective, reason-based procedures and partly to the lack of a consensus among contemporary philosophers about proper research goals and strategies. Yet with all the accomplishments of science, and in spite of disagreements among modern philosophers, nonempirical analysis and speculation have not disappeared from the research landscape. If anything, a recognition of the need for philosophic insights related to movement activity may have grown (Fahlberg & Fahlberg, 1994; Lawson, 1993; Glassford, 1987).

Reasons for this increased interest are tied to the purposes of philosophy and the potentially complementary relationship between philosophic inquiry and empirical study. Consequently, I begin this chapter with an examination of the purposes of philosophic research while drawing attention to similarities and differences between philosophy and science. This is followed by descriptions of five general methods and brief analyses of each technique's strengths and weaknesses. Exercises that will allow readers to try each one are collected at the end of the chapter.

Identifying Purposes of Philosophic Research

A fundamental goal of philosophy is to examine reality by using reflective procedures, not the empirical tools of science. Accordingly philosophers and scientists differ not so much on what they look at but more on how they study it. Both kinds of researchers are interested, for instance, in understanding exercise. Empirical scientists, however, approach this phenomenon by looking through microscopes at such things as muscle tissue, by collecting respiratory or blood pressure data, and by employing statistical procedures to determine strengths of possible causal relationships. Philosophers, on the other hand, reflect on exercise and utilize such things as ideas and ideals, meanings, lived experience, values, logical relationships, and reasons in attempting to shed some light on it.

This distinctive approach allows philosophers to answer questions that empirical methodologies cannot solve. After chemists, physiologists, sociologists, psychologists, and historians, for instance, have gathered all the information on exercise they can, questions remain about the human meanings and values associated with this phenomenon. Why should we exercise? To live longer? To live better? Both? If both, which is more important, the presence of more life per se or the existence of a certain quality of life? On what criteria would we determine quality of life, and if we can identify some of them, what are the in-principle or logical relationships between exercise and those criteria of good living?

Philosophic research is needed not because empirical methodologies are ineffective but because they are, on their own, incomplete. For example, it has long been a hope of science to uncover the various mechanisms that govern natural processes and human behavior. If this can be done, future events and behavior could be predicted and some of them might even be controlled.

Considerable progress has been made along these lines. In the realm of exercise a better empirical understanding of various physiological mechanisms, coupled with more sophisticated information on exercise as a physiological stressor, has helped us to predict and control outcomes of an active lifestyle. But human exercise is a very complex event, and this prediction and control has been tenuous at best. This is particularly so when prediction involves a complete, thinking human being in the natural world rather than an isolated physiological system in a controlled laboratory setting. Some would say that this lack of predictability is caused by the current state of empirical science and that it is only a matter of time before a far more impressive degree of control is achieved. Many philosophers would argue, however, that complete prediction is, in principle, not possible no matter how sophisticated the

---

 philosophic research — Type of research characterized by critical inquiry in which the researcher establishes hypotheses, examines and analyzes existing facts, and synthesizes the evidence into a workable theoretical model.

 Philosophy in contrast to empirical science

methods of empirical science become (Merleau-Ponty, 1964).

The reason is that exercise is an electrical-chemical-biomechanical meaningful event. To be sure, linear or chaotic electrical and chemical reactions help us understand exercise, but only to a degree. And linear or dynamical biomechanical rules shed light on various mechanisms of exercise, but again only to a degree. Inescapably (because it is people who exercise, not mere machines) there is also meaning, poignancy, interest, hope, lived experience, and idiosyncratic perception in the exercise event. These things play a role in behavior, and they cannot be fully appreciated by looking at them electrically, chemically, biomechanically, or through any other strictly empirical window. There may be no getting around it. Reflective techniques are needed to measure and analyze meanings and values as they are encountered by people.

Whether philosophers are analyzing the nature of concrete things like chairs and footballs or intangible objects like determination and fair play, their subject matter must be reflectively brought to mind. Consequently, their data, when it is being described, logically analyzed, or otherwise worked on, must be present to consciousness. It must reside in what behaviorists popularly termed "the black box." This metaphorical box was colored black because it was thought to be impenetrable.

Skinner recommended that the CNS (Central or Conceptual Nervous System) be ignored because it could never be understood well enough to be of use. Many contemporary psychologists acknowledge the importance of cognition, but they still try to reduce experience to physics, chemistry, physiology, or computer theory (Hamlyn, 1990). Even though they dare to venture inside the black box, they often refuse to allow meanings to be just meanings! As did many of their empirical predecessors, they refuse to take lived experience and its ideas seriously.

Philosophy's overall mission, it can be concluded, is to examine reality through reflective techniques. Because this is a very general characterization of philosophic research, it is useful to identify four popular subdivisions, or branches, of reflective inquiry:

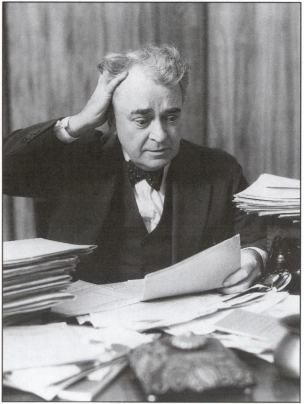

Philosophy's overall mission is to examine reality through reflective techniques.

- metaphysics
- axiology
- epistemology
- poetry

In **metaphysics** philosophers attempt to analyze the nature of things. This work runs the gamut from simple distinctions (e.g., telling sport from dance), to more complex and controversial theses (e.g., defining the nature of excellence in competitive events), and even global questions about the meaning of life itself (e.g., describing possible relationships between developing one's motor intelligence and achieving something called the good life).

Work in a second branch of philosophy called **axiology** focuses on the value of things—achievements, acquisitions, or states of affairs such as fitness, health, knowledge, and

 Four subdivisions of philosophic research: metaphysics, axiology, epistemology, and poetry

 metaphysics — The branch of philosophy that tries to explain reality. It includes the study of the nature of knowledge, reality, and the universe and its laws.

axiology — The branch of philosophy that deals with human values including ethics and aesthetics.

excellence (theories of nonmoral value). It also concentrates on human behavior such as the breaking or bending of game rules (ethics), and on art and beauty such as the qualities of certain routines in gymnastics (aesthetics). Research findings in axiology provide at least general roadmaps concerning more or less valuable movement-related destinations. Other outcomes provide theories on how we should behave toward both our neighbors and ourselves in such activities as sport, dance, exercise, games, and play.

A third branch of philosophy called **epistemology** concerns knowledge, both the ways it can be secured and the various assurances we have for holding it. Research is conducted on logic (e.g., determining the clarity and force of any apparently fixed relationships between cooperation and competition in sport); on sense perception (e.g., describing the importance of one's perspective in the lived experience of a dance, say as a performer in contrast to a spectator); and on the status of reason itself (e.g., deciding if we can trust what appear to be reasonable arguments for the superiority of playing games fairly rather than dishonestly).

A final branch of philosophy has emerged in recent times, one that some are calling **poetry** (Rosen, 1989). Paradoxically this is an antiphilosophic movement designed to liberate individuals from the claims of traditional metaphysics, ethics, and epistemology while hinting at alternatives. The liberating aspect of this research draws attention to the possible contamination of reasons given for traditional claims about, for example, the nature and value of physical activity. The hinting function suggests ways in which sport might be experienced and valued to avoid regressing to repressive metaphysics.

This brief discussion has produced five reasons for doing philosophic research. The overarching rationale points to the fact that philosophers look at reality with different tools than those used by empirical scientists. They reflect rather than actually measure and count. As a result they see aspects of things, actions, and behavior that are inaccessible to those who work only with real images and physically produced data. As researchers who reflect on reality, they take meaning or cognition itself seri-

ously and are reluctant to reduce lived experience to any of its electrical, chemical, and biological antecedents or concomitants. A recent rise of interest in philosophy may stem from a growing understanding that any failure to take meaning seriously will make it difficult if not impossible to understand fully (let alone predict and control) whole-person behavior.

Four more specific purposes of philosophic research include the need to understand the nature of things and the differences between them (metaphysics); the highest values of life, proper ways of behaving, and the qualities of art and beauty (axiology); the avenues by which humans know things and the foundations on which such knowledge rests (epistemology), and dangers of building philosophic systems and tentative suggestions about what should guide life in their stead (poetry).

This brings us to the point of considering the tools or methods needed to accomplish these purposes. Space is not sufficient here to survey the full range of techniques employed in philosophy, nor is it possible to review all the strengths and weaknesses of these diverse approaches. Consequently, the intent will be to get a general understanding of how philosophers in our field have proceeded with their research. How then do movement philosophers find a topic?

Locating a Research Problem

It is said that philosophy begins with wonder—wonder about big questions like the meaning of existence and smaller questions like the differences between games and play. In a sense, then, anything and everything is fair game for philosophers. Like all other researchers, however, these thinkers have limited time and resources.

Consequently, they must make judgments about which curiosities and wonders are worth pursuing. Issues that are personal or idiosyncratic are often judged as trivial and are assigned a lower position on research agendas. Topics of common concern or problems thought to be central to the human condition are given higher research billing. Interest-

 epistemology — The branch of philosophy that investigates the origin, nature, methods, and limits of knowledge.

 poetry — A branch of philosophy that challenges traditional philosophical reflective techniques. It suggests alternative ways of interpreting human experience and values.

ingly, many themes in our own field (e.g., sport, dance, exercise, games, and play) have fared poorly when philosophic research dockets have been approved. For instance, little attention has been given to games, sport, exercise, and physical education by philosophers across the centuries. Other, more global themes related to our field—topics like the mind-body problem, procedural or "how-to" knowledge, play, and excellence—have received more thorough treatment.

 Philosophers find their research problems in two general places—in personal experience and subsequent reflection, on the one hand, and in texts, on the other. Actual experiences with weight training, for example, may lead to questions about its nature and worth. Upon later reflection, formal questions emerge about differences between exercise and, possibly, work or play and the values of motor-active living in contrast to sedentary existence. Of course, these same issues could be encountered in some text where a philosopher has previously addressed these matters and argued for certain conclusions. In this case, analysts would begin with the text, critique it, amend it, or otherwise build upon it.

Whether a topic comes from personal experience, a text, or both, philosophers need questions to work on. It is important to notice that these questions are identified and pursued via language, by using words singly and in combinations. This presents an initial stumbling block for nonempirical researchers. Whereas exercise physiologists, for instance, can study something under a microscope and that object is usually unmistakably there for anyone who can see, philosophers bring forth their research object by uttering a word or a sentence or, more likely, a series of sentences. But language is ambiguous. A single word can mean different things to different people. A simple example will show how language inhibits the successful initiation of research and how philosophers deal with this.

Suppose that a philosopher claims to be doing research on the value of competition. Even with this rather straightforward proclamation, this individual still has considerable work left before he or she reaches the same unambiguous starting point enjoyed by the physiologist with a single object under a microscope. For instance, it could be asked, what kind of value? What precisely is meant by

competition? Competition with oneself? With others? In games? Zero sum competition where there are winners and losers? "Competition" in which everyone can be a winner (if indeed that is still competition)?

 This situation forces philosophers to begin most analyses with definitions, descriptions, clarifications, and disclaimers, particularly when they are analyzing something that is not a simple physical object—something, as we just saw, that is verbally and conceptually vague like the nature of competition. There need be nothing surreptitious about this procedure, and it does not contaminate research findings if it is done properly. The intent is merely to identify an unambiguous, though still partly unknown, object of inquiry.

The establishment of a clear research question is critical. Because most philosophers hope to shed at least some light on reality and thus want their conclusions to be considered as generally (even if incompletely and tentatively) accurate across time and culture, they expect other readers and researchers to be able to replicate their findings. The likelihood of this happening in philosophy under the best of conditions is not great, but it is even less when the original object of inquiry is not clear. Just like physiologists working independently on the same problem, philosophers need to be looking at the same thing if they hope to check the validity of one another's efforts. And just as the physiologist can choose to focus his microscope on venial rather than arterial blood flow, for example, the philosopher can choose to examine zero-sum activity rather than other actions that are also identified by the word "competition."

After a theme has been identified from personal experience, a text, or both, and after sufficient definitional spadework has been done to make sure that the topic is clear, what then do philosophers do with the material? How do they treat it?

Analyzing a Research Problem

Inductive Reasoning
Deductive Reasoning

 Where to find philosophic research problems

 How to begin an analysis

> Descriptive Reasoning
> Speculative Reasoning
> Critical and Poetic Reasoning

Unfortunately, philosophers do not agree on the best techniques for analyzing reality, and their disagreements are very serious ones. Because of that it is necessary here to introduce several methods, and readers will need to choose techniques that seem most useful to them.

In the broadest terms, philosophic methods can be divided into those that are ambitious and others that are more limited in scope. These two positions reflect conflicting judgments about the twin poles of all reflection: the thinking or reflecting itself (the research act), and the thing thought about or reflected on (the research object).

Ambitious philosophers are impressed by human powers of reasoning and believe that common biases and potentially limiting perspectives of thinking (e.g., from history, socialization, language, religion, and sense perception) can be controlled. Philosophic acts, in other words, can be objective and dispassionate or at least partially so. On this view, logic, faithful description, and even careful speculation can lead to objectively accurate conclusions. Some researchers in this optimistic school of thought (among them phenomenologists like Husserl, 1962) believe that philosophic thinking can approach, or perhaps even surpass, the precision of science.

Pessimistic researchers, on the other hand, doubt the powers of reason, see thinking as contaminated, and regard most traditional philosophic conclusions as limited, useless, or even harmful. Some of these individuals regard philosophic work as witting or unwitting rationalizations for unjust economic systems, unfair gender relationships, or individually enslaving value systems. All thinking, according to this view, proceeds from historical-, political-, and language-skewed perspectives, and no methods exist for effectively eliminating or controlling these biases.

Dramatically different judgments have also been made regarding the second half of reflection—the object thought about or reflected on. The more ambitious school of philosophy sees the world as composed of discrete classes of items—for instance, of chairs, tables, automobiles, games, play, dance, good ethics, bad ethics, and so on. Each of these things has a nature that distinguishes it from other things around it. If biases in the process of reflecting can be avoided, these and other categories of things that populate the world can be described, over time, ever more faithfully and completely. In other words, genuine philosophic progress is regarded as possible.

The more cautious philosophers, on the other hand, challenge hypotheses about the neat packaging of reality into separate classes of items. Objects in the world, on this view, are individuals; there are no essential natures of things—no neat lines that can be drawn between abstract categories like "chairness" and "tableness," games and play, or good moral behavior and its supposed counterpart. Philosophic progress makes little sense for these researchers, though it is still far better to understand that philosophic classes are arbitrarily defined parts of a continuous reality of individuals than to invent comfortable or convenient fictions.

This division in judgments about proper goals for philosophic research is reflected in the sections that follow. The tools of inductive and deductive thinking and the strategies employed by descriptive and speculative philosophers are generally representative of the more ambitious school of philosophic research. The critical and poetic techniques provide an introduction to the methods of many contemporary philosophers who see the work of philosophy as limited in scope.

Inductive Reasoning

 Inductive reasoning is thinking that moves from a limited number of specific observations to general conclusions about the thing or class of thing that was observed. It relies on the power of reason to identify common elements or similarities at an abstract level (see Metheny [1968] for a sample of research from our field that relies heavily on inductive thinking).

If we were doing some metaphysics on the nature of competition, we might select a number of events that fall safely into the realm of competition—say, contests in baseball, racquetball, swim-

 inductive reasoning — Logical process in which the researcher moves from specific observations through testing hypotheses to developing a general theory.

 Metheny, E. (1968). *Movement and meaning.* New York: McGraw-Hill.

ming, spelling, and Trivial Pursuit. We want to reason inductively from these five particular exemplars of competition to general statements about it—statements that accurately describe these events and all (genuinely competitive) past and future activities that were not used for this analysis.

Can we say anything about the number of parties or sides that must be involved in competition? These five examples suggest that at least two sides must be present for competition to take place.

Can we say anything about the nature of each side's activity? These five examples suggest that participants all face tests or problems. That is, what they are doing is not easy. It also appears that the two or more parties are facing the same kind of problem—for instance, hitting and catching baseballs in rule-defined ways, recalling "trivia" under a time limit in certain specified categories, and so on.

Can we say anything about the commitments, if any, made by the two or more competing sides? The exemplars would indicate that each party intends to solve their rule-defined problems in a superior fashion to any other teams or individuals in the game. For example, baseball players intend to score more runs than their opponents do; Trivial Pursuit players intend to fill their disc with wedges before anyone else does.

In short, the inductive process has provoked a number of claims about the nature of competition—that competition requires two or more parties, that these sides face problems and that the problems are common to all, and that each side must intend to solve their problems better than the other team(s) or individual(s) do. If these statements are valid, we now know something explicit about competition in general, something perhaps about which we were mistaken before, sensed only implicitly, or simply had never thought about.

 Inductive reasoning has its assets and liabilities. On the positive side this method places something concrete in front of the philosopher. It is a procedure that is not mystical, that utilizes data that everyone can see or reflect upon. Also, because exemplars are limited in number, it is manageable. Although it is true that the inductive process might go on indefinitely (how would

we ever know that we had finished?), the process of examining a finite number of items for common features or common elements is not technically difficult even though it can be done with differing degrees of success.

Finally, this technique is useful in distinguishing what is essential to the makeup of something and what is accidental or unnecessary. Suppose we had a group of exemplars that included four team sports and one individual activity. Focusing only on the team sports at first, we might hypothesize that competition requires that groups of individuals must face other groups of individuals. However, when we come to the individual sport, we see that the team-vs.-team phenomenon cannot be an essential feature of competition. We can then conclude that it is an option or possibility, not a requirement. We have made some progress in weeding out peripheral characteristics of our theme from central ones.

 Inductive reasoning is not foolproof. Two particular pitfalls can be mentioned here. The first involves the procedure by which the original list of exemplars is chosen. If this list is faulty—for instance, if it is incomplete, or if it includes one or more incorrect examples of the thing in question—it can produce incorrect conclusions. Had we begun our analysis of competition with a list that included only team sports, then we might have concluded inaccurately that competition requires that groups play against other groups. The second problem is with the process of seeing abstractions accurately and insightfully. This is a skill that requires different degrees of finesse and insight. For instance, some concepts concerning the nature of competition identified above may seem obvious and thus not particularly helpful. In truth there is nothing inherent in the inductive process that guarantees that the abstractions generated will be good ones, ones that tell us important and heretofore unnoticed things about competition or whatever else is being examined.

Deductive Reasoning

 Deductive reasoning is a companion technique of inductive thinking, and many philosophers adroitly and spontaneously inter-

 Three benefits of inductive reasoning

Drawbacks to inductive reasoning

deductive reasoning — Logical process in which the researcher moves from a theoretical explanation of events down to specific hypotheses about events.

mix the two. Deduction requires intellectual movement in the opposite direction from induction. Whereas inductive thinking has philosophers working from particulars to general abstractions, deduction would have us start with general claims to see what particulars follow (see Fraleigh, 1984, for examples of this kind of thinking).

These general claims or premises are of two sorts. The first are statements of fact and are often phrased, "Because such and such is true, then it follows that . . ." But premises can also be hypothetical. "If such and such is true, then it follows that . . ." We will look at a deductive line of reasoning that utilizes hypothetically stated premises based on our inductively generated concepts about the nature of competition.

If competition requires two or more parties to take a test, and

If these two or more parties must face the same test, and

If these two or more parties must be committed to passing the common test in a superior fashion, and

If taking and facing tests and being committed to superior performances are acts that can be undertaken only by conscious beings, and

If mountains are not conscious beings, then

It follows that humans cannot compete against mountains. That is, people can neither defeat mountains nor lose to them in a contest.

This conclusion may be of some interest because certain successful climbers have been quoted as saying things like, "I defeated the mountain." For many of us, such competitive-sounding statements make at least some sense. However, if the previous line of deductive reasoning is valid, we now know that such loose claims cannot refer to victories in contests. Their meaning has to lie elsewhere, perhaps in the direction of passing a severe or dangerous test that was provided, in part, by the mountain. Once again, reflective philosophic procedures (deductive ones, in this case) allowed us to clear up things about which we may have been mistaken, sensed only implicitly, or never thought about.

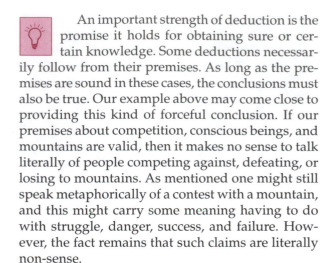

An important strength of deduction is the promise it holds for obtaining sure or certain knowledge. Some deductions necessarily follow from their premises. As long as the premises are sound in these cases, the conclusions must also be true. Our example above may come close to providing this kind of forceful conclusion. If our premises about competition, conscious beings, and mountains are valid, then it makes no sense to talk literally of people competing against, defeating, or losing to mountains. As mentioned one might still speak metaphorically of a contest with a mountain, and this might carry some meaning having to do with struggle, danger, success, and failure. However, the fact remains that such claims are literally non-sense.

A second advantage of deduction is its ability to permit speculations on the basis of unproven premises. We do not need to await confirmation of uncertain information. We can assume that it is accurate and then proceed to see what follows. Researchers who take this tack, of course, need to be frank about the tentative status of their premises. If later research confirms them, their deductions will stand. If premises are later shown to be inaccurate, then new deductions will need to be drawn.

Deduction also embodies some weaknesses. First it is difficult to find uncontested premises. Because of this fact alone, most deductive conclusions need to be held tentatively. Second, errors can be made in deduction itself even if the premises are allowed to stand. For instance, many people make ethical claims about competition based on faulty deductive thinking. Their reasoning may go something like this:

If competition requires two or more parties to face the same test with the intent of performing better than the other(s), and

If competition produces (save for occasional ties) scores that symbolize better and lesser performances, and

If at least one party must be identified with the lesser performance (i.e., as having lost),

Then it follows that competition harms one or more parties and is, at least for that reason, morally suspect.

Fraleigh, W. (1984). *Right actions in sport: Ethics for contestants*. Champaign, IL: Human Kinetics.

 Two strengths of deductive reasoning

 Two weaknesses of deduction

Although there may be some vague persuasive force to this line of reasoning, the deductive conclusions here do not necessarily follow from the premises. Something crucial is missing, and that "something" is related to important assumptions about losing, harms, and morality. Minimally, two more premises are needed—a statement to the effect that losing necessarily brings harm to people and a claim that the magnitude or quality of such harm is sufficient to raise moral concerns.

Many of us, however, would not be willing to grant the validity of these two additional premises. We would want arguments showing that losing always harms people and that the character of that harm is morally serious. This points out another weakness of deductive reasoning. It is possible to accept a conclusion as deductively valid while still rejecting that conclusion. This is done by challenging any of the premises used to generate the conclusion.

Descriptive Reasoning

Some philosophers prefer to conduct their research in less roundabout ways than those provided by inductive and deductive logic. They do not line up a series of particulars and ask themselves what they all have in common (induction), nor do they begin with a set of givens or premises to see what follows (deduction). They simply describe what they see reflectively when they examine an object of interest. This sounds disarmingly simple, almost too simple to produce anything worthwhile.

The processes of looking and faithfully describing, however, require considerable skill, and like all skills they can be done well or poorly. In addition, because human beings are not terribly attentive, tend to jump to conclusions, and often mistakenly take only one part of something for the whole, accurate, insightful, careful description can be extremely useful and enlightening.

As we have already seen with our very cursory analysis of competition, even though most of us have experienced it countless times in a variety of settings, we still may not have thought much about it. We can identify competition when we encounter it, but we may be at a loss to describe it at anything much beyond a superficial level. Imagine, however, the important things still to be discovered about competition, things that cannot be examined with the tools of empirical research but must be seen reflectively and then described.

Competition is often understood to involve disagreement, aggression, controlled fighting, striving for something that only one person or team can have but which both or all parties desire. Certainly there is more than a little truth to these descriptions, but if we are to be good philosophers we must look more closely. Does competition involve cooperation? If it is present, is it accidentally or necessarily there? Does it exist, for instance, only in ethically praiseworthy examples of sport or in all instances of competition? Does it play any crucial role in allowing competition to happen? For instance, can two or more sides in a game face the same test without cooperating in some meaningful sense?

Initially, competition seems to be associated with attempts to put other persons down, to show their inferiority, perhaps even to "blow them out" or otherwise embarrass them. But is competition compatible with friendship and even something called love? Philosophers would look more carefully and describe faithfully what they see to determine if competition has a structure that permits opposing sides to uplift one another and, if so, in what precise way. For instance, if one side in a contest provides an interesting, challenging test for the other party, is that in any sense a helpful service? Is this act of providing a challenging test compatible conceptually with what friends might do for one another? When competition goes well, when it is mutually uplifting, what is present that pushes it in this direction rather than a negative one? Is there any sense in which losing is not a putdown? What precisely is that sense? Is it possible, for example, to play well and still lose? What exactly does it mean to play well if it does not mean "to win"? The philosopher must skillfully look for concepts that effectively explain this. Optimistic philosophers believe that, if this research is done well, conclusions will coincide with findings produced independently by others who have conducted similar reflective procedures.

Descriptive methodologies place a great deal of confidence in the capacity of reason to portray reality accurately. It is important to recognize that this confidence resides in different traits and skills of human intelligence depending on the level of description attempted. If descrip-

Two levels of description

tion is intended to portray an actual lived experience—with its real perceptions, feelings, ups, and downs—then there must be a strong reliance on good memory, honesty, attention to detail, an unwillingness to embellish facts, and so on (see, e.g., Kleinman, 1968). This level of description is, in effect, making claims about what someone really experienced, and such portrayals can vary between fact and fiction.

A second level of descriptive work is disinterested in the actual subjective experience itself, such as a peak experience in basketball that occurred last week. Consequently, it relies far less on good memory, honesty, and the like. At this level, the concern is with the nature of things in principle. This level of description places confidence in the power of reason to notice important differences (see, e.g., Harper, 1972; Meier, 1980; Suits, 1978).

The danger with this methodology is not with poor memory, dishonesty, or tendencies to embellish actual events but rather with internalized biases that contaminate reason's ability to see clearly. For instance, one's religious upbringing might affect the way the world is observed. Acts of cheating may not be dealt with dispassionately and objectively. This, of course, could influence the description of same-test and different-test games.

Speculative Reasoning

 Speculation can be thought of as an extension of descriptive philosophy. As evidence and argumentation diminish for analyses of either actual subjective events (level 1 description) or the nature of things in principle (level 2 portrayals), the room for speculation increases.

This does not mean that speculation requires no argumentation whatsoever. Once again, speculating can be done well or poorly and, although speculative conclusions cannot be proven or demonstrated, they can vary in their degree of plausibility.

When looking reflectively at competition we could argue, for instance, that a mutual quest for excellence (e.g., Simon, 1991; Weiss, 1969) is the highest value of contesting. It may, in other words, be the feature that best turns competition from an activity that is, on balance, humanly harmful to one that is helpful or uplifting. Or we might claim that this highest value is a cooperative search for knowledge (Fraleigh, 1984) or a shared experience of play (Hyland, 1990). Although arguments have been rallied for each of these descriptions of what is good about competition, none of them can be regarded as conclusive. Moreover, it is likely that no amount of future research will change this situation. These value claims are plausible, perhaps even attractive, and additional arguments may be advanced at some future time to increase their plausibility or attractiveness, but no value can be shown conclusively to be the highest one, even though it is possible that one of them is. These axiological claims must, therefore, be identified as products of speculative philosophy.

 The advantage of speculative philosophy is that it broaches subjects that have human significance, that have even markedly changed human lives. For instance, people have dedicated their very existence to certain ideals and principles. Wars have been fought for a "way of life" that is grounded on the perceived superiority of some values over others. Given the apparent fact that people mold their lives around values, it may well be important to do research on such intangible things even if final proofs are not possible. The research principles here would be twofold. First, it is better to know a little (even if it is inconclusive) than to know nothing at all. And second, one can be unable to prove a claim and still be right about it.

 Disadvantages also exist. Narrow, selfish, manipulative, and even mean philosophies can masquerade as legitimate speculative statements about reality. This is, in fact, the claim made by many contemporary philosophers about much previous research in the history of philosophy. Either purposely or unknowingly, some phi-

---

 speculation — Procedure used in philosophic research that attempts to bridge the gap between description and principle. It seeks to offer plausible, though not demonstrable, conclusions or explanations for human experience and value structure.

 Advantages of speculation

 Disadvantages of speculation

losophers have spewed forth groundless opinions, biases, self-serving, and status quo-preserving visions of life in the name of philosophy. Even arguments intended to show the plausibility and attractiveness of certain claims may only play to the biased predispositions of the audience. For instance, claims about the superiority of a mutual quest for excellence may seem persuasive in a capitalistic, achievement-oriented culture in which most everyone is raised to be "all that they can be." In another society, arguments for excellence might seem odd or misplaced.

Critical and Poetic Reasoning

 As we have already seen, this brand of philosophy is based on skeptical attitudes toward the power of reason (a position called "**relativism**") and doubts about the organization of reality (a stance frequently identified as "**nominalism**"). The rise of empirical science had much to do with these concerns about philosophic acts—about thinking or reflecting. Thought processes were found to be influenced by chemicals, genes, language, and the socializing influence of family, state, and religion, to name only a few factors. Thinking and its philosophic products were therefore seen as merely relative outcomes of these and a host of other potential influences. Reason, in short, was no longer thought to be an objective, independent, cross-cultural, and a-temporal accessor of truth.

Related to the demise of reason is the judgment that reality is not as neatly organized as metaphysicians claimed it is. Abstract categories that were once thought to accurately depict reality came under attack—even categories like competitive behavior, games, play, exercise, and sport. These came to be regarded as convenient fictions that failed to represent anything that was truly "out there."

Given this brief introduction to contemporary critical/poetic philosophy and its doubts about the power of reason and the validity of philosophic cat-

egories, one might wonder what it is that philosophers thusly persuaded do. What research agenda could there possibly be for individuals who seem to have eliminated the only means of access to reflective truth (a trust in the powers of reason) and the only subject matter that would be worth scrutinizing (reality as objectively distinctive)?

Actually, at least two important research activities are undertaken by individuals in this school of thought, though it might be stretching the term unduly to call these endeavors research. Nevertheless, criticism is a debunking activity intended to show the errors of traditional philosophy. Technically termed "deconstruction," analysis attempts to reveal the futility of all metaphysical/ethical system building and point out where claims have been faulty and beliefs misplaced.

Texts are often used by deconstructionists to show where, for instance, groundless value claims have been made. One method is to show where unwarranted shifts in language and meaning have occurred—for example, the movement from "is" claims to "ought" recommendations. Here is an example from our field:

Claim #1. Exercise *is* effective in promoting both a vigorous life and a longer existence.

Claim #2. Costs of many exercises *are* minimal, and some *can* even *be* fun.

Recommendation: People *ought* to exercise.

The argument here is that facts ("is" statements) about vigor, long life, and costs still leave questions about the desirability of seeking those things (the "ought" conclusion). It makes sense to grant that exercise promotes longer life, but still ask whether we would want to pursue that. Some additional evidence is needed to warrant any "ought" recommendation. On the view of many deconstructionists, therefore, the recommendation about exercise is groundless.

 Another method is to examine texts for possible political, economic, gender, racial, historical, or other biases (see e.g., Morgan,

relativism — The theory that holds that criteria of judgment are relative, varying with the individual, time, language, and other circumstances.

nominalism — A doctrine which maintains that all abstract or general terms do not stand for real things, but exist for convenience in communication.

Gruneau, R. (1983). *Class, sports, and social development*. Amherst, MA: University of Massachusetts Press.

Kirk, D. (1992). *Defining physical education: The social construction of a school subject in postwar Britain*. London: Faimer Press.

Morgan, W.J. (1994). *Leftist theories of sport*. Urbana: University of Illinois Press.

1994, for a critical examination of such techniques and Kirk, 1992). Curriculum recommendations about exercise, competition, and play, for example, can be debunked for their provincialism or self-serving chauvinism. The strategy typically employed is one of showing the plausibility of alternate interpretations of certain biased philosophic conclusions that have been misleadingly presented as objectively valid. Sometimes possible cause and effect relationships are implied between conceptually reinforcing socioeconomic forces, on the one hand, and prevailing philosophic "truths," on the other (see, e.g., Gruneau, 1983).

Although this kind of philosophic work is largely destructive in nature, it can still be valuable. It is undoubtedly better to be suspicious of grand philosophic claims and know their shortcomings than to be blindly supportive of them. Even though this research generally does not replace defective claims with better ones, it suggests that it is an important step forward to realize that we do not (and possibly cannot) know certain things.

A constructive side to this type of philosophic research exists, however. It might best be called poetry because it cannot (without contradicting itself) make use of the reasoned argumentation and system building that it so vigorously criticizes. It is suggestive rather than explicit; it is tentative rather than sure of itself; it points to generally superior directions for living rather than laying them out systematically.

Nietzsche (1967) suggested that life should be lived without resorting to crutches of various sorts (e.g., blind religious belief or neatly packaged visions of the world) but by relying on a type of courageous freedom. Although Nietzsche did not carry out any extended discussion of relationships between game playing and his "will to power," his views lend themselves to poetic commentaries on similarities between life and games.

Hurdles that we face in games and life, it could be said, are essentially arbitrary, and when we win in either domain nothing significant has been gained or accomplished, but we can still choose to play as if the outcome mattered. If this analogy is meaningful, the poetry has done its job. However, because reason itself is held suspect, and because reality is believed not to be neatly packaged in categories, Nietzsche and other philosophers doing this kind of work would not want to make too much of the logic implicit in this analogy, nor would they want to claim that games are essentially different from other activities. It is enough to make a poetic suggestion and then move on.

 A strength of this methodology revolves around its purposes—its skepticism toward reason and its attempt to prevent people from relying on fictitious crutches and other false beliefs. It is also, for many, a scientifically palatable philosophy because it treats thinking as a very natural, in-the-world process, and describes life's purposes without resorting to myth, absolute values, mysteries, or special meanings.

A recurring difficulty is its tendency to use reason and build systems to show that reason is irredeemably corrupt and that systems are nothing but false human constructs. This requires that the products of this methodology be suggestive rather than definitive, poetic rather than systematic (Rosen, 1989). For some this is less than what philosophy can and should be.

Summary

In some ways, doing philosophy well is like performing a motor action skillfully. Alternative strategies and styles work for different people. Consequently, it is more important to get on with developing an ability to use some of them than to fret long and hard over which ones to choose, thereby delaying one's introduction to any of them.

Although the differences in philosophic methodology described here are not trivial, it is nevertheless more important to begin thinking philosophically in some manner than to wait for consensus on a perfect methodology. Philosophy, after all, is learned by doing it and receiving constructive criticism, not primarily by talking or reading about it.

 Check Your Understanding

Locating a Research Problem
(pages 280-281)

1. Suppose you are curious about whether people can exercise in the spirit of play. Un-

---

Strengths and weaknesses of poetry

fortunately, "exercise" and "play" are terms that have a multitude of meanings. Because of this, it is not clear what exactly the research question is. Thus, before you can productively begin with the project at hand, some clarifications are needed for both notions. Check with a good dictionary and reflect on your own experiences to produce a list of different concepts of exercise and play. Then, select the meanings or definitions that most nearly generated your original curiosity or that shed the most light on this aspect of human experience.

2. Suppose someone read your definitions and declared, "Those things are not exercise and play!" Is this a serious problem? Would this stop your research project in its tracks? (Remember, words are human conventions that we use to label items we encounter. A single word might be used to identify a number of different things and, conversely, a single thing might go by several terms.)

Inductive Reasoning
(pages 282-283)

3. What other generalities or abstractions can you draw from the five exemplars in this section? Can you say anything about the nature of the parties involved? For example, must they be human? What can you say about the nature of the problem faced in competition? Must it require motor skill? Is the function of motor skill in relationship to solving the game problem the same for each example of competition?

4. How would you go about picking the exemplars? How many is enough? What ground rules should be used in selecting exemplars to reduce chances for error?

Deductive Reasoning
(pages 283-285)

5. What additional deductions might you draw from this set of premises? Based on the first three premises, what can you say about competition in which one party is playing to win and the other is out for some exercise? Or one in which two parties are taking the same test at the same time (e.g., bowling), but they do not know about one another (one is bowling in California and the other in Ohio)? Or one in which two teams are playing the same game (e.g., baseball), but one side has re-

sorted to using illegal pitches?

6. If you are dissatisfied with the conclusion about people, mountains, and competition drawn in this section, what is the best method for attacking it—with the accuracy of the deduction itself, or with the validity of the premises?

Descriptive Reasoning
(pages 285-286)

7. Have you ever had a peak experience in sport—a time when your performance was qualitatively unique and delightful? Can you remember some characteristics of that event and describe them clearly and accurately?

8. It is generally believed that following game rules has a great deal to do with conducting successful competitions. But what exactly is this relationship? When you look reflectively at rule breaking, what happens in principle to competition? Are the two or more parties still taking the same test if one party breaks rules and the other does not? What would happen if rule breaking and bending were considered "part of the game"—that is, contests were held not only to determine who, for instance, could hit and catch baseballs better but, at the same time, who could break the rules of baseball more skillfully (i.e., gain an advantage without getting caught or paying too high a price for being caught)?

9. Is it likely that different philosophers, working independently but analyzing the same phenomenon, will see the same things and describe them in compatible ways? Is not one's experience of competition, for instance, a subjective/private matter and, because of that, unique and unshareable? What evidence can be produced to show that experiences are common or shared? Similarly, what evidence can be generated to suggest that experience is unique or idiosyncratic?

Speculative Reasoning
(pages 286-287)

10. How would you rank the three values of excellence, knowledge, and play in terms of their significance for achieving a good life? What additional values in competitive activity might be added to this list, and what arguments can be forwarded in their defense (see, e.g., Kretchmar, 1994)?

11. If speculative claims can never, in principle, be proven true or false, should philosophic researchers spend any time on them? Why or why not?

Critical and Poetic Reasoning
(pages 287-288)

12. Are claims about the value of competitiveness for survival in life gender biased from a uniquely male perspective, or are they rationally defensible for all human life? What about arguments to the effect that life itself is inherently competitive and that sport therefore is needed to prepare effectively for it?

13. Is your thinking capacity so contaminated by language, socialization, and other factors that you can find nothing that is objectively true? Can any steps be taken to eliminate or, at least, minimize biases?

CHAPTER 14

Research Synthesis (Meta-Analysis)

Dear Professors of Research Methods:

I'm not a good writer, but I don't like working in the laboratory either. So I'm thinking about doing a meta-analysis for my thesis. What do you think?

Experiencing writer's block,
Billy Baffled

Dear Baffled:

In his book *How to write and publish a scientific paper* (2nd ed., Philadelphia: ISI Press, 1983), Robert Day quotes James Russell Lowell in addressing your problem.

"Nature fits all her children with something to do.
He who would write and can't write, can surely review."

Writing great prose,
PRM

An analysis of the literature is a part of all types of research. The scholar is always aware of past events and how they influence current research. Sometimes, however, the literature review stands by itself as a research paper, one that involves the analysis, evaluation, and integration of the published literature. A term used to describe this is research synthesis. As mentioned in chapter 1, many journals consist entirely of literature review papers, and nearly all research journals publish review papers occasionally.

All the procedures discussed in detail in chapter 2 apply to research synthesis. The difference is that the purpose here is to use the literature for empirical and theoretical conclusions rather than to document the need for a particular research problem. A good research synthesis will result in several tangible conclusions and should spark interest in future directions for research. Sometimes a research synthesis will lead to a revision to or the proposal of a theory. The point is that a research synthesis is not simply a summary of the related literature; it is a logical type of research that leads to valid conclusions, hypothesis evaluations, and the revision and proposal of theory.

The approach to a research synthesis is like any other type of research. The researcher must clearly specify the procedures that are to be followed. Unfortunately, the literature review paper seldom specifies the procedures the author used. Thus, the basis for the many decisions made about individual papers is usually unknown to the reader. Of course, this makes an objective evaluation of a literature review nearly impossible. Questions that are important yet usually unanswered in the typical review of literature include the following:

- How thorough was the literature search? Did it include a computer search and hand search? In a computer search, what descriptors were used? Which journals were searched? Were theses and dissertations searched and included?
- On what basis were studies included or excluded from the written review? Were theses and dissertations arbitrarily excluded? Did the author make decisions about inclusion or exclusion based on the perceived internal validity of the research, on sample size, on research design, or on appropriate statistical analysis?
- How did the author arrive at a particular conclusion? Was it based on the number of studies supporting or refuting the conclusion (called vote counting)? Were these studies weighted differentially according to sample size, meaningfulness of the results, quality of the journal, and internal validity of the study?

Many more questions could be asked about the decisions made in the typical literature review paper, for good research involves a systematic method of problem solving. However, in most literature reviews the author's systematic method remains unknown to the reader, thus prohibiting an objective evaluation of these decisions.

 In recent years, several attempts have been made to solve the problems associated with literature reviews. The most notable of these attempts was made in a paper by Glass (1976) and followed up with a book by Glass et al. (1981), who proposed a technique called **meta-analysis**. The major purpose of this chapter is to present an overview of meta-analysis and the procedures developed to use in meta-analysis [but for a more general approach to research synthesis, see Cooper & Hedges (1994).]

Using Meta–Analysis to Synthesize Research

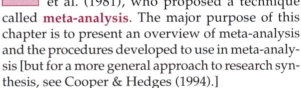

Purpose of Meta–Analysis
Examples of Meta–Analysis
Methodological Considerations
    Deciding What to Code
    Choosing Standard Deviation for the Effect Size

 Methodological questions that should be answered in a literature review

 meta–analysis — A technique of literature review that contains a definitive methodology and the quantification of the results of various studies to a standard metric that allows the use of statistical techniques as a means of analysis.

 Cooper, H., & Hedges, L.V. (Eds.) (1994). *The handbook of research synthesis.* New York: Sage Foundation.

Since Glass introduced meta-analysis in 1976, thousands of meta-analyses have been published, especially in the social, behavioral, and medical sciences. At a national conference in 1986, "Workshop on Methodological Issues in Overviews of Randomized Clinical Trials," sponsored by the National Institutes of Health, participants focused considerable attention on meta-analysis for the health-related and medical research.

Purpose of Meta-Analysis

Meta-analysis involves two procedures lacking in previous literature reviews. First, a definitive methodology is reported concerning the decisions in a literature analysis. Second, the results of various studies are quantified to a standard metric that allows the use of statistical techniques as a means of analysis. Here are the steps in a meta-analysis:

1. The identification of a problem
2. A literature search by specified means
3. A review of identified studies to determine inclusion or exclusion
4. A careful reading and evaluation to identify and code important study characteristics
5. The calculation of effect size
6. The application of appropriate statistical techniques
7. The reporting of all these steps and of the outcomes in a review paper

Of course, one of the major problems in a literature review paper is the number of studies that must be considered. To some extent, analyzing all these studies is like trying to make sense of all the data points collected on a group of subjects. However, within a study, statistical techniques are used to reduce the data to make them understandable. The procedures of meta-analysis are similar. The findings within individual studies are considered the data points to use in a statistical analysis across the findings of many studies.

How, then, can findings based on different designs, data collection techniques, dependent variables, and statistical analysis be compared? Glass addressed this issue by using an estimate he calls effect size (ES, or the symbol Δ). Note that we discussed this general concept in chapter 8 as a way of judging the meaningfulness of group differences. ES is determined by the following formula:

$$\text{ES} = \frac{M_E - M_C}{s_C} \qquad (14.1)$$

where M_E = the mean of the experimental group, M_C = the mean of the control group, and s_C = the standard deviation of the control group. Note that this formula places the difference between the experimental and control groups in control group standard deviation units. For example, if $M_E = 15$, $M_C = 12$, and $s_C = 5$, then ES $= (15 - 12)/5 = 0.60$. The experimental group's performance exceeded the control group's performance by .60 of a standard deviation. If this were done across several studies addressing a common problem, the findings of the studies would be in a common metric, ES (Δ), which could be compared. The mean and standard deviations of ES could be calculated from several studies. This would allow a statement about the average ES of a particular type of treatment.

Suppose we wanted to know whether a particular treatment affects males and females differently. In searching the literature, we find 15 studies on males comparing the treatment effects and 12 studies on females. We could calculate an ES for each of the 27 studies and the mean (and standard deviation) of the ES for males ($n = 15$) and females ($n = 12$). An independent t test could then be used to see whether the average ES differed for males and females. If the t values were significant and the average ES for the females were greater, we could conclude that the treatment had more effect on females than on males. Cooper and Hedges (1994) provide considerable detail on the methods of meta-analysis, including literature search strategies, ways to calculate ES from the statistics reported in various studies, suggestions for how and what to code from studies, and examples of the use of meta-analysis.

Steps in a meta-analysis

Certainly, meta-analysis is not the answer to all the problems associated with research synthesis. But Glass has provided an objective way to evaluate the literature. Advances (Hedges, 1981, 1982a, 1982b; Hedges & Olkin, 1980) in studying the statistical properties of ES have contributed considerably to the appropriate use of meta-analysis. The text by Hedges and Olkin (1985) provides a complete accounting of the procedures and statistical analyses appropriate for meta-analysis (also, other books have appeared on meta-analysis advocating slightly different procedures: e.g., Hunter & Schmidt, 1990). A tutorial by Thomas and French (1986) is an overview of Hedges's (and colleagues') techniques and includes examples from the study of physical activity. Some examples of meta-analyses that have appeared in the physical activity literature follow.

Examples of Meta-Analysis

Many meta-analyses have been published since 1976, including several in physical education, exercise science, and sport science. A brief overview of some of these studies should identify the value of meta-analysis.

In a meta-analysis on the effects of perceptual-motor training for improving academic, cognitive, or perceptual-motor performance, Kavale and Mattson (1983) reported a distinct lack of success for perceptual-motor training in the 180 studies included. The largest ES they found was .198, and it was associated with the 83 studies rated low in internal validity. In fact, in studies with high internal validity, the trained subjects did worse. Thus, perceptual-motor training does not appear useful for any type of outcome (academic, cognitive, or perceptual-motor) for any type of subject (normal, educable mentally retarded, trainable mentally retarded, slow learner, culturally disadvantaged, learning disabled, reading disabled, or motor disabled) at any age level (preschool, kindergarten, primary grades, middle grades, junior high school, or high school).

Sparling (1980) reported a meta-analysis of ES differences between males and females for maximal oxygen uptake ($\dot{V}O_2$max). One of the most interesting findings was that when ES was averaged across studies, it was reduced when corrections were made for the differing body compositions of males and females. When $\dot{V}O_2$max was expressed as liters per minute (l/min), 66% of the variance was explained by knowing the subject's gender; when $\dot{V}O_2$max was expressed as ml/min · kg BW (body weight), the explained variance was reduced to 49%; and when expressed as ml/min · kg FFW (fat-free weight), the explained variance was reduced to 35%. Thus, the advantage of males over females in $\dot{V}O_2$max is reduced when corrected for body weight and is reduced even more when corrected for fat-free weight.

In a meta-analysis on the effects of exercise in blood lipids and lipoproteins, Tran, Weltman, Glass, and Mood (1983) reported an analysis of 66 training studies involving a total of 2,925 subjects. They found significant relationships between training and beneficial changes in blood lipids and lipoproteins: "Initial levels, age, length of training, intensity, $\dot{V}O_2$max, body weight, and percent fat have been shown . . . to interact with exercise and serum lipids and lipoprotein changes" (p. 400).

Payne and Morrow (1993) reported a meta-analysis of the effects of exercise on children's $\dot{V}O_2$max. From 28 studies yielding 70 effect sizes, they compared cross-sectional (trained vs. untrained children) and pre- to posttraining designs. Effect sizes were large in cross-sectional studies (0.94 + 1.00) but small in training studies (0.35 + 0.82). In training studies the average improvement in $\dot{V}O_2$max was only 2 ml · kg · min^{-1}. ES for the training studies was not influenced by gender, training protocol, or the way subjects were tested on $\dot{V}O_2$max.

Hedges, L.V. (1982a). Fitting categorical models to effect sizes from a series of experiments. *Journal of Educational Statistics*, **7**, 119-137.

Hedges, L.V., & Olkin, I. (1985). *Statistical methods for meta-analysis*. New York: Academic Press.

Hunter, J.E., & Schmidt, F.L. (1990). *Methods of meta-analysis: Correcting error and bias in research findings*. Newbury Park, CA: Sage.

Thomas, J.R., & French, K.E. (1986). The use of meta-analysis in exercise and sport: A tutorial. *Research Quarterly for Exercise and Sport*, **57**, 196-204.

Payne, V.G., & Morrow, J.R. (1993). Exercise and $\dot{V}O_2$max in children: A meta-analysis. *Research Quarterly for Exercise and Sport*, **64**, 305-313.

Feltz and Landers (1983) reported a meta-analysis of the effects of mental practice on motor skill learning and performance. From 60 studies they calculated an average ES of 0.48, less than half of a standard deviation unit. They concluded that mentally practicing a motor skill is slightly better than not practicing one at all.

In studying gender differences in motor performance across childhood and adolescence, Thomas and French (1985) reported findings from 64 studies based on 31,444 subjects. They found motor performance differences to be related to age in 12 of the 20 motor tasks. These 12 tasks followed four general types of curves across age. Figure 14.1 shows one typical type of curve for three tasks (long jump, shuttle run, and grip strength). The differences are moderate (about 0.5 to 0.75 standard deviation units) before puberty but then increase dramatically during and following puberty (over 1.5 standard deviation units). They concluded that the differences before puberty were likely to be induced by environmental factors (differential treatment by parents, teachers, coaches, and peers) but that they represented an interaction of biology and environment beginning at puberty. Note the difference between the curves in Figures 14.1 and 14.2. Effect sizes for throwing performance are 1.5 standard deviation units at ages 3-4 and increase constantly across childhood and adolescence until the differences are 3.5 standard deviation units by age 18. Thomas and French suggested that differences that were so large so early in life might have some basis in biology and in the influence of cultural treatments and expectations for girls and boys.

Crews and Landers (1987) reported a meta-analysis of the relation between aerobic fitness and psychosocial stressors. They had 34 studies including 1,449 subjects and reported that reduced psychosocial stress was found in more aerobically fit subjects (ES = 0.48) when they were compared with less fit subjects or baseline measures. This effect was reliable regardless of the types of physiological or psychological measures used. In addition, none of the moderator variables (e.g., study and subject characteristics, methodological characteristics, and stressor characteristics) were important for this finding as the effect sizes were homogeneous.

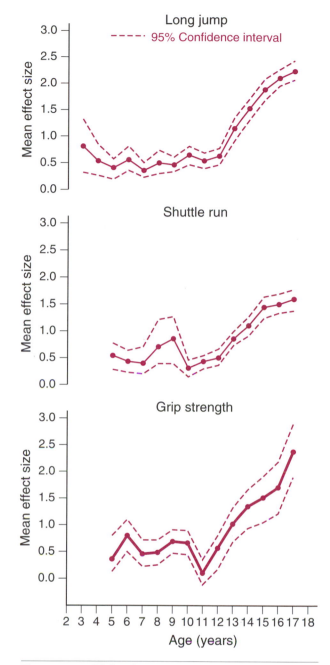

Figure 14.1   ES for three motor performance tasks. *Note.* Dotted lines are confidence intervals.

These examples have been used to illustrate the value of the meta-analysis approach. In the perceptual-motor meta-analysis, the controversial issue of the value of this type of training appears resolved: no benefit. In the

Crews, D.J., & Landers, D.M. (1987). A meta-analytic review of aerobic fitness and reactivity to psychosocial stressors. *Medicine and Science in Sports and Exercise*, **19** (suppl. 5), 120-144.

For additional detail read one of the meta-analyses in our field discussed previously.

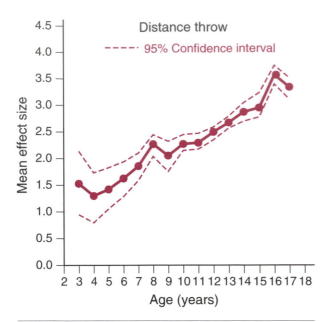

Figure 14.2 ES by age and gender for throwing for distance.

Note. Dotted lines are confidence intervals.

meta-analysis of gender differences in $\dot{V}O_2$max these large differences appear to be accounted for mainly by differences in body composition rather than any differences in underlying mechanisms. Also, exercise appears to have a positive effect on cholesterol and its components. Exercise training seems to benefit children, but the gains are relatively small by adult standards. Mental practice is better than no practice, but not by much. Gender differences in motor performance before puberty appear mainly environmentally induced, but throwing may be a skill for which biology plays a greater role before puberty. Finally, higher levels of aerobic fitness appear to be associated with lower levels of psychosocial stress.

Meta-analysis, when applied appropriately and interpreted carefully, offers a means of reducing a large quantity of studies to underlying principles. These principles can become the bases for program development, future research, and theory testing as well as various practical applications, such as practice and training.

Methodological Considerations

Thomas and French (1986) published a tutorial and example of meta-analysis, part of which is

adapted here to take you through the important steps and issues in a meta-analysis. We thank Karen French and the *Research Quarterly for Exercise and Sport* for allowing us to adapt part of this paper.

Although meta-analysis has been a widely used technique in the last few years, considerable controversy exists concerning the validity of meta-analysis (e.g., Carlberg et al., 1984; Slavin, 1984a, 1984b). Among the most severe criticisms of meta-analysis is for its combination of findings from studies representing different measurement scales, methodologies, and experimental designs. This criticism of "mixing of apples and oranges" was compounded by the results of early meta-analyses using the methods of Glass (1977), which tended to reveal few differences in ESs, even between studies in which internal validity and methodological control clearly varied. Hedges (1981, 1982a, 1982b) and Hedges and Olkin (1983, 1985) extended the original work of Glass (1977) and proposed a new set of techniques and statistical tests specifically designed to address the following questions and criticisms of meta-analysis:

- How should the process of deciding variables to code and coding systematically be organized?
- What should be used as the standard deviation when calculating an ES?
- Because sample ESs are biased estimators of the population of ESs, how can this bias be corrected?
- Should ESs be weighted for their sample size?
- Are all ESs in a sample from the same population of ESs? This is the "apples and oranges" issue: Is the sample of ESs homogeneous?
- What are appropriate statistical tests for analyzing ESs?
- If a sample of ESs includes outliers, how can they be identified?

In the following sections, we address each of these questions, summarize the theoretical basis for the statistical procedures introduced by Hedges (1981, 1982a, 1982b) and Hedges and Olkin (1983, 1985), and suggest applications of these techniques in physical education, exercise science, and sport science research.

Questions meta-analysis must address

Deciding What to Code

 One of the most difficult yet most important tasks in doing a meta-analysis is choosing variables to code and developing a scheme for coding them. Stock (1994) has provided a useful discussion of this topic. In particular the meta-analyst must realize the tradeoff between the number and importance of items to code and the time required to code. Of course, the more information that is coded about a study, the more time is required to develop a coding scheme and actually do the coding. However, omitting potentially important items to code also creates major problems as the scholar then has to go back through all studies to pick up these omitted items.

The best way to be successful in selecting items to code and a coding scheme is to know the theoretical and empirical literature on which you are doing the meta-analysis and to understand meta-analysis procedures. Stock (1994) suggest the following two important considerations when planning the coding for a meta-analysis.

 The meta-analyst is looking for items to code that are likely to influence (or be related to) the effect sizes that will be calculated. For example, when Thomas and French (1985) calculated effect sizes for gender differences in motor performance, they thought that children's ages would be related to gender differences. Specifically, they hypothesized that gender differences would become greater as children grew. Once important items to code are selected, the meta-analyst needs an organizational scheme for the items. The attachment at the end of this chapter is a coding scheme developed for her dissertation review on expertise by Sheri Parks from the Department of Human Movement Studies at the University of Queensland (Brisbane, Australia). We appreciate her permission to use the materials. Parks' coding scheme used these categories (with several subparts of each): descriptive information about the paper, type of sport/area of expertise, information about the task, type of measures used for each task, and information about the subjects.

 The material from Sheri Parks' work attached at the end of this chapter is a sample of a coding form and code book. Stock (1994)

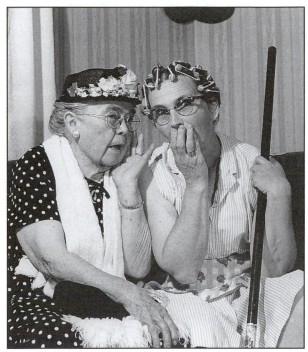

"Psst. Bertha. Let me tell you my great scheme for coding variables."

provides a generalized example of a coding form. An important issue here is how to code variables, or how to assign numbers to characteristics to be coded. Sometimes specific information is maintained—for example, if the average age of subjects from each study is important, this average age can be entered as the code. In other instances, variables will be grouped into categories for coding; for example, categories of level of expertise could be coded as 1 = internationally ranked athletic performers, 2 = nationally ranked athletic performers, 3 = college/university athletic performers, 4 = high school athletic performers. Other important issues include the training of coders and establishing and maintaining intra- and intercoder reliability.

Choosing Standard Deviation for the Effect Size

Originally, Glass et al. (1981) proposed the use of the control group's standard deviation as the most appropriate measure of group variability. From an intuitive perspective, the control group's variabil-

 Stock, W.A. (1994). Systematic coding for research synthesis. In H. Cooper & L.V. Hedges (Eds.), *The handbook of research synthesis.* New York: Sage Foundation.

How to code and classify items

Constructing a coding form and code book

ity represents the "normal" variation in an untreated population. The control group's standard deviation also has the advantage of assigning equal ESs to equal treatment means when a study contains two or more experimental groups that have heterogeneous variances. Therefore, the control group's standard deviation serves as a common standard metric from which treatment differences can be compared.

In most cases, estimates of group variance are homogeneous. Hedges (1981) argued that a pooled estimate of the variance provides a more precise estimate of the population variance. (The square root of the pooled estimate of the variance is the pooled estimate of the standard deviation.) One advantage of pooling variances is an increase in the degrees of freedom associated with the estimate of variance. The pooled estimate Hedges (1981) suggested is given in formula 14.2. Note that the variance of each group is weighted by the sample size of that group in a way that is similar to the procedure used in t tests with unequal ns. The formula is

$$s_P = \sqrt{\frac{(N_E - 1)s_E^2 + (N_C - 1)s_C^2}{N_E + N_C - 2}} \quad (14.2)$$

where N_E = the sample size of the experimental group (Group 1), N_C = the sample size of the control group (Group 2), s_E^2 = the variance of the experimental group (Group 1), and s_C^2 = the variance of the control group (Group 2).

Many studies involve tests of effects between or among categorical variables (e.g., race and gender) where there is no control condition. Early meta-analyses used an average of the standard deviations of the groups compared (Glass & Smith, 1979; Hyde, 1981; Smith, 1980). Hedges and Olkin (1985) have suggested using the weighted pooled standard deviation (s_P, formula 14.2) as the estimate of the standard deviation (for an example using gender differences in motor performance, see Thomas & French, 1985).

There are cases in which the variance for the groups is heterogeneous. Glass et al. (1981) have shown the ESs are biased when the group variances are unequal. Because parametric tests are based on the assumption of equal variances, ESs calculated from t and ANOVA may be biased if the group variances are unequal.

Researchers should evaluate whether heterogeneous variances are a common phenomenon in the area of research for the meta-analysis. We have encountered unequal variances when comparing the motor performance of children of different age levels (French & Thomas, 1985). We offer these suggestions. When the ES compares an experimental group and a control group and the group variances are unequal, use the standard deviation of the control group to calculate the ES in all studies. If the ES compares two groups (such as age or gender) in which there is no clear control condition, we believe the weighted pooled estimate (formula 14.2) suggested by Hedges (1981) is the best choice.

Calculating Effect Sizes for Within-Subject Designs

Often a researcher wants to calculate an effect size for a within-subjects design (or repeated measures effect), usually between a pre- and posttest for a treatment effect (i.e., experimental group). The appropriate formula for this effect size (Looney, Feltz, & VanVleet, 1994) is to use the pretest standard deviation in the denominator of formula 14.1. This represents the best source of untreated variance against which to standardize differences between the pre- and posttest means.

Using ES as an Estimator of Treatment Effects

Hedges (1981) has provided a theoretical and structural model for the use of ES as an estimator of treatment effects. An individual ES may be viewed as a sample statistic that estimates the population of possible treatment effects within a given experiment. Hedges has shown that the variance of an individual ES may be directly calculated from the following formula:

$$\text{var}(ES_i) = \frac{N_E + N_C}{N_E N_C} + \frac{ES_i^2}{2(N_E + N_C)} \quad (14.3)$$

where N_E = the sample size of the experimental group (Group 1), N_C = the sample size of the control group (Group 2), and ES_i = the estimate of ES. Note that the variability associated with the sample statistic, or ES, is a function of the value of the ES and the sample size. An ES based on a large sample

Thomas, J.R., & French, K.E. (1985). Gender differences across age in motor performance: A meta-analysis. *Psychological Bulletin*, **98**, 260–282.

Glass, G.V., McGaw, B., & Smith, M. (1981). *Meta-analysis in social research*. Beverly Hills, CA: Sage.

has a smaller variance than an ES based on a small sample. Therefore, ESs based on large samples are better estimates of the population parameter of treatment effects.

Hedges (1981) also demonstrated that ESs are positively biased in small samples; however, the bias is 20% or less when the sample size exceeds 20. A virtually unbiased estimate of ES can be obtained by multiplying the ES by the correction factor given in the following formula:

$$c = 1 - \frac{3}{4m - 9} \qquad (14.4)$$

where $m = N_E + N_C - 2$ when a pooled estimate is used as the standard deviation, $m = N_1 + N_2 - 2$ if a pooled estimate is used in a categorical model, or $m = N_C - 1$ when the control group standard deviation (or pretest standard deviation in the case of a within-subjects ES) is used. (This formula is correct here, but was printed incorrectly in Thomas and French [1986].)

Each ES should be corrected before averaging or further analysis. If ESs are not corrected before averaging, the average of even a large number of ESs remains biased and simply estimates an incorrect value more precisely (Hedges, 1981). Early meta-analyses in exercise and sport (Feltz & Landers, 1983; Sparling, 1980) did not correct each ES for small sample bias. The ESs reported in these studies are most likely slight overestimates.

  Although the individual ES estimate can be corrected for bias, the variability associated with the estimate remains a function of the sample size. Thus, as stated before, if other factors are equal, ESs with large samples are better estimates than ESs with small samples. Hedges (1981) and Hedges and Olkin (1985) introduced statistical techniques that weight each ES on the basis of the reciprocal of its variance (for more detail, see Thomas & French, 1986). Therefore, ESs that are more precise receive more weight in each analysis.

Testing Homogeneity

Meta-analysis has been criticized for mixing apples and oranges, or combining studies with different measurement scales, designs, and methodologies. No appropriate test existed to determine whether all the ESs were estimating the same population treatment effect until Hedges (1982a) introduced his test for homogeneity. The homogeneity statistic, H, is specifically designed to test the null hypothesis, H_0: $ES_1 = ES_2 = \ldots = ES_i$. This is equivalent to saying that all ESs tested come from the same population of ESs.

The statistic H is the weighted sum of squared deviations of ESs from the overall weighted mean. The contribution of each ES to the overall mean is weighted by the reciprocal of its variance. Effect sizes with smaller variances receive more weight in the calculation of the overall mean. Under the null hypothesis, H has a chi-square distribution with $N - 1$ degrees of freedom, where N equals the number of ESs.

When the null hypothesis is not rejected, all ESs are similar and represent a similar measure of treatment effectiveness. In this case, the researcher should report the homogeneity statistic indicating that ESs are homogeneous and use the weighted mean ES with confidence intervals for interpretation. If the null hypothesis is rejected, ESs are not homogeneous and do not represent a similar measure of treatment effectiveness, or grouping. Two methods have been proposed by Hedges (1982a) and Hedges and Olkin (1983) to examine explanatory models for ESs:

- Analysis of variance, and
- Weighted regression

The first method is analogous to ANOVA, in which the sum of squares for the total H statistic is partitioned into sum of squares between and among groups of ESs (H_B) and sum of squares within groups of ESs (H_W). Each sum of squares may be tested as a chi-square with $k - 1$ df for H_B and $N - k - 1$ df for H_W (where N = the number of ESs and k = the number of groups). Therefore, a test can be conducted for between- or among-group differences (H_B), and a test can be conducted to determine whether all ESs within a group are homogeneous (H_W). Further discussion of the categorical model is presented in Hedges (1982a) and Hedges and Olkin (1985).

The second method proposed by Hedges and Olkin (1983) to fit an explanatory model to ES data is a weighted regression technique. We have chosen to present a more detailed discussion of the regression techniques for several reasons. First, one of the meta-analyses discussed previously in

---

Thomas, J.R., & French, K.E. (1986). The use of meta-analysis in exercise and sport: A tutorial. *Research Quarterly for Exercise and Sport*, **57**, 196-204.

Two methods to examine ES models

exercise and sport has used regression techniques to analyze ES (Thomas & French, 1985). Second, it is common for a continuous variable to influence ES. Third, often more than one study characteristic influences ES. This is especially true when there are many ESs. The regression procedures can accommodate a larger number of variables in the analysis without inflating the alpha level of the statistical test. Conducting many tests using the categorical or ANOVA-like procedures results in alpha inflation. The researcher would need to report the experimentwise error rate or adjust the alpha level using the Bonferroni technique. Fourth, categorical variables can easily be dummy or effect coded and entered into the regression procedures. For example, published versus unpublished papers can be dummy coded (1 or 0) and entered into the regression. Thus, it is not necessary to conduct a separate analysis for categorical variables.

Each ES is weighted by the inverse of its variance in the weighted regression technique. Most standard statistical packages (e.g., SAS, SPSS, BMDP) have an option to perform weighted regression. Thus, the computations may be done easily on most computers.

 The sum of squares total for the regression is equivalent to the homogeneity statistic, H. It is partitioned into sum of squares regression and sum of squares error. The **sum of squares** for regression yields a test of the variance due to the predictor variables (H_R). The sum of squares regression is tested as a chi-square with $df = p$, where p equals the number of predictor variables. The sum of squares error provides a test of model specifications (H_E), or whether the ESs are homogeneous when the variance caused by the predictors is removed. The sum of squares error is tested as a chi-square with $df = N - p - 1$, where N equals the number of ESs and p equals the number of predictor variables. The test of model specification evaluates the deviation of the ESs from the regression model. A nonsignificant test of model specification indicates that the ESs do not deviate substantially from the regression model. A significant test for model specification shows that one or more ESs deviate substantially from the regression model. Ideally, the researcher wants the H_R for regression to be significant and the H_E for model specification to be nonsignificant.

When the test for model specifications is significant, one or more ESs do not follow the specified regression. Often, the ESs that do not follow the same pattern may suggest other characteristics that may be added to the model (e.g., published vs. unpublished studies). Moreover, some ESs may represent outliers (unrepresentative scores). In either case, the use of outlier techniques is helpful in identifying these ESs.

Testing for Outliers

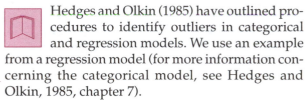 Hedges and Olkin (1985) have outlined procedures to identify outliers in categorical and regression models. We use an example from a regression model (for more information concerning the categorical model, see Hedges and Olkin, 1985, chapter 7).

Outliers in regression models may be identified by examining the residuals of the regression equation. The absolute value of the residuals is standardized to z scores by subtracting the mean and dividing by the standard deviation. Effect sizes with standardized residuals larger than 2 are often examined as potential outliers, as they fall outside 95% of the distribution.

According to Hedges and Olkin (1985), each ES makes a contribution to the regression model. The outliers identified by standardized residuals may vary depending on which ESs are in the model at the time. Hedges and Olkin have suggested computing standardized residuals multiple times with a different ES deleted from the model each time the residuals are computed. For example, if one has 10 ESs, standardized residuals would be computed 10 times with a different ES deleted from the model each time. However, some of our preliminary work has suggested that if more than 20 ESs are included in the regression model, the value of going through all possible combinations of deleting ESs from the model may be limited. Simply calculate the residuals with all the ESs in the model, standardize the residuals, and evaluate whether ESs with a z score larger than 2 might be outliers.

Accounting for Publication Bias

Journals have a tendency to accept papers that report significant findings. Thus, there may be some

---

 sum of squares — A measure of variability of scores; the sum of the squared deviations from the mean of scores.

Hedges, L.V., & Olkin, I. (1985). *Statistical methods for meta-analysis.* Orlando, FL: Academic Press.

number of studies on any topic (including one on which a meta-analysis is being done) that have not been submitted (or published if submitted) to scholarly journals. This problem has been labeled the "file-drawer" effect.

 An important question in a meta-analysis is how many of these studies are sitting around in file drawers. The meta-analyst should find every study possible, but how many studies have been done that have not been reported? Rosenthal (1979) suggested a technique for estimating how many unpublished studies with no significant effect on the variable of interest would be needed to reduce the mean ES to nonsignificance.

Other Considerations

Sometimes all the information needed to calculate an ES is not available in a research report. Both Glass et al. (1981) and Hedges and Olkin (1985) have provided ways to estimate ESs from standard statistics (e.g., t, F, and r). However, on occasion only the statement that two groups do not differ significantly will be reported. What should the meta-analyst do? To drop the study is to bias the results of the meta-analysis toward significant differences. Thomas and French (1985) inserted a *zero* ES, using the rationale that no significant differences means the differences did not reliably differ from zero. However, Thomas and French (1985) had few zero ESs. Using many zero ESs may cause problems in the analysis of homogeneity by making the studies look overly consistent. Hedges (1984) suggested a correction factor that adjusts for this problem. Regardless of the solution selected, the meta-analyst must cope with this issue and select a logical solution.

Tutorial Example of Meta-Analysis

Selection of Studies
Coded Characteristics of the Studies
Calculation of Effect Size
Test for Homogeneity
A Final Point

The following example is a subset of data from Thomas and French (1985) for gender differences in throwing velocity across age. We describe the procedures involved in each step.

Selection of Studies

To identify a set of studies that examined gender differences in motor performance, Thomas and French conducted a computer search using ERIC and Psychology Information to identify studies that compared the performance of males and females across age levels. A number of journals in exercise, sport, and psychology were searched by hand (see Thomas & French, 1985). Although the total meta-analysis had 64 studies on 20 tasks that met all the criteria for inclusion, only 5 of these studies were on throwing velocity. The studies used for this example are listed in the note to Table 14.1.

Coded Characteristics of the Studies

The age of the subjects was the primary variable that was hypothesized to be related to ES, the magnitude of which was predicted to change across age levels.

Calculation of Effect Size

Thirteen ESs were calculated from the five studies. Each ES was calculated by subtracting the mean of the female group's performance from the mean of the male group's performance and dividing by the pooled weighted standard deviation (formula 14.2). Therefore, a positive ES indicates that males throw with greater velocity than females. Each ES was multiplied by the appropriate correction factor (formula 14.4) to correct for small sample bias (Hedges, 1981). In addition, the variance of each ES and the reciprocal of the variance of each ES were calculated from formula 14.3. Table 14.1 provides a summary of these calculations.

Test for Homogeneity

The first step in the analysis of these data was to conduct the test for homogeneity to determine whether all ESs were similar. The H statistic was significant, $\chi^2(12) = 53.88$, $p < .01$. A significant por-

Rosenthal, R. (1979). The "file-drawer problem" and tolerance for null results. *Psychological Bulletin*, **86**, 638-641.

Table 14.1   Summary Information for the Five Studies

Study #	ES #	Male M	Male s	Male N	Female M	Female s	Female N	Pooled s (weighted)	Uncorrected ES	Corrected ES	Variance of ES	Inverse of the variance of ES
1	1	35.7	7.0	10	27.4	4.5	9	6.0	1.39	1.33	.258	3.88
1	2	41.4	7.8	10	30.9	3.0	9	6.0	1.74	1.66	.284	3.52
1	3	44.7	7.1	10	34.9	1.3	9	5.2	1.87	1.79	.295	3.39
2	4	35.3	7.0	12	26.2	4.2	12	5.8	1.58	1.52	.215	4.65
3	5	38.8	7.8	22	28.7	8.3	17	8.0	1.25	1.23	.124	8.08
3	6	44.3	8.3	22	31.6	8.3	17	8.3	1.53	1.50	.133	7.51
3	7	49.6	8.3	22	34.6	8.9	17	8.6	1.75	1.72	.142	7.04
3	8	77.6	10.1	22	55.9	11.3	17	10.6	2.04	2.00	.155	6.43
4	9	46.3	7.3	28	30.8	4.6	25	6.2	2.51	2.47	.133	7.50
5	10	51.5	6.6	35	34.8	4.1	35	5.5	3.03	3.00	.122	8.22
5	11	57.3	5.5	33	40.5	5.3	36	5.4	3.11	3.07	.127	7.89
5	12	63.6	7.1	39	41.6	6.5	38	6.8	3.23	3.20	.118	8.45
5	13	69.0	5.0	37	50.4	5.1	37	5.0	3.63	3.60	.144	6.94

Note. Study 1: Roberton, Halverson, Langendorfer, and Williams (1979); Study 2: Halverson, Roberton, Safrit, and Roberts (1977); Study 3: Halverson, Roberton, and Langendorfer (1982); Study 4: Maples (1977); Study 5: Glassow, Halverson, and Rarick (1965).

tion of the variance remains unexplained because that is what a significant H statistic means. The age of the subject was predicted to be related to ES; therefore, age may account for a major portion of the variance. A weighted regression was chosen as a method of analysis because age is a continuous variable. Effect size was regressed on the age of the subject. The test for regression was significant, $\chi^2(1) = 24.49, p < .01$. The test for model specification that evaluates the homogeneity of the ESs around the regression line was significant, $\chi^2(11) = 29.72$, $p < .01$. Therefore, one or more ESs deviated significantly from the regression line.

Because the test for model specification was significant, a test for outliers in the regression was conducted following the procedures discussed earlier and previously outlined by Hedges and Olkin (1985). We have tried to simplify the discussion of the outlier tests. The regression equation was calculated 13 times, and one ES was deleted from the model on each calculation. The H_R for regression and the H_E for model specification for each of the 13 regressions are given in Table 14.2. The χ_R^2 for regression and the χ_E^2 for model specification are calculated and are listed on the same line as the ES that was deleted from the model. Therefore, on the first line, the χ_R^2 for regression is 21.24 and the χ_E^2

for model specification is 29.33 when the first ES (1.33) was deleted from the regression. The absolute values of the residuals from the regression were computed and converted to z scores by subtracting the mean and dividing by the standard deviation. Rather than present the standardized residuals calculated 13 times with one ES deleted from the model each time, we present the standardized residuals for each ES with all ESs included in the regression equation in Table 14.2. The standardized residual for ES #8 (2.779) is greater than 2 and can be evaluated as a potential outlier. Furthermore, a significant reduction in the sum of squares for model specification (H_E) was found when ES #8 was deleted from the model, $\chi_R^2(10) = 11.25, p > .05$. Also, the χ_R^2 for regression increased to 42.42. Note that the χ_R^2 regression and the χ_E^2 for model specification did not change very much when the other ESs were individually deleted from the regression calculations. Thus, the ESs are homogeneous around the regression line when ES #8 is not included in the model.

Once an ES has been identified as a potential outlier, it is important to examine why it may be an outlier. An outlier could indicate other characteristics that should be added to the model. In our example, the ES identified as an outlier was consider-

Table 14.2   Standardized Residuals

ES #	Age	ES	$H_R(1)$	$H_E(10)$	Residual
1	6	1.33	21.24	29.33	−0.652
2	7	1.66	23.34	29.48	−0.801
3	8	1.79	24.25	29.11	−0.272
4	5	1.52	21.87	29.54	−1.060
5	6	1.23	16.42	28.05	−0.331
6	7	1.50	20.99	28.22	−0.266
7	8	1.71	23.88	27.91	−0.042
8	12	2.00	42.42	11.25	2.779
9	8	2.47	24.79	29.11	−0.747
10	8	3.00	25.58	23.80	1.012
11	9	3.07	22.02	26.62	0.312
12	10	3.20	18.42	27.83	−0.232
13	11	3.64	13.56	26.48	0.301

Note. With all effect sizes in the regression model, $H_R(1)$ = 24.49 and $H_E(11)$ = 29.72.

ably lower at age 12 (2.00) than those at ages 10 and 11 (3.20 and 3.64, respectively) when the ES between males and females would be expected to increase with age. Throwing velocity for the ES at age 12 was measured by a velocimeter. The study that included ESs at ages 10 and 11 used a film analysis to obtain a measure of velocity. Thus, the ES at age 12 may be lower than the ESs at 10 and 11 because of a difference in the way that throwing velocity was measured. The final model (outlier deleted) revealed that the test for regression was significant, $\chi_R^2 = 42.42$, $p < .01$, and the test for model specification nonsignificant, $\chi_E^2 = 11.25$, $p > .05$.

Figure 14.3 is a plot of the mean ESs at each age with their 95% confidence intervals, which we reported in a more comprehensive paper (Thomas & French, 1985). We chose to report the mean ES at each age. One could also use a figure with the regression line and plot each individual ES around the regression line. We felt that the mean ES with confidence interval retained a better representation of the original data. This was especially true with the other motor tasks we reported (Thomas & French, 1985), as these had a much greater number of ESs.

As you can see from Figure 14.3, gender differences in throwing velocity are large even for preschool children (1.5 standard deviation units) and increase in a linear manner during childhood and

early adolescence, when the differences are greater than 3.5 standard deviation units. Thus, boys throw with much greater velocity than girls at a very early age, and this advantage continues to increase as boys and girls age.

Although there are differences in the treatment of boys and girls, gender differences in throwing velocity as large as 1.5 standard deviation units at age 3 to 4 are unlikely to be completely environmentally caused. Thomas and French (1985) discussed other research that suggest that biological variables may contribute to the large gender difference in throwing velocity. However, the fact that the gender difference continues to increase in childhood and adolescence is probably a combination of biological and environmental influences.

One advantage of using meta-analysis to examine gender differences in motor performance across age is that the magnitude of these differences can be determined. Thomas and French (1985) calculated ESs for a number of motor tasks. No gender difference was found in performance on certain tasks. On other tasks, the gender difference was small before puberty and increased after puberty. Large gender differences in throwing velocity and throwing distance existed before puberty and increased in magnitude following puberty. Overall, the magnitude of gender differences across age was dependent on the type of task examined. These comparisons would not be possible using the traditional qualitative review of literature.

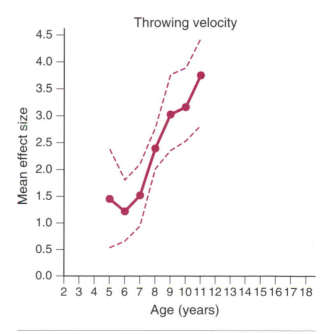

Figure 14.3   ES by age and gender for throwing velocity.

A Final Point

An issue remaining in the methodological literature on meta-analysis is the likely correlation among multiple ESs drawn from one study. For example, in our data (Table 14.1), three ESs were drawn from Study 1, four ESs from Study 3, and four ESs from Study 5. In this particular case, the ESs can be expected to be independent because each is based on the difference between female and male throwing performance at a different age level. However, one of these studies (Study 5) contained other motor performance characteristics (e.g., running and jumping) tested on the same children. Might the ESs be correlated because they are based on the same children's performance?

This problem is equivalent to the problems in a single study with multiple measures on the same subject. Certainly the variables might be correlated. The meta-analyst might select one or two alternatives. We (Thomas & French, 1985) chose to argue that previous research and theory had shown the variables to have little or no correlation; thus, they could be considered independent. If the variables are correlated, the meta-analyst should at least adjust the experimentwise error rate (see chapter 8).

Summary

A research synthesis is not just a summary of studies arranged in some kind of sequence. It should be structured, analytical, and critical and lead to specific conclusions. The meta-analysis is a definitive methodology that quantifies results and allows statistical techniques to be used as a means of analysis.

The meta-analysis explicitly details how the search was done, the sources, the choices made regarding inclusion or exclusion, the coding of study characteristics, and the analytical procedures. The basis of a meta-analysis is the effect size, which transforms differences between experimental and control groups' performances to a common metric, which is expressed in standard deviation units.

The meta-analysis technique has been widely used in recent years, including the study of physical activity. The meta-analysis offers a means of reducing large quantities of studies to underlying principles. We used a tutorial as an example of a meta-analysis to illustrate the various steps. Refinements in technique continue to be made regarding the choice of the standard deviation to be used in calculating an effect size, the weighting of effect sizes for sample bias, the test for outliers, and the statistical procedures that can be used for the analysis.

 Check Your Understanding

Select a possible problem (e.g., gender differences in running speed, effects of weight training on males and females, or influence of training at 60% of $\dot{V}O_2$max vs. 80% of $\dot{V}O_2$max). Find five studies that compare the characteristics you select (e.g., males and females). Make sure each study has the means and standard deviations for the variables of interest. Calculate the ES for each study and correct it for bias. Calculate the average ES for the five studies and their pooled standard deviations. Interpret this finding.

APPENDIX

Sample Coding Booklet for a Meta–Analysis of Sport Expertise

The following section provides a detailed account of the procedures used to code the 92 characteristics outlined for each paper of the meta-analysis in the area of expertise in sport.

Step 1

Choosing Appropriate Papers

This review is interested in any and all research which investigates expertise in sport using some form of between-group (expert-novice) comparison and addressing it using a motor behaviour approach.

Each paper must provide the means and standard deviations for each of the performance measures listed so comparisons on the basis of effect sizes can be calculated and compared to other like papers. In other words, all papers/research in this review must be of a database format.

Step 2

Providing Descriptive Information About Paper

Column 1: Article number

Each paper chosen for inclusion in analysis should be given a unique number code, and an up-to-date list of these should be kept in Appendix 1: Complete List of Articles used in this analysis.

Column 2: Year completed

Column 3: Is the research (1) published or (0) unpublished?

Column 4: Source information:

A. If published, is it from a
   - (2) refereed journal?
   - (1) nonrefereed journal?
   - (0) conference proceedings?

B. If unpublished, is it from a
   - (2) PhD dissertation?
   - (1) masters thesis?
   - (0) unpublished manuscript?

Column 5: If published, where did the research originate?

- (4) Sport science journal
- (3) Movement science journal
- (2) Mainstream psychology journal
- (1) Other source
- (0) Not applicable

Column 6: If published, name of journal

Keep a list of the journals which have been coded, i.e., 1 to 1,000, where "0" denotes the "not-applicable" option as in the case of unpublished work. This list should be kept up-to-date and included in Appendix 2.

Column 7: Affiliation

This column includes a coding for where the specific research was done (i.e., which university, which lab, which particular group of researchers). A list of the affiliations should be coded, i.e., 1 to 1,000 and included in Appendix 3.

Our thanks to Sheri Parks from the Department of Human Movement Studies, University of Queensland, Brisbane, Australia, for the use of her coding booklet.

Column 8: Internal validity ranked on a scale of

(2) Strong

(1) Moderate

(0) Weak

This is developed from the following 6 point checklist. Refer to Appendix 4 for further explanation of the rating scale for internal validity used in this analysis.

1. Did this experiment include a control group? **Y/N**

2. Did the experiment use randomization techniques to control for the following threats to internal validity?

    (2a) History and maturation—by random placement or matched pairing of subjects into each of a control and experimental group? **Y/N**

    (2b) Order effects/learning—by random ordering/presentation of the tasks? **Y/N**

3. Did the experiment establish appropriate instrumentation (or test reliability/psychometrics)? **Y/N**

4. Was the subject retention/dropout rate limited? **Y/N**

5. Were the subjects unaware of the purposes and intentions of this experiment? **Y/N**

    total yes 5-6 - strong

    total yes 2-3-4 = moderate

    total yes 0-1 - weak

Step 3

Providing Information About the Type of Sport/Area of Expertise

Column 9: Type of sport (area of expertise) studied

Keep a list of the sports/activities that have been coded, i.e., 1 to 1,000 in Appendix 5.

Column 10: Classification of sport/activity

Which cell from Higgin's 8 cell model does each sport/activity fit?

(Nature of environment (open vs. closed) * Body stability * Body transport)

Refer to Appendix 6 for further explanation of the categorizing of sports scale used in this analysis.

Column 11: Is it a (1) team sport or a (0) individual/dual sport?

Column 12: Type of motor skills involved in sport or activity:

(2) gross motor skills,

(1) fine motor skills,

(0) a combination of both gross and fine motor skills.

Step 4

Providing Information About the Task(s) Performed

Column 13: How many tasks are involved in study?

This involves counting the number of experimental tasks identified in the experiment. Many experiments will keep the same subjects and have them undergo a series of different tasks. This is acceptable, as long as the same subjects are not "reused," so to speak, in completely different research sources, as previously stated in notes for Column 4.

Column 14: Type of task

Itemize all tasks in studies, and try to group "like tasks" within a similar range of numbers, i.e., all perceptual tasks are identified by numbers 1-10, or all decision-making tasks should be identified by numbers 15-25, etc. A list of these coded tasks should be included in Appendix 7.

Column 15: Levels/conditions of the independent measure for each task

The independent measure can be defined as the variable of interest, or the part of the experiment which the researcher is manipulating (i.e., blocks of practice, occlusion condition, etc.). This can also be referred to as the experimental or treatment variable.

Column 16: Levels/conditions of the dependent measure for each task

The dependent measure can be defined as the particular performance measures used in the experiment (i.e., reaction time, error scores, etc.). This can also be considered the effect of the independent variable or the yield of the experiment.

Column 17: Scoring direction for task

Where:

(1) Higher score is better, lower is worse (i.e., performance scores)

(0) Lower score is better, higher score is worse (i.e., error scores).

Step 5

Providing Information About the Type of Measures Used in Each Task

Column 18: Ecological validity ranked on a scale of

(2) strong (total ≥ 7)

(1) moderate (total 4-6)

(0) weak (total ≤ 3)

As developed from the following 9-point checklist. Refer to Appendix 8 for further explanation of the rating scale for ecological validity used in this analysis.

1. Is the **action** involved in performing the task . . . that of the real-world sporting situation?

   (a) exactly the same as +3

   (b) somewhat the same as +2

   (c) nothing like +1

   (d) not applicable 0

2. Is the **perceptual display** offered in performing the task . . . that of the real-world sporting situation?

   (a) exactly the same as +3

   (b) somewhat the same as +2

   (c) nothing like +1

   (d) not applicable 0

3. Are the **time constraints** involved in performing the task (e.g., preparation time, decision time, performance time, etc.) . . . that of the real-world sporting situation?

   (a) exactly the same as +3

   (b) somewhat the same as +2

   (c) nothing like +1

   (d) not applicable 0

Column 19: Validity of measures ranked on a scale of

(4) Strong

(3) Moderate

(2) Weak

(1) Not mentioned or can't be interpreted on the basis of the information provided in the source

(0) If Column 20 reliability is rated as weak or not mentioned in study (1), rate validity as 0 in this column

Column 20: Reliability of measures ranked on a scale of

(2) Strong

(1) Moderate

(0) Weak

Column 21: Were the statistics & statistical procedures/analyses used appropriate, as rated on the following scale:

(2) appropriate,

(1) all right/adequate,

(0) not appropriate

Column 22: Is it a (1) lab–based or (0) field–based assessment/report?

Column 23: Is the action (1) Natural or (0) Contrived?

Column 24: Does the task duplicate normal time constraints? (1) Yes or (0) No

Column 25: If a visual display is used, is it

(2) Static?

(1) Dynamic?

(0) not applicable?

Column 26: If a visual display is used, are the stimuli

(2) task specific?

(1) alpha numeric?

(0) not applicable?

Column 27: If a visual display is used, how well does it mimic the natural situation across all modalities?

(3) Strong

(2) Moderate

(1) Weak

(0) Not applicable

Step 6

Providing Information About the Experimental Group of Subjects

Column 28: Group number code

Where groups can be one of the following:

(6) competitive at an international or Olympic level;

(5) Competitive at a national level;

(4) Competitive at a state/regional level:

(3) Participating in the sport at a recreational intramural/local level;

(2) Athletes competitive in sports other than the one of interest;

(1) Nonathletes

Column 29: Quality of definition of the group: (expert, elite, skilled, experienced, etc.)

(2) Well defined,

(1) Not enough information provided,

(0) Not defined.

Column 30: Confidence rating in performance selection:

(2) High

(1) Average

(0) Low

Column 31: How was this level determined?

(3) Previous performance record

(2) Coach's determination

(1) Other criteria

(0) Not mentioned

Column 32: Total number of subjects in group

Column 33: Gender of subjects:

(3) All Males

(2) All Females

(1) Mixed

(0) Not Stated

Column 34: Mean age of sample used in group:

(5) > 30

(4) 20-29

(3) 16-19

(2) 13-15

(1) < 12

(0) Not stated

Column 35: Mean number of years' experience with sport:

(5) > 10

(4) 7-10

(3) 4-6

(2) 2-3

(1) < 2

(0) Not stated

Column 36: Status of subjects:

(2) Paid

(1) Unpaid

(0) Not stated

Column 37: Previous experience with task:

(2) Familiar

(1) New/Novel

(0) Not stated

Column 38: Mean group performance score on task

Column 39: Group standard deviation on task

Step 7

Providing Information About the CONTROL Group of Subjects

Column 40: Group number code

Where groups can be one of the following:

(6) Competitive at an international or Olympic level

(5) Competitive at a national level

(4) Competitive at a state/regional level

(3) participating in the sport at a recreational intramural/local level

(2) Athletes competitive in sports other than the one of interest

(1) Nonathletes

Column 41: Quality of definition of the group (expert, elite, skilled, experienced, etc.)

(2) Well defined

(1) Not enough information provided

(0) Not defined

Column 42: Confidence rating in performance selection:

(2) High

(1) Average

(0) Low

Column 43: How was this level determined?

(3) Previous performance Record,

(2) coach's determination,

(1) other criteria,

(0) not mentioned

Column 44: Total number of subjects in group

Column 45: Gender of Subjects

(3) All males

(2) All females

(1) Mixed

(0) Not stated

Column 46: Mean age of sample used in group:

(5) > 30

(4) 20-19

(3) 16-19

(2) 13-15

(1) < 12

(0) Not stated

Column 47 : Mean number of years experience with sport:

(5) > 10

(4) 7-10

(3) 4-6

(2) 2-3

(1) < 2

(0) Not stated

Column 48: Status of subjects:

(2) Paid

(1) Unpaid

(0) Not stated

Column 49: Previous experience with task:

(2) Familiar

(1) New/novel

(0) Not stated

Column 50: Mean group performance score on task

Column 51: Group standard deviation on task

Step 8

Providing Information About the Intermediate Group of Subjects

Column 52: Group number code

Where groups can be one of the following:
(6) Competitive at an international or Olympic level
(5) Competitive at a national level
(4) Competitive at a state/regional level
(3) Participating in the sport at a recreational intramural/local level
(2) Athletes competitive in sports other than the one of interest
(1) Nonathletes

Column 53: Quality of definition of the group (expert, elite, skilled, experienced, etc.)

(2) Well defined
(1) Not enough information provided
(0) Not defined

Column 54: Confidence rating in performance selection

(2) High
(1) Average
(0) Low

This column attempts to address the following questions: Are these groups the best at this level? Are they only moderately competitive at this level, or do they lose first round at the Olympics, for example?

Column 55: How was this level determined?

(3) Previous performance record
(2) Coach's determination
(1) Other criteria
(0) Not mentioned

Column 56: Total number of subjects in group

Column 57: Gender of subjects:

(3) All males
(2) All females
(1) Mixed
(0) Not stated

Column 58: Mean age of sample used in group:

(5) > 30
(4) 20-29
(3) 16-19
(2) 13-15
(1) < 12
(0) Not stated

Column 59: Mean number of years' experience with sport:

(5) > 10
(4) 7-10
(3) 4-6
(2) 2-3
(1) < 2
(0) Not stated

Column 60: Status of subjects:

(2) Paid
(1) Unpaid
(0) Not stated

Column 61: Previous experience with task:

(2) Familiar
(1) New/novel
(0) Not stated

Column 62: Mean group performance score on task

Column 63: Group standard deviation on task

Step 9

Providing Information About Any Other Group of Subjects Included in Study

Column 64: Group number code

Where groups can be one of the following:

(6) Competitive at an international or Olympic level

(5) Competitive at a national level

(4) Competitive at a state/regional level

(3) Participating in the sport at a recreational intramural/local level

(2) Athletes competitive in sports other than the one of interest

(1) Nonathletes

Column 65: Quality of definition of the group (expert, elite, skilled, experienced, etc.):

(2) Well defined

(1) Not enough information provided

(0) Not defined

Column 66: Confidence rating in performance selection:

(2) High

(1) Average

(0) Low

This column attempts to address the following questions: Are these groups the best at this level? Are they only moderately competitive at this level, or do they lose first round at the Olympics, for example?

Column 67: How was this level determined?

(3) Previous performance Record

(2) Coach's determination

(1) Other criteria

(0) Not mentioned

Column 68: Total number of subjects in group

Column 69: Gender of subjects:

(3) All males

(2) All females

(1) Mixed

(0) Not stated

Column 70: Mean age of sample used in group:

(5) > 30

(4) 20-29

(3) 16-19

(2) 13-15

(1) < 12

(0) Not stated

Column 71: Mean number of years' experience with sport:

(5) > 10

(4) 7-10

(3) 4-6

(2) 2-3

(1) < 2

(0) Not stated

Column 72: Status of subjects

(2) Paid

(1) Unpaid

(0) Not stated

Column 73: Previous experience with task:

(2) Familiar

(1) New/novel

(0) Not stated

Column 74: Mean group performance score on task

Column 75: Group standard deviation on task

Step 10

Calculation of Effect Sizes & Standard Deviations

Refer to Appendix 12 for further explanation of the calculations used in this analysis.

Column 76: Experimental vs. control–effect size corrected for bias

Column 77: Experimental vs. control–variance of effect size

Column 78: Experimental vs. control–weighted effect size (inverse variance × corrected E.S)

Column 79: Experimental vs. intermediate–effect size corrected for bias

Column 80: Experimental vs. intermediate–variance of effect size

Column 81: Experimental vs. intermediate–weighted effect size (inverse variance × corrected E.S)

Column 82: Experimental vs. other–effect corrected for bias

Column 83: Experimental vs. other–variance of effect size

Column 84: Experimental vs. other–weighted effect size (inverse variance × corrected E.S)

Column 85: Control vs. intermediate–effect size corrected for bias

Column 86: Control vs. intermediate–variance of effect size

Column 87: Control vs. intermediate–weighted effect size (inverse variance × corrected E.S)

Column 88: Control vs. other–effect size corrected for bias

Column 89: Control vs. other–variance of effect size

Column 90: Control vs. other–weighted effect size (inverse variance × orrected E.S)

Column 91: Intermediate vs. other–effect size corrected for bias

Column 92: Intermediate vs. other–variance of effect size

Column 93: Intermediate vs. other–weighted effect size (inverse variance × corrected E.S)

CHAPTER **15**

Descriptive Research

Dear Professors of Research Methods:

One thing that really ticks me off about
survey research is the use of form letters.
I don't think people will respond candidly
when they are treated so impersonally. What
do you think?

Sincerely,
Likert Skaal

Dear _____:

Thank you for your letter. Opinions from knowledgeable
persons such as you are greatly appreciated. You can
be sure we will give your problem full consideration.
Have a nice day.

Candidly yours,
PRM

Descriptive research is a study of status and is widely used in education and the behavioral sciences. Its value is based on the premise that problems can be solved and practices improved through objective and thorough observation, analysis, and description. Several techniques or methods of problem solving fall into the category of descriptive research.

The most common descriptive research method is the survey, which includes **questionnaires**, personal **interviews**, phone **surveys**, and normative surveys. Developmental research is also descriptive. Through **cross-sectional** and **longitudinal studies**, researchers investigate the interaction of growth and maturation and of learning and performance variables. The **case study** is descriptive research that is widely used in a number of fields. A type of case study is the **job analysis**. Observational research and correlational studies constitute other forms of descriptive research. Through observational research one obtains quantitative and qualitative data about people and situations. Correlational studies determine and analyze relationships between variables as well as generate predictions. This chapter discusses some characteristics and basic procedures of the various types of descriptive research.

The survey is generally broad in scope. The researcher usually seeks to determine present practices (or opinions) of a specified population. The survey is used in education, psychology, sociology, and physical activity. The questionnaire, the Delphi method, the personal interview, and the normative survey are the main types of surveys.

Four Survey Techniques

The Questionnaire

Determining the Objectives

The Questionnaire

The questionnaire and the interview are the same except for the method of questioning. The proce-

---

descriptive research — Type of research concerned with status, including techniques such as surveys, case studies, and developmental research.

questionnaire — Type of paper-and-pencil survey used in descriptive research in which information is obtained by asking subjects to respond to questions rather than by observing their behavior.

interview — Survey technique similar to the questionnaire except that subjects are questioned and respond verbally rather than in writing.

survey — Technique of descriptive research that seeks to determine present practices or opinions of a specified population; can take the form of a questionnaire, interview, or normative survey.

cross–sectional study — Method of research in which samples of subjects from different age groups are selected in order to assess the effects of maturation.

longitudinal study — Research in which the same subjects are studied over a period of years.

case study — Form of descriptive research in which a single case is studied in depth to reach a greater understanding about other similar cases.

job analysis — Type of case study that determines the nature of a particular job and the types of training, preparation, skills, and attitudes necessary for success in the job.

dures for developing questionnaire and interview items are similar. Consequently, much of the discussion regarding the steps in the construction of the questionnaire also pertains to the interview.

Researchers use the questionnaire to obtain information by asking subjects to respond to questions rather than by observing their behavior. The obvious limitation to the questionnaire is that the results consist simply of what people say they do or what they say they believe or like or dislike. However, certain information can be obtained only in this manner, and so it is imperative that the questionnaire is planned and prepared carefully to ensure the most valid results. There are eight steps in the survey research process, and we discuss each in this section.

Determining the Objectives

This step may seem too obvious to mention, yet countless questionnaires have been prepared without clearly defined objectives. In fact, poor planning may account for the low esteem in which survey research is sometimes held. The investigator must have a clear understanding as to what information is needed and how each item will be analyzed. As with any research, the analysis is determined in the planning phase of the study, not after the data have been gathered.

The researcher must decide on the questionnaire's specific purposes: What information is wanted? How will the responses be analyzed? Will they merely be described by listing the percentages of subjects who responded in certain ways, or will the responses of one group be compared with those of another?

Thus, one of the most common mistakes made in constructing a questionnaire is not specifying the variables to be analyzed. In some cases, when investigators fail to list the variables, they ask questions unrelated to the objectives. In other cases, the investigator forgets to ask pertinent questions. For example, in a survey of curricular offerings in physical education, if one objective is to compare the offerings on the basis of how physical education is scheduled, investigators must ask respondents about the scheduling. If male teachers are to be compared with female teachers, then gender must be indicated, and so on. What is to be analyzed must be made clear.

Delimiting the Sample

Most researchers who use questionnaires have in mind a specific population to be sampled. Obviously, the subjects selected must be the ones who have the answers to the questions. In other words, the investigator must know who can supply what information. If information about policy decisions is desired, the subjects should be those involved in making such decisions.

Sometimes the source used in selecting the sample is inadequate. For example, some professional associations are made up of teachers, administrators, professors, and other allied professional workers. Thus, this association's membership is not a good choice as subjects for a study that is geared only for public school teachers. Unless there is some screening mechanism as to place of employment, many incomplete questionnaires will be returned because the questions were not applicable.

The representativeness of the sample is an important consideration. Stratified random sampling, as discussed in chapter 6, is sometimes used. In a questionnaire surveying the recreational preferences of a university student body, the sample should reflect the proportion of students at the different class levels. Thus, if 35% of the students are freshmen, 30% are sophomores, 20% are juniors, and 15% are seniors, then the sample should be selected according to those percentages. Similarly, if a researcher is studying school program offerings and 60% of the schools in the state have fewer than 200 students enrolled, then 60% of the sample should be from such schools.

The selection of the sample should be based on the variables specified to be studied. Certainly, this affects the generalizability of the results. If an investigator specifies that the study deals with just one sex, one educational level, or one institution, and so on, then the population is narrowly defined, and it may be easy to select a representative sample of that specific population. However, the generalizations that can be made from the results are also restricted to that specific population. On the other hand, if the researcher is aiming the questionnaire at all of a specific population (e.g., all athletic directors or all fitness instructors), then the generalizability is enhanced, but the sampling procedures become more difficult. The representativeness of the sample is more important than size.

Sample size is important from two standpoints: (a) for adequacy in representing a population and (b) for practical considerations of time and cost. Certain formulas can be used to determine adequacy of sample size (Vockell, 1983, pp. 111-118). These formulas involve probability levels and the amount of sampling error deemed acceptable. The practical considerations of time and cost need attention in the planning phase of the study. Surprisingly, students often ignore these considerations until they are forced to sit down with a calculator and tabulate the costs of printing, initial mailing (which includes self-addressed, stamped return envelopes), follow-ups, scoring, and data analysis. Sometimes the costs are so substantial that a sponsoring agency or grant must be found to subsidize the study, or else the project must be narrowed or abandoned entirely. Time is also important with regard to the variability of subjects, possible seasonal influences, and various deadlines.

Constructing the Questionnaire

The notion that constructing a questionnaire is easy is a fallacy. Questions are not simply "thought up." Anyone who prepares a questionnaire and asks someone to read it soon discovers that it is not such an easy task after all. Those questions that were so clear and concise to the writer may be confusing and ambiguous to the respondent.

One of the most valuable guidelines for writing questions is to continually ask yourself what specific objective this question is measuring. Then ask how you are going to analyze the response. While you are writing questions, it is a good idea to prepare a blank table that includes the categories of responses, comparisons, and other breakdowns of data analysis so that you can readily determine exactly how each item will be handled and how each will contribute to the objectives of the study. Next, you must select the format for the questions, some examples of which follow.

Writing Open-Ended Questions. **Open-ended questions**, such as "How do you like your job?" or "What aspects of your job do you like?" may be the easiest for the investigator to write. Such questions allow the respondent considerable latitude to express feelings and to expand on ideas. However, the several drawbacks to open-ended questions usually make them less desirable than closed questions. For example, most respondents do not like open-ended questions. For

that matter, most people do not like questionnaires because they feel they are encroachments on their time. Also, open-ended questions require more time to answer than closed questions. Another drawback is the limited control as to the nature of the response: The respondent often rambles and strays from the question. Also, such responses are difficult to synthesize and to group into categories.

Sometimes open-ended questions are used to construct closed questions. Student evaluations, or questionnaires, are often developed by having students list all the things they like and dislike about a course. From such lists, closed questions are constructed by categorizing the open-question responses.

Writing Closed Questions. **Closed questions** come in a variety of forms (some of the measurement scales were covered in chapter 11.) A few of the more commonly used closed questions are rankings, scaled items, and categorical responses.

A **ranking** forces the subject to place responses in a rank order according to some criterion. As a result, value judgments are made, and the rankings can be summed and analyzed quantitatively. An example of a rank-order response question follows.

Rank the following activities with regard to how you like to spend leisure time. Use number 1-5, with 1 being the most preferred and 5 the least preferred.

____ Reading

____ Watching television

____ Arts and crafts

____ Vigorous sports such as tennis and racquetball

____ Mild exercise activity such as walking

 Scaled items are one of the most commonly used types of closed questions. Subjects are asked to indicate the strength of their

---

open-ended question — Category of question in questionnaires and interviews that allows the respondent considerable latitude to express feelings and to expand on ideas.

closed question — Category of question found in questionnaires or interviews that requires a specific response and that often takes the form of rankings, scaled items, and categorical responses.

ranking — Type of closed question that forces the subject to place responses in a rank order according to some criterion.

scaled item — Type of closed question that requires subjects to indicate the strength of their agreement or disagreement with some statement or the relative frequency of some behavior.

agreement or disagreement with some statement or to cite the relative frequency of some behavior, as in the following example:

Indicate the frequency with which you are involved in committee meetings and assignments during the academic year.

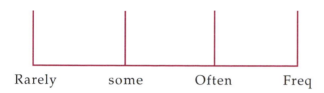

Rarely   some   Often   Freq

The Likert scale is a scale with 3 to 9 responses, in which there is an assumption of equal intervals between responses:

In a required physical education program, students should be required to take at least one dance class.

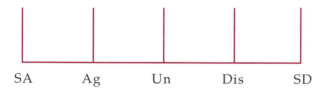

SA   Ag   Un   Dis   SD

The difference between "strongly agree" and "agree" is considered equivalent to the difference between "disagree" and "strongly disagree." Different response words can be used in scaled responses, such as "excellent," "good," "fair," "poor," "very poor," "very important," "important," "not very important," "of no importance," and so on.

Categorical responses offer the subject only two choices. Usually, the responses are "yes" and "no" or "true" and "false." An obvious limitation of categorical responses is the lack of other options such as "sometimes" or "it depends." Categorical responses do not require as much time to administer as scaled responses but also do not provide as much information as to the subject's degree of agreement or frequency of behavior.

Sometimes questions in questionnaires are keyed to the responses of other items. For example, a question might ask whether the respondent's institution offers a doctoral degree. If the subject answered "yes," then he or she would be directed to answer subsequent questions about the doctoral program. If the subject answered "no," the subject would be directed either to stop or to move on to the next section.

Borg and Gall (1989) have offered the following rules for the construction of questionnaire items:

- The items must be clearly worded so that the items mean the same to all respondents. Avoid words that have no precise meaning, such as "usually," "most," and "generally."
- Use short questions rather than long questions because they are easier to understand.
- Do not use items that have two or more separate ideas in the same question; for example, "Although everyone should learn how to swim, passing a swimming test should not be a requirement for graduation from college." This item cannot really be answered because a person might agree with the first part of the sentence but not the last or vice versa. Another example is, "Does your department require an entrance examination for master's and doctoral students?" This is confusing because the department may have such an examination for doctoral students but not for master's students or vice versa. If the response choices are only "yes" and "no," a "no" response would indicate no examination for either program, and a "yes" response would mean exams for both. This should be divided into two questions.
- Avoid using negative items such as "Physical education should not be taught by coaches." Negative items are often confusing, and the negative word is sometimes overlooked, causing the individual to answer in exactly the opposite way.
- Avoid technical language and jargon. Attempt to achieve clarity and the same meaning for everyone.
- Be careful that you do not bias the answer or lead the respondent to answer in a certain way. Sometimes questions can be stated in such a way that the person knows what is the

---

 categorical response — Type of closed question that offers the subject only two responses, such as "yes" or "no."

 Rules for constructing questionnaire items

"right" response. For example, you would know what response was expected if you encountered the question "Because teachers work so hard, shouldn't they receive higher salaries?" The same advice applies to the problem of threatening questions. If the respondent perceives certain items to be threatening, he or she will probably not return the questionnaire. A questionnaire on grading practices, for example, may be viewed as threatening because poor grading practices would indicate that the teachers are not doing a good job. Thus, a teacher who feels threatened either may not return the questionnaire or may give responses that seem to be "right answers."

Results of experiments on surveys show that very minor changes in wording, or even ordering of the alternatives, can cause differences in responses. Don Dillman, a recognized authority on the survey method, reported results of experiments on the effects of question form and survey mode on survey results at a seminar at Washington State University. As an illustration of some of the variations studied, when students were asked how many hours they studied per day, 70% said more than 2.5 hours, but when the same question was asked another way, only 23% indicated more than 2.5 hours.

Considering Appearance and Design.   Finally, the entire appearance and format of the questionnaire can have a significant bearing on the return rate. Questionnaires that appear to be poorly organized and prepared are likely to be "filed" in the wastebasket. Remember, many people have negative attitudes toward questionnaires, so anything that the researcher can do to overcome this negative attitude will enhance the likelihood of the questionnaire being answered. Some of the suggestions in this regard are merely cosmetic, such as the use of colored paper or an artistic design. Even little things, such as having dotted lines from the questionnaire item to the response options or grouping related items together, may pay big dividends.

The questionnaire should provide the name and address of the investigator. It is especially important that the instructions for answering the questions are clear and complete and that examples are provided for any items that are anticipated as being difficult to understand.

The first few questions should be easy to answer; the respondent is more likely to start answering easy questions and is also more apt to complete the questionnaire once he or she is committed. A poor strategy is to begin with questions that require considerable thought or time to gather information. In this regard, every effort should be made to make difficult questions as convenient to answer as possible. For example, questions that ask for enrollment figures, size of faculty, number of graduate assistants, and so on can often ask for responses in ranges (e.g., 1-10, 11-20, 21-30). First, you will probably group the responses for analysis purposes anyway. Second, the respondent can often answer range-type questions without having to consult the records or at least can supply the answers more quickly. An even more basic question to ask yourself is, Do I really need that information? or Does it pertain to my objectives? Unfortunately, some investigators simply ask for information off the top of their heads with no consideration as to the time required to supply the answer or as to whether the information is relevant.

A general rule is that short questionnaires are more effective than long ones. According to Borg and Gall (1989), an analysis of 98 questionnaire studies showed that, on average, each page added to a questionnaire reduced the number of returns by 0.5%. Because many people are prejudiced against questionnaires, the cover letter (which will be discussed later) and the size and appearance of the questionnaire are crucial. A lengthy questionnaire requiring voluminous information will very likely be put aside until later if not discarded immediately.

Conducting the Pilot Study

A **pilot study** is recommended for any type of research but is imperative with a survey. Actually, the designer of a questionnaire may be well advised to do two pilot studies. The first trial run consists simply of asking a few colleagues or acquaintances to read over the questionnaire. These people can provide valuable critiques about the questionnaire format, content, expression and importance of items, and whether questions should be added or deleted.

After revising the questionnaire in accordance with the criticisms obtained in the first trial run, respondents are selected who are a part of the intended population for the second pilot study. The questionnaire is administered, and the results are

---

pilot study — A preliminary study done to validate the research methodology.

subjected to item analysis (discussed in chapter 11). In some questionnaires, correlations may be run between scores on each item and the whole test to see whether the items are measuring what they are intended to measure. Responses are always examined to determine whether the items seem clear and appropriate. First, questions that are answered the same way by all respondents need to be evaluated; they probably lack discrimination. Unexpected responses may indicate that the questions are poorly worded. Some rewording and other changes might also be necessary if the subjects, who might be sensitive to some questions, do not respond to them. Furthermore, the pilot study will determine whether the instructions are adequate.

A trial run of the analysis of results should always be accomplished in the pilot study. The researcher can see whether the items can be analyzed in a meaningful way and then ascertain whether some changes may be warranted for easier analysis. This is one of the most profitable outcomes of the pilot study. Of course, if substantial changes are mandated by the results of the pilot study, another pilot study is recommended to determine whether the questionnaire is ready for initial mailing.

Writing the Cover Letter

Unquestionably, the success of the initial mailing depends largely on the effectiveness of the **cover letter** that accompanies the questionnaire. If it can explain the purposes and importance of the survey in a succinct and professional manner (and if the purposes are worthy of study), the respondent will likely become interested in the problem and will be inclined to cooperate.

An effective cover letter should also assure respondents that their privacy and anonymity will be maintained. Furthermore, the cover letter should make an appeal to the importance of the respondent's cooperation. Some use of subtle flattery may be desirable with reference to the respondent's professional status and the importance of his or her response. This must be done tactfully, however, and used only when appropriate. In this situation, the person's name and address should appear on the cover letter. A word processor should be used so that the letters look as if they were individually typed. It is insulting to try to convince persons that they have been handpicked for their expertise and valued opinions when the letters are addressed "Dear Occupant."

If the survey is endorsed by recognized agencies, associations, or institutions, specify this in the cover letter. If possible, use the organization's or institution's stationery. Respondents will be much more cooperative if some respected person or organization is supporting the study. Also acknowledge whether financial support is being given and by whom. Identify yourself by name and position. If the study is part of your thesis or dissertation, give your advisor's name. Sometimes it is advantageous if the department chairperson or the dean of the college signs the letter. To increase the response rate, contact subjects by letter, card, or telephone, asking for their participation in the survey. Provided the purposes of the study are worthwhile, offering the respondent a summary of the results is usually effective at this time. Before making this offer, give ample consideration to how much work and money such a summary will entail. However, if you do offer to provide a summary, be sure that you follow through with your promise.

Because a questionnaire imposes on a person's time, strategies involving rewards and incentives are sometimes used in an effort to amuse or involve the respondent. Some questionnaires include money (perhaps a dollar) as a token of appreciation. This may appeal to a person's integrity and evoke cooperation. Then again, you may just be out a dollar. The disadvantage is that inflation plays havoc with the effects of such rewards. A quarter may have been effective years ago, whereas one or more dollars may be required to elicit the same "sense of guilt" for not responding. Research results concerning the effectiveness of monetary incentives have been mixed. Denton and Tsai (1991) compared several sizes of monetary incentives and a raffle for a professional journal and failed to find significant benefits.

The cover letter should request that the questionnaire be returned by a certain date. (This information should also be specified on the questionnaire.) When establishing the date for the return of data, consider such things as the respondent's schedule of responsibilities, vacations, and so forth. Be reasonable in the time you allow the person to respond; however, with questionnaires it is advisable not to give the respondent too much time because of the tendency to put it aside and later forget it. One week is ample time for the respondent to answer (in addition to the mailing time).

---

cover letter — The letter attached to a survey that explains the purposes and importance of the survey.

The appearance of the cover letter is just as important as the appearance of the questionnaire. Grammatical errors, misspelled words, and improper spacing and format give the respondent the impression that the author does not attach much importance to details and that the study will probably be poorly done.

Researchers have tried a number of subtle and tactful approaches to establish rapport with the respondent. Some have tried a very solemn appeal to the monumental importance of the survey, some have attempted casual humor, and others have tried a folksy approach. Obviously, the success of any approach depends on the skill of the writer and the receptiveness of the reader. Any of these attempts can backfire.

A number of years ago, one of this book's authors (Nelson) received from the department head a note to which a letter like this was attached:

Dear Dr. _____

It has been said: "There are two kinds of information, knowing it or knowing where to find it." I asked three men you know, Doctors Eeney, Meeney, and Moe, a certain question and each said: "Sorry. I don't know his name." But they came back with the helpful suggestion--write to you.

Now for the question: What is the name of the person in your department or school who is in charge of your graduate program in physical education? . . .

Cordially yours,

Harry Homespun

The department head answered the letter; then, shortly thereafter, this letter arrived:

Dear Dr. Nelson:

Your good work in administering a graduate program is well known throughout our profession. Even though there are many knotty problems, everyone wants to upgrade the resources for graduate studies. But how? Because of your scholarly approach, my associates Doctors Eeney, Meeney, and Moe suggested that I write to you.

Knowledgeable leaders, like you, tell us of the ever-present struggle between physical education and the cultural lag. . . .

It has been said: "If you want to get something important done, ask a busy person." My associates tell me you are busier than a bird dog in tall grass. They also say that you have a high regard for excellence. . . . If you could find it convenient to return your checked copy on or before May 1, you might help reduce the cultural lag.

Cordially yours,

Harry Homespun

About a month later, another letter arrived:

Dear Dr. Nelson:

You're a great help. Your prompt reply was like a major league catcher, brilliantly fielded and efficiently returned. Many thanks.

Professional people in your position represent a storehouse of knowledge. Consequently, there is additional information which only you can supply. Please go over the enclosed checklist. . . .

Your timely help is appreciated. Your good work has preceded our correspondence. . . .

Keep up the good work.

Cordially yours,

Harry Homespun

We have, of course, omitted the main parts of the letters concerning what was being studied and what the instructions specified, but these parts were generally well done. About a year later another questionnaire arrived with the following cover letter:

Dear Dr. Nelson:

Your excellent leadership in administering graduate programs is well known throughout our profession. Because of your genuine interest in upgrading our mutual field of endeavor, my advisors Doctors Eeney, Meeney, and Moe suggested that I correspond directly with you.

Scholarly graduate administrators and advisors like you often come in contact with the problems of standards. Your considered judgment is solicited in this study to arrive at some common criteria for evaluating graduate programs. . . .

Cordially yours,

Fred Folksy

Then came another letter:

Dear Dr. Nelson:

Your prompt return of the checked statements is greatly appreciated. My advisors Doctors Eeney, Meeney, and Moe were certainly correct when they indicated you would gladly cooperate in this survey.

It has been said: "If you want to get something important done, ask a busy person." My associates tell me that you are busier than a bird dog in tall grass. . . .

If you could find it convenient to return your checked copy . . . you would help us reduce the cultural lag in our profession. . . .

Cordially yours,

Fred Folksy

It is safe to assume that these two graduate students had the same research methods course at the same institution. Most likely, in the discussion of the survey method, some examples of cover letters were given with different approaches. Professors Eeney, Meeney, and Moe would undoubtedly be embarrassed if they knew that the two students had written such nearly identical letters.

In most respects, the cover letters contained the essential information, and the topics were worthwhile. The authors were simply too heavy-handed in their attempts at a down-home approach, and their efforts to flatter the respondent regarding the respondent's expertise lacked subtlety.

Page 322 shows an example of a cover letter for a questionnaire that dealt with a potentially threatening topic. The letter effectively explains to the respondent how confidentiality will be assured. The second cover letter (page 323) focuses on the importance of the topic and on the agencies endorsing the study. It also tactfully appeals to the respondent's ego.

Sending the Questionnaire

The investigator needs to carefully consider the best time for the initial mailing. Such considerations include holidays, vacations, and especially busy times of the year. A self-addressed, stamped envelope should be included. It is almost an insult to expect respondents not only to answer your questionnaire but also to provide an envelope and a stamp to mail it back to you.

Other matters regarding the mailing of the questionnaire, such as establishing the date to be returned, have been covered in previous sections. The initial mailing represents a substantial cost to the sender. Securing a sponsor to underwrite or defray expenses and using bulk-mailing services are important considerations.

Following Up

This should not come as a big shock, but it is unlikely that you will get 100% return on the initial mailing. A follow-up letter is nearly always needed, and this can be done in many different ways. One approach is to wait about 10 days after the initial mailing and then to send a card to all nonrespondents, stressing the importance of their participation. Approximately 10 days after the card, another letter with another copy of the questionnaire and another self-addressed, stamped envelope should be sent to those who have not responded. (This is expensive, of course.) Follow-ups are effective. In a number of cases, the person has forgotten to respond, and a mere reminder will prompt a return. Other nonrespondents who had not planned to return the questionnaire may be influenced by the researcher's efforts in reiterating the significance of the study and the importance of his or her input.

The follow-up letter should be tactful. The person should not be chastised for failing to respond. The best approach is to write as though the person would have responded had it not been for some oversight or mistake by the investigator (for an example of a follow-up letter, see page 324).

Sample Cover Letter #1

Assuring confidentiality

Dear _____

    Your participation in a national survey of perceived leader behavior in physical education is needed. As a doctoral student in physical education at the University of Georgia, I am conducting this study to compare and contrast male and female faculty members' perceptions of their male and female department heads' leader behavior. This institution was randomly selected to take part in this research project. Your department head has already been contacted and expressed willingness to take part in the study. I am now asking randomly selected faculty members from your institution to become involved. Your name was one of those selected to ask to participate by answering the enclosed questionnaires.

    Participation will require approximately 15 minutes of your time to answer both questionnaires that will be used and to fill out an information sheet. The questionnaires and instructions as to how they are to be completed have been included with this letter in the hopes you will agree to be a participant. There is no evaluation intended or implied with this study. The instruments used describe the perceived leader behavior of the administrator. The analysis of the data will be utilized in group mean scores. Following the completion of the survey and the statistical analysis of the data, I will gladly send you a summary of the findings. All data will be dealt with confidentially and no institution or individual taking part in the study will be identified.

    Hopefully, you will find time in your busy schedule to participate in this study. Thank you for your time and participation. I look forward to your early response.

Sincerely,

Kay A. Johnson

Clifford G. Lewis
Major Professor

Enclosures: 5

Reprinted courtesy of C.G. Lewis.

Sample Cover Letter #2

Justifying the topic

Dear _____

    The responsibilities that I have in providing leadership in physical education for a large school district have caused me to give consideration to the approach needed to achieve acceptable objectives of physical fitness in the secondary boys' physical education program.

    Through the cooperation of the San Diego Unified School District, the School of Education and the Physical Education Department of the University of California, Los Angeles, and the Bureau of Health Education, Physical Education and Recreation of the California State Department of Education, I am undertaking a study in the area of physical fitness. Representatives of the President's Council on Physical Fitness have said this information would be most valuable for them also. The purpose of the study is to establish criteria that can be utilized in planning activities in physical education classes for secondary aged boys (12-18) to develop and maintain selected aspects of physical fitness. The selected aspects to be considered are those commonly referred to as cardiorespiratory endurance (stamina), muscular strength and endurance, and flexibility. The information gained will be used in program planning by helping to answer such questions as these: What part of the physical education lesson should be spent on specific fitness activities (such as calisthenics, interval running, weight training, etc.) and what part of the lesson should be spent on sports and games of our culture (such as basketball, volleyball, softball, track, tennis, gymnastics, dance instruction, etc.)? What guidelines should be established in planning the specifics of physical fitness work? What physical fitness activities should be used?

    A committee of exercise physiologists nominated you as a person who is qualified to comment on this topic because of your recognized position as a leader and your research in the area of physical fitness. It would be most appreciated if you would answer the enclosed questions and return them in the envelope provided at your earliest convenience. A summary of the answers will be returned to you.

Sincerely yours,

Physical Education Specialist

Sample Follow-Up Letter

Dear _____

    I sent a questionnaire regarding criteria for planning physical fitness work in physical education classes to you a few weeks ago and have not heard from you. As you can appreciate, it is important that we obtain response from everyone possible inasmuch as only a few select individuals were contacted. Our school district is planning an immediate study and updating of its physical education program based on the results of this study so it is of vital concern.

    The questionnaire was sent during the summer when you may have been away from your office. I have included another copy, however, and it would be most helpful if you could take 30–45 minutes to give your opinions on the information requested.

    Thank you so much for your cooperation.

Sincerely yours,

Physical Education Specialist

This is especially likely when the questionnaire deals with some sensitive area. For example, surveys about program offerings and grading practices are often not returned by schools with inadequate programs and poor grading practices. Thus, the obtained responses are apt to be biased in favor of the better programs and better teachers. Regardless of the nature of the survey, the results from a small return rate (e.g., 10-20%) cannot be given much credibility. People who have a particular interest in the topic being surveyed are more likely to respond than people who are less interested. These respondents are self-selected and the responses are almost invariably biased in ways that are directly related to the purposes of the research (Fowler, 1988). Green (1991) reported that subjects who responded to the initial mailing had more favorable attitudes toward the topic and also had more positive attitudes about themselves than reluctant respondents.

In fact, in most studies in which more than 20% of the questionnaires are not returned, it is recommended that a sample of the non-respondents be surveyed. Of course, this is not easy. If people have ignored the initial mailing and one or two follow-ups, the chances are not good that they will respond to another request, but it is worth a try. The preferred technique is to randomly select a small number (e.g., 5%-10%) of the nonrespondents by using the table of random numbers (this technique is sometimes called "double-dipping"). Then contact is made either by telephone or by a special cover letter (perhaps even via registered mail). After the responses have been obtained, comparisons are made between the answers of the nonrespondents and the answers of the subjects who responded initially. If the responses are similar, you can assume that the nonrespondents are not different from those who replied. If there are differences, then you should either try to get a greater percentage of the nonrespondents or be sure that these differences are noted and discussed in the research report.

To follow up on nonrespondents, one has to know who has not responded. Keeping records of those who have and have not responded may seem to fly in the face of guaranteed anonymity. However, this is not a difficult task. An identifying number written on the questionnaire or return envelope

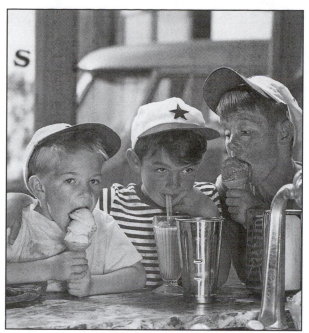

Double dipping might bring in some subjects who might not have responded otherwise.

can be used. Of course, it is recommended that you inform the respondents about the use of the number in your cover letter. You might offer an explanation such as the following:

> Your responses will be strictly confidential. The questionnaire has an identification number for mailing purposes only. With this numbering system, I can check your name off the mailing list when your questionnaire is returned. Your name will never be placed on the questionnaire.

Another approach, which works well, is to send a separate postcard (self-addressed and stamped) with the questionnaire. The card contains an identifying number and is to be mailed back separately when the person returns the questionnaire. The card simply states that the person is sending the questionnaire and therefore there is no need for the researcher to send any more reminders. This procedure assures anonymity and yet informs the researcher that the person has responded.

Analyzing the Results and Preparing the Report

These last two steps are discussed in chapter 19, which deals with the results and discussion sections of the research report. The main consideration here is that the method of analysis should be chosen in the planning phase of the study. Many questionnaires are analyzed merely by tallying the responses to the various items and reporting the percentage of the subjects that answered one way and the percentage that answered another way. Often, not much in the way of meaningful interpretation can be gained. For example, when the researcher states simply that 18% of the respondents strongly agreed with some statement, 29% agreed, 26% disagreed, 17% strongly disagreed, and 10% had no opinion, the reader's reaction may be, "So what?" Questionnaires, as well as all surveys, must be designed and analyzed with the same care and scientific insight as experimental studies.

The Delphi Method

 The **Delphi survey method** uses questionnaires but in a different manner than the typical survey. The Delphi technique uses a series of questionnaires in such a way that the respondents finally reach a consensus about the subject. It is basically a method of using expert opinion to help make decisions about practices, needs, and goals.

The procedures include the selection of the experts, or the informed persons who are to respond to the series of questionnaires. A set of statements or questions is prepared for consideration. The first stage in the Delphi technique, called a **round**, is mostly exploratory. The respondents are asked for their opinions on various issues, goals, and so on. Open-ended questions may be included that allow the subjects to express their views and opinions.

The questionnaire is then revised as a result of the first round and sent to the respondents, asking them to reconsider their answers in light of the analysis of all respondents to the first questionnaire. Subsequent rounds are carried out, and the "experts" are given summaries of previous results and asked to revise their responses if appropriate. Their consensus about the issue is finally achieved through the

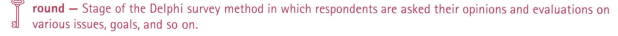

Delphi survey method — Survey technique that uses a series of questionnaires in such a way that the respondents (usually experts) reach a consensus about the subject.

round — Stage of the Delphi survey method in which respondents are asked their opinions and evaluations on various issues, goals, and so on.

series of rounds of analysis and subsequent considered judgments. Anonymity is a prominent feature of the Delphi method, and the consensus of recognized experts in the field provides a viable means of confronting important issues. For example, the Delphi method is used sometimes to determine curricular content for programs, to decide upon the most important objectives of a program, and to agree upon the best approaches to problem solving.

The Personal Interview

As mentioned earlier, the steps for the interview and the questionnaire are basically the same. The focus here is only on the differences.

Preparing for the Interview

The most obvious difference between the questionnaire and the interview is in the gathering of the data. In this respect, the interview is more valid because the responses are apt to be more reliable. Also, there are a much greater percentage of returns.

Subjects should be selected in the same manner as the questionnaire in terms of sampling techniques. Generally, the interview uses smaller samples, especially when a graduate student is doing the survey. Cooperation must be secured by contacting the subjects selected for interviewing. If some of the chosen subjects refuse to be interviewed, the researcher must consider possible bias to the results, as was done with nonrespondents in a questionnaire study.

To effectively conduct an interview takes a great deal of preparation. Graduate students sometimes have the impression that anyone can do it. The same procedures used with the questionnaire are followed in preparing the items, with which the interviewer must be very familiar. The researcher must carefully rehearse the interview techniques. One source of invalidity is that the interviewer tends to improve with experience, and thus the results of earlier interviews may differ from interviews conducted later in the study. A pilot study is very important. The interviewer can make sure the vocabulary level is appropriate and that the questions will be equally meaningful given the ages and educational backgrounds of the subjects who are surveyed.

Training is required in making initial contact and presenting the verbal cover letter by phone. At the meeting, the interviewer must establish rapport and make the person feel at ease. If a tape recorder will be used, permission must be obtained. If a tape recorder will not be used, then the interviewer must have an efficient system of coding the responses without consuming too much time and appearing to be taking dictation. The interviewer must not inject his or her own bias into the conversation and certainly should not argue with the respondent. Although the interview holds many advantages over the questionnaire with regard to the flexibility of the questioning, there is also the danger of straying from the questions and getting off the subject. The interviewer must tactfully keep the respondent from rambling, and this requires skill.

The key to getting good information is to ask good questions. We have all been impressed by watching really good interviewers on television. What makes them good? There is no single answer. Certainly, the interviewer's personality is a factor, but good interviewers have different personalities. Some are even rather obnoxious. Some are friendly and supportive with the interviewees, some seem to badger the people, and some play the devil's advocate in their questioning. Good interviewers do not ask yes-or-no questions, they do not ask multiple questions in a single question, and they try to avoid inserting their own points of view. Merriam (1988) defined four major categories of questions: hypothetical, devil's advocate, ideal position, and interpretive. Here are some examples of each:

- **Hypothetical.** "Let's suppose this is my first day of student teaching. What would it be like?"
- **Devil's advocate.** "Some people say that professional educational courses are of little value for the student teaching experience. What would you say to them?"
- **Ideal position.** "What do you think the ideal student teaching preparation program should be like?"
- **Interpretive.** "Would you say that the student teaching experience is different from what you expected?"

You may recognize these approaches from interviews you have seen on television.

The interview has the following advantages over the questionnaire:

- The interview is more adaptable. Questions can be rephrased and clarification can be sought through follow-up questions.

 Advantages of interviews over questionnaires

- The interview is more versatile with regard to the personality and receptiveness of the respondent.
- The interviewer can observe how the person responds and can thus achieve greater insight into the sensitivity of the topic and the intensity of feelings from the respondent. This can add considerably to the validity of the results as it is one of the greatest threats to validity in questionnaire studies.
- Because each person is contacted before the interview, interviews have a greater rate of return. Moreover, people tend to be more willing to talk than to fill out a questionnaire. A certain amount of ego is involved because a person who is interviewed feels more flattered than one who only receives a list of questions.

Conducting a Telephone Interview

Interviewing by telephone is becoming more prevalent. Some of the advantages of telephone interviewing over face-to-face interviewing follow:

- Telephone interviewing is less expensive than traveling to visit respondents, especially when researchers use WATS lines. One study (Graves & Kahn, 1979) reported that telephone interviews cost half as much as personal interviews.
- The interviewer can work from a central location, which facilitates the monitoring and the quality control of the interviews and provides a better opportunity for using computer-assisted interviewing techniques (Borg & Gall, 1989).
- Many people are more easily reached by telephone than by personal visitation.
- The telephone interview enables the researcher to reach a wide geographical area, which is a limitation of the personal interview. This advantage also can increase the validity of the sampling.
- There is some evidence that persons will respond more candidly to sensitive questions over the telephone than in personal interviews, in which the presence of the interviewer may inhibit some responses.

Using the microcomputer in telephone interviewing eases data collection and analysis. For example, the microcomputer displays the questions for the interviewer to ask, and then the interviewer types the subject's responses. Each response triggers the next question, so the interviewer doesn't have to turn pages and is less likely to ask inappropriate questions. Responses are stored for analysis (thus reducing scoring errors), and the stored responses can then be called out for statistical analysis.

An obvious limitation of telephone interviewing is that some people do not have telephones. This needs to be considered in sampling the poor, particularly in inner cities or rural areas. The problem of unlisted numbers can be overcome by using a table of random numbers to select the four numbers after the three-number exchange. You can reach both listed and unlisted numbers by this method. An important source of bias concerns the time when telephone surveys are done. If conducted during the day, the people most likely to be home will be biased toward homemakers, the unemployed, and the retired. Thus, the interviewers usually must work after 5:00 p.m. Also, it is estimated that one third of the people are not home on the initial call, which means call backs are necessary (sometimes as many as 10-12 times!). Dillman (1978) has provided a comprehensive discussion of the relative advantages and disadvantages of the telephone survey.

The Normative Survey

The **normative survey** is not described in most research methods textbooks. As is implied in the name, this method involves establishing norms for abilities, performances, beliefs, and attitudes. A cross-sectional approach is used in that samples of people of different ages, genders, and other classifications are selected and measured. The steps in the normative survey are generally the same as in the questionnaire, the difference being in the manner in which the data are collected. The researcher selects the most appropriate tests to measure the desired performances or abilities, such as the components of physical fitness.

 Advantages of telephone interviews

 Dillman, D.A. (1978). *Mail and telephone survey: The total design method.* New York: Wiley.

 normative survey — Survey method that involves establishing norms for abilities, performances, beliefs, and attitudes.

In any normative survey, it is important that the testing be administered in a rigidly standardized manner. Deviations in the way measurements are taken give meaningless results. The researcher collects and analyzes the data from the survey by some norming method, such as percentiles, T scores, or stanines, and then constructs norms for the different categories of age, sex, and so on.

The American Alliance for Health, Physical Education, Recreation and Dance (AAHPERD) has sponsored several normative surveys. Probably the most notable was the Youth Fitness Test (see AAHPER, 1958), conducted in response to the furor caused by the results of the Kraus-Weber test (Kraus & Hirschland, 1954), which had revealed that American children were inferior to European children in minimum muscular fitness. The Youth Fitness Test was originally given to 8,500 boys and girls in a nationwide sample. Follow-up testing was done in 1965 and 1975.

In the AAHPER normative survey, a committee determined a seven-item motor fitness test battery. The University of Michigan Survey Research Center selected a representative sample of boys and girls in Grades 5-12 and then requested the cooperation of each school. They prepared directions for giving the test items, and selected and trained physical education teachers in various parts of the country to administer and supervise the testing.

In addition, AAHPERD conducted a sport skills testing project, which established norms for skills of boys and girls of different ages in a number of sports. The National Children and Youth Fitness Study (Phase I, 1985; Phase II, 1987) was a normative survey that established norms for a health-related physical fitness test. The test battery included measures of cardiovascular condition (distance run), body composition (skinfolds), the strength and endurance of the abdominal muscles (sit-ups) and the arm and shoulder muscles (pull-ups and modified pull-ups), and the flexibility of the muscles of the posterior thigh and lower back (sit-and-reach).

Sometimes comparisons are made between the norms of different populations. In other studies, the major purpose is simply to establish norms. The primary drawbacks to any normative survey occur in test selection and the standardization of testing procedures. With many tests, there is a danger of generalizing on the basis of the test's results. For example, if one test item (such as pull-ups) is used to measure a particular component (strength), it is possible to apply the score inappropriately and make incorrect generalizations. Pull-ups, for instance, are influenced by body weight and involve primarily the arm and shoulder muscle groups. Strength in other parts of the body is not being assessed. It is incorrect to assume that a person who does well in a pull-up test would also perform well in other strength tests. Yet this assumption is often made.

This question of test selection is important in any type of research. The standardization of testing procedures is essential for establishing norms. However, when a normative survey involves several testers from different parts of the country, this becomes a source of possible measurement error. Published test descriptions simply cannot address all the aspects of test administration and the ways of handling the many problems of interpreting procedures that arise. Extensive training of testers is the answer, but this is often logistically impossible.

Developmental Research

An Overview of Longitudinal and
Cross-Sectional Designs

Four Methodological Problems of
Developmental Research

Unrepresentative Scores

Unclear Semantics

Lack of Reliability

Statistical Problems

Protecting Subjects

Summarizing Developmental Research

Developmental research implies the study of changes in behavior across years. Although much of the developmental research has focused on infancy, childhood, and adolescence, research on senior citizens and even across the total human lifespan is increasingly common.

---

developmental research — Study of changes in behavior across years.

An Overview of Longitudinal and Cross-Sectional Designs

Developmental research focuses on cross-age comparisons. For example, researchers can compare children at ages 6, 8, and 10 on how far they can jump; or, they can compare adults at 45, 55, and 65 on their knowledge of the effects of obesity on life expectancy. Both of these are developmental studies. The major distinction between developmental studies is whether researchers follow the same subjects over time (longitudinal design) or whether they select different subjects at each age level (cross-sectional design).

Longitudinal studies are powerful because the changes in behavior across the time span of interest are within the same subjects. However, longitudinal designs are time consuming. A longitudinal study of children's jumping performance at ages 6, 8, and 10 obviously requires 4 years to complete. That is probably not a wise choice of designs for a master's thesis. Longitudinal designs have additional problems besides the time required to complete them. First, over the several years of the study, some of the subjects are likely to move away when parents change jobs; or school districts may rezone attendance, causing the subjects to be spread out over several schools. In longitudinal studies of senior citizens, some may die over the course of the study. The problem with a loss of subjects is knowing whether the sample characteristics remain the same when subjects are lost. For example, when children are lost from the sample when parents change jobs, is the sample then composed of children of lower socioeconomic levels because the more affluent parents move? Furthermore, if obesity is related to longevity, are older citizens more likely to be less obese and consequently have increased knowledge because the more obese subjects with less knowledge have died? Thus, knowledge about obesity may not be changing from ages 45 to 65; rather, the sample is changing.

Another problem with longitudinal designs is that subjects become increasingly familiar with the test items, and the items may cause changes in behavior. The knowledge inventory on obesity may prompt subjects to seek information about obesity, thus changing their knowledge, attitudes, and behaviors. Therefore, the next time they complete the knowledge inventory, they have gained knowledge. However, this gain of knowledge is the result of having been exposed to the test earlier and might not have occurred without that exposure.

Cross-sectional studies are usually less time consuming to carry out. These studies test several age-groups (e.g., 6, 8, and 10) at the same point in time. Although cross-sectional studies are more time efficient than longitudinal studies, a problem called **cohorts** exists: Are all the age-groups really from the same population (group of cohorts)? Asked another way, are environmental circumstances that affect jumping performance the same today for 6-year-olds as when the 10-year-olds were 6, or have physical education programs improved over this 4-year span so that 6-year-olds receive more instruction and practice in jumping than the 10-year-olds did when they were 6? If the latter is true, then we are not looking at the development of jumping performance but rather at some uninterpretable interaction between "normal" development and the effects of instruction. The cohort problem exists in all cross-sectional studies.

An example of longitudinal developmental study is that of Halverson, Roberton, and Langendorfer (1982), who studied the throwing velocity of the overarm throw of children from early elementary school through junior high school. Thomas et al. (1983) provided an example of a cross-sectional developmental study in which they looked at the development of memory for distance information by selecting different age-groups. Then they compared the effects of a practiced strategy for remembering distance at each age level to show that the appropriate use of strategy reduces age differences in remembering distance. Each of these studies suffers from the specific defects associated with the type of developmental design. Halverson et al. (1982) had a loss of subjects over the several years of the study, whereas Thomas et al. could not establish if their younger subjects were more familiar with memory strategies than the older subjects were when they were younger.

Although both longitudinal and cross-sectional designs have some problems, they are the only means available to study development. Thus, both are needed and are important parts of the research process. These two types of designs are considered descriptive research. However, either may be con-

---

cohorts — Problem in cross-sectional design that questions whether all the age groups are really from the same population.

sidered experimental research (chapter 16); that is, an independent variable may be manipulated within an age-group. The Thomas et al. (1983) study manipulated the use of strategy within each of the three age-groups. Thus, age was a categorical variable, whereas strategy was a true independent variable. This point is addressed here because developmental research will not be covered in chapter 16 on experimental research.

Four Methodological Problems of Developmental Research

 Whether the developmental research is longitudinal or cross-sectional, several methodological problems exist (for a more detailed discussion, see Thomas, 1984).

Unrepresentative Scores

One of the most common problems is an unrepresentative score. These scores, called outliers, occur in all research but are particularly problematic at the extremes of developmental research (children and senior citizens). Outliers frequently result from shorter attention spans, distraction, and lack of motivation to do the task. The best way to handle these unrepresentative scores is to

1. plan the testing situation within a reasonable time limit that accounts for attention span,
2. set up the testing situation where distractions cannot occur, and
3. be aware of what an unrepresentative score is and retest when one occurs.

 The last thing a researcher wants to do is use unrepresentative scores. Therefore, outliers not detected at testing should be found when the distribution of the data is studied. There are several ways to test for these extreme and unrepresentative scores (e.g., see Barnett & Lewis, 1978). The developmental researcher should expect and plan to handle outliers in the data set.

Unclear Semantics

A second problem in developmental research involves semantics. Selecting the words to use in explaining the task to various age-groups of children is a formidable one. If the researcher is not careful, older children will perform better than younger children, only because they grasp the idea of what to do more quickly. Although the standard rule in good research is to give identical instructions to all the subjects, you must bend this rule for developmental studies with children. The researcher must explain the testing situation in a way the subject can understand and he or she must obtain tangible evidence that the variously aged subjects understood the testing situation before the test was conducted. To ensure the subjects do understand the testing situation, the researcher frequently has the subjects demonstrate the activity to some criterion level of performance before collecting the data.

A good example of this problem involved a group of early elementary school children taking a computer course through a continuing education program at a local college. The children were doing fine until the teacher (a college instructor of computer science) began to write instructions on the blackboard. Then everyone stopped working. Finally, one of the children whispered to the teacher, "Some of us can't read cursive." After the teacher printed the instructions in block letters, all the children happily returned to their computing work (Chronicle of Higher Education, 1983).

Lack of Reliability

 A third developmental research problem is the lack of reliability in younger children's performances. When obtaining a performance score for a child, it should be a reliable one; that is, if the child is tested again, the performance score should be about the same. Obtaining reliable performance is frequently a problem when testing younger children for many of the same reasons that outliers occur. Of course, making sure the child understands the task must be the first consideration

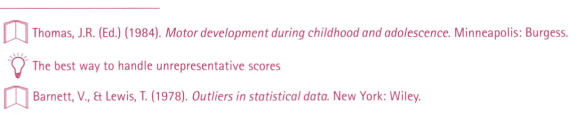

Thomas, J.R. (Ed.) (1984). *Motor development during childhood and adolescence*. Minneapolis: Burgess.

The best way to handle unrepresentative scores

Barnett, V., & Lewis, T. (1978). *Outliers in statistical data*. New York: Wiley.

Herkowitz, J. (1984). Developmentally engineered equipment and playgrounds. In J.R. Thomas (Ed.), *Motor development during childhood and adolescence*. Minneapolis: Burgess.

and maintaining motivation the second. A task made fun and enjoyable is more likely to elicit a consistent performance. This can be done by the use of cartoon figures, encouragement, and rewards (for some ideas on how cartoon figures can be used to improve motivation on many gross motor tasks, see Herkowitz, 1984). The developmental researcher should maintain frequent reliability checks during testing sessions (for appropriate techniques, see chapter 11).

Statistical Problems

The final developmental issue to mention is a statistical problem. A frequent means of making cross-age comparisons is to use ANOVA, which assumes (see chapter 8) that the groups being compared have equal variances (spread of scores about the mean). However, researchers often violate this assumption in making cross-age comparisons. Depending on the nature of the task, older children may have considerably larger or smaller variances than younger children. A developmental researcher should be aware of this potential issue and some of the solutions. In particular, pilot work using the tasks of interest in the research should provide insight into this problem.

Protecting Subjects

In chapter 5, we discussed the protection of human subjects in research. Of course, this protection also pertains to children. Parents or guardians must grant permission for minors to participate in research. Researchers should obtain this permission as they do for adult subjects, except that they give the explanation and consent forms to the parents or guardians. When minors are old enough to understand the methodology, you should also obtain their consent. This means explaining the purpose of the research in terms children can understand. Most public and private schools have their own requirements concerning approval of research studies.

The normal sequence of events involves

- planning the research;
- acquiring approval of the university's committee for protection of human subjects;
- locating and getting the approval of the school system, the school involved, and the teachers; and

- getting the approval of parents and, when appropriate, students.

You can see that this requires a good deal of paperwork. Thus, beginning the process well in advance of the time you plan to begin data collection is essential.

Summarizing Developmental Research

In summary, developmental research is an important type of study that generally involves either longitudinal or cross-sectional designs. Each design has some flaws, but each also has strengths that the other lacks. In particular, the researcher must be aware of several methodological problems existing in developmental studies. Although we present developmental studies in this chapter on descriptive research, they are frequently experimental or quasi-experimental in nature. Finally, the researcher must be especially careful in protecting the rights of children as subjects in developmental research.

The Case Study

Three Types of Case Studies
  Descriptive Studies
  Interpretive Studies
  Evaluative Studies
Considering Case Study Subjects
Characteristics of the Case Study
Gathering and Analyzing Data
Applying Case Study Research in
    Physical Activities

In the case study, the researcher strives for an in-depth understanding of a single situation or phenomenon. This technique is used in many fields, including anthropology, clinical psychology, sociology, medicine, political science, speech pathology, and various educational areas such as disciplinary problems and reading difficulties. It has been used considerably in the health sciences and to some ex-

---

Steps in acquiring approval for research studies with children

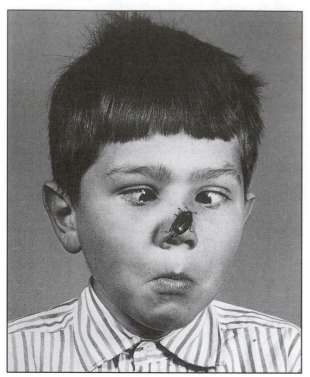

In the case study, the researcher strives for an in-depth understanding of a single situation.

tent in exercise science, sport science, and physical education.

The case study is a form of descriptive research. Whereas the survey method obtains a rather limited amount of information about many subjects, the case study gathers a large amount of information about one or a few subjects. Although the study consists of a rigorous, detailed examination of a single case, the underlying assumption is that this case is representative of many other such cases. Consequently, through the in-depth study of a single case, a greater understanding about similar cases is achieved. This is not to say, however, that the purpose of case studies is to make generalizations. On the contrary, drawing inferences about a population from a case study is not justifiable. On the other hand, the findings of a number of case studies may play a part in the inductive reasoning that is involved in the development of a theory.

The case study is not confined to the study of an individual but can be used in research involving programs, institutions, organizations, political structures, communities, and situations. The case study is used in qualitative research in dealing with critical problems of practice and extending the knowledge base of the various aspects of education, physical education, exercise science, and sport science (qualitative research is discussed in chapter 17).

Information about case study methodology is rather difficult to find. As Merriam (1988) observed, material on case study research strategies can be found everywhere and nowhere. Methodological material on case study research is scattered about in journal articles, conference proceedings, and research reports of the many different fields that use this form of research. You can usually find a brief summary of the weaknesses and strengths of the technique in most research methods textbooks. Moreover, most research methods courses do not deal with the case study except in a very cursory manner.

Consequently, most students do not consider the case study approach as a means of solving research problems, and those who do attempt case studies must either find someone to tutor them or else spend a great deal of time locating methodological material in the various journals and other sources. Frustration in trying to find substantive material about case study research in an educational setting prompted Merriam (1988) to write her interesting and informative text *Case Study Research in Education*.

Three Types of Case Studies

In many ways, case study research is similar to other forms of research. It involves the identification of the problem, the collection of data, and the analysis and reporting of results. As with other research techniques, the approach and the analysis depend on the nature of the research problem. Case studies can be descriptive, interpretive, or evaluative.

Descriptive Studies

A descriptive case study presents a detailed picture of the phenomena but does not attempt to test or build theoretical models. Sometimes, descriptive case studies are historical in nature, and sometimes they are done for the purpose of achieving a better understanding of the present status. Descriptive case studies frequently serve as an initial step or data base for subsequent comparative research and theory building (Merriam, 1988).

Merriam, S.B. (1988). *Case study research in education.* San Francisco: Jossey-Bass.

Interpretive Studies

Interpretive case studies also employ description, but the major focus is to interpret the data in an effort to classify and conceptualize the information and perhaps theorize about the phenomena. For example, a researcher might use the case study approach to better understand the cognitive processes involved in sport.

Evaluative Studies

Evaluative case studies also involve description and interpretation, but the primary purpose is to use the data to evaluate the merit of some practice, program, movement, or event. The efficacy of this type of case study relies on the competence of the researcher to use the available information to make judgments (Guba & Lincoln, 1981). The case study approach enables a more in-depth, holistic approach to the problem than may be possible with survey studies.

Considering Case Study Subjects

Subjects in a case study depend, of course, on the problem being studied. The subject (or case) may be a person (student, teacher, or coach), a program (Little League baseball), an institution (a one-room school), a project (Basic Stuff), or a concept (mainstreaming). In most studies, random sampling is not used because the purpose of a case study is not to estimate some population value but to select subjects from which one can learn the most. Chein (1981) used the term purposive sampling. Goetz and LeCompte (1984) referred to this concept as criterion-based sampling. The researcher establishes criteria necessary for being included in the study, then finds a sample that meets the criteria. Criteria may include age, years of experience, evidence of level of expertise, and situation and environment. The subject, or case, may be one classroom that meets certain criteria or a state that is involved in a specific program.

Characteristics of the Case Study

The case study involves the collection and analysis of many sources of information. In some respects, the case study has some of the same features found in historical research. Although it consists of intensive study of a single unit, it may be that the case study's ultimate worth is an insight and knowledge of a general nature and improved practices. The generalizability of a case study is ultimately related to what the reader is trying to learn from it (Kennedy, 1979). The case study approach is probably most frequently used in trying to understand why something has gone wrong.

Gathering and Analyzing Data

The case study is very flexible as to the amount and type of data that are gathered as well as to the procedures used in gathering the data. Thus, the steps in the methodology are not distinct or uniform with all case studies.

Data for case studies can be interviews, observations, or documents. It is not uncommon for a case study to employ all three types of data. A case study involving a child, for example, may include interviews with the child and the child's teachers and parents. The researcher may systematically observe the child in the class or in some other setting. Documents could include medical examination reports, physical performance test scores, achievement test results, grades, interest inventories, scholastic aptitude tests, teacher anecdotal records, and autobiographies. As noted previously, some case studies are mainly descriptive, others focus on interpretation, and others are evaluative. Some case studies propose and test hypotheses, whereas some attempt to build theories through inductive processes.

Analysis of data in a case study is a formidable task because of the nature of the data and the massive amount of information to analyze. According to Merriam (1988), analysis continues and intensifies after the data have been collected. The data must be sorted, categorized, and interpreted. As in any research, the ultimate value of a study rests on the insight, sensitivity, and integrity of the researcher, who, in the case study, is the primary instrument in the collection and analysis of the data. This is both a strength and a weakness. It is a weakness if the researcher fails to use the appropriate sources of information. The researcher can also be guilty of either oversimplifying the situation or exaggerating the actual state of affairs (Guba & Lincoln, 1981). On the other hand, a competent researcher can use the case study to provide a thorough, holistic account of a complex problem.

Applying Case Study Research in Physical Activities

Several case studies in physical education were directed by H. Harrison Clarke at the University of Oregon (Clarke & Clarke, 1970). The studies dealt with persons of low (and high) fitness levels. Most of the studies sought to discover factors that may contribute to low fitness or the substrength individual. A remarkable example of the case study approach and effective follow-up was seen in a demonstration project undertaken by Frederick Rand Roger and Fred E. Palmer (Clarke, 1968). Twenty junior high school boys with the lowest physical fitness scores were studied as to the cause of low fitness. Information used included somatotype, IQ, academic scholarship, medical history, and status. A follow-up project involved individual attention and special class meetings. Through exercises, improved health habits, medical referrals, and counseling, the students showed vast improvements in fitness, scholarship, and behavior. An example of a recent case study was in the area of pedagogy by Werner and Rink (1989), who described the teaching behaviors of four teachers.

One of the principal advantages of the case study approach is that it can be fruitful in formulating new ideas and hypotheses about problem areas, especially areas for which there is no clear-cut structure or model. The researcher selects the case study method because of the nature of the research questions being asked. The case study, when used effectively, can play an important role in contributing to knowledge in our field.

Job Analysis

A job analysis can be considered a type of case study. It is a technique designed to determine the nature of a particular job and the types of training, preparation, skills, working conditions, and attitudes necessary for success in the job.

Job analyses are regularly done in fields such as counseling and vocational training. A few such studies in physical education, exercise science, and sport science have dealt with administrative positions, intramural duties, and coaching and teaching responsibilities.

The procedures vary in conducting a job analysis. The objective is to obtain as much relevant information as possible about the job and the job requirements. One method is to observe someone in the particular occupation. Of course, this is time consuming and probably bothersome for the person in the job. Nevertheless, the procedure is recommended because the researcher can acquire a kind of vicarious on-the-job experience and gain valuable insight into the whole atmosphere connected with the occupation. A limitation to this method is the lack of sufficient time to observe all facets of the job, particularly seasonal duties and responsibilities.

Questionnaires and interviews are two effective job analysis techniques. They allow people to respond to questions about the kinds of duties they perform, the types and degree of preparation required or recommended for accomplishing their tasks, and the perceived advantages and disadvantages of their jobs.

Systematic job analysis techniques can result in highly specific and quantitative descriptions of the job. For example, a job description for an administrative position reported: (a) a breakdown in percentages of principal accountabilities, (b) number of hours per day spent sitting, standing, and walking, (c) physical effort requirements as to number of pounds lifted waist high, carried alone, and the distance carried, (d) sensory requirements of vision, hearing, and speaking, (e) mental effort requirements, (f) number of hours spent under time pressure and hours spent working rapidly, and (g) percentage of time spent indoors at a desk and in an office. Other requirements and conditions included the minimum academic degree, the necessity of working weekends and evenings, and the ability to use a computer.

The limitations of the job analysis as a research technique include the fallibility of both memory and self-reports. There may be a tendency to accent either the positive or the negative aspects of the job, depending on the time, the circumstances, and the subject. Also, there is the danger that the approach can be too mechanical, thus neglecting some of the more abstract aspects of the job and its requirements.

Clarke, H.H. (Ed.) (1968, December). *Physical Fitness Newsletter.* **14**(4).

Werner, P., & Rink, J. (1989). Case studies of teacher effectiveness in physical education. *Journal of Teaching in Physical Education*, **8**, 280-297.

Observational Research

What Behaviors Will Be Observed?

Who Will Be Observed?

Where Will the Observations Be
        Conducted?

How Many Observations Will Be Made?

When Will the Observations Be Made?

How Will the Observations Be Scored
        and Evaluated?

Using Videotape for Observation

Weaknesses in Observational Research

Observation is used in a variety of research endeavors. It provides a means of collecting data and is a descriptive method of researching certain problems. In the questionnaire and interview techniques, the researcher relies on self-reports as to how the subject behaves or what the subject believes. A weakness of self-reports is that persons may not be candid as to what they really do or feel and may give what they perceive to be socially desirable responses. An alternative descriptive research technique is for the researcher to observe subjects' behavior and use qualitative or quantitative analysis of the observations. Some educators claim that this yields more accurate data. There are, of course, several limitations to observational research.

Basic considerations in observational research include the behaviors that will be observed, who will be observed, where the observations will be conducted, and how many observations will be made. Many other considerations are connected to these basic ones. Depending on the problem and the setting, each individual investigation has its own unique procedures. Therefore, only the basic considerations can be discussed in rather general terms.

What Behaviors Will Be Observed?

This consideration relates to the statement of the problem and to the operational definitions. For example, a study on teacher effectiveness must have clearly defined observational measures of teacher

effectiveness. Definite behaviors must be observed, for example, the extent to which the teacher asks students questions. Some other aspects of teacher effectiveness include giving individual attention, demonstrating skills, dressing appropriately for activities, and starting class on time. The researcher, in determining what behaviors will be observed, must also limit the scope of the observations to make the study manageable.

Who Will Be Observed?

As with any study, the population from which samples will be drawn must be determined. Will the study focus only on elementary school teachers? Which grades? Will the study include only physical education specialists, or will it also include classroom teachers who teach physical education? There is also the question about the number of teachers who will be observed. Will the study include observations of students in addition to teachers? In other words, the researcher must describe precisely who the subjects of the study will be.

Where Will the Observations Be Conducted?

The setting for the observations must be considered in addition to the basic considerations regarding the size of the sample and the geographical area. Will the setting be unnatural or natural? Using an unnatural setting means bringing the subject to a laboratory, room, or other locale for the observations.

There are some advantages to an unnatural setting in terms of control and of freedom from distractions. For example, a one-way mirror is advantageous for observation as it removes the influence of the observer on the behavior of the subject. That behavior is affected by the presence of an observer is also shown in classroom situations. When the observer first arrives, the students (and perhaps the teacher) are curious about the observer's presence. Consequently, they may behave differently than they would if the observer were not there. The teacher may also act differently, possibly by perceiving the observer as a threat or being aware of the purpose of the observations. In any case, the researcher should not make observations on the initial visit. Allowing the subjects to become

Considerations in observational research

gradually accustomed to the observer's presence is best.

Whether the subject will be observed alone or in a group is also related to setting. In a natural setting, such as the playground or classroom, the subject may behave more typically, but there will also likely be more extraneous influences on behavior.

How Many Observations Will Be Made?

As with most measurements, the more observations, the better, due to the increased reliability gained when more trials or observations are used. However, there are obvious practical considerations with respect to feasibility; therefore, the researcher must decide on how many observations may realistically be made.

Many factors determine how many observations the researcher will make. First are the operationally defined behaviors in question and the time constraints of the study itself. For example, if you are studying the amount of activity or participation of students in a physical education class, you must consider several things. In the planning phase of the study, you must decide the type of activity unit and the number of units encompassed in the study. The number of observations for each activity is dependent on the particular stage of learning in the unit, whether in the introductory phase, the practice stage, the playing stage, and so on. This must be specified in the operational definitions, of course, but both the length of the unit and the subsequent length of each stage within each unit play major roles in determining the number of observations that are feasible.

Another factor to consider is the number of observers. If only one person is doing the observations, either the number of students (subjects) being observed or the number of observations per subject (or both) will be restricted. To attempt to generalize from observing a few subjects on a few occasions as to their "typical" behavior is hazardous.

Some types of behavior may not be manifested frequently. Sportsmanship, aggression, leadership, and other traits (as operationally defined) are not readily observable because of the lack of opportunity to display such traits (among other things). The occasion must present itself, and the elements of the situation must materialize in a way that the student has the opportunity to react. Consequently, the number of observations is bound to be extremely limited if left to chance occurrence. On the other hand, situations that are contrived to provoke certain behavior are often unsuccessful because of their artificiality.

We cannot say how many observations are necessary but can only warn against too few observations; thus, we recommend a combination of feasibility and measurement considerations. This question is readdressed in the discussion on scoring and evaluating observations.

When Will the Observations Be Made?

You can easily understand that all the basic considerations being discussed are related and overlap with one another. The determination of when to make the observations includes decisions about time of day, day of the week, phase in the learning experience, season, and other time factors.

In reference to our previous example of observing the amount of student activity in a physical education course, different results would be expected if the observations were made at the beginning of the unit than if they were made at the end. Also, allowing the subjects to get used to the situation so that the observational procedures do not interfere with normal activity is another consideration. In observing student teachers, for example, differences would certainly be expected if some were observed at the beginning of their student-teaching experience and others at the end of the semester.

Graduate students encounter major problems with regard to time and observational research. They find it difficult to spend the time necessary to make a sufficient number of observations to provide reliable results. Furthermore, graduate students usually must gather the data by themselves, making it much more time consuming than if other observers were available.

How Will the Observations Be Scored and Evaluated?

Researchers employ a number of techniques for recording observational data. Great strides have been made in recent years in this respect. The use of microcomputers and other computer-assisted event-recording methods have alleviated many of the technical problems that plagued observational research in the past. Significant advancements will undoubtedly be made in the future in the speed and accuracy of entering and analyzing data.

Some of the more commonly used procedures for recording observational data include

- narrative, or continual recording;
- tallying, or frequency counting;
- the interval method; and
- the duration method.

 The **narrative**, or **continual recording, method** involves the researcher recording in a series of sentences the occurrences he or she observes as they happen. This is the slowest and least efficient method of recording. The observer must be able to select the most important information to record because everything that occurs in a given situation cannot possibly be recorded. Probably the best use of this technique is in helping to develop more efficient recording instruments. The researcher first uses the continuous method and then develops categories for future recording from the narrative.

 The **tallying**, or **frequency counting, method** involves recording each time a certain behavior occurs. The researcher must clearly define the behavior and make the frequency counts within a certain time frame, such as the number of occurrences in 10 minutes or 30 minutes per session.

The **interval method** is used when the researcher wishes to record whether the behavior in question occurs in a certain interval of time. This method is useful when it is difficult to count individual occurrences. One of the leading standardized systems for interval recording has been the Flanders' Interaction Analysis System (Flanders, 1970), in which the observer records the behavior of the subject according to 10 specific behavior classifications within each time interval. All classroom behavior can be classified into 1 of the 10 categories. In the simplest interval system, the ob-

server merely records whether the subject exhibits the prescribed behavior in a given interval of time. Sometimes the observer selects the time intervals randomly or on some fixed basis rather than by continuous observation. Thus, they employ a form of time sampling.

The *Academic Learning Time in Physical Education* (ALT-PE) is an observational instrument developed by Siedentop and graduate students at Ohio State University (Siedentop, Birdwell, & Metzler, 1979; Siedentop, Trousignant, & Parker, 1982) for use in physical education. It entails time sampling in which a child is observed for a specified period of time, and the child's activities during that time period are coded. The recording system encompasses (a) the setting or learning environment established by the teacher; (b) the content of the instruction, such as skills, practice, knowledge, and game playing; (c) the responses of the learner whether engaged or not engaged in the content of the lesson; and (d) the difficulty of the responses when the learner is engaged in the activity.

The *Cheffers' Adaptation of the Flanders' Interaction Analysis System* **(CAFIAS)** was developed by Cheffers (1972/1973) to allow systematic observation of physical education classes and classroom situations. The CAFIAS provides a device for coding nonverbal behavior through a double category system so that any behavior can be categorized as verbal, nonverbal, or both. The CAFIAS permits the coding of the class as a whole when the entire class is functioning as one unit, when the class is divided into small groups, or when the students are working individually or independently with no teacher influence.

 Considerations in observational research

 narrative technique — Method of recording in qualitative research in which the researcher records in a series of sentences the occurrences as they happen; also called *continual recording technique*.

continual recording technique — See *narrative technique*.

tallying method — Method of recording in observational research in which the researcher records occurrence of a clearly defined behavior within a certain time frame; also called *frequency counting method*.

frequency counting method — See *tallying method*.

interval method — Method of recording in observational research, used when it is difficult to count individual occurrences, in which the researcher records whether the behavior in question occurs in a certain interval of time.

 Cheffers' Adaptation of the Flanders' Interaction Analysis System (CAFIAS) — Observational recording instrument developed by Cheffers (1972) that provides a device for coding behavior through a double category system so that any behavior can be categorized as verbal, nonverbal, or both.

The **duration method** involves some timed behavior. The researcher uses a stopwatch or other timing device to record how much time a subject spends engaged in a particular behavior. A number of studies have used this method in observing student time on-task and off-task. In the previous example about the amount of activity in a physical education class, a researcher could simply record the amount of time a student spends in actual participation or the amount of time spent standing in line or waiting to perform. The researcher usually observes a subject for a given unit of time (e.g., a class period), starting and stopping a stopwatch as the behavior starts and stops so that a cumulative time on-task (or off-task) is recorded.

Using Videotape for Observation

A potentially invaluable instrument for observational research is the videotape. Its greatest advantage is that the researcher need not worry about recording observations at the time the behavior is occurring. Furthermore, it allows the researcher to observe a number of persons at one time. For example, teachers and students can be observed simultaneously, which is difficult in normal observational techniques. In addition, the researcher can replay the videotape as needed to evaluate the behavior, and retain a permanent record.

The use of videotape does have some disadvantages. It is expensive, the filming requires a significant degree of technical competence for lighting and positioning, and it may be cumbersome at times to follow the action. The presence of a camera may also alter behavior to the extent that the subjects do not behave normally. However, if the disadvantages can be resolved, videotaping can be an effective process for observational research.

Weaknesses in Observational Research

Problems and limitations of observational research include the following:

- A primary danger in observational research lies in the operational definitions of the study. The behaviors must be carefully defined to be observable. Conse-

quently, the actions may be so restricted that they do not depict the critical behavior. For example, teacher effectiveness encompasses many behaviors, and to observe only the number of times the teacher asked questions or gave individual attention may be inadequate samples of effectiveness.

- Effectively using observation forms requires much practice. Inadequate training, therefore, represents a major pitfall in this form of research. Also, there are difficulties encountered in trying to observe too many things. Often, the observation form is too ambitious for one person to use.

- Certain behaviors cannot be evaluated as finely as some of the observation forms dictate. A common mistake is to ask the observer to make discriminations that are too precise, thus reducing the reliability of the ratings.

- The presence of the observer almost always affects the behavior of the subjects. The researcher must be aware of this and try to reduce the amount of disturbance.

- Generally, observational research is greatly expedited by having more than one observer. Failure to use more than one observer results in decreased efficiency and objectivity.

- As with other forms of descriptive research, there must be sufficient numbers of subjects and observations per subject to have adequate internal and external validity.

Unobtrusive Research Techniques

There are multiple methods of gathering information about people other than questionnaires, case studies, and observation. Webb, Campbell, Schwartz, and Sechrest (1966) discussed different approaches that they term "unobtrusive measures." Some examples they mentioned include the replacement rate for floor tiles around museum exhibits as a measure of relative popularity of exhibits. Researchers have assessed the degree of fear caused by telling ghost stories to children by observing the shrinking diameter of the circle of seated children.

---

duration method — Method of recording in observational research in which the researcher uses a stopwatch or other timing device to record how much time a subject spends engaged in a particular behavior.

Limitations of observational research

Dilation of the pupils of the eyes has been used as an index of fear and interest. Researchers have measured boredom by the amount of fidgeting movements in an audience. The rate of library withdrawals of fiction and nonfiction books has been studied to determine the impact of television in communities. Researchers have noted that children demonstrate their interest in Christmas by the size of their drawings of Santa Claus and the amount of distortion in the figures.

In some of the methods (such as those just mentioned), the experimenter is not present when the data are being produced. There are conditions, however, when the researcher is present but still acts in a nonreactive manner. In other words, the subjects are not aware that the researcher is gathering data. For example, a researcher in psychology measured the degree of acceptance of strangers among delinquent boys by measuring the distance maintained between a delinquent boy and a new boy whom the researcher introduced to the delinquent subject. Sometimes, the researcher intervenes to speed up the action or force the data but in a manner that does not attract attention to the method. In studying the cathartic effect of activity on aggression, Ryan (1970) had an accomplice behave in an obnoxious manner and then measured the amount of electric shock the subjects administered to that accomplice and to "innocent" bystanders. Other researchers have intervened by causing subjects to fail or succeed so that responses to winning and losing in competitive situations could be observed.

Levine (1990) described an interesting study on the pace of life using unobtrusive measures on people in different cities in different countries. Among the measurements used were (a) the walking speed of randomly chosen pedestrians over a distance of 100 feet, (b) the accuracy of outdoor bank clocks in a downtown area, and (c) the speed with which postal clerks fulfilled a standard request for stamps.

A similar study by Levine (1990) was done on the pace of United States cities. Four unobtrusive measures were used: (a) walking speed for 60 feet, (b) time required for bank clerks to complete a simple request, (c) talking speed of postal clerks in explaining differences between regular, certified, and insured mail, (d) and the proportion of people wearing wrist watches.

Unobtrusive measures also include a multitude of records such as birth certificates, political and judicial records, actuarial records, magazines, newspapers, archives, and inscriptions on tombstones. An interesting use of city records (Webb et al., 1966) was the analysis of city water pressure as an index of television viewing interest. Immediately after a television show, the water pressure dropped as drinks were obtained and toilets flushed. Mabley (1963) presented data on Chicago's water pressure on the day of an exciting Rose Bowl game that showed a drastic drop in pressure at the time of the game's end.

The issue of ethics arises in some forms of unobtrusive measures with regard to the invasion of privacy. Informed-consent compliance has placed considerable restraints on certain research practices, such as those that involve entrapment and experiments that aim to induce heightened anxiety.

Correlational Research

Steps in Correlational Research
Limitations of Correlational Research

Correlational research is descriptive in that it explores relationships that exist among variables. Sometimes predictions are made on the basis of the relationships, but correlation cannot determine cause-and-effect. The basic difference between experimental research and correlational research is that the latter does not cause something to happen. There is no manipulation of variables or experimental treatments administered. The basic design of correlational research is to collect data on two or more variables on the same subjects and to determine the relationships among the variables. But, of course, the researcher should have a sound rationale for exploring the relationships.

Different correlational techniques were discussed in chapter 7 through examples of situations that lend themselves to correlational research. The two main purposes for doing a correlational study are to analyze the relationships among variables and to predict.

 correlational research — Research that explores relationships among variables; sometimes involves prediction of a criterion variable.

Steps in Correlational Research

The steps in a correlational study are similar to those used in other research methods. The problem is first defined and delimited. The selection of the variables to be correlated is of critical importance. Many studies have failed in this regard. Regardless of how sophisticated the statistical analysis may be, the statistical technique can deal only with the variables that are entered, thus the saying "Garbage in, garbage out." The validity of a study that seeks to identify basic components or factors of fitness hinges on the identification of the variables to be analyzed. A researcher who wishes to discriminate between starters and substitutes in a sport is faced with the crucial task of determining which physiological or psychological variables are the important determinants of success. The researcher must lean heavily on past research in defining and delimiting the problem.

Subjects are selected from the pertinent population using recommended sampling procedures. The magnitude and even the direction of a correlation coefficient can vary greatly, depending on the sample used. Remember that correlations show only the degree of relationship between variables, not the cause of the relationship. Consequently, because of other contributing factors, one might obtain a correlation of .90 between two variables in a sample of young children and one of .10 between the same variables in adults or vice versa. Chapter 7 used examples of how factors such as age can influence certain relationships.

Another aspect of correlation is that the size of the correlation coefficient depends to a considerable extent on the spread of the scores. A sample that is fairly homogeneous in certain traits seldom will yield a high correlation between variables associated with those traits. For example, the correlation between a distance run and maximal oxygen consumption with a sample of elite track athletes will almost invariably be low because the athletes are so similar; there is not enough variability to permit a high correlation because the scores on the two measurements are too uniform. If you included some less trained subjects in the sample, the size of the correlation coefficient would increase dramatically.

In prediction studies, the subjects must be representative of the population for whom the study is directed. One of the major drawbacks to prediction studies is that the prediction formulas are often sample specific, which means that a formula's accuracy is greatest (or maybe only acceptable) when it is applied to the particular sample on whom it was developed. Chapter 11 discussed this shrinkage phenomenon as well as cross-validation, which is used to counteract shrinkage.

The collection of data requires the same careful attention to detail and standardization that all research designs do. A variety of methods for collecting data may be used, such as physical performance tests, anthropometric measurements, pencil-and-paper inventories, questionnaires, and observational techniques. The scores must be quantified, however, to be correlated.

Analysis of the data can be performed by a number of statistical techniques. Sometimes the researcher wishes to use simple correlation or multiple correlation to study how variables, either by themselves or in a linear composite of variables, are associated with some criterion performance or behavior. Factor analysis is a data-reduction method that helps determine whether relationship among a number of variables can be reduced to small combinations of factors or common components. Path analysis is a technique used to test some theoretical model about causal relationships between three or more variables.

Prediction studies usually employ multiple regression because the accuracy of predicting some criterion behavior is nearly always improved by using more than one predictor variable. Discriminant analysis is a technique used to predict group membership, and canonical correlation is a method for predicting a combination of several criterion variables from several predictor variables.

Limitations of Correlational Research

Limitations of correlational research include those of both planning and analysis. We have already pointed out the importance of the identification of pertinent variables and the selection of proper tests to measure those variables. There should be hypotheses based on previous research and theoretical considerations, rather than simply correlating a set of measurements to see what happens. The selection of an inadequate measure to use as a criterion in a prediction study is a common weakness. For example, a criterion of success in some endeavor is often difficult to operationally define.

A basic mistake in correlational research is to assume cause-and-effect rather than simply association. In prediction studies, researchers sometimes fail to use proper cross-validation procedures. As stated in chapter 7, a researcher can rely too much on statistical significance and not enough on the meaningfulness of the size of correlation coefficients.

Summary

Descriptive research encompasses many different techniques. The techniques are measures of status, although some might seek opinions or even future projections in the responses.

The most common descriptive research technique is the survey, which includes questionnaires and interviews. The two are similar except for the method of asking questions. The questionnaire is a valuable tool for obtaining information over a wide geographical area. A good cover letter is important in getting cooperation. One or two follow-ups are often necessary to secure an adequate representation. Personal interviews usually yield more valid data because of the personal contact and the opportunity to make sure that respondents understand the questions. Telephone interviews are becoming increasingly popular. They have most of the advantages of personal interviews plus flexibility to involve more subjects over a larger geographical area. The Delphi survey technique uses a series of questionnaires in such a way that the respondents eventually reach a consensus about the topic. It is frequently used to survey expert opinion in an effort to help make decisions about practices, needs, and goals.

The normative survey is designed to obtain norms for abilities, performances, beliefs, and attitudes. The various AAHPERD fitness tests developed over the years are examples of normative surveys. In all surveys, representative sampling is extremely important.

Developmental research seeks to study growth measures and changes in behavior over a period of years. In a longitudinal design the same subjects are followed over time. When different subjects are sampled at different age levels, the design is cross-sectional. Of paramount importance in developmental research is whether the subjects represent their populations and their performances. A developmental study may involve experimental treatment, with the researcher attempting to determine the interaction of some treatment with age.

In a case study, the researcher attempts to gather a lot of information about one or a few subjects (cases). Through in-depth study of a single case, a greater understanding about other similar cases is achieved. Case studies can be descriptive, interpretive, or evaluative. One of the principal advantages of the case study approach is that it can lead to the formulation of ideas and hypotheses about problem areas.

The job analysis is a type of case study in which extensive information is gathered and evaluated regarding job conditions, duties, and the types of training, preparation, skills, and attitudes that are necessary for success in a certain job.

Observational research is a descriptive technique that involves the qualitative and quantitative analysis of observed behaviors. Unlike the survey method, which relies on self-reports as to how a subject behaves, observational research attempts to study what a person actually does. Behavior is usually coded as to what occurs, when, how often, and how long. Standardized observation instruments such as the ALT-PE and the CAFIAS are frequently used. Researchers often videotape their subjects to record and store the observations for later analysis.

Some studies use unobtrusive measures in which the subjects are unaware that the researcher is gathering data. For example, instead of (or in addition to) asking a person how much he or she smokes, the researcher might count the cigarette butts in an ashtray after a certain period. Although the methods may be interesting and innovative, there may be constraints due to ethical considerations such as invasion of privacy and entrapment.

Correlational research examines relationship among variables. Sometimes the relationships are used for prediction. Although correlations are often used with experimental research, the study of relationships is descriptive in that it does not involve the manipulation of variables. A major pitfall in correlational research is to assume that because variables are related, one causes another.

 ## Check Your Understanding

1. Find a thesis (or dissertation) that uses a questionnaire to gather data. Briefly summarize the methodology, such as the procedures used in constructing and administering the questionnaire, selecting subjects, following up, and so on.
2. Locate a cross-sectional study and a longitudinal study, and answer the following questions about each:

a. Is the study descriptive or experimental?

b. What age levels are studied?

c. What are the independent and the dependent variables?

d. What statistics are used to make cross-age comparisons?

e. Do the variances (standard deviations squared) of dependent variables appear to differ across age levels? Have the authors considered this? How?

f. Does the study try to justify loss of subjects (longitudinal) or the cohort problem (cross-sectional)? How?

3. Write an abstract of a case study found in the literature. Indicate the problem, the sources of information used, and the findings.

4. Find an observational study in the literature and write a critique of the article, concentrating on the methodology.

5. Write a brief abstract of a correlational research study.

CHAPTER 16

Experimental and Quasi-Experimental Research

Dear Professors of Research Methods:

I have used a "true" experimental design and randomly assigned my subjects to groups. Does this mean that I have controlled all the threats to internal validity so I can be certain my IVs caused the changes in my dv?

Working on my design,
John Henry

Dear Mr. Henry:

Randomization (R) controls some threats to internal validity, but others can be controlled only by you. Two verses from this poem (1991) by Schuyler W. Huck (*Journal of Experimental Education*, **59**, 193-196) capture the essential point.

There once was a research design
That looked, on first glance, oh so fine.
   Yet it is stupidity
   To view its validity
As chaste due to Rs on each line.

. . . .

But what of those "internal" threats?
Are all tamed, like nicely trained pets?
   If that rings as true
   You've some learnin' to do
For Rs catch just some in their nets.

Randomly yours,
PRM

Experimental research attempts to establish cause-and-effect relationships. That is, an independent variable is manipulated to judge its effect upon a dependent variable. However, the process of establishing cause and effect is a difficult one. We have already discussed the fact that just because two variables are correlated does not mean one causes the other. However, cause and effect cannot exist unless two variables are correlated. Therefore, correlational research is frequently used before conducting experimental research. We may investigate to see whether two variables are related before trying to manipulate one to change the other.

Also, remember that cause and effect are not established by statistics. Statistical techniques can only reject the null hypothesis (establish that groups are significantly different) and identify the percent variance in the dependent variable accounted for by the independent variable or the effect size; neither of these procedures establishes cause and effect. Cause and effect can be established only by the application of logical thinking to well-designed experiments. This logical process establishes that no other reasonable explanation exists for the changes in the dependent variable except the manipulation done as the independent variable. The application of this logic is made possible by the following:

- The selection of a good theoretical frame work
- The use of appropriate subjects
- The application of an appropriate experimental design
- The use of the correct statistical model and analyses
- The proper selection and control of the independent variable
- The appropriate selection and measurement of the dependent variable
- The correct interpretation of the results

In this chapter we discuss experimental designs by explaining how you can recognize and control sources of invalidity and threats to both internal and external validity. We also explain several types of experimental designs. Before going any further into this chapter, review the following terms used throughout the discussion:

- Independent variable
- Dependent variable
- Categorical variable
- Control variable
- Extraneous variable

Sources of Invalidity

All the types of designs we discuss have strengths and weaknesses that pose threats to the validity of the research, as stated so well by Campbell and Stanley (1963):

> Fundamental . . . is a distinction between internal validity and external validity. Internal validity is the basic minimum without which any experiment is uninterpretable: Did in fact the experimental treatments make a difference in this specific experimental instance? External validity asks the question of generalizability: To what populations, settings, or treatment variables can this effect be generalized? (p. 5)

Both internal validity and external validity are important in experiments. However, they are frequently at odds in research planning and design. Gaining internal validity involves controlling all variables so that the researcher can eliminate all rival hypotheses as explanations for the outcomes observed. Yet, in controlling and constraining the research setting to gain internal validity, the researcher places the generalization (external validity) of the findings in jeopardy. In studies with strong internal validity, the answer to the question of to whom, what, or where the findings can be generalized may be very uncertain. This is

 How cause and effect can be logically established

Martens, R. (1979). About smocks and jocks. *Journal of Sport Psychology*, **1**, 94–99.

Martens, R. (1987). Science, knowledge, and sport psychology. *Sport Psychologist*, **1**, 29–55.

Siedentop, D. (1980). Two cheers for Rainer. *Journal of Sport Psychology*, **2**, 2–4.

Thomas, J.R. (1980). Half a cheer for Rainer and Daryl. *Journal of Sport Psychology*, **2**, 266–267.

Thomas, J.R., French, K.E., & Humphries, C.A. (1986). Knowledge development and sport skill performance: Directions for motor behavior research. *Journal of Sport Psychology*, **8**, 259–272.

because in ecologically valid settings (the situation as perceived by the subject), not everything is controlled and operated in the same way as in the controlled laboratory context. Thus, the researcher must decide: Is it more important to be certain that the manipulation of the independent variable caused the observed changes in the dependent variable, or is it more important to be able to generalize the results to other populations, settings, and so on? We cannot provide an easy answer to that question, which is often debated at scientific meetings and in the literature (e.g., see Martens, 1979, 1987; Siedentop, 1980; Thomas, 1980; Thomas et al., 1986).

To expect any single experiment to meet all research design considerations is unreasonable. A more realistic approach is to identify the specific goals and limitations of the research effort. Is internal validity or external validity the more important issue? Once that is decided, the researcher can plan the research with one type of validity as the major focus while maintaining as much of the other type of validity as possible. Another recourse is to plan a series of experiments in which the first experiment would have strong internal validity even at the expense of external validity. If the first experiment identified that changes in the dependent measure are the result of manipulating the independent variable, subsequent experiments could be designed with increasing external validity even at the expense of internal validity. This would allow evaluation of the treatment in settings more like the real world. [Review the discussion of basic and applied research (chapter 1; Christina, 1989) as it relates to this topic.]

Eight Threats to Internal Validity

> History
> Maturation
> Testing
> Instrumentation
> Statistical Regression

> Selection Bias
> Experimental Mortality
> Selection–Maturation Interaction
> Additional Threats

Campbell and Stanley (1963) identified eight threats to the internal validity of experiments:[1]

- **History**—events occurring during the experiment that are not part of the treatment

- **Maturation**—processes within the subjects that operate as a result of time passing (e.g., aging, fatigue, hunger)

- **Testing**—the effects of one test on subsequent administrations of the same test

- **Instrumentation**—changes in instrument calibration, including lack of agreement within and between observers

- **Statistical regression**—the fact that groups selected on the basis of extreme scores are not as extreme on a subsequent testing

- **Selection biases**—identification of comparison groups in other than a random manner

- **Experimental mortality**—loss of subjects from comparison groups for nonrandom reasons

- **Selection-maturation interaction**—specific to nonequivalent group designs where the passage of time might affect one group but not the other

If these threats are uncontrolled, the change in the dependent variable may be difficult to attribute to the manipulation of the independent variable.

History

A history threat means that some unintended event occurred during the treatment period. For example, if a study were evaluating the effects of a semester of physical education on the physical fitness of fifth graders, the fact that 60% of the children participated in a recreational soccer program would constitute a history threat to internal validity. The soc-

 Eight threats to internal validity

[1]From D.T. Campbell & J.C. Stanley (1963), *Experimental and Quasi-Experimental Designs for Research* (Chicago: Rand McNally), pp. 5-6. Copyright © 1963 by the American Educational Research Association. Used by permission of Houghton Mifflin Company.

cer program is also likely to produce benefits to physical fitness that would be difficult to separate from the benefits of the physical education program.

Maturation

Maturation as a threat to internal validity is most often associated with aging. This threat occurs frequently in designs in which one group is tested on several occasions over a long period. Elementary physical education teachers frequently encounter this source of invalidity when they give a physical fitness test in the early fall and again in the late spring. The children nearly always do better in the spring. The teacher would like to claim that the physical education program was the cause. Unfortunately, maturation is a plausible rival hypothesis for the observed increase; that is, the children have grown larger and stronger and thus probably run faster, jump higher, and throw farther.

Testing

A testing threat is the effect that taking a test once has on taking it again. For example, if a group of athletes were administered a 50-item multiple-choice test to evaluate their knowledge about steroids today and again 2 days later, the athletes would do better the second time even though no treatment intervened. Taking the test once helps in taking it again. The same effect is present in physical performance tests, particularly if the subjects are not allowed to practice the test a few times. If a class of beginners in tennis attempts to hit 20 forehand shots delivered to them from a ball machine today and again 3 days later, the subjects will usually do better the second time. They learned something from performing the test the first time.

Instrumentation

Instrumentation is a problem frequently faced in exercise science research. Suppose the researcher uses a spring-loaded device to measure strength. Unless the spring is calibrated regularly, it decreases in tension with use. Thus, the same amount of applied force will produce increased readings of strength. Instrumentation also applies to research using observers. Unless training and regular checks occur, the same observer may systematically vary his or her ratings across time or subjects (called observer drift), or different observers may not rate the same performance in the same way.

Statistical Regression

Statistical regression may occur when groups are not randomly formed but are selected on the basis of an extreme score on some measure. For example, if someone records the behavior of a group of children on a playground on an activity scale (very active to very inactive) and two groups are formed—one of very active children and one of very inactive children—statistical regression is likely to occur when the children are next observed on the playground. The children who were very active will be less active (although still active), and the very inactive children will be more active. In other words, both groups will regress (move from the extremes) toward the overall average. This phenomenon reflects only the fact that a subject's score tends to vary about her/his average performance (estimated true score). If extreme scores are used, the subject may be observed on the high (or low) side of a typical performance. The next performance is usually not as extreme. Thus, when average scores of extreme groups are compared from one time to the next, the high group on the particular attribute appears to get worse, whereas the low group appears to get better. Statistical regression is a particular problem in studies that attempt to compare extreme groups selected on some characteristic such as high anxious, fit, or skilled subjects versus low anxious, fit, or skilled subjects.

Selection Bias

Selection biases occur when groups are formed on some basis other than random assignment. Thus, when treatments are administered, the rival hypothesis is always present that any differences found are due to initial selection biases; that is, the groups were different to begin with rather than as a result of the treatments. Showing that the groups were not different at the beginning on the dependent variable does not overcome this shortcoming. Any number of other unmeasured variables on which the groups differ might explain the treatment effect. Borg and Gall (1983) asked important questions that apply to selection (or sampling) bias:

> Did the study use volunteers? Use of volunteers is common in research in the study of physical activity. Yet volunteers are often not representative of anyone but other volunteers. They may differ considerably from non-volunteers in motivation for the experimental task and setting.

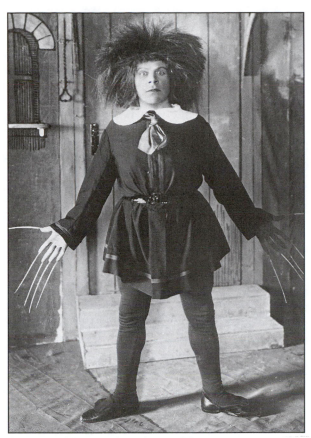

Selection bias results when subjects are extremely nonrepresentative of the population.

Are subjects extremely nonrepresentative of the population? Often we are unable to select subjects at random for our studies, but it is very useful if we at least believe (and can demonstrate) that they represent some larger group from our culture.

Recall the discussion of sampling in chapter 6, particularly the concept of a "good enough" sample.

Experimental Mortality

Experimental mortality refers to the loss of subjects from the treatment groups. Even when groups are randomly formed, this threat to internal validity may occur. Subjects may remain in an experimental group receiving a fitness program because it is fun, whereas subjects in the control group become bored, lose interest, and drop out of the study. Of course, the opposite can occur, too. Subjects may

drop out of an experimental group because the treatment is too difficult or time-consuming.

Selection-Maturation Interaction

A selection-maturation interaction occurs only in specific types of designs. In these designs, one group is identified because of some specific characteristic, whereas the other group lacks this characteristic. An example might be the differences between 6-year-olds in two school districts where one group is experimental, receiving a fitness program, and the other group is a control. If the school had different admission policies so that the 6-year-olds in the experimental group were 5 months older, it would be difficult to determine whether the fitness program or the fitness program combined with the subjects' advanced age produced the observed changes.

Additional Threats

Any of these eight threats to internal validity may reduce the researcher's ability to claim that the manipulation of the independent variable produced the changes in the dependent variable. We discuss the various experimental designs and how they control (or fail to control) the threats to internal validity later in this chapter.

One additional threat to internal validity not mentioned by Campbell and Stanley (1963) has been identified. **Expectancy** (Rosenthal, 1966) refers to experimenters or testers anticipating that certain subjects will perform better. This effect, although usually unconscious on the part of the experimenters, occurs where subjects or experimental conditions are clearly labeled. For example, testers will rate "skilled" subjects better than "unskilled" subjects regardless of treatment. This effect is also evident in observational studies in which the observers will rate posttest better than pretest performance because they expect change. Or, if the experimental and control groups are identified, observers will rate the experimental group better than the control without any treatment occurring. The expectancy effect may influence the subjects, too. For example, in a youth-sport study, coaches may actually cause poorer performance in substitutes (compared with starters) because the

---

expectancy — A threat to internal validity in which the researcher anticipates certain behavior or results to occur.

substitutes realize the coach treats them differently (e.g., the coach may show less concern about incorrect practice trials).

Four Threats to External Validity

Reactive or Interactive Effects of Testing

Interaction of Selection Bias and Experimental Treatment

Reactive Effects of Experimental Arrangements

Multiple-Treatment Interference

Campbell and Stanley (1963) have identified four threats to external validity, or the ability to generalize results to other subjects, settings, measures, and so on:[2]

- **Reactive or interactive effects of testing**—the pretest may make the subject more aware of or sensitive to the upcoming treatment. As a result, the treatment is not as effective without the pretest.

- **Interaction of selection biases and the experimental treatment**—when a group is selected on some characteristic, the treatment may work only on groups possessing that characteristic.

- **Reactive effects of experimental arrangements**—treatments that are effective in very constrained situations (e.g., laboratories) may not be effective in less constrained (more like real-world) settings.

- **Multiple-treatment interference**—when subjects receive more than one treatment, the effects of previous treatments may influence subsequent ones.

Reactive or Interactive Effects of Testing

Reactive or interactive effects of testing may be a problem in any design with a pretest. Suppose a fitness program is to be the experimental treatment. If a physical fitness test is administered to the sample first, the subjects in the experimental group might realize that their levels of fitness are low and be particularly motivated to follow the prescribed program closely. However, in an unpretested population, the program might not be as effective because the subjects would be unaware of their low levels of physical fitness.

Interaction of Selection Bias and Experimental Treatment

The interaction of selection biases and the experimental treatment may prohibit the generalization of the results to subjects lacking the particular characteristics (bias). For example, a drug education program might be quite effective in changing the attitudes toward drug use of college freshmen. This same program would probably lack effectiveness for third-year medical students because they would be very familiar with drugs and their appropriate uses.

Reactive Effects of Experimental Arrangements

Reactive effects of experimental arrangements are a persistent problem for laboratory-based research (e.g., in exercise physiology, biomechanics, motor control and learning). In these cases, is the researcher investigating an effect, process, or outcome that is specific to the laboratory and cannot be generalized to other settings? We have referred to this earlier as ecological validity. For example, in a study employing high-speed cinematography, the skill to be filmed must be performed in a certain place and joints marked for later analysis. Is the skill performed in the same way during participation in a sport? One specific type of reactive behavior has been labeled the Hawthorne effect (Brown, 1954). This refers to the fact that subjects' performances change when attention is paid to the subjects. This may be a threat to both internal and external validity, as it is likely to produce better treatment effects and reduce the ability to generalize the results.

 Four threats to external validity

[2]From D.T. Campbell and J.C. Stanley (1963), *Experimental and Quasi-Experimental Designs for Research* (Chicago: Rand McNally), pp. 5-6. Copyright © 1963 by the American Educational Research Association. Used by permission of Houghton Mifflin Company.

Multiple-Treatment Interference

Multiple-treatment interference is most frequently a problem when the same subjects are exposed to more than one level of the treatment. Suppose subjects are going to learn to move to the hitting position in volleyball using a lead step or a crossover step. We want to know which step gets the subjects in a good hitting position most quickly. If the subjects attempt both types of steps, learning one might interfere with (or enhance) learning the other. Thus, the researcher's ability to generalize the findings may be confounded by the use of multiple treatments. A better design might have been to have two separate groups, each of which learns one of the techniques.

The ability to generalize findings from research to other subjects or situations is a question of random sampling (or at least "good enough" sampling) more than any other. Do the subjects, treatments, tests, and situations represent any larger populations? Although a few of the experimental designs discussed later control certain threats to external validity, usually the researcher controls these threats by the way the sample, treatments, situations, and tests are selected.

Controlling Threats to Internal Validity

Randomization

Placebos, Blind, and Double-Blind Setups

Uncontrolled Threats to Internal Validity

Reactive or Interactive Effects

Instrumentation (Obtaining Test Reliability)

Experimental Mortality (Subject Retention)

Threats to internal and external validity are controlled in different ways and by specific techniques. In this section we describe useful approaches to solving these problems in the design of experiments. Many threats to internal validity are controlled by equating the subjects in the experimental and control groups. This is most often done by randomly assigning subjects to groups.

Randomization

As mentioned in chapter 6, randomization allows the assumption that the groups do not differ at the beginning of the experiment. The randomization process controls for history up to the point of the experiment; that is, the researcher can assume that past events are equally distributed among groups. It does not control for history effects during the experiment if experimental and control subjects are treated at different times or places. Only the researcher can make sure that no events occur in one group but not in others.

Randomization also controls for maturation, as the passage of time would be equivalent in all groups. Statistical regression is controlled because it operates only when groups are not randomly formed. Both selection biases and selection-maturation interaction are controlled because these threats occur only when groups are not randomly formed.

Sometimes ways other than random assignment of subjects to groups are used to attempt to control threats to internal validity. The matched-pair technique equates pairs of subjects on some characteristic and then randomly assigns the pairs to groups. The researcher might want very tight control on previous experience in strength training. Thus, subjects would be matched on this characteristic and then randomly assigned to the experimental and control groups.

A matched-group technique may also be used. This involves nonrandom assignment of subjects to experimental and control groups so that the group means are equivalent on some variable. This is generally regarded as an unacceptable procedure because the groups may not be equivalent on other, unmeasured variables that could affect the outcome of the research.

In within-subjects designs, the subjects are used as their own controls. This means each subject receives both the experimental and the control treatment. In this type of design, the order of treatments should be counterbalanced; that is, half the subjects should receive the experimental treatment first and then the control, and the other half should receive the control first and then the experimental treatment. If there are three levels of the independent variable (1 = control, 2 = experimental A, 3 = experimental B), the six possible combinations should be identified (1-2-3, 1-3-2, 2-1-3, 2-3-1, 3-1-2, 3-2-1) and subjects should be randomly assigned to order. As the number of treatment levels administered to the same subjects becomes larger than 3 or 4, experimenters may assign a random order of the treatments to each subject rather than counterbalancing treatments.

Placebos, Blind, and Double-Blind Setups

Other ways of controlling threats to internal validity include placebos and blind and double-blind setups. A **placebo** is used to evaluate whether the treatment effect is real or a psychological effect. Frequently, a control condition is used in which subjects receive the same attention from and interaction with the experimenter, but the treatment administered does not relate to performance on the dependent variable.

A study in which subjects do not know whether they are receiving the experimental or the control treatment is called a **blind setup** (i.e., the subject is blind to the treatment). In a **double-blind setup**, neither the subjects nor the tester knows which treatment the subjects are receiving. The triple-blind test has also been reported (Day, 1983): *The subject does not know what he or she is getting, the experimenter does not know what he or she is giving, and the investigator does not know what he or she is doing.* We can only hope the triple-blind technique finds limited use in our field.

All these techniques (except the triple-blind technique) are useful in controlling Hawthorne, expectancy, and halo effects as well as what we call the **Avis effect** (a recent version of the John Henry effect), or the fact that subjects in the control group may try harder simply because they are in the control group.

A good example of the use of these techniques for controlling psychological effects is the use of steroids to build strength in athletes. A number of studies were done to evaluate the effects of steroids. To combat the fact that athletes may get stronger because they think they should when using steroids, a placebo (another pill that looks just like the steroid) is used. The athletes are blind as to whether they receive the placebo. In a double blind, the athlete, the person dispensing the steroids (or placebo),

and the testers would all be blind to which group received the steroids. Unfortunately, until recently these procedures did not work very well in this specific type of study because taking large quantities of steroids made the athletes' urine smell bad. Thus, the athletes knew whether they were receiving the steroid or the placebo.

Uncontrolled Threats to Internal Validity

Three threats to internal validity remain uncontrolled by the randomization process.

Reactive or Interactive Effects

Reactive or interactive effects of testing can be controlled only by eliminating the pretest. However, it can be evaluated by two of the designs: randomized groups pretest/posttest and Solomon four-group (discussed later in this chapter).

Instrumentation (Obtaining Test Reliability)

Instrumentation cannot be controlled or evaluated by any design. Only the experimenter can control this threat to internal validity. In chapter 11 (measurement of research variables) we went into some detail on techniques for controlling the instrumentation threat (developing valid and reliable tests). Of particular significance is test reliability. Whether the measurement is obtained from a laboratory device (an oxygen analyzer), motor performance test (standing long jump), attitude-rating scale (feelings about drug use), observer (coding percentage of time a child is active), knowledge test (basketball strategy), or survey (available sport facilities), the answer must be consistent. This frequently involves the assessment of test reliability across situations, between and within testers or observers, and within subjects. The validity of the instrument (does it measure what it was intended to measure?) must also be established to control for instrumentation problems. The total process of establishing appropriate instrumentation for research is called psychometrics.

---

placebo — Method of controlling a threat to internal validity in which a control group receives a "false" treatment while the experimental group receives the real treatment.

blind setup — Method of controlling a threat to internal validity in which the subject does not know if he or she is receiving the experimental or control treatment.

double-blind setup — Method of controlling a threat to internal validity in which neither the subject nor the experimenter knows which treatment the subject is receiving.

Avis effect — A threat to internal validity wherein subjects in the control group may try harder just because they are in the control group.

One final point about instrumentation is called the halo effect. As we discussed in chapter 11, this occurs in ratings of several skills on the same individual. Raters seeing a skilled performance on one task are likely to rate the subject higher on subsequent tasks regardless of the level of skill displayed. In effect, the skilled behavior has rubbed off (created a "halo") on later performance. There may also be an order effect in observation. Gymnastics and swimming judges often rate earlier performers lower to "save room" on the rating scale for better performers. Because gymnastics and swimming coaches know this, they always place better performers later in the event order.

Experimental Mortality (Subject Retention)

Experimental mortality is not controlled by any type of experimental design. Only the experimenter can control this by ensuring that subjects are not lost (at all, if possible) from groups. Many of these problems can be handled in advance of the research by carefully explaining the research to the subjects and the need for them to follow through with the project. (During the experiment itself, begging, pleading, and crying sometimes work.)

Controlling Threats to External Validity

External validity is generally controlled by selecting the subjects, treatments, experimental situation, and tests to represent some larger population. Of course, random selection is the key to controlling most threats to external validity (but also recall "good enough" sampling from chapter 6). Remember, more than the subjects may be randomly selected. For example, the levels of treatment can be randomly selected from the possible levels, experimental situations can be selected from possible situations, and the dependent variable (test) could be randomly selected from a pool of potential dependent variables.

As previously noted, the idea of generalizing the situation is called ecological validity. Although the results of a particular treatment can be generalized to a larger group if the sample is representative, this generalization may apply only to the specific situation in the experiment. If the experiment is conducted under controlled laboratory conditions, then the findings may apply only under controlled laboratory conditions. Frequently, the experimenter hopes the findings will generalize to real-world exercise, sport, industrial, or instructional settings.

Whether the outcomes will generalize in this way depends largely on how the subjects perceive the study, and this influences the way subjects respond to study characteristics. The question of interest here is, Does the study have enough characteristics of real-world settings so that subjects respond as if they were in the real world? Is there ecological validity? This is not an easy question to answer, and it has resulted in a number of scholars advocating that more research in physical education, exercise science, and sport science be conducted in field settings (e.g., Costill, 1985; Martens, 1987; Thomas et al., 1986).

Reactive or interactive effects of testing can be evaluated by the Solomon four-group design. Interaction of selection biases and the experimental treatment is controlled by random selection of subjects. Reactive effects of experimental arrangements can be controlled only by the researcher (this is again the issue of ecological validity). Multiple-treatment interference may be partially controlled by counterbalancing or randomly ordering the treatments across subjects. But only the researcher can control whether the treatments will still interfere. That decision is based on knowledge about the treatment rather than the type of experimental design.

Types of Designs

Preexperimental Designs
   One-Shot Study
   One-Group Pretest-Posttest Design
   Static Group Comparison
True Experimental Designs
   Randomized-Groups Design
   Pretest-Posttest Randomized-Groups Design
   Solomon Four-Group Design
Quasi-Experimental Designs
   Time Series Design
   Reversal Design
   Nonequivalent Control Group
   Ex Post Facto Design
Other Types of Quasi-Designs
   Switched Replication Design
   Exercise Epidemiological Designs
   Single Subject Designs

This section (much of which is taken from Campbell & Stanley, 1963) is divided into three categories: preexperimental designs, true experimental designs, and quasi-experimental designs. We use the following notation:

- **R**: This signifies random assignment of subjects to groups.
- **O**: This signifies an observation or test (subscripts refer to the order of testing; i.e., O_1 is the first time a test is given and O_2 is the second).
- **T**: This signifies that a treatment is applied (the terms T_1 and T_2 on different lines refer to different treatments; terms on the same line mean that the treatment is administered more than once); a blank space means that the group is a control.
- **⋯**: A dotted line between groups means that the groups are used intact rather than being randomly formed.

Preexperimental Designs

 These three designs are called **preexperimental designs** because they control very few of the sources of invalidity. None of the designs has random assignment of subjects to groups.

1. One-Shot Study

In this design a group of subjects receives a treatment followed by a test to evaluate the treatment:

$$T \qquad O$$

This design fails all the tests of good research. All that can be said is that at a certain point in time this group of subjects performed at a certain level. In no way can the level of performance (O) be attributed to the treatment (T).

2. One-Group Pretest–Posttest Design

This design, although very weak, is better than Design 1. At least we can observe whether any change in performance has occurred:

$$O_1 \qquad T \qquad O_2$$

If O_2 is better than O_1, we can say that the subjects improved. For example, Bill Biceps (a qualified exercise instructor) conducted an exercise test at a health club. Subjects then trained 3 days per week, 40 minutes per day, at 70% of their estimated $\dot{V}O_2$max for 12 weeks. After the training period subjects retook the exercise test and significantly improved their scores. Can Mr. Biceps conclude that the exercise program caused the changes in the exercise test performance he observed? Unfortunately, this design does not allow us to say why the subjects improved. Certainly, it could be due to the treatment, but it could also be due to history. Some event other than the treatment (T) may have occurred between the pretest (O_1) and the posttest (O_2). Maturation is a rival hypothesis. The subjects may have gotten better (or worse) just as a result of the passage of time. Testing is a rival hypothesis; the increase at O_2 may be the result only of experience with the test at O_1. If the group being tested is selected for some specific reason, then any of the threats involving selection biases could occur. This design is most frequently analyzed by the dependent t test to evaluate whether significant change occurred between O_1 and O_2.

3. Static Group Comparison

This design compares two groups, one of which receives the treatment and one of which does not:

$$
\begin{array}{cc}
T & O_1 \\
\cdots & \cdots \\
& O_2
\end{array}
$$

However, the dotted line between the groups indicates that the groups were not equivalent when the study began. Most frequently, this means that the groups were selected intact rather than being randomly formed. This leaves one in the position of being unable to determine whether any differences between O_1 and O_2 are caused by T, as O_1 and O_2 might have been different only because the groups differed initially. This design is subject to invalidity because of selection biases and the selection-maturation interaction. A t test for independent groups is used to evaluate whether O_1 and O_2 differ significantly. However, even if they do differ, the difference cannot be attributed to T.

---

preexperimental design — Three types of research designs that control very few of the sources of invalidity and that do not have random assignments of subjects to groups: one-shot study, one-group pretest-posttest design, and static group comparison.

Designs 1, 2, and 3 are not valid means of answering research questions (see Table 16.1). They do not represent experiments because the change in the dependent variable cannot be attributed to manipulation of the independent variable. You will not encounter these preexperimental designs in research journals, and we hope you will not find (or produce) theses and dissertations using these designs. Designs 1, 2, and 3 represent much wasted effort because little or nothing can be concluded from the findings. If you submit studies using these designs to research journals, you are likely to receive rejection letters similar to one Snoopy (from the "Peanuts" comic strip) received: "Dear Researcher, Thank you for submitting your paper to our research journal. To save time, we are enclosing two rejection letters—one for this paper and one for the next one you send."

True Experimental Designs

These are called **true experimental designs** because the groups are randomly formed, allowing the assumption that they were equivalent at the beginning of the research. This con-

trols for past (but not present) history, maturation (which should occur equally in the groups), testing, and all sources of invalidity that are based on nonequivalency of groups (statistical regression, selection biases, and selection-maturation interaction). However, only the experimenter can make sure that nothing happens to one group (besides the treatment) and not the other (present history), that scores on the dependent measure do not vary as a result of instrumentation problems, and that the loss of subjects is not different between the groups (experimental mortality).

4. Randomized–Groups Design

Note that this design resembles Design 3 except that groups are randomly formed:

$$R \quad T \quad O_1$$
$$R \quad \quad O_2$$

If the researcher controls the threats to internal validity (no easy task) not controlled by randomization and has a sound theoretical basis for the study, then this design allows the conclusion that significant differences between O_1 and O_2 are due

Table 16.1   Preexperimental Designs and Their Control of the Threats to Validity

Validity threat	One-shot study	One-group pretest and posttest	Static group
Internal			
History	–	–	+
Maturation	–	–	?
Testing		–	+
Instrumentation		–	+
Statistical regression		?	+
Selection	–	+	–
Experimental mortality	–	+	–
Selection × maturation		–	–
Expectancy	?	?	?
External			
Testing × treatment		–	
Selection biases × treatment	–	–	–
Experimental arrangements		?	
Multiple treatments			

Note. + = strength, – = weakness,   = not relevant, ? = questionable.

From *Handbook of Research on Teaching.* Copyright 1963 by the American Educational Research Association. Reprinted with permission.

 true experimental design — Any design used in experimental research in which groups are randomly formed and that controls most sources of invalidity.

to T. An independent t test is used to analyze the difference between O_1 and O_2. This design, as depicted, represents two levels of one independent variable. It may be extended to any number of levels of an independent variable:

$$
\begin{array}{lll}
R & T_1 & O_1 \\
R & T_2 & O_2 \\
R & & O_3
\end{array}
$$

Here, three levels of the independent variable exist, where one is the control and T_1 and T_2 represent two levels of treatment. This design can be analyzed by simple ANOVA, which contrasts the dependent variable (O_1, O_2, O_3) as measured in the three groups. For example, T_1 is training at 70% of $\dot{V}O_2max$, T_2 is training at 40% of $\dot{V}O_2max$, and the control group is not training. The variables O_1, O_2, and O_3 are the measures of cardiorespiratory fitness (12-min run) in each group taken at the end of the training.

This design may also be extended into a factorial design; that is, more than one independent variable could be considered. Example 16.1 shows how this works:

Example 16.1

Independent variable 1 (IV_1) has three levels (A_1, A_2, A_3), and independent variable 2 (IV_2) has two levels (B_1, B_2). This results in six cells (A_1B_1, A_1B_2, A_2B_1, A_2B_2, A_3B_1, A_3B_2) to which subjects are randomly assigned. At the end of the treatments, each cell is tested on the dependent variable (O_1, O_2, O_3, O_4, O_5, O_6). This design is analyzed by a 3×2 factorial ANOVA that tests the effects of IV_1 (F_A), IV_2 (F_B) and their interaction (F_{AB}).

This design may also be extended to an increased number of independent variables (three, four, or more) and retain all the controls for internal validity previously discussed. Sometimes this design is used with a categorical independent variable. Looking again at Example 16.1, suppose that IV_2 (B_1, B_2) represented two age levels. Clearly, the levels of B could not be randomly formed. The design would appear as follows:

$$
\begin{array}{cccc}
 & R & A_1 & O_1 \\
B_1 & R & A_2 & O_2 \\
 & R & A_3 & O_3 \\
\hline
 & R & A_1 & O_4 \\
B_2 & R & A_2 & O_5 \\
 & R & A_3 & O_6
\end{array}
$$

The levels of A are randomly formed within B, but the levels of B cannot be randomly formed. This no longer qualifies completely as a true experimental design but is frequently used in the study of physical activity. This design is analyzed in a 3×2 ANOVA, but the interpretation of results must be done more conservatively.

Any of the versions of Design 4 may also have more than one dependent variable. Although the consideration of the design remains the same, the statistical analysis becomes multivariate. Where two or more levels of one independent variable exist but several dependent variables are present, discriminant analysis is the appropriate multivariate statistic. In the factorial versions of this design (two or more independent variables), if multiple dependent variables are used, then MANOVA is typically the most appropriate analysis, although practical concerns (e.g., subject numbers) or theoretical matters may dictate alternative statistical analyses.

5. Pretest–Posttest Randomized–Groups Design

In this design the groups are randomly formed, but both groups are given a pretest as well as a posttest. This design is labeled as follows:

$$R \quad O_1 \quad T \quad O_2$$
$$R \quad O_3 \quad\quad O_4$$

The major purpose of this type of design is to determine the amount of change produced by the treatment; that is, does the experimental group change more than the control group? This design threatens the internal validity of testing, but the threat is controlled, as the comparison of O_3 to O_4 in the control group includes the testing effect as well as the comparison of O_1 to O_2 in the experimental group. Thus, although the testing effect cannot be evaluated in this design, it is controlled.

This design is used frequently in the study of physical activity, but its analysis is rather complex. There are at least three common ways to do a statistical analysis of this design. First, a factorial repeated measures ANOVA can be used. One factor (between subjects) is the treatment versus no treatment, whereas the second factor is pretest versus posttest (within subjects or repeated measures). However, the interest in this design is usually the interaction: Do the groups change at different rates from pretest to posttest? If you choose a repeated measures ANOVA for this design (in our opinion the best choice), pay close attention to our discussion of repeated measures in chapter 8 (univariate issues in repeated measures) and chapter 9 (multivariate issues in repeated measures). A second analysis is to use simple ANCOVA with the pretest for each group (O_1 and O_3) used to adjust the posttest (O_2 and O_4). Recall that there are some problems with using the pretest as a covariate (see discussion of ANCOVA in chapter 8). Finally, the experimenter could subtract each subject's pretest value from the posttest value (called a **difference score**) and perform a simple ANOVA (or, with only two groups, an independent t test) using each subject's difference score as the dependent variable. Each of these techniques has strengths and weaknesses, but you will find all three used in the literature.

In this design the important question is, Does one group change more than the other group? Although this issue is frequently called the analysis of difference scores, a more appropriate label is the assessment of change. Clearly, in a learning study the change is expected to be gain. But in an exercise physiology study, the change might be decreased performance caused by fatigue. Regardless, the issues are the same. How can this change be assessed appropriately?

The easiest answer is to obtain a change score by subtracting the pretest from the posttest. Although this is intuitively attractive, it does have some problems. First, these change scores tend to be unreliable. Second, the level of initial values applies: Subjects who begin low in performance can improve more easily than those who begin with high scores. Thus, initial score is negatively correlated with the change score. How would you like your tennis performance evaluated on change if your initial score was high (e.g., 5 successful forehand drives out of 10 trials) compared with a friend who began with a low score (e.g., 1 out of 10 successful hits)? If you improved to 7 out of 10 on the final test and your friend improved to 5 out of 10 (the level of your initial score), your friend has improved twice as much as you have (a gain of 4 versus 2 successful hits). Yet your performance is still considerably better and it was more difficult for you to improve.

The issues involved in the proper measurement of change are complex, and we cannot treat these issues here. However, much has been written on this topic. We suggest you read Schmidt (1988, chapter 11) about this problem in motor learning and performance or, for complete coverage, see Harris (1963).

This design may also be extended into more complex forms. First, more than two (pretest and posttest) repeated measures can be used. This is common in the areas of motor learning and control. Two randomly formed groups of subjects might be measured 20, 30, or 40 or more times as they learn a task. The two groups might differ in the information they are given. The design is a 2 (Groups) × 30 (Trials), and a 2 × 30 ANOVA with repeated measures on the second factor (Trials) might be the statistical analysis. Remember from chapter 8 that meeting the assumptions for a repeated measures ANOVA with many repeated measures is very difficult. Thus, in designs like these, trials may be blocked (e.g., several trials averaged, reducing the number of repeated measures) or one of the multivariate repeated measures analyses can be used (see chapter 9).

Sometimes the design is extended in other ways. For example, we could take the design in Example

---

difference score — A score which represents the difference (gain) from pretest to posttest.

16.1 (a 2×3 factorial) and add a third factor of a pretest and a posttest. This would result in a three-way factorial with repeated measures on the third factor. All the versions of this design are subject to the first threat to external validity: reactive or interactive effects of testing. The pretest may make the subject more sensitive to the treatment and thus reduce the ability to generalize the findings to an unpretested population.

6. Solomon Four–Group Design

This design is the only true design to specifically evaluate one of the threats to external validity: reactive or interactive effects of testing. The design is depicted as follows:

$$
\begin{array}{llll}
R & O_1 & T & O_2 \\
R & O_3 & & O_4 \\
R & & T & O_5 \\
R & & & O_6
\end{array}
$$

This combines Designs 4 and 5. The purpose is explicitly to determine whether the pretest results in increased sensitivity of the subjects to the treatment. This design allows a replication of the treatment effect (is $O_2 > O_4$ and is $O_5 > O_6$), an assessment of the amount of change due to the treatment [is $(O_2 - O_1) > (O_4 - O_3)$], an evaluation of the testing effect (is $O_4 > O_6$), and an assessment of whether the pretest interacts with the treatment (is $O_2 > O_5$). Thus, this is a very powerful experimental design. Unfortunately, it is also an inefficient design as twice as many subjects are required. This results in very limited use, especially among graduate students doing theses and dissertations. In addition, no good way exists to analyze this design statistically. The best alternative (this one does not use all the data) is a 2×2 ANOVA set up as follows:

	No T	T
Pretested	O_4	O_2
Unpretested	O_6	O_5

Thus, IV_1 has two levels (pretested and not pretested), and IV_2 has two levels (treatment and no treatment). In the ANOVA, the F ratio for IV_1 establishes the effects of pretesting, the F for IV_2 establishes the effects of the treatment, and the F for interaction evaluates the external validity threat of interaction of the pretest with the treatment. Table 16.2 summarizes the control of threats to validity for the true experimental designs.

Table 16.2   True Experimental Designs and Their Control of the Threats to Validity

Validity threat	Randomized groups	Pretest-posttest randomized groups	Solomon four-group
Internal			
History	+	+	+
Maturation	+	+	+
Testing	+	+	+
Instrumentation	+	+	+
Statistical regression	+	+	+
Selection	+	+	+
Experimental mortality	+	+	+
Selection × maturation	+	+	+
Expectancy	?	?	?
External			
Testing × treatment	–	+	+
Selection biases × treatment	?	?	?
Experimental arrangements	?	?	?
Multiple treatments			

Note. + = strength, – = weakness,   = not relevant, ? = questionable.

Quasi-Experimental Designs

Not all research in which an independent variable is manipulated fits clearly into one of the true experimental designs. As researchers attempt to increase external and ecological validity, the careful and complete control of the true designs becomes increasingly difficult if not impossible. The purpose of **quasi-experimental designs** is to fit the design to settings more like the real world while still controlling as many of the threats to internal validity as possible. The use of these types of designs in physical education, exercise science, and sport science and in other areas (e.g., education, psychology, and sociology) has increased considerably in recent years. Perhaps the most authoritative text on quasi-experimental designs is that by Cook and Campbell (1979).

7. Time Series Design

This design has only one group but attempts to show that the change that occurs when the treat-ment is interjected differs from the times when it is not. This design may be depicted as follows:

$$O_1 \quad O_2 \quad O_3 \quad O_4 \quad T \quad O_5 \quad O_6 \quad O_7 \quad O_8$$

The basis for claiming that the treatment causes the effect is that a constant rate of change can be established from O_1 to O_4 and from O_5 to O_8 but that this rate of change varies between O_4 and O_5 where T has been administered. For example, in Figure 16.1, lines A, B, and C suggest that the insertion of the treatment (T) results in a visible change across observations, whereas lines D, E, F, and G indicate that the treatment has no reliable effect.

The typical statistical analyses previously discussed do not fit time series designs very well. For example, a repeated measures ANOVA with appropriate follow-ups applied to line C in Figure 16.1 might indicate that all observations (O_1 to O_8) differ significantly even though we can visibly see a change in the rate of increase between O_4 and O_5. We do not present the details, but regression techniques can be used to test both the slopes and the intercepts in time series designs.

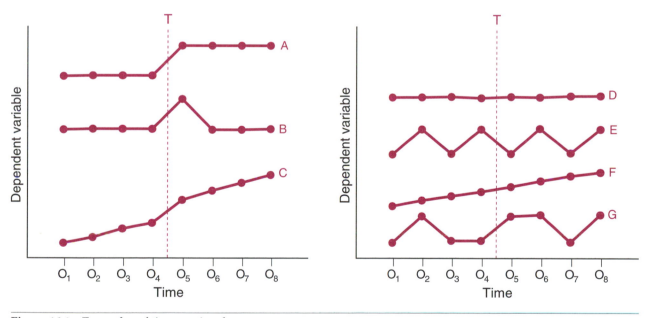

Figure 16.1   Examples of times series changes.

D.T. Campbell and J.C. Stanley, *Experimental and Quasi-Experimental Designs for Research.* Copyright © 1963 by Houghton Mifflin Company. Reprinted with permission.

 quasi-experimental design — Research designs in which the experimenter tries to fit the design to more "real-world" settings while still controlling as many of the threats to internal validity as possible.

Cook, T.D., & Campbell, D.T. (1979). *Quasi-experimentation: Design and analysis issues for field settings.* Chicago: Rand-McNally.

This type of design appears to control for a number of the threats to internal validity. For example, maturation would appear to be constant between observations. Testing effects can also be evaluated, although they could be difficult to separate from maturation. Selection biases also appear to be controlled because the same subjects are used at each observation. Of course, history, instrumentation, and mortality are controlled only to the extent that the researcher controls them. See a humorous example of a time series design on pages 359-360.

8. Reversal Design

This type of design is used increasingly in school settings and is depicted as follows:

$$O_1 \quad O_2 \quad T_1 \quad O_3 \quad O_4 \quad T_2 \quad O_5 \quad O_6$$

The purpose here (as with the time series) is to determine a baseline measure (O_1 and O_2), evaluate the treatment (change between O_2 and O_3), evaluate a no treatment time period (O_3 to O_4), evaluate the treatment again (O_4 to O_5), and evaluate a return to a no treatment condition (O_5 to O_6). This design is sometimes called A B A B A (or sometimes just A B) where A = baseline condition and B = treatment condition.

In Figure 16.2, lines such as A, B, and C suggest that the insertion of the treatment is effective, whereas lines such as D, E, and F do not support a treatment effect. Statistical analyses for reversal designs also need to be regression tests of the slopes and intercepts of the lines among various observations.

9. Nonequivalent Control Group

This design is frequently used in real-world settings where groups cannot be randomly formed. The design is as follows:

$$\begin{array}{ccc} O_1 & T & O_2 \\ \cdots\cdots\cdots \\ O_3 & & O_4 \end{array}$$

You will recognize this as Design 5 without randomization. Frequently, researchers will compare O_1 to O_3 and declare the groups equivalent if this comparison is not significant. Unfortunately, just because the groups do not differ on the pretest does not mean they are not different on any number of unmeasured characteristics that could affect the outcome of the research. If the groups differ when compared (O_1 versus O_3), ANCOVA is usually employed to adjust O_2 and O_4 for initial differences. Although this design is frequently used, we believe that Designs 7 and 8 are much stronger quasi-experimental designs for investigating intact situations.

10. Ex Post Facto Design

In its simplest case, this is Design 3 but with the treatment not under the control of the experimenter. For example, we frequently compare the characteristic of athletes versus nonathletes, high fit versus low fit individuals, female versus male performers, and expert performers versus novice performers. In effect, we are searching for variables that dis-

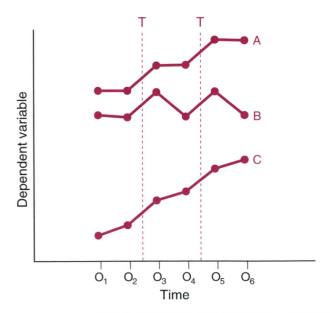
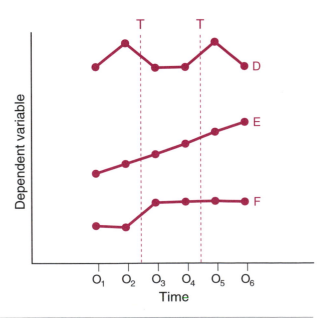

Figure 16.2 Examples of changes across time in reversal designs.

7 ± 2: Miller Must Have Been An Assistant Professor

Jerry R. Thomas

Summary.—**Miller's magical number for memory span (7 ± 2) is humorously brought to task because of its inability to predict the everyday performance of teenagers, graduate students, and full professors. Explanations are provided for the deficits in memory performance of these subgroups during lifespan development.**

Miller's (1956) classic paper identifying the memory span as 7 ± 2 items must have omitted using full professors as subjects, at least based on an *n* of 1, namely me. I have frequently heard clinical psychologists accused of going into psychology to study their own problems. Maybe that is a more valid explanation than bringing Miller's work to task. For years my graduate students have said that I study memory for movement because (a) I have little or no memory, and (b) I lose my spatial orientation just walking around the block. However, I prefer to think that Miller's results only apply to a subsample of the population—6- to 10-yr.-old children, college students, and new assistant professors. Six- to 10-yr.-old children never forget anything you promised to do (or even things you said may . . .). However, as soon as they approach the teen years, their memory spans drop to less than 1 unit of information.

Teenagers cannot remember to make their beds as they are getting out of them. Evidently, nothing ever happens to teenagers at school, although I prefer to think that they just cannot recall anything that happened. When these teenagers with little memory capacity go to college, an amazing transition in memory occurs. Between the freshman and senior years, the young adults' memory capacity increases to at least 7 ± 2 units of information. Loosely defined, this means *they know everything*; conversely, parents know nothing.

After working a few years and coming back to graduate school, memory facility is somewhat reduced. Graduate students have a memory capacity of 3 ± 1 units of information: (a) They know that they are graduate students; (b) They remember to pick up their graduate assistantship paycheck; (c) They remember to attend their graduate seminars. The ± 1 refers to the fact that they occasionally remember to do the reading for the seminar (+ 1) but they sometimes forget to come to class (– 1).

As soon as graduate students receive their PhDs, Miller's magical number (7 ± 2) is again a good predictor of memory—new assistant professors know everything. However, movement through the academic ranks gradually reduces capacity to remember until the average capacity of full professors (and parents) is reached, 2 ± 1 units of information. A full professor can remember (a) he or she is a full professor and (b) his or her paycheck comes regularly. The ± 1 refers to the fact that the full professor sometimes remembers that he or she has graduate students (+ 1) but occasionally forgets to pick up the regular paycheck (– 1).

Based on the failure of this model to meet the assumptions of stage theory (i.e., one should never regress to an earlier stage), we must assume that this uneven transition in memory states (see Fig. 1) is environmentally induced.

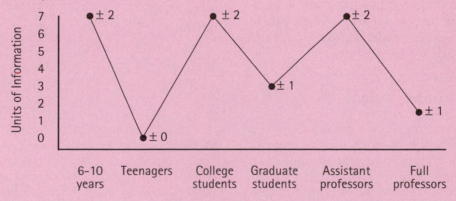

Figure 1.   Maximum number of units of information retained in memory across the lifespan.

But how can the environment cause these wide variations in memory performance? First, I believe we have to assume that Miller is correct about the structural maximum of memory performance because the deficits are not confined to a single point in the lifespan (i.e., teenagers, graduate students, full professors). The question of interest then becomes, *what causes such a serious depression in memory performance for teenagers, graduate students, and full professors?* Given my extensive study of memory as well as personal experience with all the stages, I can deduce the answer.

For teenagers the drop to about 0 memory with no variance is an interaction of carbonated soft drinks, junk food, and other boys or girls (whichever sex the teenager in question is not). This interaction is not a simple one and has an indirect effect, that is, this interaction causes pimples and the need for braces, both of which are very distracting in and of themselves. Taken in combination with Mom saying, "Wash your face" and "Brush your teeth," all of the teenager's memory capacity is occupied.

The deficit that occurs for graduate students is easy to explain. Three factors are involved. First, the graduate student is expected to work full-time (either as a research or teaching assistant) for one-third or less of normal pay, a very distracting and disconcerting circumstance. Second, the graduate student is expected to study and do research day and night. One's major professor assumes graduate students do not need sleep. Finally, the graduate student's major professor is continually nagging him or her to read this paper, collect these data, write this paper, and work on his or her dissertation. In combination, these items reduce memory capacity.

But why does the full professor who seems to have everything going for him or her show such poor memory performance? Full professors have a living wage (according to some), cars that run, houses with real furniture, tenure, graduate students to do the work, and time to play golf and tennis. What could possibly explain the deficit in memory performance? Answering that question is the easiest of all:
GRADUATE STUDENTS AND TEENAGERS!

Reference

Miller, G. (1956). The magical number seven, plus or minus two: Some limits on our capacity for processing information. *Psychological Review,* **63**, 81-97

From "7 ± 2: Miller Must Have Been an Assistant Professor" by J.R. Thomas, 1987, *NASPSPA Newsletter,* **12**(1), pp. 10-11. Adapted with permission.

criminate among these groups. Our interest usually resides in questions like, Did these variables influence the way these groups became different? Of course, this design cannot answer this question, but it may provide interesting insight and characteristics for manipulation in other experimental designs. This design is also often called a causal comparative design. Table 16.3 summarizes the threats to validity of quasi-experimental designs 7 to 10 and of design 11, which we discuss below.

Other Types of Quasi-Designs

The previously mentioned quasi-designs have been frequently reported in research on the study of physical activity. However, several additional designs have considerable potential but have seen less use in our research. We hope the following presentations will increase interest and use of these designs.

11. Switched Replication Design

This design (Cook & Campbell, 1979) can be either true or quasi depending on whether levels are subjects or groups.

Levels (Subjects or Group)	Trials				
	1	2	3	4	5
1	O_1 T	O_2	O_3	O_4	O_5
2	O_6	O_7 T	O_8	O_9	O_{10}
3	O_{11}	O_{12}	O_{13} T	O_{14}	O_{15}
4	O_{16}	O_{17}	O_{18}	O_{19} T	O_{20}

If subjects are randomly assigned to levels 1 to 4, the design is a true one. If levels 1 to 4 are different "intact" groups (e.g., tennis players—college, high school, and two age levels of youth leagues), then the design is quasi. Any number of levels beyond two can be used, but the number of trials must be one greater than the number of levels.

Table 16.3   Quasi-Experimental Designs and Their Control of the Threats to Validity

Validity threat	Time series	Nonequivalent control	Reversal	Ex post facto	Switched replication
Internal					
History	–	–	–	?	?
Maturation	+	+	+	?	+
Testing	+	+	+		+
Instrumentation	?	+	+		?
Statistical regression	+	?	+		+
Selection	+	+	+	–	?
Experimental mortality	+	+	+		?
Selection × maturation	+	–	+	–	+
Expectancy	?	?	?	?	+
External					
Testing × treatment	–	–	?	–	?
Selection biases × treatment	?	?	?	?	?
Experimental arrangements	?	?	?	?	+
Multiple treatments			?		+

Note. + = strength, – = weakness,   = not relevant, ? = questionable.

Donald T. Campbell and Julian C. Stanley, *Experimental and Quasi-Experimental Designs for Research.* Copyright © 1963. Reprinted with permission of Houghton Mifflin Company.

This design has two strong features: The treatment is replicated several times, and long-term treatment effects can be evaluated. There is no standard statistical analysis for this design, but various ANOVAs with repeated measures could be used. Or the design might be analyzed by fitting regression lines to each level and testing how the slopes and intercepts change.

Many opportunities exist to use this design in our field, yet it is seldom used. This design might be particularly useful in research on sport teams where teams could be different levels or where different players within a team could be assigned to the various levels. (Thanks to Sandy Braver, Department of Psychology at Arizona State University, for this idea.)

12. Exercise Epidemiological Designs

The interest in exercise epidemiology has grown considerably both in our field and in other health-related areas (e.g., medicine). Epidemiology describes the level of need and demand related to health services. In particular, exercise epidemiology research focuses on the value of physical activity on prevention and rehabilitation issues in health. Research in this area often identifies both the overall need and those of greatest need. In chapter 7 we

mentioned that statistical techniques used in exercise epidemiology can assess the relation of physical activity to risk factors (thus, the ratios we discussed).

There are two general types of designs in exercise epidemiology: case-control studies (also called case-comparison studies) and cohort studies. Case-control studies select individuals from some source (e.g., hospitals, rehabilitation programs, clinics) who have been diagnosed as having a disorder and compare them to cases who do not have the disorder (selected from similar circumstances as those having the disorder). The problem with case-control studies is the researcher does not know the population proportion represented by the selected cases and controls.

Cohort studies are of two general types: groups of subjects that have been exposed to the cause of the disorder versus those who have not with the relative frequency of the exposure/nonexposure known; or a sample of cohorts is selected from the population and using standardized procedures, subjects are grouped in cases and noncases relative to the disorder. In case-control and cohort designs, studies may be

- **retrospective**—the researcher looks backwards from the effects to the preceding causes. For example, a group of men who

Three types of case-control and cohort designs

have had heart attacks during the past 10 years but have not died are compared with an age-matched group who died following heart attacks during this same period. The groups are compared on their amount of physical activity in the 5 years preceding their heart attacks.

- **prospective**—the researcher identifies an event or cause at one point and follows a group of subjects who become disordered or who recovered from the event over some specified period. Our field has often looked at individuals who have experienced heart attacks and evaluated the effects of degree of adherence to an exercise rehabilitation program on future risk factors.

- **cross-sectional**—the researcher measures potential causes and effects at a common point and estimates their relationship. For example, are people who are involved in an exercise program likely to have lower cardiovascular risk factors than those not exercising regularly?

13. Single Subject Designs

In our field single subject designs are most often used in clinical settings. Examples include observing physical education instruction, pursuing sport psychology work with athletes, studying an outstanding performer (e.g., Olympic athlete), or looking at the motor function of an impaired individual (e.g., reaching and grasping by a Parkinson's patient). A subject in this type of study is typically measured repeatedly on the task of interest. Many trials are needed to evaluate the influence of the treatment. During some periods a baseline measure is obtained, and during other periods a treatment is administered. The focus is often on subject variability as well as average values. Quasi-designs 7, 8, and 11 all work as single subject designs and group designs. When used with single subjects, these designs are often called A B or A B A B designs. In this instance A refers to the baseline condition (no treatment) and B refers to when the treatment is being administered. Sometimes more than one treatment is administered to the same subject. As in research using a group of subjects, counterbalancing the treatment order to separate treatment effects is important. Possible questions include the following:

- Does the treatment produce the same effect each time?
- Are the effects of the treatment cumulative, or does the subject return to baseline following each treatment period?

- Does the subject's response to the treatment become less variable over multiple treatment periods?
- Is the subject's magnitude of response less sensitive to multiple applications of the treatment?
- Do varying intensities, frequencies, and lengths of treatment produce varying responses?

Other quasi-experimental designs exist, but the ones discussed here are the most commonly used. Of course, quasi designs never quite control internal validity as well as do true designs, but they do allow us to conduct investigations either when true designs cannot be used or when the use of a true design significantly reduces external validity.

Summary

In experimental research one or more independent variables (the treatment) are manipulated to assess the effects on one or more dependent variables (the response measured). Research studies are concerned with both internal and external validity. Internal validity pertains to controlling factors as required so that the results can be attributed to the treatment. Threats to internal validity include history, maturation, testing, instrumentation, statistical regression, selection biases, experimental mortality, selection-maturation interaction, and expectancy.

External validity is the ability to generalize the results to other subjects and to other settings. Four threats exist to external validity: reactive or interactive effects of testing, the interaction of selection biases and the experimental treatment, reactive effects of experimental arrangements, and multiple-treatment interference. Having high degrees of both internal and external validity is nearly impossible. The rigid controls needed for internal validity make it difficult to generalize the results to the real world. Conversely, studies with high external validity are usually weak in internal validity. Random selection of subjects and random assignment to treatments are the most powerful means of controlling most threats to internal and external validity.

Preexperimental designs are weak in that they can control few sources of invalidity. True experimental designs are characterized by random formulation of groups, which allows the assumption that the groups were equivalent at the beginning of the study. The randomized groups, the pretest-posttest randomized groups, and the Solomon four-group designs are examples of true experimental designs.

Quasi-experimental designs are often used when it is difficult or impossible to use true experimental designs or when a true design significantly limits external validity. Time series designs, the reversal design, the nonequivalent control group design, and the ex post facto design are the most commonly used. The switched replication design, exercise epidemiology designs, and single subject designs are potentially useful but less frequently used quasi-experimental designs.

 Check Your Understanding

Locate two research papers in refereed journals in your area of interest. One paper should have a true experimental design and the other a quasi-experimental design.

1. Describe the type of design. Draw a picture of it, using the notation from this chapter.
2. How many independent variables are there? How many levels of each? What are they?
3. How many dependent variables? What are they?
4. What type of statistical analysis was used? Explain how it fits the design.
5. Identify the threats to internal validity that are controlled and uncontrolled. Explain each.
6. Identify the controlled and uncontrolled threats to external validity. Explain each.

CHAPTER 17

Qualitative Research

Dear Professors of Research Methods:

I am planning to write a thesis on the interaction between a teacher and her students. I intend to use the qualitative research method in which I will observe and interview the teacher and students over several months. My friend claims that because I am good in statistics I should use a quantitative approach, such as a survey. What do you think?

In a qualitative-quantitative quandary,
Quag Meyer

Dear Quag:

Research is a means of solving problems. The formulation of the method to be used in a research study should depend primarily on the question that is being asked. One should not let the method determine the nature of the study. Remember the adage that if one only has a hammer then every problem is viewed as a nail. Some of the most important research questions are best approached via qualitative methodology. One of Yogi Berra's "laws" proclaims: "You can observe a lot just by watching." Participant observation can yield valuable insights and perspectives concerning the interactions of people in a particular setting. Go for it.

Methodologically yours,
PRM

Qualitative research in physical education, exercise science, and sport science is relatively new. Researchers in education began adapting ethnographic research design to educational settings in the United States in the 1970s (Goetz & LeCompte, 1984), and significant qualitative research in physical education and sport science has been conducted steadily since the 1980s. In 1989, Locke was invited to write an essay/tutorial on qualitative research that was published in the Review and Commentary section of the *Research Quarterly for Exercise and Sport*.

The qualitative method of research is not new, however, in other fields. It has been employed in anthropology, psychology, and sociology for many years. This general form of research has been called various names, including ethnographic, naturalistic, interpretive, grounded, phenomenological, subjective, and participant observational. Although the approaches are all slightly different, each "bears a strong **family resemblance** to the others" (Erickson, 1986, p. 119).

For those of you who are unfamiliar with the term qualitative research, it might be beneficial to review your courses or readings in anthropology. Nearly everyone has heard of classic ethnographic studies (even if you have never heard them referred to as ethnographic), such as the famous cultural research Margaret Mead conducted when she lived in the Samoan Islands in the South Pacific. Mead interviewed the Samoans at length about their society, their traditions, and their beliefs. This is an example of qualitative research. You do not need to live among natives in a remote, exotic land to do it, however. The qualitative research we refer to in this chapter is done mainly in everyday settings, such as schools, gymnasiums, sport facilities, fitness centers, and hospitals.

It could be argued that the term *qualitative research* may be too restrictive in that it seems to denote the absence of anything quantitative; however, this is certainly not the case. Nonetheless, qualitative research seems to be the term used most often in our field. Our discussion of qualitative research focuses on the interpretive method as opposed to the so-called thick, rich description that characterized early research in anthropology, psychology, and sociology. This latter approach involves a very long and detailed account of the entity or incident and was espoused by Franz Boas, who is considered the "father" of cultural anthropology. In rejecting the armchair speculation that typified the late-19th-century work, Boas insisted that the researcher not only collect his or her own data but that it be reported with as little comment or interpretation as possible (cited in Kirk & Miller, 1986).

We believe that the most significant feature of qualitative research is the interpretive content rather than an overconcern about procedure. Erickson (1986) argues that the technique of narrative description (sometimes referred to as "writing like crazy") does not necessarily mean that the research being conducted is interpretive or qualitative. It is not our intention to present a comprehensive review of qualitative research. One reason is that we do not have the space to do so, as this text is designed primarily to survey various methods of research. Despite our assertion that qualitative research is quite new in our field, a comprehensive review would still be a major undertaking because we would need to draw from many related fields. Whereas 30 years ago there was almost nothing in print in the area of qualitative methodology, there is now a tremendous amount of literature in the form of books, articles, and monographs. Moreover, there is considerable disagreement among qualitative researchers concerning their methodologies and theoretical presuppositions that would need to be addressed. You can gain a solid appreciation regarding the scope of qualitative research, the different approaches to data collection, and their theoretical foundations by consulting, for example, Jacob (1987, 1988) and the references in essays such as those of Erickson (1986) and Locke (1989). Readable single-source texts include those of Bogdan and Biklen (1992), Goetz and LeCompte (1984), and Lincoln and Guba (1985). Another suggested reading is a qualitative study in

---

family resemblance theory — Theory in philosophic research in which, in an attempt to unify components of a concept, the researcher recognizes that though the components lack specific shared characteristics, they share a system of overlapping features.

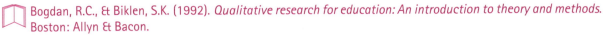

Bogdan, R.C., & Biklen, S.K. (1992). *Qualitative research for education: An introduction to theory and methods.* Boston: Allyn & Bacon.

Lincoln, Y.S., & Guba, E.G. (1985). *Naturalistic inquiry.* Newbury Park, CA: Sage.

Rovegno, I. (1994). Teaching within a curricular zone of safety: School culture and the situated nature of student teachers' pedagogical content knowledge. *Research Quarterly for Exercise and Sport, 65,* 269-279.

pedagogy in physical education by Inez Rovegno (1994).

The Quantitative–Qualitative Quandary

Much has been written on the debate over the comparative merits of quantitative and qualitative approaches to problem solving, so we do not discuss it here. Locke (1989) observed that the debate in our field comes at a point where the same dispute is winding down in other areas. So, instead of relating some arguments about which method is better, let us simply contrast some basic differences between quantitative and qualitative research.

Qualitative research is often depicted as the antithesis of the more traditional quantitative methods, such as experimental and survey research. Quantitative research methods typically involve precise measurements, rigid control of variables (often in a laboratory setting), and statistical analyses. Qualitative research methods generally include field observations, case studies, ethnography, and narrative reports (Linn, 1986). Bogdan and Biklen (1992) provide a detailed contrast of characteristics of qualitative and quantitative research regarding terms, key concepts, theoretical and academic affiliations, goals, design, samples, data, and the nature of research proposals in each paradigm.

Quantitative research tends to focus on analysis (i.e., taking apart and examining components of a phenomenon), whereas qualitative research seeks to understand the meaning of an experience to the participants in a specific setting and how the components mesh to form a whole. Some basic characteristics of quantitative and qualitative research are contrasted in Table 17.1. Patton (1987) uses two responses to a questionnaire item to illustrate the depth, detail, and meaning in qualitative methods. In the quantitative approach, a teacher was asked to respond to a statement: "Accountability as practiced in our school system creates an undesirable atmosphere of anxiety among teachers." The choices were strongly agree, agree, disagree, and strongly disagree. She checked "strongly agree." However, her response to an open-ended question about the accountability approach revealed a much more intense, negative feeling about the system. She stressed the atmosphere of fear among the teachers and the strong political motives imbedded in the system. She described her feelings of frustration, bitterness, and hatred and condemned accountability as totally counterproductive.

Qualitative research focuses on the "essence" of the phenomena. The view of the world varies with one's perception and is highly subjective. The objectives are primarily description, understanding, and meaning. The researcher does not manipulate variables through experimental treatments but takes more interest in process than in product. The researcher observes and gathers data in the field, that is, the natural setting. There are no preconceived hypotheses, which characterize quantitative research. Rather, qualitative research strives to develop hypotheses from the observations. In other words, qualitative research emphasizes induction, whereas quantitative research largely emphasizes deduction.

In quantitative research, the researcher tries very hard to keep out of the data-gathering process by

Table 17.1   Contrasting Characteristics of Qualitative and Quantitative Research

Research component	Qualitative	Quantitative
Hypothesis	Inductive	Deductive
Sample	Purposive, small	Random, large
Setting	Natural, real world	Laboratory
Data gathering	Researcher is primary instrument	Objective instrumentation
Design	Flexible, may change	Determined in advance
Data Analysis	Descriptive, interpretive	Statistical methods

Bogdan, R.C., & Biklen, S.K. (1992). *Qualitative research for education: An introduction to theory and methods.* Boston: Allyn & Bacon.

using laboratory measurements, questionnaires, and other so-called objective instruments. The quantitative data are then usually analyzed by statistical formulas, with computations performed by computers. However, the researcher is the primary instrument for data collection and analysis in qualitative research, which is very subjective in this sense. The researcher is interacting with the subjects, and the researcher's sensitivity and perception are crucial in procuring and processing the observations and responses.

Procedures in Qualitative Research

Define the Problem

Formulate Hypotheses and Theoretical Framework

Collect the Data

    Training and Pilot Work

    Subject Selection

    Entering the Setting

    Methods of Collecting Data

       Interviews

       Focus Groups

       Observation

       Action Research

       Other Recording Devices

Analyze the Data

    Sorting, Analyzing, and Categorizing Data

    Interpreting Data and Constructing a Theory

       Quantitative Analysis

       Triangulation of Data

       Theory Construction

Write the Report

It should go without saying that there are many variations in the way qualitative research is done. Consequently, the procedures outlined in this section should be viewed simply as an attempt to provide an orientation for readers who are unfamiliar with qualitative research. As with any type of research, the novice will benefit most from reading completed studies that have used particular methods.

Define the Problem

We will not spend much time defining the problem because we have talked about this step before, and it does not differ appreciably from that of other research methods. We emphasized that several possible methods can be used for any research problem. The different methods can yield different information about the problem. Thus, when the researcher decides to use qualitative research as opposed to some other design, the decision is based on what he or she wants to know about the problem (for more discussion on this point, review chapter 1).

Formulate Hypotheses and Theoretical Framework

In highlighting some differences between quantitative and qualitative research, we stated that qualitative research usually builds hypotheses and theories in an inductive manner, that is, as a result of the observations. Quantitative research often begins with research hypotheses that are subsequently tested. Thus, not having stated hypotheses in the first part (or chapter) is common for a qualitative study. As explained by Goetz and LeCompte (1984), although research ultimately may hope to discover causal relationships, ethnographers commonly avoid assuming a priori relationships. However, some studies are designed to confirm or refine hypotheses developed in previous research. In such studies, hypotheses are stated in the first part of the report. The researcher then modifies, refines, confirms, or rejects them.

Collect the Data

Several components are involved in collecting data for qualitative research, just as in quantitative research. Training and pilot work are still necessary, and so is selecting subjects appropriately. In addition, you need to enter the field setting and become as unobtrusive as possible in your collection of data.

Training and Pilot Work

In qualitative research the investigator is the instrument for collecting and analyzing the data. It is imperative, then, that the researcher is adequately prepared. Certainly course work, fieldwork reports, and interaction with one's advisor are helpful, but ultimately the only way to become competent is through hands-on experience. In the classic anthropological tradition, fieldwork is essentially unteachable (Erickson, 1986), although clinical experience is usually acquired through projects under the direction of an advisor.

As always, pilot work is essential, and fieldwork experience in a setting similar to that of the proposed study is recommended. If the researcher has experience in the field setting (e.g., as an instructor, a coach, or a player), it will be helpful in most respects. However, Locke (1989) made a good point while describing the phases of a qualitative study about familiarity, in that it tends to spawn "an almost irresistible flood of personal judgments" (p. 7) that, if not recognized and controlled, could become a significant threat to the integrity of the data.

Subject Selection

Basically, the selection of subjects for a qualitative study is the same as described for the case study in chapter 15. Qualitative research studies do not attempt to make inferences from their subjects to some larger population. Rather, the subjects are selected because they have certain characteristics. Obviously, there are pragmatic reasons concerning the location and the availability of subjects because in nearly every case numerous other sites and subjects with similar characteristics exist.

 Probability sampling is not used, simply because there is no way to estimate the probability that each subject has of being selected and no assurance that each subject has some chance of being included (Chein, 1981). Instead, the selection of subjects in qualitative research is purposive, which in essence means that a sample is selected from which one can learn the most. The researcher may be looking for subjects with certain levels of expertise or experience. Goetz and LeCompte (1984) used the term **criterion-based sampling**, in which the researcher establishes certain criteria or standards that must be met before a subject can be included in the investigation. In essence, then, the selection of subjects in qualitative research involves consideration of where to observe, when to observe, whom to observe, and what to observe (Burgess, 1982).

Entering the Setting

The researcher must have access to the field setting to conduct a qualitative study. Moreover, the researcher must be able to observe and interview the subjects at the appropriate time and location. These mundane details may seem somewhat trivial in the overall scheme of things in the mystical world of research, but nothing is more important than site

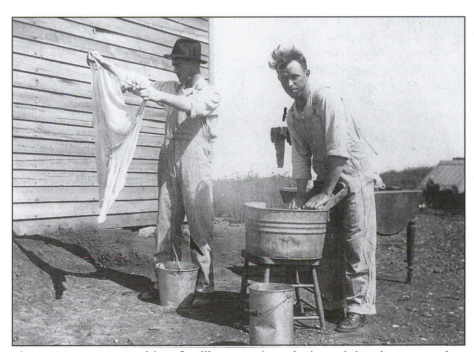

The only way to become competent with unfamiliar procedures is through hands-on experience.

criterion-based sampling — See *purposive sampling*.

entry. In any type of research you must have access to the data, whether it be source material in historical research or subjects in an experimental or a survey study. However, the problem can be of greater magnitude in qualitative research than in most other methods. The quantitative researcher is simply borrowing the subjects for a short time for some measurements or taking a little class time to administer a questionnaire. In qualitative research, the investigator is often at the site for weeks or months. This "outsider" is listening, watching, coding, and videotaping, as well as imposing on the time of the teacher (or coach, or whomever) and the students (players and participants) for interviews.

We are intentionally exhausting this topic because it is so important. Obviously, it takes diplomacy, personality, and artful persuasion to gain site entry. Frankly, some people just cannot do this. Even when entry is achieved, some studies have failed because the investigator "rubbed people the wrong way" and the subjects were not motivated to cooperate fully. Thus, the negotiation of gaining access to the subjects in their naturalistic setting is important and complex. It starts with the first contact by telephone or letter, extends through data collection, and continues after the researcher has left the site (Erickson, 1986).

Before we discuss some aspects of data collection, we should elaborate a little more on the topic of cooperation with the subjects. Rapport is everything. The subjects must feel that they can trust you, or else they will not give you the information you seek. Obviously, formal informed consent must be obtained and the stipulations embodied in the whole concept of informed consent must be observed.

Qualitative research involves a number of ethical considerations simply because of the intensive personal contact with the subjects. Thus, the subjects need to know that provisions will be followed to safeguard their rights of privacy and to guarantee anonymity. If, for some reason, it is impossible to keep information confidential, this must be made clear. The researcher must give a great deal of thought to these matters before collecting data and must be able to explain the purpose and significance of the study effectively and convey the importance of subject cooperation in language that the subjects can understand. One of the largest obstacles in the quest for natural behavior and candor on the part of the subjects is their suspicion that the researcher will be evaluating them. The researcher must be

very convincing in this regard. The most successful studies are those in which the subjects feel as though they are a part of the project. In other words, a collaborative relationship should be established.

Methods of Collecting Data

The most common sources of data collection in qualitative research are interviews, observations, and researcher-designed instruments (Goetz & LeCompte, 1984). The methodology is planned and pilot-tested before the actual study. Creswell (1994) places the data-collecting procedures into four categories: observations, interviews, documents, and audiovisual materials. He provides a concise table of the four methods, the options within each type, the advantages of each type, and the limitations of each (p. 150).

The researcher will typically have some type of framework (subpurposes perhaps) that determines and guides the nature of the data collection. For example, one phase of the research might pertain to the manner in which expert and nonexpert sport performers perceive various aspects of a game. This phase could involve having the subject describe his or her perceptions of what is taking place in a specific scenario. A second phase of the study might focus on the interactive thought processes and decisions of the two groups of subjects while they are playing. The data for this phase could be obtained from filming the subjects in action and then interviewing the subjects while they are watching their performances on videotape. Still another aspect of the study could be directed at the knowledge structure of the subjects, which could be determined by a researcher-constructed instrument.

Interviews.   The interview is undoubtedly the most common source of data in qualitative studies. The person-to-person format is most prevalent, but occasionally group interviews are conducted. Interviews range from the highly structured style—in which questions are determined before the interview—to the open-ended, conversational format. In qualitative research, the highly structured format is used primarily to gather sociodemographic information. For the most part, however, interviews are more open-ended and less structured (Merriam, 1988). Frequently, the interviewer will ask the same questions of all the subjects, but the order of the questions, the exact wording, and the type of follow-up questions may vary considerably.

Four categories of data-collecting procedures

It requires skill and experience to be a good interviewer. We emphasized earlier that the researcher must first establish rapport with the subjects. If the subjects do not trust the researcher, they will not open up and describe their true feelings, thoughts, and intentions. Complete rapport is established over time as people get to know and trust one another. However, one facet of skill in interviewing is being able to ask questions in such a way that the respondent feels that he or she can talk freely.

Kirk and Miller (1986) described their field research in Peru, where they tried to learn how much urban, lower-middle-class people knew about coca, the organic sources of cocaine. Coca is legal and widely available there. In their initial attempts to ask the people to tell them about coca, they received the same culturally approved answers from all the subjects. It was only after they changed their style of asking less sensitive questions (e.g., How did you find out you didn't like coca?) that the Peruvians opened up and elaborated on their knowledge of (and sometimes their personal commitment to) coca. Kirk and Miller made a good point about asking the right questions and the value of using different approaches. Indeed, this is a basic argument for the validity of qualitative research.

Skillful interviewing takes practice. Ways to develop such skill include videotaping one's own performance in conducting an interview, observing experienced interviewers, playing roles, and critiquing peers. It is very important that the interviewer appear nonjudgmental. This can be difficult in situations in which the subject's views are quite different from those of the interviewer. The interviewer must be alert to both verbal and nonverbal messages and be flexible in rephrasing and pursuing certain lines of questioning. The researcher must be able to ask questions so that the subject understands what is being asked. One must use words that are clear and meaningful to the respondent. Above all, the interviewer has to be a good listener.

The use of a tape recorder is undoubtedly the most common method of recording interview data as it has the obvious advantage of preserving the entire interview for later analysis. Although some subjects may experience nervousness in talking while being taped, this uneasiness usually disappears in a short time. The main drawback with tape recording is equipment malfunctioning. This is vexing and frustrating when it happens during the interview, but it is devastating when it happens af-terward when you are trying to replay and analyze the interview. Certainly, it is wise always to have fresh batteries and to make sure the recorder is working properly early in the interview. It is also recommended that halfway through the interview you stop and play back some tape to see whether the person is speaking into the microphone loudly and clearly enough and whether you are getting the data. The subjects (especially children) love to hear themselves speak, so playing back the tape for them also serves as motivation. Remember, however, that machines can always malfunction.

Videotaping seems to be the best method because you not only hear what the subject said but also preserve nonverbal behavior. Videotape is not used much because it is awkward and intrusive. However, it will probably become more prevalent as technical advances continue to be made.

Taking notes during the interview is another common method. Sometimes it is used in addition to recording, primarily when the interviewer wishes to denote certain points of emphasis or make additional notations. Taking notes without taping prevents one from being able to record all that is said. It also keeps the interviewer very busy, interfering with one's thoughts and observations while the subject is talking. In highly structured interviews and when using some type of formal instrument, the interviewer can more easily take notes by checking and writing short responses.

The least preferred technique is trying to remember and write down afterward what was said in the interview. The drawbacks are many, and this method is seldom used.

Focus Groups.   Another type of qualitative research technique can employ interviews with a small group of people on a specific topic. It can be an efficient technique in that the researcher can gather information about several people in one session. The group is usually homogeneous, such as a group of school children, an athletic team, or a group of teachers.

 In his 1988 book *Focus Groups as Qualitative Research*, Morgan discusses the social science applications of focus groups in qualitative research. Patton (1987) argues that **focus group** interviews may provide quality controls in that participants tend to provide checks and balances on each other that can serve to curb false or extreme views. Focus group interviews are usually

---

 focus groups — The application of qualitative research methodology with a small group of individuals concerning a specific topic.

enjoyable for the participants, and there may be less fear of the interviewer evaluating the individual because of the group setting. The group members get to hear what others in the group have to say, which may stimulate the individuals to rethink their own views.

In the focus group interview, the researcher is not trying to persuade the group to reach consensus. It is an interview. Taking notes can be difficult, but a tape recorder or videotape may solve that problem. Certain group dynamics such as power struggles and reluctance to state views publicly are limitations of the focus group interview. One is also limited in the number of questions that can be asked in one session. Obviously, the focus group should be used in combination with other data-gathering techniques.

Observation.   Earlier studies relied on direct observation with note taking and coding of certain categories of behavior. More recently, videotaping has been the method of choice. The videotape can observe all of a subject's behavior and preserve it for later analysis. If desired, sounds associated with the observations can simultaneously be recorded, as can comments by the researcher. The newer cameras are lightweight and capable of obtaining remarkably clear pictures in natural lighting.

One major drawback to observation methods is obtrusiveness. A stranger with a camera or pad and pencil is recording people's natural behavior. A key word here is "stranger." The task of a qualitative researcher is to make sure that the subjects become accustomed to having the researcher (and video camera) around. For example, the researcher may want to practice or pretend to film in the setting for at least a couple of days before the initial filming.

In an artificial setting, researchers can use one-way mirrors and observation rooms. In a natural setting, the limitations that stem from the presence of an observer can never be ignored. Locke (1989) has observed that most naturalistic field studies are reports of what goes on when a visitor is present. The important question is, How important and limiting is this? Locke suggested ways of suppressing reactivity, such as both being in the setting long enough so that the visitor is no longer considered a novelty and being as unobtrusive as possible in everything from dress to choice of location in a room.

Action Research.   A type of observational research, **action research** refers to the application of a research approach to local problems such as within a classroom. The primary difference between action research and "regular" research is the extent to which findings can be generalized. Action research does not attempt to infer beyond the local situation.

Although both quantitative and qualitative approaches are used in action research, the qualitative paradigm lends itself very well to the local scenario. The very essence of qualitative research is the search to find out "what is going on here." It involves the systematic study of the perceptions and experiences of individuals within the context of the local setting. The researcher can observe and participate in actual program activities. Often direct observation and firsthand presence allow the researcher to see interactions, complexities, and dynamic processes from a more holistic perspective, which can lead to better understanding and greater insights about the situation or program.

Other Recording Devices.   There are many sources of data in qualitative research. We have mentioned researcher-constructed behavior-coding inventories. Self-reports of knowledge and attitude are occasionally used. Their use is limited, simply because of the inherent limitations of such formal self-reports with regard to a truly qualitative study. We also mentioned the use of scenarios, which are usually developed by the researcher. The subject's responses provide his or her perceptions, interpretations, and awareness of the total situation and the interplay of the actors in the scenario.

Other recording devices include notebooks, narrative field logs, and diaries, in which researchers records their reactions, concerns, and speculations. Printed materials such as course syllabi, team rosters, evaluation reports, subject notes, and photographs of the setting and situations are examples of document data used in qualitative research.

Analyze the Data

Data analysis in qualitative research is quite different from conventional quantitative research. First, analysis is done during and after data collection. During data collection the researcher sorts and organizes data and speculates and develops tentative

---

action research — The practical application of research techniques in dealing with problems in a specific setting. There is no intention of generalizing the results.

hypotheses to guide him or her to other sources and types of data. Qualitative research is often done in a manner somewhat similar to multiple experiment research, in which discoveries made during the study shape each successive phase of the study. Thus, simultaneous data collection and analysis allow the researcher to work more effectively. Analysis then becomes more intensive after the data have been collected (Merriam, 1988). Another difference between quantitative and qualitative data analysis is that qualitative data are generally presented through words, descriptions, and images, whereas quantitative analysis is typically presented through numbers.

The analysis of data in a qualitative study can take different forms, depending on the nature of the investigation and the defined purposes. Consequently, one cannot go into great depth in discussing analysis without tying it to a specific study. Therefore, we summarized the general phases of analysis synthesized from descriptions in several qualitative research texts. The general phases include sorting and analysis during data collection, analysis and categorization, and interpretation and theory construction.

Sorting, Analyzing, and Categorizing Data

The simultaneous collection and analysis of data are an important feature of qualitative research. It enables researchers to focus better on certain questions and, in turn, to direct the data collection more effectively. Although the researchers have specific questions in mind when the data collection begins, they will probably shift their focus as the data unfold.

Researchers need to keep in close touch with the data. It is a foolish mistake to wait until after the data are collected to analyze them. Decisions must be made concerning scope and direction, or the researchers may be left with data that are unfocused, repetitious, and overwhelming in the sheer volume of material that needs to be processed (Merriam, 1988). Also, there could be gaps because the researchers are so close to the data that they may not realize that some needed evidence was not collected.

Researchers typically write many observer comments to stimulate critical thinking about what they are observing. They should not be merely human recording machines. They should try out new ideas

and consider how certain data relate to the large theoretical, methodological, and substantive issues (Bogdan & Biklen, 1992). However, Goetz and LeCompte (1984) recommend that researchers should periodically review the research proposal to make sure the investigation is not straying too far from the original questions that must be addressed in the final report.

Analysis is the process of making sense out of one's data. Goetz and LeCompte (1984) have recommended that researchers read the data again before analysis to ensure completeness and generate analytic categories. This is the beginning of the stages of organizing, abstracting, integrating, and synthesizing, which ultimately permit researchers to report what they have seen and heard. They may develop an outline to search for patterns that can be transformed into categories.

The qualitative researcher faces a formidable task in sorting the data for content analysis. Obviously, there are many types of categories that can be devised with any given set of data, depending on the problem being studied. For example, a researcher could categorize observations of a physical education class in terms of the teacher's management style; another category could relate to social interaction among the students; another category could deal with sex differences in behavior or treatment; and one could be based on verbal and nonverbal instructional behaviors. Categories can range in complexity from relatively simple units of behavior types to conceptual typologies or theories (Merriam, 1988).

Researchers use different techniques for sorting data. Index cards and file folders have been widely used for years. Computers can be programmed to store, sort, and retrieve data. First, interview transcripts, notes, and observations are entered into the computer. Then, after themes (categories) have been designated, the researcher can retrieve sets of data that have been sorted by category. Miles and Huberman (1994) provide extensive criteria for choosing computer programs for qualitative data analysis.

Data categorization is a key facet of true qualitative research. Instead of using mere description, the researcher may use descriptive data as examples of the concepts that are being advanced. The data need to be studied and categorized so that the researcher can retrieve and analyze information across categories as part of the inductive process.

Miles, M.B., & Huberman, A.M. (1994). *Qualitative data analysis: A sourcebook of new methods* (2nd ed.). Thousand Oaks, CA: Sage.

Interpreting Data and Constructing a Theory

When the data have been organized and sorted, the researcher then attempts to merge them into a holistic portrayal of the phenomenon. An acknowledged goal of qualitative research is to vividly reconstruct what happened during the fieldwork. This is accomplished through the **analytic narrative**. This may consist of a descriptive narrative organized chronologically or topically. In our concept of qualitative research, however, we support the position voiced by Goetz and LeCompte (1984) that researchers who merely describe fail to do justice to their data. As Peshkin (1993) observes, "Pure, straight description is a chimera; accounts that attempt such a standard are sterile and boring" (p. 24). Goetz and LeCompte maintain that, by leaving readers to their own conclusions, one risks misinterpretation and perhaps trivialization of the data by readers who are unable to make the implied connections. They further suggest (p. 196) that the researcher who can find no implications beyond the data should never have undertaken the study in the first place.

The analytic narrative is the foundation of qualitative research. Researchers (especially novices) are often reluctant to take the bold action needed to assign meaning to the data. Erickson (1986) has suggested that to stimulate analysis early in the process one should force oneself to make an assertion, choose an excerpt from the field notes that substantiates the assertion, and then write a **narrative vignette** that portrays the validity of the assertion. In the process of making decisions concerning the event to report and the descriptive terms to use, the researcher becomes more explicitly aware of the perspectives that are emerging from the data. This awareness thus stimulates and facilitates further critical reflection.

The narrative vignette is one of the fundamental characteristics of qualitative research. As opposed to the typical analysis sections in quantitative research studies (which are about as interesting as watching paint dry), the vignette captures the reader's attention, thereby helping the researcher make his or her point. It gives the reader a sense of "being there." A well-written description of a situation can convey a sense of holistic meaning that is definitely advantageous in providing evidence for the researcher's various assertions. In characterizing qualitative research, Locke (1989) has stated that the researcher can describe the physical education scene so vividly that "you can smell the lockers and hear the thud of running feet" (p. 4). Griffin and Templin (1989) provide the following example of a vignette:

> The second period physical education class at Big City Middle School is playing soccer. The teacher has placed two piles of sweatshirts at each end of a large open field to serve as goals. There are no field markings. Four boys run up and down the field following the ball. Several other students stand silently in their assigned positions until the ball comes near, then they move tentatively toward the ball to kick it away. Three girls stand talking in a tight circle near the far end of the field. They are startled when the ball rolls into their group, and two boys yell at them to get out of the way. They do and then regroup after the ball and the boys go to the other side of the field. Two boys, who have not touched the ball during the class, engage in a playful wrestling match near one goal. The teacher stands in the center of the field with a whistle in his mouth. He hasn't said anything since he divided students into teams at the beginning of class. He has blown the whistle twice to call fouls. The students play around him as if he were not there. A bell rings, and all the students drop their pinneys where they are and start toward the school building. Belatedly, the teacher blows his whistle to end the game and begins to move around the field picking up pinneys.
>
> After class, as we walk back to the building, the teacher says, "These kids are wild. If you can just run off some of their energy, they don't get into so much trouble in school. This group especially, not too many smarts (taps his temple), don't get into much game strategy." (He sees a boy and girl from the class standing near the door of the girls' locker room talking.) He yells, "Johnson, get your butt to the shower and stop bothering the ladies." He smiles at me. "You've got to be on them all the time." He looks up and sighs, "Well, two [classes] down, three to go." (p. 399)

---

 analytic narrative — A short, interpretive description of an event or situation used in qualitative research.

 narrative vignette — Component of qualitative research reports that gives detailed descriptions of an event, including what people say, do, think, and feel in that setting.

We caution you, however, that Locke and other scholars do not hold that richness of detail alone is what makes a narrative vignette valid. Siedentop (1989) has warned that whether data are to be trusted should not be based on the narrative skills of the researcher. According to Erickson (1986), a valid account is not simply a description but an analysis: "A story can be an accurate report of a series of events, yet not portray the meaning of the actions from the perspectives taken by the actors in the event. . . . It is the combination of richness and interpretive perspective that makes the account valid" (p. 150). Vignettes are not left to stand by themselves. The researcher should make interpretive connections between narrative vignettes and other forms of description, such as direct quotations and quantitative materials.

Direct quotes from interviews with the subjects taken from field notes and audiotapes or videotapes are another form of vignette that enriches the analysis and furnishes documentation for the researcher's point of view. Direct quotes from different individuals may serve to demonstrate agreement (or disagreement) about some phenomenon. Direct quotations from the same people on different occasions may provide evidence that certain events are typical or could demonstrate a pattern or trend in perceptions over time.

For example, Nelson (1988), trying to illustrate differences in the thought processes of students taught by expert and novice teachers, used quotes to document her assertion that students of novice teachers tended to think about procedures and organization more than content:

Interviewer: What are you thinking at this point in the lesson?

Student: I didn't know what to do. I thought we were going to run around the gym.

Student: I was thinking are we all going to be in the same group. (p. 58)

In contrast, students' thoughts during classes taught by experts were more related to the lesson content:

Interviewer: What are you thinking at this point in the lesson?

Student: He was showing us how it [heart rate] would change after we did aerobics.

Student: I was thinking about how to . . . uh, make sure I was adding correctly to get the right score and everything like that. (p. 59)

It is usually emphasized in qualitative research that one should communicate one's perspective clearly to the reader. The narrative's function is to present the researcher's interpretive point in a clear and meaningful manner.

Quantitative Analysis.   Although we have tended to emphasize the differences between qualitative and quantitative research, we do not want you to conclude that there are no (or should not be any) quantitative features in a qualitative study (and vice versa). Actually, qualitative research can use a wide range of quantitative analyses, from simple frequency tables to multivariate statistical techniques.

Frequency tables are not uncommon at all (e.g., Garcia, 1994). Raw frequencies of occurrences are used to reduce data. This is especially appropriate in studies that use some type of observational instrument that codes designated categories of behavior. The frequencies are often converted to percentages to show the extent of certain behaviors or to make comparative statements.

Frequency data in qualitative research are often nominal measures. Thus, contingency tables are sometimes used to show data patterns. Nonparametric statistics are usually the most appropriate type of statistical analysis because of the difficulty in making the necessary assumptions for parametric statistics. Miles and Huberman (1994) describe hundreds of techniques that can be used in coding, analyzing, and interpreting qualitative data. In his commentary on Locke's 1989 study, Schutz (1989) argued that there are many mathematical and nonmathematical ways of analyzing qualitative data. He cited the "systematic network analysis" strategy proposed by Bliss and colleagues as being a viable nonmathematical method that produces a pictorial representation (tree diagram) of the manner by which coded categories are related "which are independent

Garcia, C. (1994). Gender differences in young children's interactions when learning fundamental motor skills. *Research Quarterly for Exercise and Sport*, **65**, 213-225.

Miles, M.B., & Huberman, A.M. (1994). *Qualitative data analysis: A sourcebook of new methods* (2nd ed.). Thousand Oaks, CA: Sage.

Schutz, R.W. (1989). Qualitative research: Comments and controversies. *Research Quarterly for Exercise and Sport*, **60**, 30-35.

and which are conditional on the choice of others" (p. 33). Among the mathematical procedures, Schutz highlighted loglinear analysis as having relevance for qualitative data analysis. Although qualitative variables are nominally scaled, the frequency of occurrence lends itself to quantitative analysis by contingency tables and to subsequent procedures similar to factorial ANOVA. "The loglinear analysis transforms the relative frequencies to logarithms which yield an additive model similar to the additivity of the Sum of Squares in ANOVA" (Schutz, 1989, p. 34).

The main point we are trying to make here is that qualitative research does not exclude quantitative analysis. One of the negative features or outcomes of arguments that support or defend particular methods is that the reader fails to see points of **convergence** among different methods. The researcher should always be alert and amenable to using any methods that could yield meaningful information. Remember, the major purpose of any analysis is to make the most sense out of the data.

Triangulation of Data. The term **triangulation**, borrowed from the field of surveying, refers to the use of more than one source of data to substantiate a researcher's conclusion. Triangulation provides a means by which qualitative researchers test the strength of their interpretations. It is a means used to establish validity and reliability in qualitative research (see chapter 11). Basically, triangulation is a way of increasing confidence in one's findings. Intuitively, it makes sense that the more evidence one has, the more likely one's conclusions are valid. Triangulation is not a simple concept. There are different types of triangulation, and in some cases triangulation can act to increase error rather than reduce it.

Denzin, cited in Fielding and Fielding (1986), classified triangulation into four types:

- Data
- Investigator
- Method
- Theory

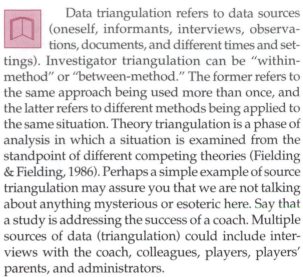

Data triangulation refers to data sources (oneself, informants, interviews, observations, documents, and different times and settings). Investigator triangulation can be "within-method" or "between-method." The former refers to the same approach being used more than once, and the latter refers to different methods being applied to the same situation. Theory triangulation is a phase of analysis in which a situation is examined from the standpoint of different competing theories (Fielding & Fielding, 1986). Perhaps a simple example of source triangulation may assure you that we are not talking about anything mysterious or esoteric here. Say that a study is addressing the success of a coach. Multiple sources of data (triangulation) could include interviews with the coach, colleagues, players, players' parents, and administrators.

Generally, triangulation is valuable because of the increased quality control achieved by combining methods, observers, and data sources. However, it is naive to think that merely combining different kinds of data will "unproblematically add up to produce a more complete picture" (Hammersley & Atkinson, 1983, p. 199). There is the definite likelihood that multiple methods may serve to magnify error. In other words, each method has some error associated with it, and some methods have more than others. This has a multiplying effect. The different methods must be weighed and considered in terms of their relative biases and limitations. Moreover, although theoretical triangulation can provide a more complete picture, it does not necessarily reduce bias. Thus, an important aspect of triangulation is to consider the relationships of the different kinds of data to counteract the threat to validity of each.

The concept of convergence is embodied in triangulation. Convergence is what you might imagine triangulation would accomplish. It is analogous to robustness in factor analysis in that, if the same results appear with different methodological techniques, it probably is not simply the product of the method. Convergence strengthens the evidence.

---

 convergence — Consistency of results across two or more methodological techniques.

 triangulation — Term borrowed from the field of surveying that refers to the use of more than one source of data to substantiate a researcher's conclusion.

 Four types of data triangulation

 Fielding, N.G., & Fielding, J.L. (1986). *Linking data.* Beverly Hills, CA: Sage.

 Hammersley, M., & Atkinson, P. (1983). *Ethnography: Principles in practice.* London: Tavistock.

Theory Construction. Our use of the terms **theory** and **theorizing** should not unduly alarm graduate students and discourage them from undertaking qualitative research. We are not talking about developing a model on the scale of the theory of relativity here. Theorizing, according to Goetz and LeCompte (1984), is a cognitive process of discovering abstract categories and the relationships among those categories. A theory is an explanation of some aspect of practice that permits the researcher to draw inferences about future events. This process is a fundamental tool to develop or confirm explanations. One processes information, compares the findings with past experience and sets of values, and then makes decisions. The decisions may not be correct, so one may then need to revise the theory or model in such cases.

Data analysis depends on theorizing. The tasks of theorizing are "perceiving; comparing, contrasting, aggregating, and ordering; establishing linkages and relationships; and speculating" (Goetz & LeCompte, 1984, p. 167). Perceiving involves the consideration of all sources of data and all aspects of the phenomena being studied. Of course, this takes place during data collection as well as afterward. The perceptual process of determining which specific factors to analyze guides the collection of data.

The tasks of comparing, contrasting, aggregating, and ordering are primary functions in qualitative research. The researcher decides which units are similar and dissimilar and what is important about the differences and similarities. Analytic description cannot occur until the researcher builds the categories of like and unlike properties and carries out a systematic content analysis of the data. Establishing linkages and relationships constitutes a kind of detective work that qualitative researchers do in the theorizing process. The researcher uses both inductive and deductive methods of establishing relationships "while developing a theory or hypothesis that is grounded in the data" (Goetz & LeCompte, 1984, p. 172).

Speculation is often depicted as the key to hypothesizing and developing theories. It requires the researcher to play with the data and make inferences. The researcher must go beyond the data and predict what will happen in the future. Speculation is a basic component of the inductive process. **Negative case selection** is also used in theorizing. In this procedure, the researcher looks for exceptions to the hypothesized construct. The exceptions require either a reformulation of the hypothesis, a redefinition of the phenomenon, or a qualification of the circumstances.

Establishing hypotheses requires evidence to make an educated guess about some phenomenon. The researcher tests the hypothesis and then modifies and refines it until the hypothesis either is rejected or is accepted as a suitable explanation. Taylor and Bogdan (1984) have set forth some steps in analytic induction. The researcher roughly defines the phenomenon and formulates an explanatory hypothesis that may be based on the data, the literature, or the researcher's experience and intuition. The researcher tests the hypothesis with one or more cases. Negative cases are also sought to disprove the hypothesis. Whenever the data do not fit the hypothesis, the researcher reformulates the hypothesis or redefines the phenomenon. This process continues until the hypothesis seems to hold up over a broad range of cases. Tested hypotheses evolve into theories, which are generalizable and can explain various phenomena.

A theory based on and evolving from data is called a **grounded theory** (Glaser & Strauss, 1967). In applied research, grounded theories are considered the best at explaining observed phenomena, understanding relationships, and drawing inferences about future activities.

Write the Report

There is no standard (or "correct") format for a qualitative research report, just as there are no formats that are rigorously obeyed for any other type of research. Here we simply mention some main

---

theory — Explanation of some aspect of practice that permits the researcher to draw inferences about future happenings.

theorizing — Cognitive process of discovering abstract categories and the relationships among those categories.

negative case selection — Procedure used in theorizing in which the researcher looks for exceptions to the hypothesized construct that require either a reformulation of the hypothesis, a redefinition of the phenomenon, or a qualification of the circumstances.

grounded theory — A theory based on and evolving from data.

components of a qualitative research report and their placement in the report. Your department or university may have a definite order of components that you must follow.

The components of a qualitative study are similar to those of other conventional research reports. The first part introduces the problem and provides background and related literature. A description of method is an integral part of the report. Although this section is not as extensive in a journal article as in a thesis, it is usually much more extensive than in other forms of research. The reasons are obvious. The methodology is integrally related to the analysis and is also important in terms of validity and reliability.

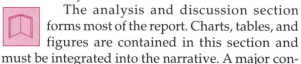 The analysis and discussion section forms most of the report. Charts, tables, and figures are contained in this section and must be integrated into the narrative. A major con-

tributor to the bulk of this section is the description contained in a qualitative study. As we said earlier, narrative vignettes and direct quotations are basic to this type of research. The qualitative study strives to provide enough detail to show the reader that the author's conclusions make sense (Firestone, 1987). The author is faced with a delicate problem in terms of finding a balance between the rich descriptive materials and the analysis and interpretation. Some writers include too much description to illustrate their points, and some use too little. Researchers have suggested that 60-70% of the report be descriptive material and that 30-40% should be devoted to the conceptual framework (Merriam, 1988). Definitely, some balance is needed, and the task requires judgment in deciding which evidence to include to illustrate one's ideas.

It is doubtful that any graduate student is under the false impression that doing qualitative research

---

Funny Things That Happened During the Collection of Qualitative Data

1. On two occasions, reported to gymnasium (carrying camera, TV monitor, tape recorder, and notes) to find door locked. Had to walk all the way around the building—once in the rain.

2. Reported to school to collect data to find classes wouldn't be held because of
   a. a doughnut sale
   b. teacher was ill (twice)
   c. Christmas music rehearsal

3. Interview with teacher interrupted by principal due to crisis over a parent and a charity clothing sale. Interview postponed.

4. Tape recorder became inoperable during interview.

5. Tape recorder became inoperable while transcribing. Had to repeat interviews.

6. Group tape-recording session had to be rescheduled because of complete loss of control when a third-grade student belched into the microphone.

7. Had to buy own camera because department's camera was inoperable.

8. Broke own camera. Repair took two weeks.

9. Had to use participating school's TV monitor but couldn't find proper cord. Interviews had to be rescheduled.

10. While the grad student was making backup tapes, the VCR with original data tape was stolen. Police nabbed the culprit and data were recovered, but the graduate student was comatose.

Firestone, W.A. (1987). Meaning in method: The rhetoric of quantitative and qualitative research. *Educational Researcher, 16*(7), 16-21.

is a quick-and-easy technique. To emphasize this point, we call your attention to page 378, which lists some of the trials and tribulations that befell one doctoral student while she was attempting to collect data.

Establishing Internal and External Validity in Qualitative Research

Internal Validity
External Validity

All types of research must address the concepts of internal and external validity. Lincoln and Guba (1985) have suggested that the term **truth value** be used instead of internal validity and that the term **transferability** be used for external validity. In previous chapters we have emphasized that some types of research designs are stronger in internal validity. Furthermore, the two concepts may work in opposition: Tight controls to increase internal validity reduce the generalizability of the findings and, conversely, designs that strive for external validity suffer from threats to internal validity.

Internal Validity

Although experimental laboratory research is often depicted as the epitome of internal validity, some researchers contend that qualitative research possesses equally or higher internal validity. Merriam (1988) has stated that internal validity deals with the question of how one's findings match reality. In other words, do the findings capture what is really there? Reality is viewed as holistic, multidimensional, and ever-changing. Thus, the qualitative re-

searcher is primarily interested in perspectives rather than truth per se (Taylor & Bogdan, 1984). Ratcliff (1983) has argued that there are only notions of validity and that committing oneself to a particular notion of validity can lead to a **Type III error** (solving the wrong problem) or a **Type IV error** (solving a problem that is not worth solving).

Goetz and LeCompte (1984) have taken a more conventional approach to internal validity. They believe that qualitative research faces some of the same threats to internal validity as other types of research. History, for example, is seen as a threat to qualitative research. The researcher should try to establish baseline data and determine which data remain stable over time and which data change. Systematic replication and comparisons with baseline data can help control not only for the threat of history but also for that of maturation.

Observer effects represent a significant threat to internal validity in qualitative research. Observer effects must be considered in light of specific contexts. The threat can be greatly reduced by the first-hand presence of the researcher over time. Unobtrusiveness, honesty, and constructive personal relationships with the subjects will enhance internal validity. Locke (1989) has emphasized that qualitative researchers should learn to be wary of subjects who occasionally do not tell the truth (for any of several reasons) and thus the researcher must become skilled at penetrating false data.

Selection and regression problems face the qualitative researcher just as in experimental research. The qualitative researcher does not usually have any treatment effects to isolate, but he or she must analyze the data carefully in light of the specificity of the participants. Spurious conclusions can result from bias and contamination of the data. The researcher needs to examine the data carefully and make good use of corroborative sources of data and thorough analytical techniques. Merriam (1988) listed six basic strategies to ensure internal validity:

- Triangulation
- Plausibility checks of taking data and interpretations back to the subjects

---

truth value — In qualitative research, the term analogous to internal validity in experimental research.

transferability — In qualitative research, the term analogous to external validity in experimental research.

Type III error — Solving the wrong problem.

Type IV error — Solving a problem that is not worth solving.

Taylor, S.J., & Bogdan, R. (1984). *Introduction to qualitative research methods* (2nd ed.). New York: Wiley.

Six basic strategies to ensure internal validity in qualitative research

- Long-term data collection and repeated observations
- Peer examination and evaluation of one's findings
- Involving the participants in all phases of the research
- Clarifying the researcher's own bias and theoretical orientation at the outset of the study

External Validity

The generalizability of external validity has often been questioned because of the small number of subjects and the lack of random sampling in the typical qualitative research study. Some qualitative researchers have attempted to meet this criticism in the traditional sense with multicase or cross-case methods (Yin, 1984). On the other hand, Erickson (1986) maintained that generalizable knowledge is inappropriate for qualitative research and that one should concentrate on "concrete universals" arrived at through specific cases and then compare them with the specifics of other similar cases. What one learns from a specific situation is transferable.

One of the strongest intuitive arguments for external validity in qualitative research is the concept of **user generalizability**. The user (reader) evaluates the findings of the carefully described and interpreted study and asks what things apply to his or her situation. Thus, it is the consumer of the research, not the author, who does the generalizing (Peshkin, 1993). This is a common practice in medicine and law. Thus, generalizing is left to those who can apply the findings to their own situations. Locke (1989) stated that, given the rich conceptual description, most readers can easily recognize which situations apply to their own and that the strong recognition of application by the readers is in no way an inferior measure of external validity. Goetz and LeCompte (1984) used the term transferability to refer to the degree to which the qualitative researcher uses and communicates the theoretical frameworks, definitions, and research techniques that are accessible to and understood by other researchers in the same or related fields.

Concluding Remarks

The relatively recent attention given qualitative research in the fields of physical education, exercise science, and sport science (along with the lively discussions and arguments between qualitative and quantitative advocates) is viewed by some to be an insult to the integrity and tradition of qualitative research. Qualitative research is not some brand-new, unsubstantiated method of inquiry. Interpretive, participant observational fieldwork has been used in the social sciences as a research method for over 80 years (Erickson, 1986). Siedentop (1989), commenting on this fact, stated that ethnographic methodology has long been accepted and even honored. He then asked why there is the current flap about qualitative research in physical education.

One point of contention is that qualitative research does not report evidence of validity and reliability in the traditional sense. Kirk and Miller (1986) have stated that because qualitative research is based on different assumptions about reality and uses a different paradigm, there should be different conceptualizations of validity and reliability. To the qualitative researcher, reality is assumed to be holistic, multidimensional, and fluid rather than a single, fixed, objective phenomenon waiting to be discovered (Merriam, 1988):

Unlike experimental designs where validity and reliability are accounted for before the investigation, rigor in a qualitative study derives from the researcher's presence, the nature of the interaction between researcher and participants, the triangulation of data, the interpretation of perceptions, and rich, thick description. (p. 120)

Yin, R.K. (1984). *Case study research: Design and methods.* Newbury Park, CA: Sage.

user generalizability — Concept in which the user (reader) evaluates the findings of the carefully described and interpreted study and asks what things apply to his or her situation.

Peshkin, A. (1993). The goodness of qualitative research. *Educational Researcher*, **22**(2), 23-29.

Siedentop, D. (1989). Do the lockers really smell? *Research Quarterly for Exercise and Sport*, **60**, 36-41.

Answers to questions about what is happening here may seem trivial at first glance. On further inspection, however, we see that it is not, as everyday life is, largely invisible to us because of familiarity and its contradictions. Often we do not realize the patterns of our actions as we perform them. Anthropologist Clyde Kluckhohn said that the fish would be the last creature to discover water. Locke (1987) added that the last person to understand the dynamics of a gym class might well be a physical educator. What is happening can become visible and can be documented systematically.

We should point out that qualitative research is by no means confined to the area of pedagogy. Getting that impression is easy because of the ever-increasing volume of literature on qualitative research in educational journals and textbooks. Qualitative research has a great deal of application in the study of the sociological aspect of sport. Bain (1989) observed that two of the earliest qualitative research studies published in the *Research Quarterly for Exercise and Sport* were on this topic. Sage (1989) cited several qualitative studies on sports dealing with Little League baseball, bodybuilding, soccer, surfing, and coaching.

In a provocative essay dealing with the science of human behavior, Martens (1987) questioned the basic assumptions of orthodox science. A longtime critic of the conventional experimental approach to sport psychology as the only way to conduct research, Martens presented a convincing argument and appeal for qualitative paradigms and the emphasis on experiential knowledge.

This chapter has focused on interpretive qualitative research. Bain (1989) discussed another approach called **critical theory**, whereby the main difference between the two approaches is found in the research goals. Interpretive research is largely free of value, whereas critical theory research is based on value. In other words, in critical theory the aim is to give the research subjects the insight necessary to make choices that will improve their lives. Bain also stated that critical research is usually grounded in feminism, neo-Marxism, or the empowering pedagogy of Freire. Each of these theoretical perspectives challenges the status quo and strives for greater equality. Very little research in critical theory has been done in exercise and sport science and physical education. However, a number of obvious issues in sport regarding women, race, and exploitation of athletes would lend themselves to this form of research.

The debates between the quantitative and the qualitative researchers will undoubtedly continue, but it is hoped that they will rise above name calling (e.g., the "number crunchers" vs. the "navel gazers") and address the issues and problems in a professional and constructive manner. Actually, the boundaries between quantitative and qualitative methodologies sometimes get blurred and break down when subjected to scrutiny. It seems advantageous for the discipline and profession, and for research in general, to capitalize on the strengths of both methods rather than to argue about the differences. The quantitative researcher must make many qualitative decisions regarding the question, design, measurements, analytical procedures, and interpretations to emphasize. Similarly, the qualitative researcher often finds certain quantitative summaries, classifications, and analyses to be useful (Linn, 1986). Kidder and Fine (cited in Merriam, 1988) stated that there is nothing mysterious about combining quantitative and qualitative measures. This is, in fact, a form of triangulation that enhances the validity and reliability of one's study. Sage (1989) pointed out that there is a growing maturity in physical education, exercise science, and sport science with regard to drawing

---

Locke, L.F. (1987). The question of quality in qualitative research. In J.K. Nelson (Ed.), *Proceedings of the Fifth Measurement and Evaluation Symposium* (pp. 31-36). Baton Rouge: Louisiana State University Press.

Bain, L.L. (1989). Interpretive and critical research in sport and physical education. *Research Quarterly for Exercise and Sport*, **60**, 21-24.

Martens, R. (1987). Science, knowledge, and sport psychology. *Sport Psychologist*, **1**, 29-55.

critical theory — A value-based form of qualitative research that helps individuals make constructive choices.

Sage, G.H. (1989). A commentary on qualitative research as a form of inquiry in sport and physical education. *Research Quarterly for Exercise and Sport*, **60**, 25-29.

Merriam, S.B. (1988). *Case study research in education.* San Francisco: Jossey-Bass.

concepts, theories, and methods from all the social sciences as well as the humanities.

Qualitative research is a legitimate means of addressing certain questions in our field. There has been a remarkable growth of increasingly sophisticated methods to guide qualitative researchers. We should take advantage of the work done in other fields and try to extend the boundaries of knowledge by our own contributions. Locke (1989) has provided a fitting concluding statement regarding the place of qualitative research in our field: It should be done, it will be done, and it is important that it be done well.

Page 383 exemplifies a scale that can be used in evaluating the quality of qualitative research studies. It was developed by Linda Bain and presented at the 1992 national convention of the American Alliance for Health, Physical Education, Recreation and Dance.

Summary

Qualitative research methods include field observations, case studies, ethnography, and narrative reports. The researcher gathers data in the natural setting such as the gymnasium, the classroom, the fitness center, or the sport facility.

Qualitative research does not have the preconceived hypotheses that characterize quantitative research. Inductive reasoning is stressed, whereby the researcher seeks to develop hypotheses from observations. The focus is on the "essence" of the phenomena. The researcher should exhibit sensitivity and perception when collecting and analyzing the data.

We stressed the importance of gaining access to the data in the field setting. Establishing rapport and gaining the subjects' trust are essential. The most common methods of collecting data are observations and interviews. Data should be analyzed during and after collection. The researcher must sort and organize the data and develop tentative hypotheses that lead to other sources and types of data.

Data analysis involves organizing, abstracting, integrating, and synthesizing. The analytic narrative is the foundation of qualitative research. The narrative vignette gives the reader a sense of being present for the observation; it conveys a sense of holistic meaning to the situation. It is not unusual for a qualitative study to include quantitative analysis.

Triangulation of data is used to establish validity and reliability. Data triangulation includes multiple sources of data, different investigators, and different methods. In theory triangulation, the situation is examined from different theoretical standpoints.

The qualitative researcher often attempts to construct a theory through the inductive process to explain relationships among categories of data. A theory that evolves from data is called a grounded theory. In the written report, the qualitative researcher must achieve a balance between the rich description and the analysis and interpretation.

Internal validity and external validity are important concepts in qualitative research just as they are in other research methods. Internal validity is the ability of the researcher to capture "what is really there." One of the most effective tools in achieving internal validity is the intensive firsthand presence of the researcher over an extended period. Triangulation of data, unobtrusiveness, honesty, and constructive personal relationships with the subjects all contribute significantly to internal validity.

One of the strongest arguments for external validity of qualitative research is user generalizability. In other words, the reader of the study evaluates the descriptions and analysis and determines what things apply to his or her situation.

Qualitative research is a viable approach to solving problems in our field. It applies to pedagogy in physical education, to exercise science, and to sport science. Answers to the question "what is happening here?" can best be obtained in natural settings through the systematic observation and interaction methodology of qualitative research.

 Check Your Understanding

Locate a qualitative study and write an abstract of approximately 300 words on the methods used in gathering the data (observations, interviews, etc.) and in presenting the results (narrative vignettes, quotes, tables, etc.).

Evaluating the Quality of Qualitative Research

Linda L. Bain
California State University, Northridge
AAHPERD, Indianapolis
April 8, 1992

Definition of the Problem

_____ Purpose is clearly stated

_____ Focuses on a significant issue

_____ Seeks to understand meaning of experiences for the participants

_____ Provides holistic view of the setting

Data Collection

_____ Researcher has training in methods used

_____ Pilot work done in similar setting using similar methods

_____ Rationale provided for selection of the sample

_____ Researcher has trusting, collaborative relationship with participants

_____ Methods for data collection are unobtrusive

_____ Data collection procedures provide thorough description of events

_____ Sufficient time spent in field

Data Analysis

_____ Analysis done during and after data collection

_____ Triangulation of data sources and search for convergence

_____ Search for negative cases

_____ Provides interpretation and theory as well as description of events

_____ Provides opportunity for participants to corroborate interpretation

_____ Arranges for peer evaluation of procedures and interpretation

Preparation of Report

_____ Complete description of setting

_____ Complete description of procedures

_____ Includes description of researcher's values and assumptions

_____ Uses vignettes and quotes to support conclusions and interpretation

General Assessment

_____ Internal validity: How much confidence do you have in the quality of the description and interpretation of events in the particular research setting?

_____ External validity: What is your assessment of the extent to which the results of this study apply to a different setting with which you are familiar?

IV
PART

Writing the Research Report

P art I discussed the research proposal, its purpose, and the structure of the different parts. Parts II and III provided the details needed to understand and conduct research, including statistics, measurement, and types of research. This section completes the research process with instructions on how to prepare the research report. You may also want to refer to chapter 2, which discussed some rules and recommendations for writing the review of literature, for this is an important part of the research report.

Chapter 18 briefly examines all the parts of the research proposal that have already been discussed. In addition, we offer some of our thoughts about the nature of the meeting to review the research proposal.

The final two chapters focus on the final written research report. Up until now we have tried to explain how to understand other research and how to plan your own research. Chapter 19 helps you organize and write the results and discussion sections (or chapters). We also explain how to prepare tables, figures, and illustrations and where to place them in the research report.

Finally, in chapter 20 we suggest ways of using journal and traditional styles to organize and write theses and dissertations. We also present a brief section on writing for scientific journals and a short discourse on preparing and giving oral and poster presentations.

The Research Proposal

Dear Professors of Research Methods:

What if I have my thesis proposal meeting, and my chair and committee do not like what I want to do? What should I do, and how can I handle it?

Really nervous,
Robert Rejection

Dear Rejection:

Our friend (at least until we published this), Dr. Richard Nelson at Pennsylvania State University, developed a letter that is appropriate for your use [revised from *NASPSPA Newsletter*, 1979, **4**(3)] with your chair and committee:

Dear Thesis Chair and Committee:

I regret to inform you that your rejection of my thesis proposal did not place among my rejections this year that I have determined to be acceptable. During the current year I have received an unusual number of high-quality rejections (in class and from other professors, as well as from my significant other) and as a consequence the competition for the limited number of rejections available has been intense. I have sought the advice of several other highly qualified graduate students (and derelicts) to evaluate my rejections, and yours was ranked very low. Upon written request, I will forward to you copies of the reviews of your rejection.

Although I was unable to accept this rejection, I thank you for submitting it and assure you I shall be pleased to consider future rejections which you may wish to submit.

Methodologically yours,
PRM

The research proposal contains the definition, scope, and significance of the problem and the methodology that will be used to solve it. If the journal style format for preparing the thesis or dissertation (advocated in this book but reviewed in detail in chapter 20) is used, then the proposal consists of the introduction and method sections, appropriate tables, figures, and appendices (e.g., score sheets, cover letters, questionnaires, sample informed-consent forms, and pilot study data). In a four-section thesis or dissertation (introduction, method, results, and discussion), the proposal consists of the first two sections. In studies using a five-section format, in which the review of literature is the second, the proposal encompasses the first three sections.

One of the goals of this book has been to help prepare a student to develop a research proposal. We have already discussed the contents of the proposal. Chapters 2, 3, and 4 in this text pertain specifically to the body of the research proposal. Other chapters relate to various facets of planning a study with regard to the hypotheses, measurements, designs, and statistical analyses. This chapter attempts to bring the proposal together. We also devote space to the proposal meeting and committee actions. Finally, we touch on basic considerations involved in grant proposals, specifically, how they differ from thesis and dissertation proposals.

Developing a Good Introduction

The student's most important task is to convince the committee (whether it be the proposal committee, a journal reviewer, or a reviewing committee for a granting agency) that the problem is important and worth investigating. The first section of the proposal should do this, and it should also attract the reader's interest to the problem. The review of literature provides background information and a critique of the previous research done on the topic, pointing out weaknesses, conflicts, and areas needing study. A concise statement of the problem informs the reader of the exact purpose, that is, what the researcher intends to do.

Hypotheses are advanced on the basis of previous research and perhaps some theoretical model. Furthermore, operational definitions serve to inform the reader exactly how the researcher is using certain terms. Operational definitions must be observable and must generally relate to the dependent

and independent variables. Basic assumptions are also stated and serve to specify certain conditions and premises that must exist for the study to proceed. Limitations are possible shortcomings or influences that are acknowledged by the researcher and are generally the result of the delimitations to the study that the investigator imposes. The first section concludes with a statement about the significance of the study, which can be judged from either a basic or an applied research standpoint. The significance section emphasizes contradictory findings and limitations of previous research and the ways in which the proposed study will contribute to further knowledge about the research topic.

Chapter 2 of this book concerned the literature review and included a discussion on the inductive and deductive reasoning processes used in developing the problem and formulating hypotheses. Chapter 3 covered the other parts typically required in the introduction section or chapter of a proposal.

Innumerable hours are involved in preparing the first section (introduction) of the proposal, especially with respect to the literature search and the formulation of the problem. The student usually depends heavily on an advisor and on completed studies for examples of format and description. Before we continue, however, we need to mention that you should write your proposal in the future tense. You will state that so many subjects will be selected and that certain procedures will be carried out. Theoretically, if the proposal is carefully planned and well written, you need only change from future to past tense to have the first two sections or chapters of the thesis or dissertation. Realistically, however, numerous revisions will probably be made between the proposal and the final version. To reiterate, the importance of the study and its contribution to the profession is the main focus of the first section in the proposal, and this constitutes the basis for approval or disapproval.

Describing the Method

The method section of the proposal frequently draws the most questions from committee members in the proposal meeting. In the method section or chapter, the student must clearly describe how the data will be collected to solve the problem set forth in the first section. The student needs to specify who the subjects will be and how they will be chosen, how many subjects will participate, any special characteristics of importance, how the subjects' rights and privacy will be protected, and how informed consent will be obtained. Measurements are detailed, and the validity and reliability of these measures are documented. Next, the procedures are described. If, for example, the study is a survey, the student discusses the steps in developing the instrument and cover letter, mailing the questionnaires, and following up. If the study is experimental, the treatments (or experimental programs) are described explicitly along with the control procedures that will be exercised. Finally, the student must explain the experimental design and planned statistical analysis of the data.

Periodically, we have emphasized the importance of conducting pilot studies before gathering data. If pilot work has been done, it should be described and the results reported. Often the committee members have major concerns about such questions as whether the treatments can produce meaningful changes, whether the measurements are accurate and can reliably discriminate between subjects, and whether the investigator can satisfactorily perform the measurements and administer the treatments. The pilot study should provide answers to these questions.

We recommended in chapter 4 that the student use the literature to help determine the methodology. Answers to questions about whether certain treatment conditions are sufficiently long, intense, and frequent to produce anticipated changes in behavior can be defended by results of previous studies.

The Proposal Process

What to Expect of the Proposal Committee
How to Prepare the Formal Proposal
What Happens at the Proposal Meeting

We have reiterated the contents of the proposal: the introduction (including the review of literature) and the methods to be used. The proposed purpose—in conjunction with pertinent background information, plausible hypotheses, operational definitions, and delimitations—is the factor that will determine whether the study is worthwhile. Consequently, the first section (or chapter) is instrumental in stimu-

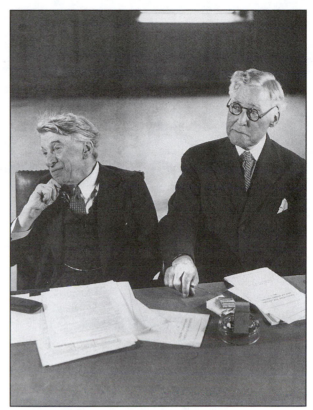

The typical proposal committee (as seen through the eyes of a student, of course).

lating interest in the problem and establishing the rationale and significance of the study. The committee's decision to approve or disapprove rests primarily with the persuasiveness exhibited in the first section.

Actually, the basic decision about the topic's merit should already have been made before the proposal meeting. The student should consult with the advisor and most (if not all) of the committee members to reach a consensus about the study's worth before the proposal meeting is scheduled. If you cannot convince the majority of the committee that your study is worthwhile, do not convene a formal proposal meeting. You may have a problem if you get your proposal returned with a checklist such as that on page 390.

What to Expect of the Proposal Committee

Let us digress a moment to discuss the composition of the proposal committee. The structure of committees and the number of committee members will vary from one institution to another. It is probably safe to say that most thesis committees consist of at least three members and most dissertation com-

Interim Thesis/Dissertation Evaluation

Dear _____:

Greetings! I regret that my busy schedule prohibits me from rendering a detailed written evaluation of your thesis/dissertation. However, I have checked the appropriate actions or comments that apply to your proposal.

_____ If at first you don't succeed, try, try again.

_____ Don't sell your research methods textbook (Thomas & Nelson, of course); you'll need to take the course again.

_____ You were not required to write your paper in a foreign language (Burmese, or whatever it was).

_____ I couldn't read beyond the third page; one does not have to eat a whole pie to know it is bad.

_____ I hear they are hiring at Sam's Diner.

_____ May I have your permission to use your proposal as an example next semester when I teach research methods?

_____ Have you paid your tuition and fees yet? If not . . .

_____ Please call my secretary and arrange an appointment with me. Consider taking a tranquilizer before you arrive.

_____ I have been serving on thesis/dissertation committees for over 15 years and can now honestly say that I've seen it all.

mittees at least five. The major and minor professors are included in these numbers, although the master's student is often not required to have a minor. Other members should be chosen on the basis of their knowledge about the subject or their expertise in other aspects of the research, such as design and statistical analysis. Sometimes the institution or department specifies a certain number of the committee who must be from inside or outside the department. Usually no limit is placed on the maximum number of committee members allowed.

In regard to the topic of premeeting support, we strongly recommend that the student, with the help and advice of the major professor, get general approval and support for the problem itself from at least two of the three thesis committee members (or three of the five dissertation committee members). This support is tentative, of course, and final approval is contingent on the refinements that might be needed and on the adequacy of the methodology.

Do not wait until the formal committee meeting to plan the study. This should be completed beforehand. In this regard, some graduate programs have so-called preproposal meetings for brainstorming

and informally reaching an agreement on the efficacy of the proposed topic. This kind of meeting functions to garner support from the committee before a great deal of time and effort are wasted on a fruitless endeavor. The student prepares and distributes an outline of the purpose and basic procedures before the meeting. The student should have spent considerable time in consultation with the advisor (and probably at least another committee member) and should have searched the literature sufficiently to be adequately prepared to present a sound case for the study. The preproposal meeting is not just a "bull" session in which the student is fishing for basic ideas. At the same time, the informality of the occasion does allow a good interchange of ideas and suggestions.

How to Prepare the Formal Proposal

The formal proposal should be carefully prepared. If the proposal contains errors of grammar, spelling, and format, committee members may conclude that the student lacks the interest, motivation, or competence to do the proposed research. With the availability of microcomputers and word processors, no reason exists for a student to present a poorly prepared proposal. Also, spell-checking routines, available with most word-processing software, should always be used. Remember, however, that a spell-checker will not identify the use of an incorrect word that is spelled correctly, as the following poem by Jerrold H. Zar illustrates:

I have a spelling checker.
It came with my PC.
It plane lee marks four my review
Miss steaks aye can knot see.

Also you should be aware that most campuses have high-quality printers available that a student may use for printing good copies of proposals to be distributed to committee members.

Committee members should not ignore errors in proposals with the idea that the student will correct these later. Doing so may lead the student to assume that carelessness is acceptable in data collection or in the final written thesis or dissertation. Copies of the proposal should be given to the committee members well before the meeting. The department or university usually specifies the advance number of days.

What Happens at the Proposal Meeting

In the typical proposal meeting, the student is asked to briefly summarize the rationale for the study, its significance, and the methodology (good visual aids enhance this presentation). The remainder of the session consists of questioning by the committee members. If the topic is acceptable, the questions concern mainly the methods and the competence of the student who will conduct the study. The student should exhibit tactful confidence in presenting the proposal. A common mistake students make is to be so humble and pliable that they agree to every suggestion made, even those that radically change the study. The advisor should help ward off these "helpful" suggestions, but the student must also be able to respectfully defend the scope of the study and the methodology. If adequate planning has gone into the proposal, the student (with the assistance of the major professor) should be able to recognize useful suggestions and defend against those that seem to offer minimal aid.

A projected schedule of what procedures will be accomplished when is commonly required for grant proposals. This may or may not be required for a thesis or dissertation proposal. Regardless of whether a time frame is formally required, it is definitely something that a student should address. A common mistake in planning for a thesis or dissertation is underestimating how long each phase of the study will take. Students tend to assume, like Pollyanna, that everyone involved (subjects, helpers, committee members, typists, and university personnel) will drop everything else they are doing to accommodate their study. Moreover, they assume that all phases of the study will proceed without a hitch. Unfortunately, it just doesn't work that way. The simple logistics of accomplishing each aspect of the study are usually more complicated and time-consuming than anticipated. Much grief can be avoided if the student will carefully and realistically project how long the various steps in the research process will take (and then add some more time).

Once the proposal is approved, most institutions treat it as a contract in that the committee expects the study to be done in the manner specified in the proposal. Moreover, the student can assume that if the study is conducted and analyzed as planned and is well written, it will be approved. If any unforeseen changes are required during the course of the study, they must be approved by the advisor. Substantial changes usually must be reviewed by some or all of the committee members.

Preparing and Presenting Qualitative Research Proposals

The content, procedures, and expectations for the proposal that we have discussed so far largely pertain to quantitative theses and dissertations. Although many similarities exist in the kinds of information presented in quantitative and qualitative research proposals, some salient differences should be mentioned.

Preparing the proposal is much easier if all committee members are familiar with qualitative research. However, if one or more members do not understand the nature of

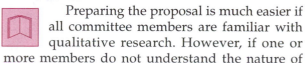
Locke, L.F., Spirduso, W.W., & Silverman, S.J. (1993). *Proposals that work: A guide for planning dissertations and grant proposals* (3rd ed.). Newbury Park, CA: Sage.

Marshall, C., & Rossman, G.B. (1989). *Designing qualitative research.* Newbury Park, CA: Sage.

qualitative research and the methodological differences between quantitative and qualitative paradigms, problems may arise. The student who is contemplating doing a qualitative study is strongly urged to read Locke, Spirduso, and Silverman's *Proposals That Work* (1993) or *Designing Qualitative Research* by Marshall and Rossman (1989).

One of the problems that the qualitative researcher may face concerns the possible shifts in focus and methods that may occur during the study. Earlier, we likened the proposal to a contract, whereby the committee members expect the student to carry out the study as specified in the proposal. Unlike quantitative research, however, qualitative research typically undergoes changes in the focus of the research question and/or the sources of data, the methodology, and the analysis of data. This aspect of qualitative research demands an "open contract" (Locke et al., 1993).

Another difference between the quantitative and qualitative proposal is the literature review. In qualitative research, closely related studies may be purposefully omitted when planning the study because the researcher does not want to be influenced by the views and perceptions of others. Still another difference is the need for the qualitative researchers to address their own values, biases, and perceptions in order to more clearly understand the context of the research setting.

All committee members, whether familiar or unfamiliar with qualitative research, will be interested in methodological concerns: Where will the study take place? Who will be the subjects? How will the researcher gain access to the site? What data sources will be used? Does the researcher possess the needed research skills? What pilot work has been done? How will ethical concerns be handled? What strategies will be employed in collecting, sorting, categorizing, and analyzing the data?

It should be apparent by now that there are differences in the quantitative and qualitative proposal format and in the nature of the proposal process. These differences must be recognized and accepted. As with any type of research, the major professor plays a vital role in preparing the student (and, in some cases, preparing the committee members), in showing support, and in helping the student get out of "tight spots." Most of all, the student, with the support of the major professor, must be able to assure the committee that the study will be carried out in a competent and scholarly manner.

Writing Proposals for Granting Agencies

All sources of grants, whether governmental agencies or private foundations, require research proposals so that they can decide which projects to fund and how much to award. The granting agencies nearly always publish guidelines for applicants to follow in preparing proposals.

A well-written proposal is everything. The researcher rarely gets a chance to explain or to defend the purpose or procedures. Thus, the decision is based entirely on the written proposal. The basic format for a grant proposal is similar to the thesis or dissertation proposal. However, some additional types of information are required, as are some procedural deviations.

We cannot emphasize too strongly the importance of following the guidelines. Granting agencies tolerate little (if any) deviation from their directions. All sections of the application must be addressed and deadlines strictly followed. Frequently, a statement of intent to submit a proposal is required a month or so before the proposal is filed.

Grant proposals include

- an abstract of the proposed project,
- a statement of the problem, and
  its relevance to one of the granting agency's specified priorities,
- the methodology to be followed,
- a time frame,
- a budget, and
- the vitae of the investigators.

A limited review of literature is often required to demonstrate familiarity with previous research. Occasionally, the funding agency will impose some restrictions on design and methods. For example, it is not uncommon for an agency to prohibit control groups if the treatment is hypothesized to be effective. In other words, the agency may not want anyone to be denied treatment. This can pose some problems for the researcher in scientifically evaluating the outcomes of the project.

Because every granting agency has stipulations regarding the types of programs it can and cannot fund, a detailed budget is required, as is a justification for each budget item. A time frame is usually expected so that the reviewers can see how the

---

Parts of a grant proposal

project will be conducted and when the various phases will be accomplished. This time frame provides the reviewers with information about the depth and scope of the study, justification for the length of time that support is requested, the contributions of the various personnel, and when the granting agency can expect progress reports.

The competence of the researcher has to be documented. Each researcher must attach a vita and often a written statement pertaining to appropriate preparation, experience, and accomplishments. The adequacy of facilities and sources of support must also be addressed. Letters of support are occasionally encouraged. These are included in the appendix. Numerous copies of the proposal are usually required. The proposal is evaluated by a panel of reviewers in accordance with certain criteria regarding the contribution to knowledge, relevance, significance, and soundness of design and methodology.

The preparation of a grant proposal is a time-consuming and exacting process. Several types of information are specified, and time is needed to gather the information and state it in the manner prescribed by the guidelines. One is advised to begin preparing the proposal as soon as the guidelines are available.

Finally, it is usually wise to contact the granting agency before preparing and submitting a proposal. Seldom are proposals funded that are submitted without some prior contact with the granting agency. Finding out the agency's interests and needs is a timesaving venture for the researcher. Often, a visit to, or an extended phone conversation with, the research officer is advisable. It helps to look at proposals previously funded by the agency or seek guidance from researchers who have been funded.

Submitting Internal Proposals

Many colleges and universities (particularly larger research universities) offer internal funding for graduate student research. Although these grants usually are not large, they do offer funds for research. These typically require a two- to five-page proposal that has the support of the major professor and often the department chair. The contents usually include an abstract, a budget, and a short narrative focusing on the proposed methodology and why the research is important. Notices that internal funding is available are routinely posted or advertised around the college or university. A good place to find out is at the office of your graduate school or vice president for research.

Summary

The research proposal describes the definition, scope, and significance of a problem and the methodology to be used to study it. The proposal is essentially the plan for the study. The introduction provides the background and literature for the problem, the problem statement, hypotheses, definitions, assumptions and limitations, and the significance of the study. The method section describes the subjects, instrumentation, procedures, and design and analysis.

These two chapters are presented by a student to his or her research committee as the plan for inquiry. The student's committee determines the worth of the study, suggests needed alterations, and ultimately must agree that the study should be done. The proposal must be carefully prepared with appropriate pilot work so that the committee is convinced that the student can complete the research plan.

Proposals to granting agencies are similar but are typically required to have specific lengths and formats. Students are advised to talk with outside agencies and more experienced grant writers before preparing and submitting proposals. Many colleges and universities have internal grants for which graduate students can apply to support thesis and dissertation research.

 Check Your Understanding

Find out the steps for writing a thesis or dissertation proposal at your school. List them in chronological order (e.g., select a major professor and committee, prepare a proposal, and get the proposal approved). Explain the process at each step.

CHAPTER 19

Results and Discussion

Dear Professors of Research Methods:

My thesis advisor constantly criticizes me for little things such as misplacing a decimal point. For example, I reported that two means were significantly different ($F = 112.45$, $p < .01$), when it should have been $F = 1.1245$, which was not significant. Now I have to rewrite my entire discussion section. Doesn't she know that to err is human?

Sincerely,
F as in Frustration

Dear F:

Although a decimal may be a trivial matter to you, a misplaced decimal can have a tremendous impact on the results in your thesis as well as in other areas of one's life. Imagine the blow to your bank account if the bank recorded a $10.00 check as $100.00. To err is human, but as some scholar once observed, if your eraser wears out faster than the lead in your pencil, you are overdoing it.

Methodologically yours,
PRM

At the end of chapter 4 we promised we would discuss the final sections of the thesis or dissertation. Those sections are the **results** and discussion. Results are what you have found, and discussion explains what the results mean. In theses and dissertations, the results and discussion usually are separate sections, although they are sometimes combined (particularly in multi-experiment papers). We discuss these sections here as separate parts of the research report.

How to Write the Results Section

The results section is the most important part of the research report. The introduction and literature review indicate why you conducted the research, the method explains how you did it, and the results section presents your contribution to knowledge, that is, what you found. The results should be concise and effectively organized and should include appropriate tables and figures.

Because there is no one correct way to present the results section, the results may be organized in various ways. The best way may be to address each of the tested hypotheses; on other occasions, the results may be organized around the independent or dependent variables of interest. Occasionally, you may want to show first that certain standard and expected effects have been replicated before you go on to discuss other findings. For example, in developmental studies of motor performance tasks, older children typically perform better than younger ones. The researcher may want to report the replication of this effect before discussing the other results. When looking at the effects of training on several dependent variables, you may first want to establish that a standard dependent variable known to respond to training did, in fact, respond. For example, before looking at the effects of cardiovascular training as potentially reducing cognitive stress, you need to show that a change occurred in cardiovascular response as a result of the training.

Some items should always be reported in the results. The means and standard deviations for all dependent variables under the important conditions should be included. These are basic descriptive data that allow other researchers to evaluate your findings. The main descriptive data should be presented in one table if possible. Sometimes only the means and standard deviations of important findings are included in the results. However, all the remaining means and standard deviations should be included in the appendix.

The results section should also use tables and figures to display appropriate findings. Figures are particularly useful for percentage data, interactions, or summarizing related findings. Only the important tables and figures should be included in the results; those remaining should be placed in the appendix.

Statistical information should be summarized in the text where possible. Statistics from ANOVA and MANOVA should always be summarized in the text and complete tables relegated to the appendix. Make sure, however, that you include the appropriate statistical information in the text. For example, when giving the F ratio, report the degrees of freedom, the probability, and possibly the effect size: $F(1,36) = 6.23$, $p < .02$, $ES = 0.65$. Above all, the statistics reported should be meaningful. Day (1983) reported a classic case that read "33-1/3% of the mice used in this experiment were cured by the test drug; 33-1/3% of the test population were unaffected by the drug and remained in a moribund condition; the third mouse got away" (p. 35).

Sometimes tables are a better way to present this information. If the perfect scientific paper is ever written, the results section will read, "The results are shown in Table 1" (Day, 1983, p. 36). However, this does not mean that the results section should consist mostly of tables and figures. It is disconcerting to have to thumb through eight tables and figures placed between two pages of text. But even worse is to have to turn 50 pages to the appendix to find a necessary table or figure. Read what you have written. Are all the important facts there? Have you provided more information than the reader can absorb?

Do not be redundant and repetitive. A common error is to include a table or figure in the results and then repeat it in the text. It is appropriate to describe tables and figures in a general way or to point out particularly important facts, but do not repeat every finding. Also, be sure you do not call tables figures, and vice versa. However, as Day (1983) has reported, some writers are so concerned with reducing verbiage that they lose track of antecedents, particularly "it":

"The left leg became numb at times and she walked it off. . . . On her second day, the knee

---

results — Chapter or section of a research report that describes what the researcher found.

was better, and on the third day it had completely disappeared." The antecedent for both *its* was presumably "the numbness," but I rather think that the wording in both instances was a result of dumbness. (p. 36)

What to Include in the Discussion Section

Although the results are the most important part of the research report, the discussion is the most difficult to write. There are no cute tricks or clear-cut ways to organize the discussion, but there are some rules that define what to include:

- Discuss your results—not what you wish they were but what they are.
- Relate your results back to the introduction, previous literature, and hypotheses.
- Explain how your results fit within theory.
- Interpret your findings.
- Recommend or suggest applications of your findings.
- Summarize and state your conclusions with appropriate supporting evidence.

Your discussion should point out where data both support and fail to support the hypotheses and important findings. But do not confuse significance with meaningfulness in your discussion. In fact, be especially careful to point out where they may not coincide. In particular, the discussion should point out factual relationships among variables and situations,

---

Writing the Discussion

Problem Statement: Why did the chicken cross the road?

Method: One chicken observed by several individuals

Results: Said chicken crossed the road

Discussion: Following are the explanations given for the chicken crossing the road.

Plato—For the greater good

Karl Marx—It was a historical inevitability

Timothy Leary—That's the only kind of trip the Establishment would let the chicken take

Oliver North—National security was at stake

B.F. Skinner—Because the internal influences which had pervaded its senses from birth had caused it to develop in such a fashion that it would tend to cross roads, even while believing these actions to be of its own free will

Jean-Paul Sartre—In order to act in good faith and be true to itself, the chicken found it necessary to cross the road

A. Einstein—Whether the chicken crossed the road or the road crossed the chicken depends on your frame of reference

Aristotle—To actualize its potential

Buddha—If you can ask this question, you deny your own chicken-nature

Darwin—It was the next logical step after coming down from the trees

Emily Dickinson—Because it could not stop for death

Ralph Waldo Emerson—It didn't cross the road, it transcended it

Ernest Hemingway—To die, in the rain

Socrates—The question is unanswerable as it contains within it some untenable assumptions

Shakespeare—To cross or not to cross, that is the question

Environmental activist—Is that a free-range chicken

Health nut—Is that chicken skinless, boneless, and hormone-free

Graduate student—Was that regular or extra-crispy

 Information to include in the discussion

thus leading to a presentation of the significance of the research. Of course, this is an essential place not to confuse cause and effect with correlation.

The discussion should end on a positive note, possibly a summarizing statement of the most important finding and its meaning. Never end your **discussion with a variation of the "old standby of graduate students":** *More research is needed.* **Who would have thought otherwise?**

The discussion should also point out any methodological problems that occurred in the research. However, a methodological cop-out to explain the results is unacceptable. *If you did not find predicted outcomes and you resort to methodological failure as an explanation, you did not do sufficient pilot work.*

Graduate students sometimes want their results to sound wonderful and to solve all the problems of the world. Thus, in their discussions they often make claims well beyond what their data indicate. Your major professor and committee are likely to know a lot about your topic and therefore are unlikely to be fooled by these claims. They can see the data and read the results. They know what you have found and the claims that can be made. A much better strategy is to make your points effectively in your discussion and not try to generalize these points into grandiose ideas that will solve humanity's major problems. Write so that your limited contribution to knowledge is highlighted. If you

make broader claims, knowledgeable readers are likely to discount the importance of your legitimate findings. Your discussion should not sound like the "Calvin and Hobbes" cartoon (Bill Watterson) in which Calvin said, "I used to hate writing assignments, but now I enjoy them. I realized that the purpose of writing is to inflate weak ideas, obscure poor reasoning, and inhibit clarity."

Another point about writing your discussion is to write so that reasonably informed and intelligent people can understand what you have found. Do not use a thesaurus to replace your normal vocabulary with multisyllabic words and complex sentences. Your writing should not look like the examples below. By translating you can probably recognize these sentences as some well-known sayings.

Your discussion can generally be guided by the following questions taken from the *Publication Manual of the American Psychological Association* (APA, 1994, p. 19):

- What have I contributed here?
- How has my study helped to resolve the original problem?
- What conclusions and theoretical implications can I draw from my study?

The responses to these questions are the core of your contribution, and readers have a right to clear

In Other Words

1. As a case in point, other authorities have proposed that slumbering canines are best left in a recumbent position.

2. It has been posited that a high degree of curiosity proved lethal to a feline.

3. There is a large body of experimental evidence which clearly indicates that smaller members of the genus Mus tend to engage in recreational activity while the feline is remote from the locale.

4. From time immemorial, it has been known that the ingestion of an "apple" (i.e., the pome fruit of any tree of the genus Malus, said fruit being usually round in shape and red, yellow, or greenish in color) on a diurnal basis will with absolute certainty keep a primary member of the health care establishment from one's local environment.

5. Even with the most sophisticated experimental protocol, it is exceedingly unlikely that you can instill in a superannuated canine the capacity to perform novel feats of legerdemain.

6. A sedimentary conglomerate in motion down a declivity gains no addition of mossy material.

7. The resultant experimental data indicate that there is no utility in belaboring a deceased equine.

It would be a good idea to get a copy of the APA manual (or the style manual used in your department).
American Psychological Association. (1994). *Publication manual of the American Psychological Association* (4th ed.). Washington, DC: Author.

and direct answers. If after reading your discussion the reader asks, "So what?" then you have failed in your research reporting.

How to Handle Multiple Experiments in a Single Report

Graduate students are conducting more research that involves multiple experiments. These experiments may ask several related questions about a particular problem or may be built on one another with the outcomes of the first leading to questions for the second. This is a positive trend, but it sometimes leads to problems within the traditional (chapter structure) thesis or dissertation format. Chapter 20 discusses the journal and traditional formats for organizing theses and dissertations.

Multiple experiments in journal format typically involve a general introduction and literature review. This is followed by a presentation of each experiment with its own short introduction and review, method, results, and discussion (sometimes the results and discussion may be combined). It concludes with a general discussion of the series of experiments and their related findings.

Within the traditional framework, multiple experiments are probably best handled by separate chapters. The first chapter includes the introduction, theoretical framework, literature review, a general statement of the research problem, and related definitions and delimitations. Subsequent chapters describe each experiment. Each of these chapters includes a brief introduction, a discussion of the specific problem and hypotheses, and the method, results, and discussion sections. The final chapter is a general discussion in which the experiments are tied together. It contains the features of the discussion previously presented.

How to Use Tables and Figures

Preparing Tables

Examples of Poor and Good Tables

Improving Tables
Preparing Figures and Illustrations

Preparing tables and figures is a difficult task. Howard Wainer (1992) wrote one of the best papers on this topic. We begin with a quotation he used.

 Drawing graphs, like motor-car driving and love-making, is one of those activities which almost every educator thinks can be done well without instruction. The results are of course usually abominable. [paraphrased, with my [Wainer's] apologies, from Margerison, 1965]

Wainer suggests that tables and figures should allow the reader to answer questions at three levels:

- Basic: Extraction of data
- Intermediate: Trends in parts of the data should be evident
- Advanced: Overall questions involving deep structure of the data (seeing trends and comparing groupings) should be available

These questions can be thought of as an ordered effect:

1. Variables by themselves (data)
2. One variable in relation to another
3. The overall comparisons and relationships in the data

Preparing Tables

Getting information from a table is like extracting sunlight from a cucumber (Farquhar & Farquhar, 1891).

Remember, tables are for communicating to the reader, not storing data. The first question is, Do you need a table? There is no easy answer, but two characteristics are important: Is the material more easily understood in a table? And does the table interfere with reading the results? Once you decide you need a table (not all numbers require tables), follow these basic rules:

- Like characteristics should read vertically in the table.
- Headings of tables should be clear.

 Wainer, H. (1992). Understanding graphs and tables. *Educational Researcher*, **21**(1), 14-23.

 Rules for building tables

- The reader should be able to understand the table without referring to the text.

Examples of Poor and Good Tables

Table 19.1 is an example of a useless table that could be more easily presented in the text. This table can be handled in one sentence: "The experimental group ($M = 17.3$, $s = 4.7$) was significantly better than the control group ($M = 12.1$, $s = 3.9$), $t(28) = 3.31$, $p < .05$." Table 19.2 is also unnecessary. From the 10 comparisons among group means, only 1 was significant. The values in the table are the equivalent of t tests. This table can also be presented in one sentence: "The Scheffé test was used to make comparisons among the age-group means, and the only significant difference was between the youngest (7-year-olds) and oldest (15-year-olds) groups, $t = 8.63$, $p < .05$."

We have borrowed an example of a useful table (see Table 19.3) from Safrit and Wood (1983). As you can see, like characteristics appear vertically. Also,

Table 19.1   Useless Table Number 1

Means, Standard Deviations, and t Test for Distance Cartwheeled While Blindfolded				
Groups	N	M	s	t
Experimental	15	17.3 m	4.7 m	
				3.31*
Control	15	12.1 m	3.9 m	

*$p < .05$.

Table 19.2   Useless Table Number 2

Scheffé's Test for Difference Among Age Levels in Ability to Wiggle Their Ears				
Age	7	9	11	13	15
7	–	1.20	1.08	1.79	8.63*
9		–	1.32	1.42	1.57
11			–	1.58	1.01
13				–	0.61
15					–

*$p < .05$.

 More rules for developing tables

an extensive amount of text would be required to present these same results, yet they are easy to understand in this brief table.

Improving Tables

The most important question is how to improve tables so that they are more useful, more informative, and easier to interpret. Wainer (1992) offers three good rules when developing tables.

- The columns and rows should be ordered so that they make sense. For example, the row elements are often placed in alphabetical order according to the label for the row (e.g., names, places). This is seldom useful. Order the rows either naturally

Table 19.3   Example of a Useful Table

Characteristics of Users and Nonusers HRFT Pilot Survey		
	Users	Nonusers
Gender		
Male	4 (36.4%)	33 (62.3%)
Female	7 (63.6%)	20 (37.7%)
Age		
20–25	1 (09.1%)	2 (03.8%)
25–30	1 (09.1%)	8 (15.1%)
30–35	5 (45.5%)	9 (17.0%)
35–40	1 (09.1%)	7 (13.2%)
40 and over	3 (27.2%)	27 (50.9%)
Type of school		
Elementary	1 (09.1%)	18 (34.0%)
Middle	0 (00.0%)	18 (34.0%)
Junior-senior high	1 (09.1%)	0 (00.0%)
High	9 (81.8%)	17 (32.0%)
Student population		
0–100	0 (00.0%)	0 (00.0%)
100–500	1 (09.1%)	17 (33.3%)
500–1,000	0 (00.0%)	16 (31.4%)
1,000–1,500	1 (09.1%)	1 (02.0%)
Over 1,500	9 (81.8%)	17 (33.3%)

From "The Health-Related Fitness Test Opinionnaire: A Pilot Survey," by M.J. Safrit and T.M. Wood, 1983, *Research Quarterly for Exercise and Sport*, **54**, p. 205. Copyright 1983. Reproduced with permission from the American Alliance for Health, Physical Education, Recreation and Dance, Reston, VA 22091.

(e.g., time is ordered from the past to the future) or by size (e.g., put the biggest or smallest value first—largest mean value or frequency).

- When values go to multiple decimal places, round them off. Two digits are about the most that people can understand, that can be measured with precision, or that anyone cares about. For example, what does a $\dot{V}O_2$max value mean when carried to four decimal places? We don't understand it, we can't measure it that precisely, and no one cares. Sometimes attempts at precision become humorous, bringing to mind the report that the average American family has 2.4 children. (We thought children came only in whole units!) A single child is the smallest (most discrete) unit of measurement available.

- Use and pay attention to the summaries of rows and columns. The summary data, often provided as the last row or column, are important because these values (sometimes sums, means, or medians) provide a standard of comparison (or usualness). Often setting these values apart in some way (e.g., bold type) is valuable.

So let us try these procedures on a table. In our research methods class, we often assign students to find a table in *Research Quarterly for Exercise and Sport* and improve it by applying Wainer's suggestions. Our graduate students have not been hesitant about finding tables from "our scholarly work" to improve. (Professors: It's not only our work. Offer your students one of your published figures or tables. They will improve it, too.) A good example from a paper by Thomas, Salazar, and Landers (1991) that appeared in *RQES* was provided by James D. George (our thanks to Jim for allowing us to use his work), one of our doctoral students (at the time) at Arizona State University. The example on page 402 shows the data as presented by Thomas, Salazar, and Landers. The one on page 403 is George's rearrangement. Observing the improvements in data presentation and understanding is easy. First, the data in the column of "ES Info" has been reordered with all the "yes" responses followed by all the "no" responses (it might be just as well to remove the "no" responses and list the authors' names at the bottom of the table). Then the next column of *N* (sample size) has been ordered from smallest to largest. Finally, an additional label (Study's most important effects) was inserted under the "Primary ES" column to clarify the meaning of those three columns.

How do these changes relate to Wainer's three questions? The revised table makes clear the sample size and ES information (question 1) for each study (but so did the original table). At the level of questions 2 and 3, however (trends, relations, and overall structure), the revised table is a considerable improvement. For example, you can more easily observe that sample size and ES are unrelated; that is, neither studies with large samples nor small samples are more likely to produce larger or smaller treatment effects (as estimated by ES).

Another example of the mindless reporting of numbers is with statistical values. Just because computer printouts carry the statistics (e.g., *F*, *r*) and probabilities (*p*) to five or more places beyond the decimal does not mean the numbers should be reported to that level. Two or (at most) three places are adequate. However, this can result in rather odd probabilities: $t(22) = 14.73$, $p < .000$. Now, $p < .000$ means no chance of error; this cannot occur because, if there is no chance of error, how can it be a probability? What happened is that the exact probability was something like $p < .00023$ and the researcher rounded it back to $p < .000$. You cannot do this. As indicated earlier, we believe it is more appropriate to report the exact probability (e.g., $p < .001$) and whether this probability exceeded the alpha set for the experiment (e.g., $p < .05$). However, a 1 or a higher number must always be the last term in the probability. The previous example, $p < .00023$, if reported to three decimals, should read $p < .001$.

Although the mindless use of numbers frequently occurs, sometimes other items are reported that are just as mindless. In reviewing for a research journal, one of us encountered a study in which children were given a 12-week treatment. The author reported the mean age and standard deviation of the children before and after the 12-week treatment. Not surprisingly, the children had all aged 12 weeks. The author also calculated a *t* test between the pre- and the posttreatment means for age that was, of course, significant. That is, the fact that the children had aged 12 weeks during the 12-week period was a reliable finding.

Preparing Figures and Illustrations

Many suggestions about table construction also apply to figures and illustrations because a figure is only another way to present a table. Before using a table or a figure, ask, Does the reader need the actual numbers, or is a picture of the results more useful? A more important question may be, Do you need either? Can the data be presented more concisely and easily in the text? Figures and tables do not add scientific validity to your research report.

A Fine Table Made Better

The Original Table

Table 2.   Data on articles in Volume 59, 1988

First Author	ES Info	N^c	Primary ES*		
Doody	no				
Kamen[b]	yes	9	0.64	0.72	0.14
Alexander	yes	26–48	0.33	0.73*	0.39
Era	yes	5–6	0.50*	0.10	1.42*
Kokhonen	yes	9–12	−1.97*	−2.64*	−1.78*
Farrell	yes	45–368	0.77*	−0.51*	0.37*
Heinert	no				
Kamen	no[a]	10	1.14	0.81	0.90
Ober	no				
Simard	yes	7	−1.59*	0.52	−2.71*
Berger	no				
Stewart	no				
Abernethy	no				
Etnyre	no				
Nelson[b]	yes	13	0.73	1.76	0.85
Wesson	no				
Housh	yes	20	−0.53*	−2.11*	0.25*
Hutcheson	yes	34	−0.06	0.63*	−0.30*

*Comparison of Ms forming ES was significant, $p < .05$.

[a]No significant main effects.

[b]The main effect is significant, but no information is provided regarding the significance of the post hoc comparison.

[c]Per comparison group.

A Fine Table Made Better

The Better Way

Table 2.   Data on articles in Volume 59, 1988

First Author	ES Info	N^c	Primary ES* (Study's most important effects)		
Era	yes	5–6	0.10	0.50*	1.42*
Simard	yes	7	−2.71*	−1.59*	0.52
Kamen[a]	yes	9	0.14	0.64	0.72
Kamen	yes[b]	10	0.81	0.90	1.14
Kokhonen	yes	9–12	−2.64*	−1.97*	−1.78*
Nelson[b]	yes	13	0.73	0.85	1.76
Housh	yes	20	−2.11*	−0.53*	0.25*
Hutcheson	yes	34	−0.30*	−0.06	0.63*
Alexander	yes	26–48	0.33	0.39	0.73*
Farrell	yes	45–368	−0.51*	0.37*	0.77*
Abernethy	no				
Berger	no				
Doody	no				
Etnyre	no				
Heinert	no				
Ober	no				
Stewart	no				
Wesson	no				

[a]Per comparison group.

[b]Comparison of Ms forming ES

[c]The main effect is significant, but no information is provided regarding the significance of the post hoc comparison.

[d]No significant main effects.

*ES was significant, $p < .05$.

In fact, they may only clutter the results. Day (1983) suggested a reasonable means for deciding whether to use a table or a figure: "If the data show pronounced trends making an interesting picture, use a graph. If the numbers just sit there, with no exciting trend in evidence, a table should be satisfactory" (p. 56).

Several other considerations are important in preparing figures. Selection of the type of figure is somewhat arbitrary, but some distinctions make the choice of one type of figure more appropriate than another (see Table 19.4). To evaluate whether you've used a figure appropriately, make sure it

- does not duplicate text,
- contains important information,
- does not have visual distractions,
- is easy to read,
- is easy to understand, and
- is consistent with other figures in the text.

Figures are useful in presenting interactions and data points that change over time (or across multiple trials). Of course, the dependent variable is placed on the y-axis and some independent or categorical variable on the x-axis. If you have more than one independent variable, how do you decide which to put on the x-axis? We have already partially answered that question. If time or multiple trials are used, put them on the x-axis. For example, if a study found an interaction on the dependent variable between age level (7-, 9-, 11-, 13-, and 15-year-old males) and the treatment (experimental versus control), age with five levels is usually the more appropriate choice for the x-axis. Note that

Table 19.4   Charts and Diagrams

	Bar and column charts—bars (horizontal) are best for comparing amounts; arrange by size, small to large or large to small; columns (vertical) are good for comparing amounts over time, especially if trends are evident; shading may be used to distinguish, or stack bars or columns.
	Curve graphs—best for showing change over time; time is horizontal with quantity vertical; allows more than one curve to be compared; sometimes area between curves can be shaded to show amount of change; shading, broken lines, symbols, or colored lines may be used to distinguish lines.
	Dot graph—shows patterns of individual scores where each dot represents a score on both the vertical and horizontal axis; different dots or dot symbols may be used to distinguish groups.
	Flow charts—shows relationships in process; often useful for demonstrating steps in a process where more than one option exists (e.g., if yes, then this; if no, then this).
	Pie chart—circle for pie equals 100%; maximum of five or six segments; best at showing proportions of segments; order segments from large to small starting at 12:00 o'clock; highlight segments with shadings making smallest segment the darkest.
	Schematics—relations between variables or concepts (e.g., overlap in two correlated variables).

Developed from White, J.V. (1984). *Using charts and graphs: 1000 ideas for visual persuasion*. New Providence, NJ: R.R. Bowker Co.

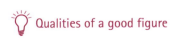

Qualities of a good figure

this is a general rule, but specific circumstances may dictate otherwise. A good example of the use of a figure to present an interaction is shown in Figure 19.1. Note that both age and time are independent variables, so time is placed on the *x*-axis.

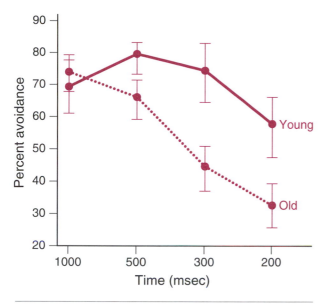

Figure 19.1   Appropriate use of a figure to depict an interaction.

From "Exercise and the Aging Brain," by W.W. Spirduso, 1983, *Research Quarterly for Exercise and Sport*, **54**, p. 211. Copyright 1983. Reproduced with permission from the American Alliance for Health, Physical Education, Recreation and Dance, Reston, VA 22091.

Figure 19.2 is a good example of a useless figure. The results can be summarized in two sentences: "During acquisition, all three groups reduced their frequency of errors but did not differ significantly from one another. At retention, Experimental Group 2 further reduced its number of errors, whereas Experimental Group 1 and the Controls remained at the same level." Also, when results of different groups follow a similar pattern, a figure frequently appears cluttered.

One final consideration is the construction of the *y*-axis. In general, between 8 and 12 intervals encompassing the range of means is useful. Do not extend the *y*-axis outside the range of means. This wastes space. Again, consider whether you need a figure at all. Sometimes theses and dissertations include drawings such as that in Figure 19.3. Looking at that figure, you immediately see a strong and significant interaction between knowledge of results (KR) and goal setting. Now look at the *y*-axis, on which the dependent variable is shown. Note that the scores are given to the nearest hundredth

of a second. Actually, there is less than a half-second (< 500 msec) difference among the four groups on a task in which average performance is about 18 seconds (18,000 msec). In fact, this interaction is not significant and clearly accounts for little variance. It should merely be reported as nonsignificant with no figure included. The researcher made the interaction appear important by the scale used on the *y*-axis.

Sometimes multiple figures reporting data across several independent variables are used. For example, a comparison of Chinese, African, and U.S. boys and girls in five age groups might be reported on running speed. A single figure would be cluttered with all this data, so several figures (one for each continent of origin, each age, or each gender) might be used. The *y*-axis on each figure should have the same 8 to 12 points for running speed. Otherwise, visual comparisons of the data are difficult.

Illustrations (photographs and line drawings) are also used in research reporting. Most frequently, illustrations are of experimental arrangements and equipment. They should not be used when the equipment is of a standard design or make; a brief description will suffice. Any unusual arrangement

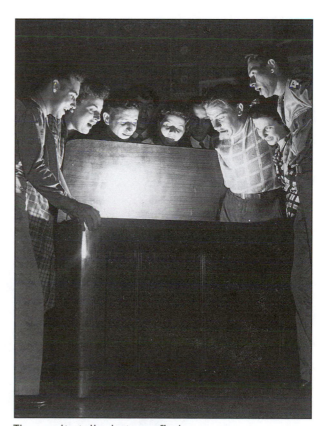

The results tell what you find.

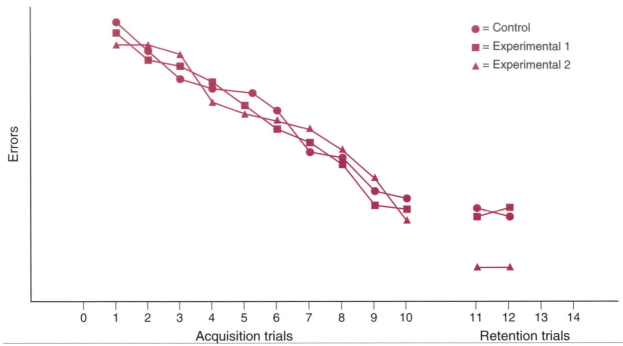

Figure 19.2   Example of a useless figure.

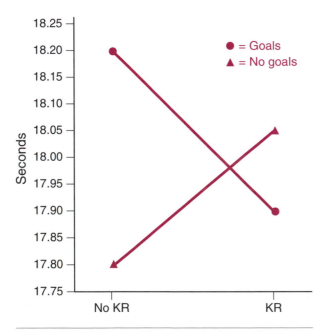

Figure 19.3   A nonsignificant interaction made to appear significant by the scale of the dependent variable.

or novel equipment should be described and either a picture or line drawing included. If specifications and relationships are important to include within the illustration rather than in the text, a line drawing is preferable because it can be more easily labeled.

Remember, tables, figures, and illustrations are generally appropriate for the results chapter but not for the discussion. An exception to this rule is a report of multiple experiments in which the general discussion section could contain a table or figure to display common findings or a summary across several experiments.

To review, when determining where tables, figures, and illustrations should appear—in the text or in the appendix—consider the following recommendations:

- Put important tables, figures, and illustrations in the text and all others in the appendix.
- Try not to clutter the results with too many tables, figures, and illustrations.
- Do not put summary tables for ANOVA and MANOVA in the results. Place the important statistics from these tables in the text and put the tables in the appendix.

Remember that all journals have prescribed formats and styles for articles submitted to them

Where to include figures and tables

(e.g., those of the American Psychological Association or *Index Medicus*). These instructions for authors usually include directions for preparing tables and figures. Many of these decisions are arbitrary. Read and look at what you have written, then use common sense. Select the tables, figures, and illustrations that are needed to read and understand the results. Everything else goes into the appendix. The appropriate use of tables, figures, and illustrations can add to the interest, understanding, and motivation of the reader.

Summary

The results and discussion sections are written after the data have been collected and analyzed. The results tell what you found; the discussion explains what the results mean. The results are the most important part of the research. They represent the unique findings of your study and your contribution to knowledge. The discussion ties the findings back to the literature review, theory, and empirical findings from other studies. Your findings should be interpreted in the discussion. In journal format, the results and discussion are sections in the body of the paper (more on this in chapter 20). In the traditional format, the results are chapter 3 and the discussion is chapter 4. However, in multiple experiment studies, each experiment may best be reported in a separate section (or chapter) with its own brief introduction, method, results, and discussion. This is often followed by a section (or chapter) of general discussion of the multiple experiments.

Tables should be used in the discussion to summarize and present data when they are more effective than text presentation. Figures and illustrations are also used in the results, most frequently to demonstrate more dramatic findings. Careful construction of tables and figures is important in communicating information to the reader.

Check Your Understanding

Select a research report of interest from a refereed journal in your area of interest. Read the paper, but concentrate on the results and discussion. Answer the following questions in a brief report.

1. Results:
   a. How is the results section organized?
   b. Compare the order of reported findings with the introduction, literature review, and statement of the problem. Do you see any relationships?
   c. How else might the results have been organized? Would this have been better or worse? Why?

2. Tables, figures, and illustrations:
   a. Are there any? How many of each?
   b. Why are they used? Could the data have been reported more easily in the text? When either a table or figure is used, would the other have been as good? Better? Why?
   c. Can you restructure one of the tables or figures to improve it?

3. Discussion:
   a. How is the discussion organized?
   b. Are all results discussed?
   c. Is the discussion accurate in terms of the results?
   d. Are previous findings and theory woven into the discussion?
   e. Are all conclusions and supporting evidence clearly presented?
   f. Did the authors use any methodological cop-outs?

CHAPTER 20

Ways of Reporting Research

Dear Professors of Research Methods:

I am planning my thesis defense with my major professor and committee. Do you have any advice about the meeting?

Anticipating all alternatives,
Anxious Annie

Dear AA:

Over the years we have developed the Thomas and Nelson Top Ten Things Not to Say or Do at Your Thesis Defense as follows:

10. Have your mother present at the start of the meeting to show baby pictures of you and rave about how smart you are.
9. Wear dark glasses. Inscrutability is unnerving.
8. To recoup your photocopying costs, sell T-shirts that have some tasteful slogan such as "People who live in glass houses shouldn't pick their noses."
7. Answer every question with a question and insert "you know" two or three times in every sentence.
6. Call all male committee members "Big Guy."
5. Do the moon walk while showing your slides.
4. Yell "Yes!" and lead the spectators in a wave when you think you have given a good answer.
3. When a committee member is speaking to you, open your mouth and stare incredulously at him until he loses his train of thought.
2. Periodically, act very agitated and complain to an imaginary friend, named Boomer, about the committee picking on you.

(Drum roll!) And the Number One Thing Not to Say or Do at Your Thesis Defense is:

1. When asked a difficult question, suddenly perform the Heimlich Maneuver on the committee member next to you. Claim she was choking on a doughnut.

Looking forward to your next defense,
PRM

Our favorite author, Day (1983), provides an appropriate introduction to this chapter on ways of reporting research with the following quotation:

> Scientific research is not complete until the results have been published. Therefore, a scientific paper is an essential part of the research process. Therefore, the writing of an accurate, understandable paper is just as important as the research itself. Therefore, the words in the paper should be weighed as carefully as the reagents in the laboratory. Therefore, the scientists must know how to use words. Therefore, the education of a scientist is not complete until the ability to publish has been established. (p. 158)

 Chapter 18 covered the research proposal: how to write the introduction, the literature review, the problem statement, and the methodology for the thesis or dissertation. Chapter 19 explained how to organize and write the results and discussion sections. Effectively coordinating all this information into a thesis or a dissertation is the topic of concern in this chapter. We present both the journal style of organization, which we (Thomas, Nelson, & Magill, 1986) have advocated, and the traditional chapter style. In addition, we include information about writing for publication in research journals, preparing abstracts, and presenting papers orally (including in a poster format). After you've read the chapter, you might read *Quest* (Vol. 39, August 1987). This issue focuses on graduate programs in physical education, exercise science, and sport science. The entire issue is quite informative to potential master's and doctoral students. Articles of particular interest are by Newell (p. 88), Massengale (p. 97), Spirduso (p. 103), Thomas (p. 114), Spirduso and Lovett (p. 129), and King and Bandy (p. 153). Additional articles in this issue focus on specific types of graduate programs (e.g., teacher preparation and sport management).

Basic Writing Guidelines

Again we quote Day (1983). His unwritten rule—although because he wrote it maybe it is no longer

unwritten (somewhere in that statement is a limited amount of logic)—is this: "Write your thesis to please your major professor, if you can figure out what turns him (or her) on" (p. 125). Once this basic principle is understood, we can offer some guidelines. But in case of doubt or conflict, return to that basic principle.

- Collect all the documents that outline university, graduate school, and departmental policy for theses and dissertations. Then actually read these documents, as someone at some level will eventually check to see whether you have followed them.
- Review the theses and dissertations of past graduate students whose work is well regarded by your institution. Identify common elements in their work, and pattern your work after theirs.
- Allow twice as much time as you think you will need. Remember Murphy's Law, "Whatever can go wrong will go wrong," and its special version, "When several things can go wrong, the one that will go wrong is the one that will cause the greatest harm."

The thesis and dissertation have basically the same parts found in any scientific paper: an introduction and a literature review, method, results, and discussion sections. In chapter format each of these parts becomes a chapter. Sometimes the introduction and the literature review are separate chapters, leading to five rather than four chapters. This format may vary in historical papers (see chapter 12) or multiple experiments (see chapter 19) or when your major professor says it should.

A Brief Word About Acknowledgments

 A section seldom mentioned in articles and books on preparing theses and dissertations is that of **acknowledgments** You should ac-

---

 See *Quest*, **39** (August 1987) for more information on graduate programs in physical education, exercise science, and sport science.

 Guidelines for writing a successful thesis or dissertation

acknowledgments — Section of a scholarly paper that credits individuals important to the development of the work.

knowledge those people without whom the research would have been impossible. However, acknowledgments, as prepared by graduate students, take some odd turns. We saw one in which a woman acknowledged her ex-husband. She said that if he had not been so difficult to live with, she would never have gone back to the university and done graduate work. By doing that she found an area in which she had a tremendous interest, and this represented a significant change in her life. That is about the only positive statement we have ever heard about ex-spouses. Some other funny acknowledgments follow:

- My parents, husband, and children provided inspiration and support throughout, but I was able to complete my thesis anyway.
- My major professor, Dr. I.M. Published, coordinated the work and made an occasional contribution.
- Professor B.A. Snobb wants everyone to know he had nothing to do with this thesis.
- Finally, we would like to thank our proofreader, I.D. Best, without whose hell; thes document wld net be pausible.

More seriously, you can acknowledge appropriate individuals, but keep the list short and to the point and do not be mushy. As in other areas, use correct English. In their acknowledgments, graduate students often use "wish" when they mean "want," as in "I wish to acknowledge I.B.A. Fink." Does that mean they might have acknowledged him if his contribution had not been so lousy? The graduate student really wants to acknowledge him. But more appropriately, why not just say it: "I acknowledge I.B.A. Fink."

Thesis and Dissertation Format: Traditional Versus Journal

A Case for the Journal Format
Limitations of Chapter Style
Structure of the Journal Format
    Preliminary Materials
    Body of the Thesis or Dissertation
    Appendixes
        More Thorough Literature Review

Additional Method Information
Additional Results Information
Other Additional Materials
One-Page Vita
Examples of Theses and Dissertations
    Using Journal Format

We devote considerable space here to the journal format for thesis and dissertation writing. Our material is partially reproduced from an article we wrote with a colleague (Thomas, Nelson, & Magill, 1986). We acknowledge the contribution of Dr. Richard Magill from Louisiana State University, and we appreciate *Quest* (Human Kinetics) allowing us to adapt the article for this book.

Graduate education in the United States, especially at the doctoral level, was modeled after graduate education in Germany. The German university spirit of the search for knowledge and the concomitant emphasis on productive research were transplanted in large measure in America (Rudy, 1962). Although there have been some changes over the years in the requirements for the doctoral degree, the basic aims and expectations have in essence remained unaltered. The doctoral degree is conferred in recognition of a candidate's scholarship and research accomplishments in a specific field of learning through an original contribution of significant knowledge and ideas (Boyer, 1973).

Stated more simply, research is the foundation of the doctoral program, and the dissertation is the most distinctive aspect of the doctoral degree. It has been reported that the dissertation occupies an average of 39% of the time devoted to obtaining the degree in the fields of biochemistry, electrical engineering, psychology, physics, sociology, and zoology (Porter, Chubin, Rossini, Boeckmann, & Connally, 1982).

A Case for the Journal Format

The major purpose of the thesis and the dissertation is to contribute new knowledge with scientific merit (American Psychological Association, 1959; Berelson, 1960; Porter & Wolfe, 1975). A purpose typically cited in university bulletins is that it provides evidence of competency in planning, conducting, and reporting research. In terms of program objectives, the study is a valuable learning experience in that the thesis and the dissertation are functional exercises in executing the steps in the scientific method of problem solving. Even "ABDs" ("all-but-dones," or persons completing all work for the PhD except the dissertation) acknowledge the contribution that dissertations make to science and the scientific method (Jacks, Chubin, Porter & Connally, 1983).

The importance of the dissemination of research results as an integral part of the research process is well established. It follows that one of the purposes of the thesis or dissertation is to serve as a vehicle to carry the results of independent investigation undertaken by the graduate student. Thus, the dissertation or thesis becomes part of the dissemination process. Porter et al. (1982) reported that dissertations do make substantial contributions to the knowledge base and that authors' published dissertations are cited more often than other papers they write.

Despite the potential contribution that the thesis and dissertation can make to a field of study, the fact remains that only about one third to one half of the dissertations (and even fewer theses) become available to the profession through publications (McPhie, 1960; Porter et al., 1982). There are, of course, several reasons why a thesis or dissertation is never published. For one, despite the emphasis placed on research by the institutions, many students do not consider research an important aim. Porter et al. (1982) reported that 24% of the doctoral recipients surveyed expressed this feeling. Arlin (1977) went so far as to claim that most educators never do another piece of published research after they complete the master's thesis or doctoral dissertation. In addition, job placements fix varying degrees of importance on research and publication. There is also the inescapable fact that not all theses and dissertations are worthy of publication.

Conceivably, another contributing factor in the low rate of publication is the traditional style and format often used in the thesis or dissertation. Granted, the highly motivated new PhD will spend the time and effort to rewrite the dissertation into the proper format for journal review, but the less motivated student may not. The point is, why should dissertations and theses be written in a format that requires rewriting before publication if a vital part of the research process is publication of the research study (Day, 1983)?

We contend that the traditional format of dissertations and theses is archaic. Doctoral students (especially those working with productive major professors) may have several scholarly refereed publications by the time the PhD is awarded. Should such people, who have shown that their previous work has scientific merit, be required to go through the ritual of writing a dissertation involving separate chapters that spell out every detail of the research process? It seems more logical to us to have the body of the dissertation prepared in the appropriate format and style for submission to a journal, which is the acceptable model for communicating results of research and scholarly works in much of the arts, sciences, and professions. We suggest a format that accomplishes this purpose by restructuring the thesis and dissertation and explaining the contents of the various parts.

Limitations of Chapter Style

Conventional theses and dissertations typically contain four or five chapters. Traditionally, the chapters are intended to reflect the scientific method for solving problems: developing the problem and formulating the hypotheses, gathering the data, and analyzing and interpreting the results. These steps are usually embodied in chapters such as the introduction (which sometimes contains the literature review; at other times the literature review is a separate chapter), and the method, results, and discussion sections.

The thesis and dissertation also have several introductory pages as prescribed by the institution, usually consisting of the title page, acknowledgments, abstract, table of contents, and lists of figures and tables. At the end of the study are the references and one or more appendices that contain items such as subject consent forms, tabular materials not presented in the text, more detailed descriptions of procedure, instructions to subjects, and raw data. A brief biographical sketch (the vita) is usually the last entry in the conventional thesis and dissertation.

The chapter format is, of course, steeped in scholastic tradition. In defense of this tradition, the discipline required to accomplish the steps involved in the scientific method is usually viewed as an educationally beneficial experience. Moreover, for the master's student, the thesis is normally the first research effort, and there may be merit in formally addressing such steps as operationally defining terms, delimiting the study, stating the basic assumptions, and justifying the significance of the study.

A more serious limitation of the chapter style relates to the dissemination of the results of the study, that is, publishing the manuscript in a research journal. Considerable rewriting is usually required to publish a thesis or dissertation because journal formats differ from those of theses and dissertations prepared in chapter format. Granted, the information for the journal article is provided in the thesis and the dissertation, but a considerable amount of deleting, reorganizing, and consolidating is necessary to transform the study to journal format.

With regard to the dissertation, the student usually would like to publish this product of months (years) of time and painstaking effort. But in terms of expediency, the chapter format is decidedly counterproductive. The rewriting required may be made more difficult by the fact that the typical new PhD recipient immediately begins a new job that demands considerable time and energy. Unless the new PhD is motivated, the transformation of the conventional dissertation style to journal format may be delayed, sometimes indefinitely. Porter et al. (1982) claimed that new PhDs who fail to publish within 2 years subsequent to the awarding of the degree are unlikely to publish later.

The master's thesis is even more unlikely to be published. One reason is that the master's student generally does not consider publishing unless the major professor suggests it. Furthermore, the master's student may not be as well prepared to write for publication as the doctoral student. Thus, the burden for publication is on the major professor, who understandably is often unwilling to spend the additional time necessary to supervise (or do) the rewriting. Thus, most theses are not submitted for publication. Ironically, the time-honored, scholarly style of the thesis and dissertation in chapter format actually impedes an integral part of the research process: the dissemination of results.

Structure of the Journal Format

To develop a better model for theses and dissertations, the limitations of the chapter format for reporting must be overcome while maintaining the concept of a complete research report. The format we suggest has three major parts. Preliminary materials include such items as the title page, acknowledgments, and abstract. The body of the thesis and dissertation is a complete manuscript prepared in journal form. Included are the standard parts of a research report, such as the introduction, method, results, discussion, references, figures, and tables. The appendices often include a more thorough literature review, additional detail about method, and additional results not placed in the body of the thesis or dissertation. However, the journal format, as we describe it, is more appropriate for reporting descriptive (e.g., surveys and correlational studies) and experimental research. The format requires some adjustments for reporting analytical research (e.g., historical and philosophical studies and meta-analysis) and qualitative studies.

Thus, parts of the thesis and dissertation using the journal format would include the following:

1.0 **Preliminary materials**

    1.1 Title Page
    1.2 Acknowledgments
    1.3 Abstract
    1.4 Table of contents
    1.5 List of tables
    1.6 List of figures

2.0 **Body of the thesis or dissertation**

    2.1 Introduction
    2.2 Method
    2.3 Results
    2.4 Discussion
    2.5 References
    2.6 Tables
    2.7 Figures

3.0 **Appendices**

    3.1 Extended literature review
    3.2 Additional methodology
    3.3 Additional results
    3.4 Other additional materials

4.0 **One-page vita**

How can this format overcome the limitations of the chapter style? For both master's and doctoral students, a manuscript (body of the thesis or dissertation) is developed that is ready for journal submission. All that remains is to add the title page and abstract, and the paper can be sent to a suitable journal.

The advantage of this format for doctoral students should be apparent. Because PhDs who fail to publish their dissertations within 2 years are unlikely to publish afterwards, encouraging publication by a more functional format is worthwhile. Especially when we consider that dissertations appear to make an important contribution to knowledge, the evaluation and subsequent publication of that knowledge through refereed journals is an important step to accomplish. Although master's theses are not as likely as dissertations to be published, any format that encourages the publication of quality thesis work is desirable.

One final point before proceeding to the structure of the journal format: Your graduate school probably requires that the thesis or dissertation follow a standard style manual (or at least the style of a journal). The three most common are the *Publication Manual of the American Psychological Association, Index Medicus*, and *The Chicago Manual of Style*. This format adapts nicely to any of these style manuals. University regulations usually do not specify a particular style, but frequently an academic department may adopt one or two specific styles. If the journal format is to be used, a department might want to allow more than one style. For example, many journals reporting exercise physiology and biomechanical studies use *Index Medicus*. Journals publishing articles in motor learning/control/development, sport psychology and sociology, and professional preparation frequently use the APA manual. Journals that publish history and philosophy-of-sport articles may use *The Chicago Manual of Style*. It would be of considerable benefit for the graduate student to have the flexibility of choosing the style recommended by the journal to which the paper will be submitted.

Preliminary Materials

Most of this information will be required by the institution and usually appears at the beginning of the thesis or dissertation. Generally included are the title page, committee approval form, acknowledgments, dedication, abstract, table of contents, list of tables, and list of figures. Special considerations involved in preparing these specific pages are covered in other parts of this book. However, we recommend a slight change in the length of the abstract. Many institutions require that the abstract follow the form for *Dissertation Abstracts International*, which sets a 300-word maximum for the abstract length. Journals (and the style manuals mentioned previously) typically require abstracts between 100 and 150 words. If the thesis or dissertation writer keeps the abstract between 100 and 150 words, it can serve both requirements.

Body of the Thesis or Dissertation

This section should be a complete research report using the appropriate style for the journal to which it is to be submitted (or the style required by the department in which the work was done). Included are the introduction and literature review, method, results, discussion, references, tables, and figures. The author should keep the length within the bounds set by the journal. This is typically 15-25 pages for single experiments. Most journals allow additional pages for multiple experiments or unusually complex articles. To accomplish this, the student and major professor must be rigorous in keeping the paper to a length that a journal will consider. In our experience maintaining an acceptable length is the most difficult goal to achieve using this format.

The thesis or dissertation author should consult several sources in preparing the body of the paper. One source is the journal to which submission is anticipated. Guidelines to authors and instructions regarding the appropriate style manual are typically published in journals (e.g., see each issue of *Research Quarterly for Exercise and Sport*). The author should read a number of similar papers in the selected journal to see how specific issues are handled (tables, figures, unusual citations, multiple experiments). In addition, the thesis or dissertation author should carefully follow the style manual that has been selected.

Of course, the ultimate goal of this part of the thesis or dissertation is to enable the paper to be submitted to a journal as soon as possible. Improved format and better writing will not aid poor quality research. On the other hand, quality research can easily be hidden by a poor format that makes rewriting difficult, poor reporting that omits important information, or weak and boring writing that makes reading tedious. "Thus the scientist must not only 'do' science; he (or she) must 'write' science. Although good writing does not lead to the publication of bad science, bad writing can and often does prevent or delay the publication of good science" (Day, 1983, p. x). Research is not recognized in any formal sense as having been conducted until it has been shared with and evaluated by the academic community. As an additional point, there is no law (that we can locate) saying that the thesis or the

American Psychological Association. (1994). *Publication manual of the American Psychological Association* (4th ed.). Washington, DC: Author.

National Library of Medicine. (1995). *Index Medicus*. Bethesda, MD: Author.

University of Chicago Press. (1993). *The Chicago manual of style* (14th ed.). Chicago: Author.

dissertation must be written in such a way that the reader has difficulty staying awake.

Appendices

In the conventional format, the appendices primarily serve as a depository for nonessential information. To a degree this still characterizes what should be put in the appendices when using the journal format, but some additional features give them unique worth. Usually, the number and content of the appendices are determined by the collective agreement of the student, the advisor, and the supervisory committee. In the journal format we suggest four sections that provide a basis from which to develop the appendices. There may be other sections that could be included. However, we see these four as essential components of all appendices.

Each appendix should begin with a description of what is in a particular section and how that information relates to the body of the thesis or dissertation. This enables the reader to get the most use of the information in the section.

More Thorough Literature Review. A very important and useful component of the appendices is a review of literature. The introduction in the body of the thesis or dissertation includes a discussion of related research, but it does so only with regard to presenting a minimum amount of information to establish an appropriate background for the one or more studies that follow. One purpose of the thesis or dissertation is to allow the student an opportunity to demonstrate a knowledge of the research literature related to the topic. In the body of the journal format, there is limited opportunity for the demonstration because journals typically have concise introductions. A comprehensive literature review should be included as the first appendix to provide an appropriate mechanism for the student to demonstrate knowledge of the relevant literature. We recommend that this review also be written in journal style.

At least two additional purposes are served by including this literature review as an appendix. First, it provides an opportunity to have this information available for the student's committee members, some of whom may not be sufficiently familiar with the literature related to the thesis or dissertation. Second, if properly developed, the literature review can go directly to a journal for publication.

The literature review contained in the appendices can take several forms, the most popular of which is probably the comprehensive narrative that synthesizes and evaluates research. This review links various studies and establishes a strong foundation on which to build the research. It also reveals how the research represented by the thesis or dissertation extends the existing body of knowledge related to the student's research topic.

A second form the appendix literature review could take is a meta-analysis, which is a quantitative literature review that synthesizes previous research by analyzing results of many research studies by specified statistical methods (e.g., chapter 14). An example of a meta-analysis related to the study of physical activity can be seen in an article by Thomas and French (1985).

Additional Method Information. A second important component of the appendices is the presentation of additional methodological information not included in the body of the thesis or dissertation. Journals encourage authors to provide method information that is brief yet sufficient to describe essential details related to the subjects, apparatus, and procedures used in the research. The disadvantage of journal articles is that often sufficient information is not provided to enable someone to replicate the study. In the journal format for the thesis or dissertation, this useful additional information becomes an appendix. Information suitable for this section includes more detailed subject characteristics, more comprehensive experimental design information, fuller descriptions (and perhaps photographs) of tests or testing apparatus, copies of tests, inventories or questionnaires, and specific instructions given to the subjects.

Additional Results Information. The third appendix should include information that is not essential for inclusion in the results section of the body of the thesis or dissertation. Journal editors typically want only summary statements about the analyses and a minimum number of figures and tables. Thus, considerable material concerning the results can be placed in the appendix, such as all means and standard deviations, ANOVA tables, multiple correlation tables, validity and reliability information, and additional tables and figures.

Providing this type of information serves several purposes. First, it provides evidence to your com-

Thomas, J.R., & French, K.E. (1985). Gender differences across age in motor performance: A meta-analysis. *Psychological Bulletin*, **98**, 260-282.

mittee and advisor that the data descriptions and analyses were properly done. Second, the student's committee members are given an opportunity to evaluate the statistical analyses and interpretations from the body of the thesis or dissertation. Third, other researchers are provided access to more detailed data and statistical information should they want it. For example, a researcher may want to include this thesis or dissertation in a meta-analysis. Because the additional results presented in the appendix may have many future uses, their importance to the total thesis or dissertation cannot be overestimated.

Other Additional Materials.   A fourth appendix could include information that is not appropriate for the body of the thesis or dissertation or the other appendices, such as human subjects committee approval form, individual subject's consent form, sample data recording forms, and perhaps the raw data from each subject. Also, detailed descriptions of any pilot work done before the study could be included in this or a separate appendix.

As can be seen from these descriptions, the appendices in the journal format of a thesis or dissertation provide a mechanism for including information not contained in the journal article that may be significant for the student, the student's committee, and other researchers. It also provides a means for elaborating on some information in the journal article. Moreover, the comprehensive literature review provides the student with another possible publication. As a result, the appendices become meaningful components of the total thesis or dissertation.

One-Page Vita

Many colleges and universities request that the last page of the thesis or dissertation be a one-page vita about the student. This should be a professional version of a vita including items like education and previous work experience.

Examples of Theses and Dissertations Using Journal Format

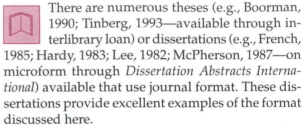 There are numerous theses (e.g., Boorman, 1990; Tinberg, 1993—available through interlibrary loan) or dissertations (e.g., French, 1985; Hardy, 1983; Lee, 1982; McPherson, 1987—on microform through *Dissertation Abstracts International*) available that use journal format. These dissertations provide excellent examples of the format discussed here.

The information in an unpublished thesis or dissertation remains the exclusive domain of a few individuals. We established earlier that a vital part of the research process is the dissemination of knowledge. We maintain that a style and format should not impede this process. The proposed journal format accomplishes the traditional objectives of the thesis or dissertation, yet facilitates the dissemination of knowledge.

Helpful Hints for Successful Journal Writing

We highly recommend the third edition of a work to which we have frequently referred here: *How to Write and Publish a Scientific Paper* (Day, 1988). In our opinion, this book is the researcher's best resource in preparing a paper for submission to a research journal. The book is short (<200 pages), informative, readable, and funny. Although the small section here cannot replace Day's more thorough treatment, we do offer a few suggestions.

Boorman, M.A. (1990). *Effect of age and menopausal status on cardiorespiratory fitness in masters women endurance athletes.* M.S. thesis, Arizona State University, Tempe.

French, K.E. (1985). *The relation of knowledge development to children's basketball performance.* Unpublished doctoral dissertation, Louisiana State University, Baton Rouge.

Hardy, C.J. (1983). *The mediational role of social influence in the perception of exertion.* Unpublished doctoral dissertation, Louisiana State University, Baton Rouge.

Lee, T.D. (1982). *On the locus of contextual interference in motor skill acquisition.* Unpublished doctoral dissertation, Louisiana State University, Baton Rouge.

Tinberg, C.M. (1993). *The relation of practice time to coaches' objectives, players' improvement, and level of expertise.* M.S. thesis, Arizona State University, Tempe.

Day, R.D. (1988). *How to write and publish a scientific paper* (3rd ed.). Phoenix: Oryx Press.

First, decide to which journal the research paper is to be submitted. Carefully read its guidelines (select a recent issue, as these items may change from older issues) and follow the recommended procedures. Guidelines usually explain the journal's publication style; how to prepare tables, figures, and illustrations; where to submit papers (and how many copies); acceptable lengths; and sometimes estimated review time. Nearly all journals require that manuscripts not be submitted elsewhere simultaneously. To do so is unethical.

Journals follow a standard procedure for papers submitted. One of your authors (Thomas) was editor-in-chief of *Research Quarterly for Exercise and Sport* for 6 years (1983-1989). Here is what happens to a manuscript between submission to the editor and return to the author (the average time of this process for *RQES* is 50-70 days):

1. The editor checks to see whether the paper is within the scope of the journal, is of appropriate length, and uses correct style. If any of these characteristics are inappropriate, it may be returned to the author.
2. The editor looks through the paper to determine that all appropriate materials are included (e.g., abstract, tables, and figures).
3. The editor reads the abstract, looks at the key words, and evaluates the reference list to identify potential reviewers.
4. Depending on the journal's size, there may be section editors (*RQES* has 10 sections, e.g., biomechanics, pedagogy, physiology, and psychology) or a board of associate editors. The editor places the paper in the appropriate section or with an appropriate associate editor.
5. The editor (sometimes in consultation with section or associate editors) assigns reviewers (usually two or three).
6. The reviewers and section editor (or associate editor) receive copies of the paper with review forms. They have a specific date by which they should complete the review.
7. The reviewers mail their reviews to the section editor (or associate editor), who evaluates the paper and the reviews and makes a recommendation to the editor.
8. The editor reads the paper, the reviews, and the evaluations and writes the author concerning the paper's status. Usually the editor will outline the major reasons for the decision.

Smaller, more narrowly focused journals may not have section or associate editors, so reviews go directly to the editor, who decides. These decisions usually fall into three general categories (some journals have levels of the categories):

- Accept (sometimes with varying degrees of revision)
- Unacceptable (sometimes called rejected without bias), which means you can revise the paper and the editor will have it evaluated again
- Reject, which usually means the journal will no longer consider your paper

Review criteria are fairly common and are discussed in chapter 2. Rates for decisions to publish vary by the quality of the journal and the area of the paper and are frequently available. *Research Quarterly for Exercise and Sport* accepts about 25% of the papers submitted (see each June issue for a more detailed description).

If this is your first paper, seek some advice from a more experienced author. This may be your major professor or another faculty member. Often papers are rejected because they fail to provide important information. More experienced authors will pick up on this immediately. Journal editors and reviewers do not have time to teach you good scientific reporting. Not everyone is fond of journal editors. One wag was reported to have said, "Editors have only one good characteristic—if they can understand a scientific paper, anyone can!" Another said, "Editors are, in my opinion, a low form of life—inferior to the viruses and only slightly above academic deans" (Day, 1983, p. 80). Teaching good reporting is the responsibility of your major professor, research methods courses, and books such as this one, but it is your responsibility to acquire the skill.

Do not be discouraged if your paper is rejected. All of us have had papers rejected. Carefully evaluate the reviews and determine whether the paper can be salvaged. If it can, then rewrite it, taking into account the reviewers' and the editor's criticisms, and submit it to another journal. Do not send the paper out to another journal without evaluating the reviews and making appropriate revisions. Often another journal will use the same reviewers, who

---

Steps in the journal review process

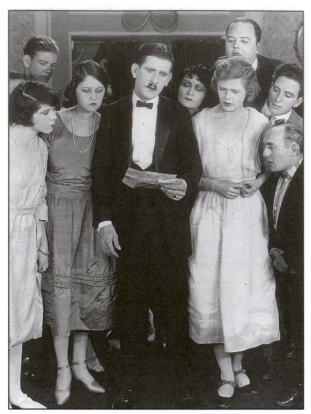

Don't be discouraged if your paper is rejected.

will not be happy if you didn't take their original advice. If your research and paper cannot be salvaged, learn from your mistakes.

 Reviewers and editors will not always agree in what they say about your paper. This is frustrating because sometimes they tell you different things. Recall also that editors may select reviewers for different reasons. For example, in a sport psychology study that develops a questionnaire, the editor may decide that one or more content reviewers and a statistical reviewer are needed to evaluate the work. You would not expect the content and statistical reviewers to discuss the same issues. Studies have been done of the peer review system for scholarly journals. For example, Morrow, Bray, Fulton, and Thomas (1992) reported that the *Research Quarterly for Exercise and Sport* had an average reviewer agreement of .37 based on 363 manuscripts between 1987 and 1991. They reported that other behavioral journals had reviewer agreements from a high of .70 in the *American Psychologist* to a low range of .17 to .40 for a group of medical journals. Whether reviewer agreement is to be expected is debatable. [For a good overview of the

peer review process, see *Behavioral and Brain Sciences*, **14**(1), 1991.] Our advice to you as a graduate student is to seek help from your advisor and other faculty in making revisions when you receive reviews of a paper you have submitted.

Occasionally, you may feel you have received an unfair review. If so, write back to the editor, point out the biases, and ask for another assessment by a different reviewer. Editors are generally open to this type of correspondence if it is handled in a professional way. However, opening with the sentence "Look what you and the stupid reviewers said" is unlikely to achieve success (for a humorous example see page 419). Recognize that appealing to the editor is less likely to be successful if two or more reviewers have agreed on the important criticisms. Editors cannot be expert in every area, and they must rely on reviewers. If you find yourself resorting to this tactic very often, the problem is likely in your work. You do not want to end up like Snoopy in "Peanuts" (C. Schulz), who received this note from the journal to which he had submitted a manuscript: "Dear Contributor, We are returning your manuscript. It does not suit our present needs. P.S. We note that you sent your story by first-class mail. Junk mail may be sent third-class."

As a final point in this part, we have noted the infrequency with which most scientific papers are read (of course, none of ours fall into that category). Some writers have speculated that only two to four people read the average paper completely. Is it possible that organizing the scientific paper differently might promote an increased audience? The answer might lie in a paper published in *Omni* magazine, reproduced here on page 420. The author, B. A. Realist (G. Benford), proposed a new format to aid potential authors of scientific papers.

Writing Abstracts

Thesis or Dissertation Abstracts
Abstracts for Published Papers
Conference Abstracts

Whether you are writing for a journal, using the chapter or journal format for preparing a thesis or

---

For a good overview of the peer review process, see *Behavioral and Brain Sciences*, **14**(1), 1991.

A Letter We've All Wanted to Write

Dear Sir, Madam, or Other:

Enclosed is our latest version of MS#85-02-22-RRRR, that is, the re-re-re-revised revision of our paper. Choke on it. We have again rewritten the entire manuscript from start to finish. We even changed the #@*! running head! Hopefully we have suffered enough by now to satisfy even you and your bloodthirsty reviewers.

I shall skip the usual point-by-point description of every single change we made in response to the critiques. After all, it is fairly clear that your reviewers are less interested in details of scientific procedure than in working out their personality problems and frustrations by seeking some kind of demented glee in the sadistic and arbitrary exercise of tyrannical power over hapless authors like ourselves who happen to fall into their clutches. We do understand that, in view of the misanthropic psychopaths you have on your editorial board, you need to keep sending them papers, for if they weren't reviewing manuscripts they'd probably be out mugging old people or clubbing baby seals to death.

Some of the reviewer's comments we couldn't do anything about. For example, if (as reviewer C suggested) several of my recent ancestors were indeed drawn from other species, it is too late to change that. Other suggestions were implemented, however, and the paper has improved and benefited. Thus, you suggested that we shorten the manuscript by 5 pages, and we were able to accomplish this very effectively by altering the margins and printing the paper in a different font with a smaller typeface. We agree with you that the paper is much better this way.

Our perplexing problem was dealing with suggestions 13 through 28 by reviewer B. As you may recall (that is, if you even bother reading the reviews before writing your decision letter), that reviewer listed 16 works that he/she felt we should cite in this paper. These were on a variety of different topics, none of which had any relevance to our work that we could see. Indeed, one was an essay on the Spanish-American War from a high school literary magazine. The only common thread was that all 16 were by the same author, presumably someone whom reviewer B greatly admires and feels should be more widely cited. To handle this, we have modified the Introduction and added, after the review of relevant literature, a subsection entitled "Review of Irrelevant Literature" that discusses these articles and also duly addresses some of the more asinine suggestions in the other reviews. We hope that you will be pleased with this revision and will finally recognize how deserving of publication this work is. If not, then you are an unscrupulous, depraved monster with no shred of human decency. You ought to be in a cage. If you do accept it, however, we wish to thank you for your patience and wisdom throughout this process and to express our appreciation of your scholarly insights. To repay you, we would be happy to review some manuscripts for you; please send us the next manuscript that any of these reviewers submits to your journal.

Assuming you accept this paper, we would also like to add a footnote acknowledging your help with this manuscript and pointing out that we liked the paper much better the way we originally wrote it, but that you held the editorial shotgun to our heads and forced us to chop, reshuffle, restate, hedge, expand, shorten, and in general convert a meaty paper into stir-fried vegetables. We couldn't or wouldn't have done it without your input.

Sincerely,

Trying to Publish but Perishing Anyway

From *Bulletin of the Canadian Society for Psychomotor Learning and Sport Psychology* (June, 1991). Adapted with permission.

Writing a Scientific Paper

Everyone knows that scientists write badly—everybody, that is, except scientists. They think they're merely being precise and orderly, and everyone else on the planet is either (a) illiterate, (b) sloppy, (c) a humanist, or (d) all of the above (Ref. 1). In some cases, of course, the individual scientist is not well acquainted with the English language. (In the opinion of English scientists, this explains the frequently unintelligible papers of Americans.)

The scientist is, by his reliance on the passive voice, hobbled, leading to sentences like this one, in which the subject is acted upon with lumpy nouns, without ever saying exactly whom the action is done by, so that the sentences get longer and longer as you read and never seem to end, even when there is clearly nothing more to say in the sentence, at which point the reader sometimes gets a meager little semicolon; this gives him a rest, so that he can go on and read another long phrase without really learning anything more, because the writer's hand has kept on moving even though his brain has long since been disengaged.

What to do? Trying to straighten a scientist's syntax is like trying to unsnarl week-old spaghetti, with some exceptions (see Ref. 2). It is far better to change the packaging of the sentences. Scientific papers are written like elaborate lab reports—first A, then B, on to C, plodding on to the conclusion. Such papers assume the reader is fascinated by the pearls of wisdom that ooze through the barnacle-laden sentences. The sad truth is that hardly anyone ever reads a paper all the way through. A study by a British physics journal shows that the average number who finish the whole paper is 0.5—and that includes the author. Apparently, most scientists can't bear to reread their own work, much less read anyone else's.

In this paper a new scheme for paper organizing is proposed. It does not rely on weaning scientists away from the passive-voice construction, like that last one. Instead it relies on the way scientists actually read and on their motivation for reading papers.

While reading a scientific paper, scientists are led by two needs: (a) ego and (b) desire for information. Our research shows that ego always dominates. Therefore, papers should be organized to satisfy this. The preferred approach, one that makes the most of these insights, is as follows:

1. *Title*
2. *Author's name*
3. *References*. These must contain a broad spectrum of sources, mostly to ensure the greatest probability of naming the reader. Use as many multiauthor papers as possible to maximize the number of people who can be mentioned. A scientist will *always* pay greater attention to colleagues who cite him, if only to find where in the text he gets mentioned. Thus, the best strategy is to cite everybody you can, but then place the citations in the most unlikely places in the paper. Then the scientists have to read all or most of the paper carefully to find mention of them. They might even discover what the paper is about. A really high-risk alternative is to cite someone in the list of references but not in the text. Then he or she will read the whole paper, twice. The disadvantage, of course, is that the scientist will be livid with rage and frustration.
4. *Acknowledgments*. An important ego feeding ground. Thank the big names in your field, even if your sole contact with them was over coffee at some conference 3 years ago. The list should be lavish, implying close connections with the movers and shakers, but avoid mentioning dead people. They can do you no more good, and their rivals are still around. Finally, if space permits, include those who actually helped you. This part of the acknowledgments is purely optional.
5. *Grant reference*. Your grant-monitoring officer will always look for this. So stick it in early. Also, others will want to know what agency got suckered into paying for this stuff, so they can hit it up for grant money themselves.
6. *Introduction*. Here you explain what you plan to do. Promise a lot. Few will actually read the main text (see #8) to find out whether you actually do it. Fewer still will care.
7. *Conclusions*. Always overstate your results. Claim certainty where you have only the vaguest of suspicions.
8. *Main text*. With any luck, there will be no need to write this section. Everyone will have turned to the next paper to resume the search for his or her own name.

References

1. "Professorial Pathology," by E.U. Reka, A.B. Surd, and I.M. Pedant, *Journal of Academic Backstabbing*, Vol. 3, 1980.
2. *Explaining Asimov* (12 volumes), by the National Academy of Sciences, 1981.

From "How to Write a Scientific Paper," by B.A. Realist [G. Benford], *Omni*, March 1982, p. 130. Reprinted by permission of *Omni*, © 1982, Omni Publications International, Ltd.

dissertation, or are readying a conference paper, you will need to include an abstract. Abstracts for each purpose require slightly different orientations, but nearly all have constraints on length and form.

Thesis or Dissertation Abstracts

The abstract for your thesis or dissertation will probably have several specific constraints, including those of length, form, style, and location. First, consult your university or graduate school regulations, then follow these carefully. With dissertations, this nearly always includes the form for submission to *Dissertation Abstracts International*. The exact headings, length, and margins are provided in a handout available from your graduate school office. In writing the abstract, consider who will read it. It will be located in computer searches by the title and key words. (The importance of these was discussed in chapters 2 and 3.) Write the abstract so that anyone reading it can decide whether to look at the total thesis or dissertation. Clearly identify the theoretical framework, the problem, the subjects, the measurements, and your findings. Do not use all the space writing about your sophisticated statistical analyses or minor methodological problems. Keep jargon to a minimum. People in related areas will be reading this to see if your work is relevant to theirs. One of us ran across the following sentence in a dissertation abstract recently. Due to jargon (and some would argue our poor vocabulary), we could not interpret the sentence:

> Amalgamating the decision maker's inputs is a new and unique decision model that can be classified as a fuzzily parametered, multi-staged, forward and backward chained, Displaced Ideal, two-dimensional attribute model of business-level strategic objectives and the functional-level strategies that realize those objectives.

Abstracts for Published Papers

An abstract for a published paper is much shorter, usually, between 100 and 150 words. The important consideration is to get to the point: What was the problem? Who were the subjects? What did you find? The most useless statement encountered in

these abstracts is "Results were discussed." Would anyone have expected that results would not be discussed?

Conference Abstracts

Abstracts for conferences are slightly different. Usually you are allowed a little more space because the reviewers must be convinced to accept your paper for presentation. In these abstracts, you should follow these procedures:

1. Write a short introduction to set up the problem statement.
2. State the problem.
3. Describe the methodology briefly, including
   a. subjects,
   b. instrumentation,
   c. procedures, and
   d. design and analysis.
4. Summarize the results.
5. Explain why the results are important.

Below is a humorous example of an abstract developed by one of your authors (Thomas, 1989).

Writing a Scientific Paper

Please use the following style for all abstracts.

I.M. Tenured and U.R. Promoted, JR's South Fork School of Hard Knocks, Dallas, TX 00001

How Motor Skill Research Can Get You a Merit Raise

Current research suggests that merit raises are directly related to the number of papers faculty present and publish and inversely related to the quality of the research . . .

. . . The long-term effect is to increase the number of journals, conferences, and full professors.

The results and their importance are a critical part of a conference abstract. If you do this in a nondescript way, the reviewer may conclude that you have not completed the study. This generally leads to rejection. The conference planners cannot turn

Procedures for writing conference abstracts

down other completed research when it is possible that yours will not be finished.

Finally, most conferences require that the paper be presented before publication. So, if you have a paper in review at a journal, submitting it to a conference that is 8-12 months away could be hazardous. Also, many conferences require that the paper not have been previously presented. Be aware of this, and follow regulations. Violating these guidelines will never enhance your professional status, and other scholars will quickly become aware of it.

Making Oral and Poster Presentations

How to Give Oral Presentations
Using a Poster Presentation to Its Best Advantage

Once your conference paper is accepted, you are faced with presenting it. The presentation will be conducted either orally or in a poster session.

How to Give Oral Presentations

Oral presentations usually cause panic among graduate students and new faculty members. First, there is no way to get over this except to give several papers. But you can help assuage the feeling of apprehension. Usually the time allowed for oral research reports is 10-20 minutes, depending on the conference. You will be notified of the time limit when your paper is accepted. Because you must stay within the time limit and there is no way to present a complete report within this limit, what do you do? We suggest that you present the essential features of the report using the following divisions for a 15-minute presentation:

- Introduction that cites a few important studies: 3 minutes
- Statement of the problem: 1 minute (use slides or an overhead)

> ### Thomas and Nelson's Five Laws of Oral Presentations
>
> 1. Something always goes wrong with the slide projector. More specifically,
>   a. unless you check it beforehand, it will not work;
>   b. either the electrical cord or the slide control cord (or both) will be too short;
>   c. any slide not checked immediately before the presentation will be in upside down;
>   d. if the projector has worked perfectly for the three previous presenters, the bulb will burn out during your presentation;
>   e. every slide will require that the projector be refocused;
>   f. a person getting up to leave after the previous paper will knock over the slide projector.
> 2. You will only drop your slide tray when you have the top off.
> 3. The screen will be too small for the room.
> 4. Your paper will be the last one scheduled during the conference. This will result in only the moderator, you, and the previous presenter being there, the latter of whom will leave on completing his or her paper. Or conversely, your paper will be scheduled at 7:30 a.m., at which time you will be hung over and everyone else will still be in bed.
> 5. At your first presentation, the most prestigious scholar in your field will show up, be misquoted by you, and ask you a question.

- Method: 3 minutes (slides or an overhead are helpful)
- Results: 3 minutes (slides or overheads of tables and figures; figures are usually better because tables are hard to read)
- Discussion: 2 minutes (slides or overheads of main points)
- Questions and discussions: 3 minutes

Total: 15 minutes

The most frequent errors in oral presentations are spending too much time on method and presenting results poorly. Proper use of slides (or overheads) is the key to an effective presentation, particularly in the results. Place a brief statement of the problem on a slide, and show it while you talk.

---

 oral presentation — Method of presenting a paper in which the author speaks before a group of colleagues at a conference following this format: introduction, statement of the problem, method, results, discussion, questions.

 How to use your time in an oral presentation

A slide of the experimental arrangements reduces much of the verbiage in method. Always use slides to illustrate the results. A picture of the results (particularly figures and graphs) is much more effective than either tables or a verbal presentation. Keep the figures and graphs simple and concise. Tables and figures prepared for a written paper are seldom effective when converted for visual presentations. They typically contain too much information and are not large enough. Have a pointer available to indicate significant features. Finally, remember Thomas and Nelson's Five Laws of Oral Presentations (page 422). The way to avoid most of the problems associated with these laws is self-evident. One that may not be so obvious is practicing your presentation. We gather graduate students and faculty who are presenting papers at upcoming conferences and conduct practice sessions. Everyone presents her or his paper and has it timed. Then the audience asks questions and offers suggestions to clarify presentations and visual aids. Practice sessions improve the quality of the graduate students' presentations and strengthen their confidence.

Using a Poster Presentation to Its Best Advantage

The poster session is another way to present a conference paper. This involves the use of a large room in which presenters place summaries of their research on the wall or poster stands. The session is scheduled for a specific period, during which presenters stand by their work while anyone interested walks around, reads the material, and discusses items of interest with the presenters.

We prefer this format to oral presentations. The audience can look at the papers in which they are interested and have more detailed discussions with the authors. Within 75 minutes in a large room, 15-40 poster presentations can be made available. In contrast, 15-minute oral presentations allow only five presentations in 75 minutes. In addition, the audience must sit through several papers, often losing interest or creating a disturbance by arriving or leaving.

The presenter at a poster session should follow these guidelines:

- Know how much space is available for your materials (exact dimensions).
- Provide the necessary equipment for attaching your materials to the wall or poster board (even when the conference has indicated that supplies will be available).
- Mount your posters on contrasting backgrounds so they will be easily visible and will not blend into the backboards.
- Use figures and graphs where possible (as opposed to text and tables).
- Use large lettering for all text, numbers, and labels.

Clearly label the six parts of the poster presentation: introduction, statement of the problem, method, results (with figures and graphs), discussion and conclusions, and important references.

Summary

The journal format for theses and dissertations has the advantage of being in the form for journal publication, one of the main ways used to evaluate scholarly work. Yet it retains the essential characteristics of the complete reporting that is so valued in the thesis and dissertation. This format comprises preliminary materials (e.g., title page, abstract), the body (e.g., introduction, method, results, discussion), and a set of appendices (e.g., extended literature review, additional results). The goal of this reporting style is to promote rapid publication of quality research.

Abstracts are frequently used as a form for submitting papers to scholarly meetings so they can be evaluated for possible presentation. Usually the abstract is limited in length and form according to the format prescribed by the scholarly group to whom it is submitted. If the abstract paper is accepted for presentation, the form may be oral or poster. Oral presentations usually last 10 to 20 minutes, and poster presentations are typically limited to a specific display space.

 Check Your Understanding

1. Writing: Select a study from a journal and write a 150-word abstract in APA style (or whatever style your department uses).

 Guidelines for poster presentations

2. Oral presentations: To emphasize the importance of time limits on oral presentations, we suggest that the professor organize the following presentations in class:
   a. Have each student select a published research study and present a 2-minute summary.
   b. Do the same with another study, but give a 5-minute summary.

3. Poster presentation: Have each student prepare a poster presentation of a research study from a journal. Put the posters around the classroom walls. Have students critique each poster (or some percentage of posters for larger classes).

Statistical Tables

Table A.1   Table of Random Numbers

22 17 68 65 84	68 95 23 92 35	87 02 22 57 51	61 09 43 95 06	58 24 82 03 47
19 36 27 59 46	13 79 93 37 55	39 77 32 77 09	85 52 05 30 62	47 83 51 62 74
16 77 23 02 77	09 61 87 25 21	28 06 24 25 93	16 71 13 59 78	23 05 47 47 25
78 43 76 71 61	20 44 90 32 64	97 67 63 99 61	46 38 03 93 22	69 81 21 99 21
03 28 28 26 08	73 37 32 04 05	69 30 16 09 05	88 69 58 29 99	35 07 44 75 47
93 22 53 64 39	07 10 63 76 35	87 03 04 79 88	08 13 13 85 51	55 34 57 72 69
78 76 58 54 74	92 38 70 96 92	52 06 79 79 45	82 63 18 27 44	69 66 92 19 09
23 68 35 26 00	99 53 93 61 28	52 70 05 48 34	56 65 05 61 86	90 92 10 70 80
15 39 25 70 99	93 86 52 77 65	15 33 59 05 28	22 87 26 07 47	86 96 98 29 06
58 71 96 30 24	18 46 23 34 27	85 13 99 24 44	49 18 09 79 49	74 16 32 23 02
57 35 27 33 72	24 53 63 94 09	41 10 76 47 91	44 04 95 49 66	39 60 04 59 81
48 50 86 54 48	22 06 34 72 52	82 21 15 65 20	33 29 94 71 11	15 91 29 12 03
61 96 48 95 03	07 16 39 33 66	98 56 10 56 79	77 21 30 27 12	90 49 22 23 62
36 93 89 41 26	29 70 83 63 51	99 74 20 52 36	87 09 41 15 09	98 60 16 03 03
18 87 00 42 31	57 90 12 02 07	23 47 37 17 31	54 08 01 88 63	39 41 88 92 10
88 56 53 27 59	33 35 72 67 47	77 34 55 45 70	08 18 27 38 90	16 95 86 70 75
09 72 95 84 29	49 41 31 06 70	42 38 06 45 18	64 84 73 31 65	52 53 37 97 15
12 96 88 17 31	65 19 69 02 83	60 75 86 90 68	24 64 19 35 51	56 61 87 39 12
85 94 57 24 16	92 09 84 38 76	22 00 27 69 85	29 81 94 78 70	21 94 47 90 12
38 64 43 59 98	98 77 87 68 07	91 51 67 62 44	40 98 05 93 78	23 32 65 41 18
53 44 09 42 72	00 41 86 79 79	68 47 22 00 20	35 55 31 51 51	00 83 63 22 55
40 76 66 26 84	57 99 99 90 37	36 63 32 08 58	37 40 13 68 97	87 64 81 07 83
02 17 79 18 05	12 59 52 57 02	22 07 90 47 03	28 14 11 30 79	20 69 22 40 98
95 17 82 06 53	31 51 10 96 46	92 06 88 07 77	56 11 50 81 69	40 23 72 51 39
35 76 22 42 92	96 11 83 44 80	34 68 35 48 77	33 42 40 90 60	73 96 53 97 86
26 29 13 56 41	85 47 04 66 08	34 72 57 59 13	82 43 80 46 15	38 26 61 70 04
77 80 20 75 82	72 82 32 99 90	63 95 73 76 63	89 73 44 99 05	48 67 26 43 18
46 40 66 44 52	91 36 74 43 53	30 82 13 54 00	78 45 63 98 35	55 03 36 67 68
37 56 08 18 09	77 53 84 46 47	31 91 18 95 58	24 16 74 11 53	44 10 13 85 57
61 65 61 68 66	37 27 47 39 19	84 83 70 07 48	53 21 40 06 71	95 06 79 88 54
93 43 69 64 07	34 18 04 52 35	56 27 09 24 86	61 85 53 83 45	19 90 70 99 00
21 96 60 12 99	11 20 99 45 18	48 13 93 55 34	18 37 79 49 90	65 97 38 20 46
95 20 47 97 97	27 37 83 28 71	00 06 41 41 74	45 89 09 39 84	51 67 11 52 49
97 86 21 78 73	10 65 81 92 59	58 76 17 14 97	04 76 62 16 17	17 95 70 45 80
69 92 06 34 13	59 71 74 17 32	27 55 10 24 19	23 71 82 13 74	63 52 52 01 41
04 31 17 21 56	33 73 99 19 87	26 72 39 27 67	53 77 57 68 93	60 61 97 22 61
61 06 98 03 91	87 14 77 43 96	43 00 65 98 50	45 60 33 01 07	98 99 46 50 47
85 93 85 86 88	72 87 08 62 40	16 06 10 89 20	23 21 34 74 97	76 38 03 29 63
21 74 32 47 45	73 96 07 94 52	09 65 90 77 47	25 76 16 19 33	53 05 70 53 30
15 69 53 82 80	79 96 23 53 10	65 39 07 16 29	45 33 02 43 70	02 87 40 41 45
02 89 08 04 49	20 21 14 68 86	87 63 93 95 17	11 29 01 95 80	35 14 97 35 33
87 18 15 89 79	85 43 01 72 73	08 61 74 51 69	89 74 39 82 15	94 51 33 41 67
98 83 71 94 22	59 97 50 99 52	08 52 85 08 40	87 80 61 65 31	91 51 80 32 44
10 08 58 21 66	72 68 49 29 31	89 85 84 46 06	59 73 19 85 23	65 09 29 75 63
47 90 56 10 08	88 02 84 27 83	42 29 72 23 19	66 56 45 65 79	20 71 53 20 25
22 85 61 68 90	49 64 92 85 44	16 40 12 89 88	50 14 49 81 06	01 82 77 45 12
67 80 43 79 33	12 83 11 41 16	25 58 19 68 70	77 02 54 00 52	53 43 37 15 26
27 62 50 96 72	79 44 61 40 15	14 53 40 65 39	27 31 58 50 28	11 39 03 34 25
33 78 80 87 15	38 30 06 38 21	14 47 47 07 26	54 96 87 53 32	40 36 40 96 76
13 13 92 66 99	47 24 49 57 74	32 25 43 62 17	10 97 11 69 84	99 63 22 32 98

10 27 53 96 23	71 50 54 36 23	54 31 04 82 98	04 14 12 15 09	26 78 25 47 47
28 41 50 61 88	64 85 27 20 18	83 36 36 05 56	39 71 65 09 62	94 76 62 11 89
34 21 42 57 02	59 19 18 97 48	80 30 03 30 98	05 24 67 70 07	84 97 50 87 46
61 81 77 23 23	82 82 11 54 08	53 28 70 58 96	44 07 39 55 43	42 34 43 39 28
61 15 18 13 54	16 86 20 26 88	90 74 80 55 09	14 53 90 51 17	52 01 63 01 59
91 76 21 64 64	44 91 13 32 97	75 31 62 66 54	84 80 32 75 77	56 08 25 70 29
00 97 79 08 06	37 30 28 59 85	53 56 68 53 40	01 74 39 59 73	30 19 99 85 48
36 46 18 34 94	75 20 80 27 77	78 91 69 16 00	08 43 18 73 68	67 69 61 34 25
88 98 99 60 50	65 95 79 42 94	93 62 40 89 96	43 56 47 71 66	46 76 29 67 02
04 37 59 87 21	05 02 03 24 17	47 97 81 56 51	92 34 86 01 82	55 51 33 12 91
63 62 06 34 41	94 21 78 55 09	72 76 45 16 94	29 95 81 83 83	79 88 01 97 30
78 47 23 53 90	34 41 92 45 71	09 23 70 70 07	12 38 92 79 43	14 85 11 47 23
87 68 62 15 43	53 14 36 59 25	54 47 33 70 15	59 24 48 40 35	50 03 42 99 36
47 60 92 10 77	88 59 53 11 52	66 25 69 07 04	48 68 64 71 06	61 65 70 22 12
56 88 87 59 41	65 28 04 67 53	95 79 88 37 31	50 41 06 94 76	81 83 17 16 33
02 57 45 86 67	73 43 07 34 48	44 26 87 93 29	77 09 61 67 84	06 69 44 77 75
31 54 14 13 17	48 62 11 90 60	68 12 93 64 28	46 24 79 16 76	14 60 25 51 01
28 50 16 43 36	28 97 85 58 99	67 22 52 76 23	24 70 36 54 54	59 28 61 71 96
63 29 62 66 50	02 63 45 52 38	67 63 47 54 75	83 24 78 43 20	92 63 13 47 48
45 65 58 26 51	76 96 59 38 72	86 57 45 71 46	44 67 76 14 55	44 88 01 62 12
39 65 36 63 70	77 45 85 50 51	74 13 39 35 22	30 53 36 02 95	49 34 88 73 61
73 71 98 16 04	29 18 94 51 23	76 51 94 84 86	79 93 96 38 63	08 58 25 58 94
72 20 56 20 11	72 65 71 08 86	79 57 95 13 91	97 48 72 66 48	09 71 17 24 89
75 17 26 99 76	89 37 20 70 01	77 31 61 95 46	26 97 05 73 51	53 33 18 72 87
37 48 60 82 29	81 30 15 39 14	48 38 75 93 29	06 87 37 78 48	45 56 00 84 47
68 08 02 80 72	83 71 46 30 49	89 17 95 88 29	02 39 56 03 46	97 74 06 56 17
14 23 98 61 67	70 52 85 01 50	01 84 02 78 43	10 62 98 19 41	18 83 99 47 99
49 08 96 21 44	25 27 99 41 28	07 41 08 34 66	19 42 74 39 91	41 96 53 78 72
78 37 06 08 43	63 61 62 42 29	39 68 95 10 96	09 24 23 00 62	56 12 80 73 16
37 21 34 17 68	68 96 83 23 56	32 84 60 15 31	44 73 67 34 77	91 15 79 74 58
14 29 09 34 04	87 83 07 55 07	76 58 30 83 64	87 29 25 58 84	86 50 60 00 25
58 43 28 06 36	49 52 83 51 14	47 56 91 29 34	05 87 31 06 95	12 45 57 09 09
10 43 67 29 70	80 62 80 03 42	10 80 21 38 84	90 56 35 03 09	43 12 74 49 14
44 38 88 39 54	86 97 37 44 22	00 95 01 31 76	17 16 29 56 63	38 78 94 49 81
90 69 59 19 51	85 39 52 85 13	07 28 37 07 61	11 16 36 27 03	78 86 72 04 95
41 47 10 25 62	97 05 31 03 61	20 26 36 31 62	68 69 86 95 44	84 95 48 46 45
91 94 14 63 19	75 89 11 47 11	31 56 34 19 09	79 57 92 36 59	14 93 87 81 40
80 06 54 18 66	09 18 94 06 19	98 40 07 17 81	22 45 44 84 11	24 62 20 42 31
67 72 77 63 48	84 08 31 55 58	24 33 45 77 58	80 45 67 93 82	75 70 16 08 24
59 40 24 13 27	79 26 88 86 30	01 31 60 10 39	53 58 47 70 93	85 81 56 39 38
05 90 35 89 95	01 61 16 96 94	50 78 13 69 36	37 68 53 37 31	71 26 35 03 71
44 43 80 69 98	46 68 05 14 82	90 78 50 05 62	77 79 13 57 44	59 60 10 39 66
61 81 31 96 82	00 57 25 60 59	46 72 60 18 77	55 66 12 62 11	08 99 55 64 57
42 88 07 10 05	24 98 65 63 21	47 21 61 88 32	27 80 30 21 60	10 92 35 36 12
77 94 30 05 39	28 10 99 00 27	12 73 73 99 12	49 99 57 94 82	96 88 57 17 91
78 83 19 76 16	94 11 68 84 26	23 54 20 86 85	23 86 66 99 07	36 37 34 92 09
87 76 59 61 81	43 63 64 61 61	65 76 36 95 90	18 48 27 45 68	27 23 65 30 72
91 43 05 96 47	55 78 99 95 24	37 55 85 78 78	01 48 41 19 10	35 19 54 07 73
84 97 77 72 73	09 62 06 65 72	87 12 49 03 60	41 15 20 76 27	50 47 02 29 16
87 41 60 76 83	44 88 96 07 80	85 05 83 38 96	73 70 66 81 90	30 56 10 48 59

Table A.1 is taken from Table XXXIII of Fisher, *Statistical Methods for Research Workers*, published by Oliver and Boyd, Ltd., Edinburgh.

Table A.2   The Standard Normal Curve

z	One tail π beyond	One tail π remainder	Two tail π beyond	Two tail π remainder	z	One tail π beyond	One tail π remainder	Two tail π beyond	Two tail π remainder
0.00	0.5000	0.5000	1.0000	0.0000	0.45	0.3264	0.6736	0.6527	0.3473
0.01	0.4960	0.5040	0.9920	0.0080	0.46	0.3228	0.6772	0.6455	0.3545
0.02	0.4920	0.5080	0.9840	0.0160	0.47	0.3192	0.6808	0.6384	0.3616
0.03	0.4880	0.5120	0.9761	0.0239	0.48	0.3156	0.6844	0.6312	0.3688
0.04	0.4840	0.5160	0.9681	0.0319	0.49	0.3121	0.6879	0.6241	0.3759
0.05	0.4801	0.7199	0.9601	0.0399	0.50	0.3085	0.6915	0.6171	0.3829
0.06	0.4761	0.5239	0.9522	0.0478	0.51	0.3050	0.6950	0.6101	0.3899
0.07	0.4721	0.5279	0.9442	0.0558	0.52	0.3015	0.8985	0.6031	0.3969
0.08	0.4681	0.5319	0.9362	0.0638	0.53	0.2981	0.7019	0.5961	0.4039
0.09	0.4641	0.5359	0.9283	0.0717	0.54	0.2946	0.7054	0.5892	0.4108
0.10	0.4602	0.5398	0.9203	0.0797	0.55	0.2912	0.7088	0.5823	0.4177
0.11	0.4562	0.5438	0.9124	0.0876	0.56	0.2877	0.7123	0.5755	0.4245
0.12	0.4522	0.4378	0.9045	0.0955	0.57	0.2843	0.7157	0.5687	0.4313
0.13	0.4483	0.5517	0.8966	0.1034	0.58	0.2810	0.7190	0.5619	0.4381
0.14	0.4443	0.5557	0.8887	0.1113	0.59	0.2776	0.7224	0.5552	0.4448
0.15	0.4404	0.5596	0.8808	0.1192	0.60	0.2743	0.7257	0.5485	0.4515
0.16	0.4364	0.5636	0.8729	0.1271	0.61	0.2709	0.7291	0.5419	0.4581
0.17	0.4325	0.5675	0.8650	0.1350	0.62	0.2676	0.7324	0.5353	0.4647
0.18	0.4286	0.5714	0.8493	0.1507	0.63	0.2643	0.7357	0.5276	0.4713
0.19	0.4247	0.5753	0.8493	0.1507	0.64	0.2611	0.7389	0.5222	0.4778
0.20	0.4207	0.5793	0.8415	0.1585	0.65	0.2578	0.7422	0.5157	0.4843
0.21	0.4168	0.5832	0.8337	0.1663	0.66	0.2546	0.7454	0.5093	0.4907
0.22	0.4129	0.5871	0.8259	0.1741	0.67	0.2514	0.7486	0.5029	0.4971
0.23	0.4090	0.5910	0.8181	0.1819	0.6745	0.25	0.75	0.50	0.50
0.24	0.4052	0.5948	0.8103	0.1897	0.68	0.2483	0.7517	0.4965	0.5035
0.25	0.4013	0.5987	0.8026	0.1974	0.69	0.2451	0.7549	0.4902	0.5098
0.26	0.3974	0.6026	0.7949	0.2051	0.70	0.2420	0.7580	0.4839	0.5161
0.27	0.3936	0.6064	0.7872	0.2128	0.71	0.2389	0.7611	0.4777	0.5223
0.28	0.2897	0.6103	0.7795	0.2205	0.72	0.2358	0.7642	0.4715	0.5285
0.29	0.3859	0.6141	0.7718	0.2282	0.73	0.2327	0.7673	0.4654	0.5346
0.30	0.3821	0.6179	0.7642	0.2358	0.74	0.2296	0.7704	0.4593	0.5407
0.31	0.3783	0.6217	0.7566	0.2434	0.75	0.2266	0.7734	0.4533	0.5467
0.32	0.3745	0.6255	0.7490	0.2510	0.76	0.2236	0.7764	0.4473	0.5527
0.33	0.3707	0.6293	0.7414	0.2586	0.77	0.2206	0.7794	0.4413	0.5587
0.34	0.3669	0.6331	0.7339	0.2661	0.78	0.2177	0.7823	0.4354	0.5646
0.35	0.3632	0.6368	0.7263	0.2737	0.79	0.2148	0.7852	0.4295	0.5705
0.36	0.3594	0.6406	0.7188	0.2812	0.80	0.2119	0.7881	0.4237	0.5763
0.37	0.3557	0.6443	0.7114	0.2886	0.81	0.2090	0.7910	0.4179	0.5821
0.38	0.3520	0.6480	0.7039	0.2961	0.82	0.2061	0.7939	0.4122	0.5878
0.39	0.3483	0.6517	0.6965	0.3035	0.83	0.2033	0.7967	0.4065	0.5935
0.40	0.3446	0.6554	0.6892	0.3108	0.84	0.2005	0.7995	0.4009	0.5991
0.41	0.3409	0.6591	0.6818	0.3182	0.8416	0.20	0.80	0.40	0.60
0.42	0.3372	0.6628	0.6745	0.3255	0.85	0.1997	0.8023	0.3953	0.6047
0.43	0.3336	0.6664	0.6672	0.3328	0.86	0.1949	0.8051	0.3898	0.6102
0.44	0.3300	0.6700	0.6599	0.3401	0.87	0.1922	0.8078	0.3843	0.6157

	One tail		Two tail			One tail		Two tail	
z	π beyond	π remainder	π beyond	π remainder	z	π beyond	π remainder	π beyond	π remainder
0.88	0.1894	0.8106	0.3789	0.6211	1.32	0.0934	0.9066	0.1868	0.8132
0.89	0.1867	0.8133	0.3735	0.6265	1.33	0.0918	0.9082	0.1835	0.8165
0.90	0.1841	0.8159	0.3681	0.6319	1.34	0.0901	0.9099	0.1802	0.8198
0.91	0.1814	0.8186	0.3628	0.6372	1.35	0.0885	0.9115	0.1770	0.8230
0.92	0.1788	0.8212	0.3576	0.6424	1.36	0.0869	0.9131	0.1738	0.8202
0.93	0.1762	0.8238	0.3524	0.6476	1.37	0.0853	0.9147	0.1707	0.8293
0.94	0.1736	0.8264	0.3472	0.6528	1.38	0.0838	0.9162	0.1676	0.8324
0.95	0.1711	0.8289	0.3421	0.6579	1.39	0.0823	0.9177	0.1645	0.8355
0.96	0.1685	0.8315	0.3371	0.6629	1.40	0.0808	0.9192	0.1615	0.8385
0.97	0.1660	0.8340	0.3320	0.6680	1.41	0.0793	0.9207	0.1585	0.8415
0.98	0.1635	0.8365	0.3271	0.6729	1.42	0.0778	0.9222	0.1556	0.8444
0.99	0.1611	0.8389	0.3222	0.6778	1.43	0.0764	0.9286	0.1527	0.8473
1.00	0.1587	0.8413	0.3173	0.6827	1.44	0.0749	0.9251	0.1499	0.8501
1.01	0.1562	0.8438	0.3125	0.6875	1.45	0.0735	0.9265	0.1471	0.8529
1.02	0.1539	0.8461	0.3077	0.6923	1.46	0.0721	0.9279	0.1443	0.8567
1.03	0.1515	0.8485	0.3030	0.6970	1.47	0.0708	0.9292	0.1416	0.8584
1.04	0.1492	0.8508	0.2983	0.7017	1.48	0.0694	0.9306	0.1389	0.8611
1.05	0.1469	0.8531	0.2937	0.7063	1.49	0.0681	0.9319	0.1362	0.8638
1.06	0.1446	0.8554	0.2891	0.7109	1.50	0.0668	0.9332	0.1336	0.8664
1.07	0.1423	0.8577	0.2846	0.7154	1.51	0.0655	0.9345	0.1310	0.8690
1.08	0.1401	0.8599	0.2801	0.7199	1.52	0.0643	0.9357	0.1285	0.8715
1.09	0.1379	0.6621	0.2757	0.7243	1.53	0.0630	0.9370	0.1260	0.8740
1.10	0.1357	0.8643	0.2713	0.7287	1.54	0.0618	0.9382	0.1236	0.8764
1.11	0.1335	0.8665	0.2670	0.7330	1.55	0.0606	0.9394	0.1211	0.8789
1.12	0.1314	0.8686	0.2627	0.7373	1.56	0.0594	0.9406	0.1188	0.8812
1.13	0.1292	0.8708	0.2585	0.7415	1.57	0.0582	0.9418	0.1164	0.8836
1.14	0.1271	0.8729	0.2543	0.7457	1.58	0.0571	0.9429	0.1141	0.8859
1.15	0.1251	0.8749	0.2501	0.7499	1.59	0.0559	0.9441	0.1118	0.8882
1.16	0.1230	0.8770	0.2460	0.7540	1.60	0.0548	0.9452	0.1096	0.8904
1.17	0.1210	0.8790	0.2420	0.7580	1.61	0.0537	0.9463	0.1074	0.8926
1.18	0.1190	0.8810	0.2380	0.7620	1.62	0.0526	0.9474	0.1052	0.8948
1.19	0.1170	0.8830	0.2340	0.7660	1.63	0.0516	0.9484	0.1031	0.8969
1.20	0.1151	0.8049	0.2301	0.7699	1.64	0.0505	0.9495	0.1010	0.8990
1.21	0.1131	0.8869	0.2263	0.7737	1.645	0.05	0.95	0.10	0.90
1.22	0.1112	0.8888	0.2225	0.7775	1.65	0.0495	0.9505	0.0989	0.9011
1.23	0.1093	0.8907	0.2187	0.7813	1.66	0.0485	0.9515	0.0969	0.9031
1.24	0.1075	0.8925	0.2150	0.7890	1.67	0.0475	0.9525	0.0949	0.9051
1.25	0.1056	0.8944	0.2113	0.7887	1.68	0.0465	0.9535	0.0930	0.9070
1.26	0.1038	0.8962	0.2077	0.7923	1.69	0.0455	0.9545	0.0910	0.9090
1.27	0.1020	0.8980	0.2041	0.7959	1.70	0.0446	0.9554	0.0891	0.9109
1.28	0.1003	0.8997	0.2005	0.7995	1.71	0.0436	0.9564	0.0873	0.9127
1.282	0.10	0.90	0.20	0.80	1.72	0.0427	0.9573	0.0854	0.9146
1.29	0.0985	0.9015	0.1971	0.8029	1.73	0.0418	0.9582	0.0836	0.9164
1.30	0.0968	0.9032	0.1936	0.8064	1.74	0.0409	0.9591	0.0819	0.9181
1.31	0.0951	0.9049	0.1902	0.8098	1.75	0.0401	0.9599	0.0801	0.9199

(continued)

Table A.2   (continued)

	One tail		Two tail			One tail		Two tail	
z	π beyond	π remainder	π beyond	π remainder	z	π beyond	π remainder	π beyond	π remainder
1.76	0.0392	0.9608	0.0784	0.9216	2.20	0.0139	0.9661	0.0278	0.9722
1.77	0.0384	0.9616	0.0767	0.9233	2.21	0.0136	0.9864	0.0271	0.9729
1.78	0.0375	0.9625	0.0751	0.9249	2.22	0.0132	0.9868	0.0264	0.9736
1.79	0.0367	0.9633	0.0734	0.9266	2.23	0.0129	0.9871	0.0257	0.9743
1.80	0.0359	0.9641	0.0719	0.9281	2.24	0.0125	0.9875	0.0251	0.9749
1.81	0.0352	0.9649	0.0703	0.9297	2.25	0.0122	0.9878	0.0244	0.9756
1.82	0.0344	0.9656	0.0688	0.9312	2.26	0.0119	0.9881	0.0238	0.9762
1.83	0.0336	0.9664	0.0672	0.9328	2.27	0.0116	0.9884	0.0232	0.9768
1.84	0.0329	0.9671	0.0658	0.9342	2.28	0.0113	0.9887	0.0226	0.9774
1.85	0.0322	0.9678	0.0643	0.9357	2.29	0.0110	0.9890	0.0220	0.9780
1.86	0.0314	0.9686	0.0629	0.9371	2.30	0.0107	0.9893	0.0214	0.9786
1.87	0.0307	0.9693	0.0615	0.9385	2.31	0.0104	0.9896	0.0209	0.9791
1.88	0.0301	0.9699	0.0601	0.9399	2.32	0.0102	0.9898	0.0203	0.9797
1.89	0.0294	0.9706	0.0588	0.9412	2.326	0.01	0.99	0.02	0.98
1.90	0.0287	0.9713	0.0574	0.9426	2.33	0.0099	0.9901	0.0198	0.9802
1.91	0.0281	0.9719	0.0561	0.9439	2.34	0.0096	0.9904	0.0193	0.9807
1.92	0.0274	0.9726	0.0549	0.9451	2.35	0.0094	0.9906	0.0188	0.9812
1.93	0.0268	0.9732	0.0536	0.9464	2.36	0.0091	0.9909	0.0183	0.9817
1.94	0.0262	0.9738	0.0524	0.9476	2.37	0.0089	0.991	0.0178	0.9822
1.95	0.0256	0.9744	0.0512	0.9488	2.38	0.0087	0.9913	0.0173	0.9827
1.960	0.025	0.975	0.05	0.95	2.39	0.0084	0.9916	0.0168	0.9832
1.97	0.0244	0.9756	0.0488	0.9512	2.40	0.0082	0.9918	0.0164	0.9836
1.98	0.0239	0.9761	0.0477	0.9523	2.41	0.0080	0.9920	0.0160	0.9840
1.99	0.0233	0.9767	0.0466	0.9534	2.42	0.0078	0.9922	0.0155	0.9845
2.00	0.0228	0.9772	0.0455	0.9545	2.43	0.0075	0.9925	0.0151	0.9849
2.01	0.0222	0.9778	0.0444	0.9556	2.44	0.0073	0.9927	0.0147	0.9853
2.02	0.0217	0.9783	0.0434	0.9566	2.45	0.0071	0.9929	0.0143	0.9857
2.03	0.0212	0.9788	0.0424	0.9576	2.46	0.0069	0.9931	0.0139	0.9861
2.04	0.0207	0.9793	0.0414	0.9586	2.47	0.0068	0.9932	0.0135	0.9865
2.05	0.0202	0.9798	0.0404	0.9596	2.48	0.0066	0.9934	0.0131	0.9869
2.054	0.02	0.98	0.04	0.96	2.49	0.0064	0.9936	0.0128	0.9872
2.06	0.0197	0.9803	0.0394	0.9606	2.50	0.0062	0.9938	0.0124	0.9876
2.07	0.0192	0.9808	0.0385	0.9615	2.51	0.0060	0.9940	0.0121	0.9879
2.08	0.0188	0.9812	0.0375	0.9625	2.52	0.0059	0.9941	0.0117	0.9883
2.09	0.0183	0.9817	0.0366	0.9634	2.53	0.0057	0.9943	0.0114	0.9886
2.10	0.0179	0.9821	0.0357	0.9643	2.54	0.0055	0.9945	0.0111	0.9889
2.11	0.0174	0.9826	0.0349	0.9651	2.55	0.0054	0.9946	0.0108	0.9892
2.12	0.0170	0.9830	0.0340	0.9660	2.56	0.0052	0.9948	0.0105	0.9895
2.13	0.0166	0.9834	0.0332	0.9668	2.57	0.0051	0.9949	0.0102	0.9898
2.14	0.0162	0.9838	0.0324	0.9676	2.576	0.005	0.995	0.01	0.99
2.15	0.0158	0.9842	0.0316	0.9684	2.58	0.0049	0.9951	0.0099	0.9901
2.16	0.0154	0.9846	0.0308	0.9692	2.59	0.0048	0.9952	0.0096	0.9904
2.17	0.0150	0.9850	0.0300	0.9700	2.60	0.0047	0.9953	0.0093	0.9907
2.18	0.0146	0.9854	0.0293	0.9707	2.61	0.0045	0.9955	0.0091	0.9909
2.19	0.0143	0.9857	0.0285	0.9715	2.62	0.0044	0.9956	0.0088	0.9912

Table A.2   *(continued)*

	One tail		Two tail			One tail		Two tail	
z	π beyond	π remainder	π beyond	π remainder	z	π beyond	π remainder	π beyond	π remainder
2.63	0.0043	0.9957	0.0085	0.9915	3.25	0.0006	0.9994	0.0012	0.9986
2.64	0.0041	0.9959	0.0083	0.9917	3.291	0.0005	0.9995	0.001	0.999
2.65	0.0040	0.9960	0.0080	0.9920	3.30	0.0005	0.9995	0.0010	0.9990
2.70	0.0035	0.9965	0.0069	0.9931	3.35	0.0004	0.9996	0.0008	0.9992
2.75	0.0030	0.9970	0.0060	0.9940	3.40	0.0003	0.9997	0.0007	0.9993
2.80	0.0026	0.9974	0.0051	0.9949	3.45	0.0003	0.9997	0.0006	0.9994
2.85	0.0022	0.9978	0.0044	0.9956	3.50	0.0002	0.9998	0.0005	0.9995
2.90	0.0019	0.9981	0.0037	0.9963	3.55	0.0002	0.9998	0.0004	0.9996
2.95	0.0016	0.9984	0.0032	0.9968	3.60	0.0002	0.9998	0.0003	0.9997
3.00	0.0013	0.9987	0.0027	0.9973	3.65	0.0001	0.9999	0.0003	0.9997
3.05	0.0011	0.9989	0.0023	0.9977	3.719	0.0001	0.9999	0.0002	0.9998
3.090	0.001	0.999	0.002	0.998	3.80	0.0001	0.9999	0.0001	0.9999
3.10	0.0010	0.9990	0.0019	0.9981	3.891	0.00005	0.99995	0.0001	0.9999
3.15	0.0008	0.9992	0.0016	0.9984	4.000	0.00003	0.99997	0.00006	0.99994
3.20	0.0007	0.9993	0.0014	0.9988	4.265	0.00001	0.99999	0.00002	0.99998

From *Biometrika Tables for Statisticians*, Vol. 1, 3rd ed., by E.S. Pearson and H.O. Hartley, 1966, London: Cambridge University Press. Adapted with permission of the Biometrika Trustees.

Table A.3   Critical Values of Correlation Coefficients

	Level of significance for one-tailed test						Level of significance for one-tailed test				
	.05	.025	.01	.005	.0005		.05	.025	.01	.005	.0005
	Level of significance for two-tailed test						Level of significance for two-tailed test				
$df - N - 2$	.10	.05	.02	.01	.001	$df - N - 2$	.10	.05	.02	.01	.001
1	.9877	.9969	.9995	.9999	1.000	16	.4000	.4683	.5425	.5897	.7084
2	.9000	.9500	.9800	.9900	.9990	17	.3887	.4555	.5285	.5751	.6932
3	.8054	.8783	.9343	.9587	.9912	18	.3783	.4438	.5155	.5614	.6787
4	.7293	.8114	.8822	.9172	.9741	19	.3687	.4329	.5034	.5487	.6652
5	.6694	.7545	.8329	.8745	.9507	20	.3598	.4227	.4921	.5368	.6524
6	.6215	.7067	.7887	.8343	.9249	25	.3233	.3809	.4451	.4869	.5974
7	.5822	.6664	.7498	.7977	.8982	30	.2960	.3494	.4093	.4487	.5541
8	.5494	.6319	.7155	.7646	.8721	35	.2746	.3246	.3810	.4182	.5189
9	.5214	.6021	.6851	.7348	.8471	40	.2573	.3044	.3578	.3932	.4896
10	.4973	.5760	.6581	.7079	.8233	45	.2428	.2875	.3384	.3721	.4648
11	.4762	.5529	.6339	.6835	.8010	50	.2306	.2732	.3218	.3541	.4433
12	.4575	.5324	.6120	.6614	.7800	60	.2108	.2500	.2948	.3248	.4078
13	.4409	.5139	.5923	.6411	.7603	70	.1954	.2319	.2737	.3017	.3799
14	.4259	.4973	.5742	.6226	.7420	80	.1829	.2172	.2565	.2830	.3568
15	.4124	.4821	.5577	.6055	.7246	90	.1726	.2050	.2422	.2673	.3375
						100	.1638	.1946	.2301	.2540	.3211

Table A.3 is taken from Table VII of Fisher & Yates, *Statistical Tables for Biological, Agricultural and Medical Research* published by Longman Group Ltd., 1974.

Table A.4   Transformation of r to Z_r

r	Z_r	r	Z_r	r	Z_r	r	Z_r	r	Z_r
.000	.000	.200	.203	.400	.424	.600	.693	.800	1.099
.005	.005	.205	.208	.405	.430	.605	.701	.805	1.113
.010	.010	.210	.213	.410	.436	.610	.709	.810	1.127
.015	.015	.215	.218	.415	.442	.615	.717	.815	1.142
.020	.020	.220	.224	.420	.448	.620	.725	.820	1.157
.025	.025	.225	.229	.425	.454	.625	.733	.825	1.172
.030	.030	.230	.234	.430	.460	.630	.741	.830	1.188
.035	.035	.235	.239	.435	.466	.635	.750	.835	1.204
.040	.040	.240	.245	.440	.472	.640	.758	.840	1.221
.045	.045	.245	.250	.445	.478	.645	.767	.845	1.238
.050	.050	.250	.255	.450	.485	.650	.775	.850	1.256
.055	.055	.255	.261	.455	.491	.655	.784	.855	1.274
.060	.060	.260	.266	.460	.497	.660	.793	.860	1.293
.065	.065	.265	.271	.465	.504	.665	.802	.865	1.313
.070	.070	.270	.277	.470	.510	.670	.811	.870	1.333
.075	.075	.275	.282	.475	.517	.675	.720	.875	1.354
.080	.080	.280	.288	.480	.523	.680	.829	.880	1.376
.085	.085	.285	.293	.485	.530	.685	.838	.885	1.398
.090	.090	.290	.299	.490	.536	.690	.848	.890	1.422
.095	.095	.295	.304	.495	.543	.695	.858	.895	1.447
.100	.100	.300	.310	.500	.549	.700	.867	.900	1.472
.105	.105	.305	.315	.505	.556	.705	.877	.905	1.499
.110	.110	.310	.321	.510	.563	.710	.887	.910	1.528
.115	.116	.315	.326	.515	.570	.715	.897	.915	1.557
.120	.121	.320	.332	.520	.576	.720	.908	.920	1.589
.125	.126	.425	.337	.525	.583	.725	.918	.925	1.623
.130	.131	.330	.343	.530	.590	.730	.929	.930	1.658
.135	.136	.335	.348	.535	.597	.735	.940	.935	1.697
.140	.141	.340	.354	.540	.604	.740	.950	.940	1.738
.145	.146	.345	.360	.545	.611	.745	.962	.945	1.783
.150	.151	.350	.365	.550	.618	.750	.973	.950	1.832
.155	.156	.355	.371	.555	.626	.755	.984	.955	1.886
.60	.161	.360	.377	.560	.633	.760	.996	.960	1.946
.165	.167	.365	.383	.565	.640	.765	1.008	.965	2.014
.170	.172	.370	.388	.570	.648	.770	1.020	.970	2.092
.175	.177	.375	.394	.575	.655	.775	1.033	.975	2.185
.180	.182	.380	.400	.580	.662	.780	1.045	.980	2.298
.185	.187	.385	.406	.585	.670	.785	1.058	.985	2.443
.190	.192	.390	.412	.590	.678	.790	1.071	.990	2.647
.195	.198	.395	.418	.595	.685	.795	1.085	.995	2.994

From *Statistical Methods*, 2nd ed., (p. 427), by A.L. Edwards, 1967, New York: Holt, Rinehart and Winston, Inc. Copyright 1967 by Allen L. Edwards.

Table A.5   Critical Values of t

	Level of significance for one-tailed test					
	.10	.05	.025	.01	.005	.0005
	Level of significance for two-tailed test					
df	.20	.10	.05	.02	.01	.001
1	3.078	6.314	12.706	31.821	63.657	636.619
2	1.886	2.920	4.303	6.965	9.925	31.598
3	1.638	2.353	3.182	4.541	5.841	12.941
4	1.533	2.132	2.776	3.747	4.604	8.610
5	1.476	2.015	2.571	3.365	4.032	6.859
6	1.440	1.943	2.447	3.143	3.707	5.959
7	1.415	1.895	2.365	2.998	3.499	5.405
8	1.397	1.860	2.306	2.896	3.355	5.041
9	1.383	1.833	2.262	2.821	3.250	4.781
10	1.372	1.812	2.228	2.764	3.169	4.587
11	1.363	1.796	2.201	2.718	3.106	4.437
12	1.356	1.782	2.179	2.681	3.055	4.318
13	1.350	1.771	2.160	2.650	3.012	4.221
14	1.345	1.761	2.145	2.624	2.977	4.140
15	1.341	1.753	2.131	2.602	2.947	4.073
16	1.337	1.746	2.120	2.583	2.921	4.015
17	1.333	1.740	2.110	2.567	2.898	3.965
18	1.330	1.734	2.101	2.552	2.878	3.922
19	1.328	1.729	2.093	2.539	2.861	3.883
20	1.325	1.725	2.086	2.528	2.845	3.850
21	1.323	1.721	2.080	2.518	2.831	3.819
22	1.321	1.717	2.074	2.508	2.819	3.792
23	1.319	1.714	2.069	2.500	2.807	3.767
24	1.318	1.711	2.064	2.492	2.797	3.745
25	1.316	1.708	2.060	2.485	2.787	3.725
26	1.315	1.706	2.056	2.479	2.779	3.707
27	1.314	1.703	2.052	2.473	2.771	3.690
28	1.313	1.701	2.048	2.467	2.763	3.674
29	1.311	1.699	2.045	2.462	2.756	3.659
30	1.310	1.697	2.042	2.457	2.750	3.646
40	1.303	1.684	2.021	2.423	2.704	3.551
60	1.296	1.671	2.000	2.390	2.660	3.460
120	1.289	1.658	1.980	2.358	2.617	3.373
∞	1.282	1.645	1.960	2.326	2.576	3.291

Table A.5 is taken from Table III of Fisher & Yates; *Statistical Tables for Biological, Agricultural and Medical Research* published by Longman Group UK Ltd., 1974.

Table A.6   Critical Values of F

n_1, degrees of freedom (for greater mean square)

Each cell gives the 0.05 critical value (top, black) and the 0.01 critical value (bottom, red).

n_2	1	2	3	4	5	6	7	8	9	10	11	12	14	16	20	24	30	40	50	75	100	200	500	∞
1	161 / 4,052	200 / 4,999	216 / 5,403	225 / 5,625	230 / 5,764	234 / 5,859	237 / 5,928	239 / 5,981	241 / 6,022	242 / 6,056	243 / 6,082	244 / 6,106	245 / 6,142	246 / 6,169	248 / 6,208	249 / 6,234	250 / 6,258	251 / 6,286	252 / 6,302	253 / 6,323	253 / 6,334	254 / 6,352	254 / 6,361	254 / 6,366
2	18.51 / 98.49	19.00 / 99.00	19.16 / 99.17	19.25 / 99.25	19.30 / 99.30	19.33 / 99.33	19.36 / 99.34	19.37 / 99.36	19.38 / 99.38	19.39 / 99.40	19.40 / 99.41	19.41 / 99.42	19.42 / 99.43	19.43 / 99.44	19.44 / 99.45	19.45 / 99.46	19.46 / 99.47	19.47 / 99.48	19.47 / 99.48	19.48 / 99.49	19.49 / 99.49	19.49 / 99.49	19.50 / 99.50	19.50 / 99.50
3	10.13 / 34.12	9.55 / 30.82	9.28 / 29.46	9.12 / 28.71	9.01 / 28.24	8.94 / 27.91	8.88 / 27.67	8.84 / 27.49	8.81 / 27.34	8.78 / 27.23	8.76 / 27.13	8.74 / 27.05	8.71 / 26.92	8.69 / 26.83	8.66 / 26.69	8.64 / 26.60	8.62 / 26.50	8.60 / 26.41	8.58 / 26.35	8.57 / 26.27	8.56 / 26.23	8.54 / 26.18	8.54 / 26.14	8.53 / 26.12
4	7.71 / 21.20	6.94 / 18.00	6.49 / 16.69	6.39 / 15.98	6.26 / 15.52	6.16 / 15.21	6.09 / 14.98	6.04 / 14.80	6.00 / 14.66	5.96 / 14.54	5.93 / 14.45	5.91 / 14.37	5.87 / 14.24	5.84 / 14.15	5.80 / 14.02	5.77 / 13.93	5.74 / 13.83	5.71 / 13.74	5.70 / 13.69	5.68 / 13.61	5.66 / 13.57	5.65 / 13.52	5.64 / 13.48	5.63 / 13.46
5	6.61 / 16.26	5.79 / 13.27	5.41 / 12.06	5.19 / 11.39	5.05 / 10.97	4.95 / 10.67	4.88 / 10.45	4.82 / 10.27	4.78 / 10.15	4.74 / 10.05	4.70 / 9.96	4.68 / 9.89	4.64 / 9.77	4.60 / 9.68	4.56 / 9.55	4.53 / 9.47	4.50 / 9.38	4.46 / 9.29	4.44 / 9.24	4.42 / 9.17	4.40 / 9.13	4.38 / 9.07	4.37 / 9.04	4.36 / 9.02
6	5.99 / 13.74	5.14 / 10.92	4.76 / 9.78	4.53 / 9.15	4.39 / 8.75	4.28 / 8.47	4.21 / 8.26	4.15 / 8.10	4.10 / 7.98	4.06 / 7.87	4.03 / 7.79	4.00 / 7.72	3.96 / 7.60	3.92 / 7.52	3.87 / 7.39	3.84 / 7.31	3.81 / 7.23	3.77 / 7.14	3.75 / 7.09	3.72 / 7.02	3.71 / 6.99	3.69 / 6.94	3.68 / 6.90	3.67 / 6.88
7	5.59 / 12.25	4.74 / 9.55	4.35 / 8.45	4.12 / 7.85	3.97 / 7.46	3.87 / 7.19	3.79 / 7.00	3.73 / 6.84	3.68 / 6.71	3.63 / 6.62	3.60 / 6.54	3.57 / 6.47	3.52 / 6.35	3.49 / 6.27	3.44 / 6.15	3.41 / 6.07	3.38 / 5.98	3.34 / 5.90	3.32 / 5.85	3.29 / 5.78	3.28 / 5.75	3.25 / 5.70	3.24 / 5.67	3.23 / 5.65
8	5.32 / 11.26	4.46 / 8.65	4.07 / 7.59	3.84 / 7.01	3.69 / 6.63	3.58 / 6.37	3.50 / 6.19	3.44 / 6.03	3.39 / 5.91	3.34 / 5.82	3.31 / 5.74	3.28 / 5.67	3.23 / 5.56	3.20 / 5.48	3.15 / 5.36	3.12 / 5.28	3.08 / 5.20	3.05 / 5.11	3.03 / 5.06	3.00 / 5.00	2.98 / 4.96	2.96 / 4.91	2.94 / 4.88	2.93 / 4.86
9	5.12 / 10.56	4.26 / 8.02	3.86 / 6.99	3.63 / 6.42	3.48 / 6.06	3.37 / 5.80	3.29 / 5.62	3.23 / 5.47	3.18 / 5.35	3.13 / 5.26	3.10 / 5.18	3.07 / 5.11	3.02 / 5.00	2.98 / 4.92	2.93 / 4.80	2.90 / 4.73	2.86 / 4.64	2.82 / 4.56	2.80 / 4.51	2.77 / 4.45	2.76 / 4.41	2.73 / 4.36	2.72 / 4.33	2.71 / 4.31
10	4.96 / 10.04	4.10 / 7.56	3.71 / 6.55	3.48 / 5.99	3.33 / 5.64	3.22 / 5.39	3.14 / 5.21	3.07 / 5.06	3.02 / 4.95	2.97 / 4.85	2.94 / 4.78	2.91 / 4.71	2.86 / 4.60	2.82 / 4.52	2.77 / 4.41	2.74 / 4.33	2.70 / 4.25	2.67 / 4.17	2.64 / 4.12	2.61 / 4.05	2.59 / 4.01	2.56 / 3.96	2.55 / 3.93	2.54 / 3.91
11	4.84 / 9.65	3.98 / 7.20	3.59 / 6.22	3.36 / 5.67	3.20 / 5.32	3.09 / 5.07	3.01 / 4.88	2.95 / 4.74	2.90 / 4.63	2.86 / 4.54	2.82 / 4.46	2.79 / 4.40	2.74 / 4.29	2.70 / 4.21	2.65 / 4.10	2.61 / 4.02	2.57 / 3.94	2.53 / 3.86	2.50 / 3.80	2.47 / 3.74	2.45 / 3.70	2.42 / 3.66	2.41 / 3.62	2.40 / 3.60
12	4.75 / 9.33	3.88 / 6.93	3.49 / 5.95	3.26 / 5.41	3.11 / 5.06	3.00 / 4.82	2.92 / 4.65	2.85 / 4.50	2.80 / 4.39	2.76 / 4.30	2.72 / 4.22	2.69 / 4.16	2.64 / 4.05	2.60 / 3.98	2.54 / 3.86	2.50 / 3.78	2.46 / 3.70	2.42 / 3.61	2.40 / 3.56	2.36 / 3.49	2.35 / 3.46	2.32 / 3.41	2.31 / 3.38	2.30 / 3.36
13	4.67 / 9.07	3.80 / 6.70	3.41 / 5.74	3.18 / 5.20	3.02 / 4.86	2.92 / 4.62	2.84 / 4.44	2.77 / 4.30	2.72 / 4.19	2.67 / 4.10	2.63 / 4.02	2.60 / 3.96	2.55 / 3.85	2.51 / 3.78	2.46 / 3.67	2.42 / 3.59	2.38 / 3.51	2.34 / 3.42	2.32 / 3.37	2.28 / 3.30	2.26 / 3.27	2.24 / 3.21	2.22 / 3.18	2.21 / 3.16
14	4.60 / 8.86	3.74 / 6.51	3.34 / 5.56	3.11 / 5.03	2.96 / 4.69	2.85 / 4.46	2.77 / 4.28	2.70 / 4.14	2.65 / 4.03	2.60 / 3.94	2.56 / 3.86	2.53 / 3.80	2.48 / 3.70	2.44 / 3.62	2.39 / 3.51	2.35 / 3.43	2.31 / 3.34	2.27 / 3.26	2.24 / 3.21	2.21 / 3.14	2.19 / 3.11	2.16 / 3.06	2.14 / 3.02	2.13 / 3.00
15	4.54 / 8.68	3.68 / 6.36	3.29 / 5.42	3.06 / 4.89	2.90 / 4.56	2.79 / 4.32	2.70 / 4.14	2.64 / 4.00	2.59 / 3.89	2.55 / 3.80	2.51 / 3.73	2.48 / 3.67	2.43 / 3.56	2.39 / 3.48	2.33 / 3.36	2.29 / 3.29	2.25 / 3.20	2.21 / 3.12	2.18 / 3.07	2.15 / 3.00	2.12 / 2.97	2.10 / 2.92	2.08 / 2.89	2.07 / 2.87
16	4.49 / 8.53	3.63 / 6.23	3.24 / 5.29	3.01 / 4.77	2.85 / 4.44	2.74 / 4.20	2.66 / 4.03	2.59 / 3.89	2.54 / 3.78	2.49 / 3.69	2.45 / 3.61	2.42 / 3.55	2.37 / 3.45	2.33 / 3.37	2.28 / 3.25	2.24 / 3.18	2.20 / 3.10	2.16 / 3.01	2.13 / 2.96	2.09 / 2.89	2.07 / 2.86	2.04 / 2.80	2.02 / 2.77	2.01 / 2.75
17	4.45 / 8.40	3.59 / 6.11	3.20 / 5.18	2.96 / 4.67	2.81 / 4.34	2.70 / 4.10	2.62 / 3.93	2.55 / 3.79	2.50 / 3.68	2.45 / 3.59	2.41 / 3.52	2.38 / 3.45	2.33 / 3.35	2.29 / 3.27	2.23 / 3.16	2.19 / 3.08	2.15 / 3.00	2.11 / 2.92	2.08 / 2.86	2.04 / 2.79	2.02 / 2.76	1.99 / 2.70	1.97 / 2.67	1.96 / 2.65
18	4.41 / 8.28	3.55 / 6.01	3.16 / 5.09	2.93 / 4.58	2.77 / 4.25	2.66 / 4.01	2.58 / 3.85	2.51 / 3.71	2.46 / 3.60	2.41 / 3.51	2.37 / 3.44	2.34 / 3.37	2.29 / 3.27	2.25 / 3.19	2.19 / 3.07	2.15 / 3.00	2.11 / 2.91	2.07 / 2.83	2.04 / 2.78	2.00 / 2.71	1.98 / 2.68	1.95 / 2.62	1.93 / 2.59	1.92 / 2.57

19	4.38	3.52	3.13	2.90	2.74	2.63	2.55	2.48	2.43	2.38	2.34	2.31	2.26	2.21	2.15	2.11	2.07	2.02	2.00	1.96	1.94	1.91	1.90	1.88
	8.18	5.93	5.01	4.50	4.17	3.94	3.77	3.63	3.52	3.43	3.36	3.30	3.19	3.12	3.00	2.92	2.84	2.76	2.70	2.63	2.60	2.54	2.51	2.49
20	4.35	3.49	3.10	2.87	2.71	2.60	2.52	2.45	2.40	2.35	2.31	2.28	2.23	2.18	2.12	2.08	2.04	1.99	1.96	1.92	1.90	1.87	1.85	1.84
	8.10	5.85	4.94	4.43	4.10	3.87	3.71	3.56	3.45	3.37	3.30	3.23	3.13	3.05	2.94	2.86	2.77	2.69	2.63	2.56	2.53	2.47	2.44	2.42
21	4.32	3.47	3.07	2.84	2.68	2.57	2.49	2.42	2.37	2.32	2.28	2.25	2.20	2.15	2.09	2.05	2.00	1.96	1.93	1.89	1.87	1.84	1.82	1.81
	8.02	5.78	4.87	4.37	4.04	3.81	3.65	3.51	3.40	3.31	3.24	3.17	23.07	2.99	2.88	2.80	2.72	2.63	2.58	2.51	2.47	2.42	2.38	2.36
22	4.30	3.44	3.05	2.82	2.66	2.55	2.47	2.40	2.35	2.30	2.26	2.23	2.18	2.13	2.07	2.03	1.98	1.93	1.91	1.87	1.84	1.81	1.80	1.78
	7.94	5.72	4.82	4.31	3.99	3.76	3.59	3.45	3.35	3.26	3.18	3.12	3.02	2.94	2.83	2.75	2.67	2.58	2.53	2.46	2.42	2.37	2.33	2.31
23	4.28	3.42	3.03	2.80	2.64	2.53	2.45	2.38	2.32	2.28	2.24	2.20	2.14	2.10	2.04	2.00	1.96	1.91	1.88	1.84	1.82	1.79	1.77	1.76
	7.88	5.66	4.76	4.26	3.94	3.71	3.54	3.41	3.30	3.21	3.14	3.07	2.97	2.89	2.78	2.70	2.62	2.53	2.48	2.41	2.37	2.32	2.28	2.26
24	4.26	3.40	3.01	2.78	2.62	2.51	2.43	2.36	2.30	2.26	2.22	2.18	2.13	2.09	2.02	1.98	1.94	1.89	1.86	1.82	1.80	1.76	1.74	1.73
	7.82	5.61	4.72	4.22	3.90	3.67	3.50	3.36	3.25	3.17	3.09	3.03	2.93	2.85	2.74	2.66	2.58	2.449	2.44	2.36	2.33	2.27	2.23	2.21
25	4.24	3.38	2.99	2.76	2.60	2.49	2.41	2.34	2.28	2.24	2.20	2.16	2.11	2.06	2.00	1.96	1.92	1.87	1.84	1.80	1.77	1.74	1.72	1.71
	7.77	5.57	4.68	4.18	3.86	3.63	3.46	3.32	3.21	3.13	3.05	2.99	2.89	2.81	2.70	2.62	2.54	2.45	2.40	2.32	2.29	2.23	2.19	2.17
26	4.22	3.37	2.98	2.74	2.59	2.47	2.39	2.32	2.27	2.22	2.18	2.15	2.10	2.05	1.99	1.95	1.90	1.85	1.82	1.78	1.76	1.72	1.70	1.69
	7.72	5.53	4.64	4.14	3.82	2.59	3.42	3.29	3.17	3.09	3.02	2.96	2.86	2.77	2.66	2.58	2.50	2.41	2.36	2.28	2.25	2.19	2.15	2.13
27	4.21	3.35	2.96	2.73	2.57	2.46	2.37	2.30	2.25	2.20	2.16	2.13	2.08	2.03	1.97	1.93	1.88	1.84	1.80	1.76	1.74	1.71	1.68	1.67
	7.68	5.49	4.60	4.11	3.79	3.56	3.3.9	3.26	3.14	3.06	2.98	2.93	2.83	2.74	2.63	2.55	2.47	2.38	2.33	2.25	2.21	2.16	2.12	2.10
28	4.20	3.34	2.95	2.71	2.56	2.44	2.36	2.29	2.24	2.19	2.15	2.12	2.06	2.02	1.96	1.91	1.87	1.81	1.78	1.75	1.72	1.69	1.67	1.65
	7.64	5.45	4.57	4.07	3.76	3.53	3.36	3.23	3.11	3.03	2.95	2.90	2.80	2.71	2.60	2.52	2.44	2.35	2.30	2.22	2.18	2.13	2.09	2.06
29	4.18	3.33	2.93	2.70	2.54	2.43	2.35	2.28	2.22	2.18	2.14	2.10	2.05	2.00	1.94	1.90	1.85	1.80	1.77	1.73	1.71	1.68	1.65	1.64
	7.60	5.42	4.54	4.04	3.73	3.50	3.33	3.20	3.08	3.00	2.92	2.87	2.77	2.68	2.57	2.49	2.41	2.32	2.27	2.19	2.15	2.10	2.06	2.03
30	4.17	3.32	2.92	2.69	2.53	2.42	2.34	2.27	2.21	2.16	2.12	2.09	2.04	1.99	1.93	1.89	1.84	1.79	1.76	1.72	1.69	1.66	1.64	1.62
	7.56	5.39	4.51	4.02	3.70	3.47	3.30	3.17	3.06	2.98	2.90	2.84	2.74	2.66	2.55	2.47	2.38	2.29	2.24	2.16	2.13	2.07	2.03	2.01
32	4.15	3.30	2.90	2.67	2.51	2.40	2.32	2.25	2.19	2.14	2.10	2.07	2.02	1.97	1.91	1.86	1.82	1.76	1.74	1.69	1.67	1.64	1.61	1.59
	7.50	5.34	4.46	3.97	3.66	3.42	3.25	3.12	3.01	2.94	2.86	2.80	2.70	2.62	2.51	2.42	2.34	2.25	2.20	2.12	2.08	2.02	1.98	1.96
34	4.13	3.28	2.88	2.65	2.49	2.38	2.30	2.23	2.17	2.12	2.08	2.05	2.00	1.95	1.89	1.84	1.80	1.74	1.71	1.67	1.64	1.61	1.59	1.57
	7.44	5.29	4.42	3.93	3.61	3.38	3.21	3.08	2.97	2.89	2.82	2.76	2.66	2.58	2.47	2.38	2.30	2.21	2.15	2.08	2.04	1.98	1.94	1.91
36	4.11	3.26	2.86	2.63	2.48	2.36	2.28	2.21	2.15	2.10	2.06	2.03	1.98	1.93	1.87	1.82	1.78	1.72	1.69	1.65	1.62	1.59	1.56	1.55
	7.39	5.25	4.38	3.89	3.58	3.35	3.18	3.04	2.94	2.86	2.78	2.72	2.62	2.54	2.43	2.35	2.26	2.17	2.12	2.04	2.00	1.94	1.90	1.87
38	4.10	3.25	2.85	2.62	2.46	2.35	2.26	2.19	2.14	2.09	2.05	2.02	1.96	1.92	1.85	1.80	1.76	1.71	1.67	1.63	1.60	1.57	1.54	1.53
	7.35	5.21	4.34	3.86	3.54	3.32	3.15	3.02	2.91	2.82	2.75	2.69	2.59	2.51	2.40	2.32	2.22	2.14	2.08	2.00	1.97	1.90	1.86	1.84
40	4.08	3.23	2.84	2.61	2.45	2.34	2.25	2.18	2.12	2.07	2.04	2.00	.195	1.90	1.84	1.79	1.74	1.69	1.66	1.61	1.59	1.55	1.53	1.51
	7.31	5.18	4.31	3.83	3.51	3.29	3.12	2.99	2.88	2.80	2.73	2.66	2.56	2.49	2.37	2.29	2.20	2.11	2.05	1.97	1.94	1.88	1.84	1.81
42	4.07	3.22	2.83	2.59	2.44	2.32	2.24	2.17	2.11	2.06	2.02	1.99	1.94	1.89	1.82	1.78	1.73	1.68	1.64	1.60	1.57	1.54	1.51	1.49
	7.27	5.15	4.29	3.80	3.49	3.26	3.10	2.96	2.86	2.77	2.70	2.64	2.54	2.46	2.35	2.26	2.17	2.08	2.02	1.94	1.91	1.85	1.80	1.78
44	4.06	3.21	2.82	2.58	2.43	2.31	2.23	2.16	2.10	2.05	2.01	1.98	1.92	1.88	1.81	1.76	1.72	1.66	1.63	1.58	1.56	1.52	1.50	1.48
	7.24	5.12	4.26	3.78	3.46	3.24	3.07	2.94	2.84	2.75	2.68	2.62	2.52	2.44	2.32	2.24	2.15	2.06	2.00	1.92	1.88	1.82	1.78	1.75

Table A.6   *(continued)*

n_1 degrees of freedom (for greater mean square)

Values given as *.05 level* / *.01 level*.

n_2	1	2	3	4	5	6	7	8	9	10	11	12	14	16	20	24	30	40	50	75	100	200	500	∞
46	4.05/7.21	3.20/5.10	2.81/4.24	2.57/3.76	2.42/3.44	2.30/3.22	2.22/3.05	2.14/2.92	2.09/2.82	2.04/2.73	2.00/2.66	1.97/2.60	1.91/2.50	1.87/2.42	1.80/2.30	1.75/2.22	1.71/2.13	1.65/2.04	1.62/1.98	1.57/1.90	1.54/1.86	1.51/1.80	1.48/1.76	1.46/1.72
48	4.04/7.19	3.19/5.08	2.80/4.22	2.56/3.74	2.41/3.42	2.30/3.20	2.21/3.04	2.14/2.90	2.08/2.80	2.03/2.71	1.99/2.64	1.96/2.58	1.90/2.48	1.86/2.40	1.79/2.28	1.74/2.20	1.70/2.11	1.64/2.02	1.61/1.96	1.56/1.88	1.53/1.84	1.50/1.78	1.47/1.73	1.45/1.70
50	4.03/7.17	3.18/5.06	2.79/4.20	2.56/3.72	2.40/3.41	2.29/3.18	2.20/3.02	2.13/2.88	2.07/2.78	2.02/2.70	1.98/2.62	1.95/2.56	1.90/2.46	1.85/2.39	1.78/2.26	1.74/2.18	1.69/2.10	1.63/2.00	1.60/1.94	1.55/1.86	1.52/1.82	1.48/1.76	1.46/1.71	1.44/1.68
55	4.02/7.12	3.17/5.01	2.78/4.16	2.54/3.68	2.38/3.37	2.27/3.15	2.18/2.98	2.11/2.85	2.05/2.75	2.00/2.66	1.97/2.59	1.93/2.53	1.88/2.43	1.83/2.35	1.76/2.23	1.72/2.15	1.67/2.06	1.61/1.96	1.58/1.90	1.52/1.82	1.50/1.78	1.46/1.71	1.43/1.66	1.41/1.64
60	4.00/7.08	3.15/4.98	2.76/4.13	2.52/3.65	2.37/3.34	2.25/3.12	2.17/2.95	2.10/2.82	2.04/2.72	1.99/2.63	1.95/2.56	1.92/2.50	1.86/2.40	1.81/2.32	1.75/2.20	1.70/2.12	1.65/2.03	1.59/1.93	1.56/1.87	1.50/1.79	1.48/1.74	1.44/1.68	1.41/1.63	1.39/1.60
65	3.99/7.04	3.14/4.95	2.75/4.10	2.51/3.62	2.36/3.31	2.24/3.09	2.15/2.93	2.08/2.79	2.02/2.70	1.98/2.61	1.94/2.54	1.90/2.47	1.85/2.37	1.80/2.30	1.73/2.18	1.68/2.09	1.63/2.00	1.57/1.90	1.54/1.84	1.49/1.76	1.46/1.71	1.42/1.64	1.39/1.60	1.37/1.56
70	3.98/7.01	3.13/4.92	2.74/4.08	2.50/3.60	2.35/3.29	2.23/3.07	2.14/2.91	2.07/2.77	2.01/2.67	1.97/2.59	1.93/2.51	1.89/2.45	1.84/2.35	1.79/2.28	1.72/2.15	1.67/2.07	1.62/1.98	1.56/1.88	1.53/1.82	1.47/1.74	1.45/1.69	1.40/1.62	1.37/1.56	1.35/1.53
80	3.96/6.96	3.11/4.88	2.72/4.04	2.48/3.56	2.33/3.25	2.21/3.04	2.12/2.87	2.05/2.74	1.99/2.64	1.95/2.55	1.91/2.48	1.88/2.41	1.82/2.32	1.77/2.24	1.70/2.11	1.65/2.03	1.60/1.94	1.54/1.84	1.51/1.78	1.45/1.70	1.42/1.65	1.38/1.57	1.35/1.52	1.32/1.49
100	3.94/6.90	3.09/4.82	2.70/3.98	2.46/3.51	2.30/3.20	2.19/2.99	2.10/2.82	2.03/2.69	1.97/2.59	1.92/2.51	1.88/2.43	1.85/2.36	1.79/2.26	1.75/2.19	1.68/2.06	1.63/1.98	1.57/1.89	1.51/1.79	1.48/1.73	1.42/1.64	1.39/1.59	1.34/1.51	1.30/1.46	1.28/1.43
125	3.92/6.84	3.07/4.78	2.68/3.94	2.44/3.47	2.29/3.17	2.17/2.95	2.08/2.79	2.01/2.65	1.95/2.56	1.90/2.47	1.86/2.40	1.83/2.33	1.77/2.23	1.72/2.15	1.65/2.03	1.60/1.94	1.55/1.85	1.49/1.75	1.45/1.68	1.39/1.59	1.36/1.54	1.31/1.46	1.27/1.40	1.25/1.37
150	3.91/6.81	3.06/4.75	2.67/3.91	2.43/3.44	2.27/3.14	2.16/2.92	2.07/2.76	2.00/2.62	1.94/2.53	1.89/2.44	1.85/2.37	1.82/2.30	1.75/2.20	1.71/2.12	1.64/2.00	1.59/1.91	1.54/1.83	1.47/1.72	1.44/1.66	1.37/1.56	1.34/1.51	1.29/1.43	1.25/1.37	1.22/1.33
200	3.89/6.76	3.04/4.71	2.65/3.88	2.41/3.41	2.26/3.11	2.14/2.90	2.05/2.73	1.98/2.60	1.92/2.50	1.87/2.41	1.83/2.34	1.80/2.28	1.74/2.17	1.69/2.09	1.62/1.97	1.57/1.88	1.52/1.79	1.45/1.69	1.42/1.62	1.35/1.53	1.32/1.48	1.26/1.39	1.22/1.33	1.19/1.28
400	3.86/6.70	3.02/4.66	2.62/3.83	2.39/3.36	2.23/3.06	2.12/2.85	2.03/2.69	1.96/2.55	1.90/2.46	1.85/2.37	1.81/2.29	1.78/2.23	1.72/2.12	1.67/2.04	1.60/1.92	1.54/1.84	1.49/1.74	1.42/1.64	1.38/1.57	1.32/1.47	1.28/1.42	1.22/1.32	1.16/1.24	1.13/1.19
1000	3.85/6.66	3.00/4.62	2.61/3.80	2.38/3.34	2.22/3.04	2.10/2.82	2.02/2.66	1.95/2.53	1.89/2.43	1.84/2.34	1.80/2.26	1.76/2.20	1.70/2.09	1.65/2.01	1.58/1.89	1.53/1.81	1.47/1.71	1.41/1.61	1.36/1.54	1.30/1.44	1.26/1.38	1.19/1.28	1.13/1.19	1.08/1.11
∞	3.84/6.64	2.99/4.60	2.60/3.78	2.37/3.32	2.21/3.02	2.09/2.80	2.01/2.64	1.94/2.51	1.88/2.41	1.83/2.32	1.79/2.24	1.75/2.18	1.69/2.07	1.64/1.99	1.57/1.87	1.52/1.79	1.46/1.69	1.40/1.59	1.35/1.52	1.28/1.41	1.24/1.36	1.17/1.25	1.11/1.15	1.00/1.00

■ = .05 level; ■ = .01 level.

From *Statistical Methods*, 7th ed., (pp. 480–483), by G.W. Snedecor and W.G. Cochran, 1980, Ames, Iowa: The Iowa State University Press. Copyright 1980 by The Iowa State University Press. Reprinted with permission.

Table A.7   Critical Values of the Studentized Range Statistic

df for S_{ω^2}	$1-\alpha$	k = number of means or steps between ordered means								
		2	3	4	5	6	7	8	9	10
1	.95	18.0	27.0	32.8	37.1	40.4	43.1	45.4	47.4	49.1
	.99	90.0	135	164	186	202	216	227	237	246
2	.95	6.09	8.3	9.8	10.9	11.7	12.4	13.0	13.5	14.0
	.99	14.0	19.0	22.3	24.7	26.6	28.2	29.5	30.7	31.7
3	.95	4.50	5.91	6.82	7.50	8.04	8.48	8.85	9.18	9.46
	.99	8.26	10.6	12.2	13.3	14.2	15.0	15.6	16.2	16.7
4	.95	3.93	5.04	5.76	6.29	6.71	7.05	7.35	7.60	7.83
	.99	6.51	8.12	9.17	9.96	10.6	11.1	11.5	11.9	12.3
5	.95	3.64	4.60	5.22	5.67	6.03	6.33	6.58	6.80	6.99
	.99	5.70	6.97	7.80	8.42	8.91	9.32	9.67	9.97	10.2
6	.95	3.46	4.34	4.90	5.31	5.63	5.89	6.12	6.32	6.49
	.99	5.24	6.33	7.03	7.56	7.97	8.32	8.61	8.87	9.10
7	.95	3.34	4.16	4.69	5.06	5.36	5.61	5.82	6.00	6.16
	.99	4.95	5.92	6.54	7.01	7.37	7.68	7.94	8.17	8.37
8	.95	3.26	4.04	4.53	4.89	5.17	5.40	5.60	5.77	5.92
	.99	4.74	5.63	6.20	6.63	6.96	7.24	7.47	7.68	7.87
9	.95	3.20	3.95	4.42	4.76	5.02	5.24	5.43	5.60	5.74
	.99	4.60	5.43	5.96	6.35	6.66	6.91	7.13	8.32	7.49
10	.95	3.15	3.88	4.33	4.65	4.91	5.12	5.30	5.46	5.60
	.99	4.48	5.27	5.77	6.14	6.43	6.67	6.87	7.05	7.21
11	.95	3.11	3.82	4.26	4.57	4.82	5.03	5.20	5.35	5.49
	.99	4.39	5.14	5.62	5.97	6.25	6.48	6.67	6.84	6.99
12	.95	3.08	3.77	4.20	4.51	4.75	4.95	5.12	5.27	5.40
	.99	4.32	5.04	5.50	5.84	6.10	6.32	6.51	6.67	6.81
13	.95	3.06	3.73	4.15	4.45	4.69	4.88	5.05	5.19	5.32
	.99	4.26	4.96	5.40	5.73	5.98	6.19	6.37	6.53	6.67
14	.95	3.03	3.70	4.11	4.41	4.64	4.83	4.99	5.13	5.25
	.99	4.21	4.89	5.32	5.63	5.88	6.08	6.26	6.41	6.54
16	.95	3.00	3.65	4.05	4.33	4.56	4.74	4.90	5.03	5.15
	.99	4.13	4.78	5.19	5.49	5.72	5.92	6.08	6.22	6.35
18	.95	2.97	3.61	4.00	4.28	4.49	4.67	4.82	4.96	5.07
	.99	4.07	4.70	5.09	5.38	5.60	5.79	5.94	6.08	6.20
20	.95	2.95	3.58	3.96	4.23	4.45	4.62	4.77	4.90	5.01
	.99	4.02	4.64	5.02	5.29	5.51	5.69	5.84	5.97	6.09
24	.95	2.92	3.53	3.90	4.17	4.37	4.54	4.68	4.81	4.92
	.99	3.96	4.54	4.91	5.17	5.37	5.54	5.69	5.81	5.92
30	.95	2.89	3.49	3.84	4.10	4.30	4.46	4.60	4.72	4.83
	.99	3.89	4.45	4.80	5.05	5.24	5.40	5.54	5.56	5.76
40	.95	2.86	3.44	3.79	4.04	4.23	4.39	4.52	4.63	4.74
	.99	3.82	4.37	4.70	4.93	5.11	5.27	5.39	5.50	5.60
60	.95	2.83	3.40	3.74	3.98	4.16	4.31	4.44	4.55	4.65
	.99	3.76	4.28	4.60	4.82	4.99	5.13	5.25	5.36	5.45
120	.95	2.80	3.36	3.69	3.92	4.10	4.24	4.36	4.48	4.56
	.99	3.70	4.20	4.50	4.71	4.87	5.01	5.12	5.21	5.30
∞	.95	2.77	3.31	3.63	3.86	4.03	4.17	4.29	4.39	4.47
	.99	3.64	4.12	4.40	4.60	4.76	4.88	4.99	5.08	5.16

Table A.8   Critical Values of Chi-Square

df	.99	.98	.95	.90	.80	.70	.50	.30	.20	.10	.05	.02	.01	.001
					Probability under H_0 that $\chi^2 \geqslant$ chi-square									
1	.00016	.00063	.0039	.016	.064	.15	.46	1.07	1.64	2.71	3.84	5.41	6.64	10.83
2	.02	.04	.10	.21	.45	.71	1.39	2.41	3.22	4.60	5.99	7.82	9.21	13.82
3	.12	.18	.35	.58	1.00	1.42	2.37	3.66	4.64	6.25	7.82	9.84	11.34	16.27
4	.30	.43	.71	1.06	1.65	2.20	3.36	4.88	5.99	7.78	9.49	11.67	13.28	18.46
5	.55	.75	1.14	1.61	2.34	3.00	4.35	6.06	7.29	9.24	11.07	13.39	15.09	20.52
6	.87	1.13	1.64	2.20	3.07	3.83	5.35	7.23	8.56	10.64	12.59	15.03	16.81	22.46
7	1.24	1.56	2.17	2.83	3.82	4.67	6.35	8.38	9.80	12.02	14.07	16.62	18.48	24.32
8	1.65	2.03	2.73	3.49	4.59	45.53	7.34	9.52	11.03	13.36	15.51	18.17	20.09	26.12
9	2.09	2.53	3.32	4.17	5.38	6.39	8.34	10.66	12.24	14.68	16.92	19.68	21.67	27.88
10	2.56	3.06	3.94	4.86	6.18	7.27	9.34	11.78	13.44	15.99	18.31	21.16	23.21	29.59
11	3.05	3.61	4.58	5.58	6.99	8.15	10.34	12.90	14.63	17.28	19.68	22.62	24.72	31.26
12	3.57	4.18	5.23	6.30	7.81	9.03	11.34	14.01	15.81	18.55	21.03	24.05	26.22	32.91
13	4.11	4.76	5.89	7.04	8.63	9.93	12.34	15.12	16.98	19.81	22.36	25.47	27.69	34.53
14	4.66	5.37	6.57	7.79	9.47	10.82	13.34	16.22	18.15	21.06	23.68	26.87	29.14	26.12
15	5.23	5.98	7.26	8.55	10.31	11.72	14.34	17.32	19.31	22.31	25.00	28.26	30.58	37.70
16	5.81	6.61	7.96	9.31	11.15	12.62	15.34	18.42	20.46	23.54	26.30	29.63	32.00	39.29
17	6.41	7.26	8.67	10.08	12.00	13.53	16.34	19.51	21.62	24.77	27.59	31.00	33.41	40.75
18	7.02	7.91	9.39	10.86	12.86	14.44	17.34	20.60	22.76	25.99	28.87	32.35	34.80	42.31
19	7.63	8.57	10.12	11.65	13.72	15.35	18.34	21.69	23.90	27.20	30.14	33.69	36.19	43.82
20	8.26	9.24	10.85	12.44	14.58	16.27	19.34	22.78	25.04	28.41	31.41	35.02	37.57	45.32
21	8.90	9.92	11.59	13.24	15.44	17.18	20.34	23.86	26.17	29.62	32.67	36.34	38.93	46.80
22	9.54	10.60	12.34	14.04	16.31	18.10	21.34	24.94	27.30	30.81	33.92	37.66	40.29	48.27
23	10.20	11.29	13.09	14.85	17.19	19.02	22.34	26.02	28.43	32.01	35.17	38.97	41.64	49.73
24	10.86	11.99	13.85	15.66	18.06	19.94	23.34	27.10	29.55	33.20	36.42	40.27	42.98	51.18
25	11.52	12.70	14.61	16.47	18.94	20.87	24.34	28.17	30.68	34.38	37.65	41.57	44.31	52.62
26	12.20	13.41	15.38	17.29	19.82	21.79	25.34	29.25	31.80	35.56	38.88	42.86	45.64	54.05
27	12.88	14.12	16.15	18.11	20.70	22.72	26.34	30.32	32.91	36.74	40.11	44.14	46.96	55.48
28	13.56	14.85	16.93	18.94	21.59	23.65	27.34	31.39	34.03	37.92	41.34	45.42	48.28	56.89
29	14.26	15.57	17.71	19.77	22.48	24.58	28.34	32.46	35.14	39.09	42.56	46.69	49.59	58.30
30	14.95	16.31	18.49	20.60	23.36	25.51	29.34	33.53	36.25	40.26	43.77	47.96	50.89	59.70

Table A.8 is taken from Table IV of Fisher & Yates; *Statistical Tables for Biological, Agricultural and Medical Research* published by Longman Group UK Ltd., 1974.

Table A.9   Values of Spearman r_s
for the .05 and .01 Levels of Significance

N	.05	.01	N	.05	.01
6	.886	–	19	.462	.608
7	.786	–	20	.450	.591
8	.738	.881	21	.438	.576
9	.683	.833	22	.428	.562
10	.648	.818	23	.418	.549
11	.623	.794	24	.409	.537
12	.591	.780	25	.400	.526
13	.566	.745	26	.392	.515
14	.545	.716	27	.385	.505
15	.525	.689	28	.377	.496
16	.507	.666	29	.370	.487
17	.490	.645	30	.364	.478
18	.476	.625			

Reprinted, by permission, from E.G. Olds, 1938, "Distributions of sums of squares of rank differences for small
numbers of individuals," *Annals of Mathematical Statistics*
9: 133-148, and E.G. Olds, 1949, "The 5% significance
levels for sums of squares of rank differences and a
correction," *Annals of Mathematical Statistics* 20:117-118.

A Brief Historical Overview of Research in Physical Activity in the United States

Early Physical Education Research

Postwar Research

All of the types of research we have been talking about didn't just happen randomly by chance. Research has systematically evolved in the United States since the mid-1800s. We present here a chronicle of that evolutionary process. Our information came from several secondary sources (Hackensmith, 1966; Lee, 1983; Leonard & Affleck, 1947; Van Dalen & Bennet, 1971). Particularly helpful were Lee's summaries of research (see Lee, 1983, chaps. 6, 9, 13, and 16).

The subdisciplines in the study of physical activity (e.g., biomechanics, exercise physiology, motor behavior, sport psychology, sport sociology, sport pedagogy, adapted physical activity, sport history, sport philosophy) all trace their beginnings to varying times and fields of study. Not until the 1960s did research in these subdisciplines coalesce under a common area, the study of physical activity. The following account represents the general field of physical education that developed into the study of physical activity. In addition to knowing the history of the field of physical activity, graduate students should have more detailed knowledge and an analysis of the intellectual history of their specific subdiscipline. Massengale and Swanson (Eds.) (1996) provide a history of the subdisciplines of adapted physical education, exercise physiology, biomechanics, motor behavior (including motor learning, control and development), sport psychology, sport pedagogy, sport sociology, history, and philosophy.

Early Physical Education Research

The beginnings of systematic research in physical education in the United States closely followed the establishment in 1854 of the first department of hygiene and physical education at Amherst College. Although John Hooker was the first director of this department, the appointment of Edward Hitchcock (MD, Harvard Medical School, 1853) as director in 1861 represents the beginnings of research efforts in physical education. Dr. Hitchcock frequently made anthropometric measurements and used chin-ups to assess arm strength. Over the next 20 years, the list of measurements taken was extended considerably. The tabulation of these measurements was first published in the *Anthropometric Manual*

(1887; revised editions in 1889, 1893, and 1900), which represents one of the first data-based research publications of physical education in the United States.

Then, Dudley Sargent, who received his MD from Yale Medical School in 1878, established a private gymnasium in New York, where he began applying a series of bodily measurements to participants. Two years later, he was appointed assistant professor at Harvard and director of the new Hemenway Gymnasium. All entering freshmen were given an examination, including both strength tests and anthropometric measures. Dr. Sargent collected more than 50,000 anthropometric measures on individuals during his career. In fact, lifelike statues of typical American youths were constructed on the basis of his measurements and displayed at the 1893 Chicago World's Fair. This might be listed as the first formal research presentation in physical education in the United States. Sargent also led in the development of strength testing, and he used these tests to determine membership of Harvard's athletic teams. Following Sargent's lead, several women's colleges (Bryn Mawr, Mount Holyoke, Radcliffe, Rockford, Vassar, and Wellesley) established programs of anthropometric measurements and strength tests of students in the 1880s.

When a new gymnasium was constructed at Johns Hopkins in 1883, Edward Hartwell (PhD, Johns Hopkins; MD, Medical College of Ohio) was appointed its director. There, in 1897, he began the use of survey research in physical education through his evaluations of gymnastics in the United States.

To measure throwing, running speed, and distance jumped, Dr. Luther Gulick devised the very first achievement test in 1890. Called the Pentathlon Test, it was initially created for the Athletic League of the YMCAs of America but was further developed in the early 1900s for the Public School Athletic League in New York.

In the late 1800s and early 1900s, several books reported, summarized, or influenced early research in physical education. Among those were Blaikie's *How to Get Strong and How to Stay So* (1879), which reported Sargent's early work and influenced Harvard (Blaikie was a Harvard alumnus) to employ Sargent. In Berlin in 1885, DuBois-Reymond published *Physiology of Exercise*, which was translated into English in *Popular Science Monthly*. Following Sargent's lead in anthropometric measure-

Massengale, J.D., & Swanson, R.A. (Eds.) (1996). *History of exercise and sport sciences.* Champaign, IL: Human Kinetics.

ment, Seaver published *Anthropometric and Physical Examinations* in 1896.

The beginning of the 20th century saw a continuing interest in physical education research. In particular, an interest arose in tests of physical achievement and cardiovascular efficiency. Physicians (both inside and outside the physical education profession) showed increased interest in classifying people for exercise intensity based on cardiovascular function. At Springfield College (Massachusetts), James McCurdy (1895-1935) began studying changes occurring during adolescence in heart function and blood pressure. The first of the widely used cardiovascular efficiency tests was developed in 1917 by Schneider at Connecticut Wesleyan College and was used in World War I for evaluating the fitness of aviators.

Physical achievement testing advanced considerably in the early 1900s, and in 1922 the American Physical Education Association set up a committee under McCurdy's direction to develop motor ability tests. The two most recognized tests of the 1920s were Sargent's Physical Test of Man and Roger's Physical Fitness Index. By the 1930s many schools and colleges were administering physical achievement tests. In fact, this increase in motor performance and fitness testing probably led to the establishment in 1930 of *Research Quarterly* by the American Physical Education Association (for a review of the history of *RQ*, see Park, 1980). This was the first journal established specifically to report research in physical education.

The American Academy of Physical Education was established in 1926 with the purpose of electing outstanding scholars and leaders in the field to a limited and select membership. The Academy attempts to use the research knowledge developed by scholars in the field to influence the direction that the study of physical activity takes. The organization continues today under the name American Academy of Kinesiology and Physical Education with a maximum at one time of 125 elected Fellows. Since 1926 more than 350 outstanding scholars have been elected to membership.

In the 1930s, tests and measurements became the most active research area in physical education. Many physical fitness and motor ability tests were developed and widely used in both public schools and colleges and universities. Names of particular importance in test development were David Brace and C.H. McCloy.

The progressive education movement (1930s), frequently characterized as "teach what the child wants to learn," had a significant impact on both academic education and physical education. Physical educators concentrated on making the curriculum fun. This resulted in questionnaire research designed to discover what children liked to do. However, a statement by McCloy (1960) seemed to put everything into perspective: "I hope the next fifty years will cause physical education to . . . seek for facts, proved objectively; to question principles based on average opinions of people who don't know but are all anxious to contribute their average ignorance to form a consensus of uninformed dogma" (p. 91).

As testing became more popular in the schools during the 1930s, the use of true-false knowledge tests for physical education activities increased considerably. With the advent of new statistical techniques, both physical and knowledge tests were provided with increased scientific rigor and standards for physical education. Sometimes, however, the emphasis on numbers got out of hand: "We lived in one long orgy of tabulation. . . . Mountains of fact were piled up, condensed, summarized, and interpreted by the new quantitative technique. The air was full of normal curves, standard deviations, coefficients of correlation, regressive equations" (Rugg, 1941, p. 182).

Postwar Research

The outbreak of World War II brought renewed interest in physical fitness as large numbers of the men drafted did not meet the minimum standards for physical fitness. In fact, one third of the men examined were found unfit for service, and even those accepted generally lacked adequate levels of physical fitness. Many physical education leaders were assigned to test and condition servicemen. Thus, many advances were made in both testing and training in exercise physiology.

World War II also led to the development of the area known today as motor learning and control. Many psychologists were involved in developing pilot training programs. Considerable motor coordination is involved in learning to control an airplane, and this led to many studies of motor skill

Park, R.J. (1980). The *Research Quarterly* and its antecedents. *Research Quarterly for Exercise and Sport, 51,* 1-22.

performance and learning. Unfortunately, when the war ended, most of the interest in motor skill acquisition was lost as experimental psychologists returned to their interest in cognitive performance.

The 1950s brought a renewed interest in physical fitness. The 1953 publication of the Kraus-Weber test results revealed the poor record of American children when compared to European children. Although the test does not assess many of the factors considered important in fitness today (e.g., cardiovascular endurance and strength), the fact that nearly 60% of the American children failed compared to less than 9% of the European children attracted national attention. As a result, President Eisenhower called a special White House conference in 1956. This conference and several subsequent ones led to the establishment of the President's Council on Youth Fitness and the development of the AAHPERD Fitness Test. This boosted research in exercise physiology, tests, and measurements.

In the 1960s, research in physical education began to expand rapidly. Franklin Henry's historic memory drum theory (Henry & Rogers, 1960) launched a renewed interest in motor learning and control. Henry (1964) contributed further with his paper about physical education as a discipline. This led to the identification of a knowledge base for physical education that was frequently called human movement or physical activity. Research expanded dramatically as exercise physiology, biomechanics, motor learning and control, motor development, sport psychology, and sport sociology began to develop as subdisciplines and to produce knowledge about movement. The *Research Quarterly* was expanded, and such new journals as *Medicine and Science in Sport* and the *Journal of Motor Behavior* emerged.

The 1970s saw a continued interest in research in the study of physical activity, but renewed interest evolved in research within the professional base of physical education. Observational techniques were developed and refined that allowed accurate assessment of teaching behavior and student-teacher interaction. The area of classroom observation called "research on teaching" in education was developed for use in the gymnasium and playing fields in physical education. Research on curriculum theory in physical education, measurement and evaluation, and the history of sport and physical education received fresh attention.

Many researchers from the discipline of physical activity began to establish specific professional groups outside the traditional affiliations these researchers had held in AAHPERD. Such groups as the American College of Sports Medicine, the North American Society for Sport History, the North American Society for the Psychology of Sport and Physical Activity, and several others contributed to the research base. Responding to these inroads into membership and activities, AAHPERD created various academies, elevated the Research Consortium to the research arm of the alliance, and changed the name of *Research Quarterly* on its 50th anniversary to *Research Quarterly for Exercise and Sport*. In its first issue under the new name (Safrit, 1980), the editor and the advisory committee had solicited papers from the various subdisciplines in the study of physical activity: biomechanics, exercise physiology, psychology of sport, measurement and research design, sociology of sport, motor development, and motor behavior.

This increased emphasis on research in both the study of physical activity and the professional base of physical education can lead only to increased knowledge and higher scholarly standards. While the discipline based on the study of physical activity continues to undergo growing pains and an identity crisis (e.g., What shall we call ourselves—kinesiology, exercise and sport science, movement science?), quality graduate programs, research, and scholarship are evident. For example, a special issue of *Quest* was published in the fall of 1987 devoted completely to graduate education. New scholarly journals have evolved, particularly associated with specialized subareas of the discipline (e.g., *Journal of Exercise and Sport Psychology, Journal of Sport Sociology, Pediatric Exercise Science*).

School- and community-based exercise and sport skill programs are now refining their goals (developing physical fitness and motor skills) based on a solid knowledge of physical activity and on increased sophistication in planning and teaching children and adults. New scholarly journals have evolved in these areas, such as the *Journal of Teaching in Physical Education*, to accommodate the growth in knowledge produced. Each of these factors should result in a more knowledgeable, physically fit, and skillful population during the next 20 to 30 years.

Computers in Research and Scholarship

Using Personal Computers in Statistical Analysis and Scholarly Writing

Using Statistical Packages on Larger Mainframe Computers

Using Computers in Measuring Movement

In the two previous editions (1985, 1990) we have provided computer programs (1985) or the commands (1990) to use a commercial package (SPSSPC and SPSSX) for statistical analyses. That effort has not turned out to be very useful as the new editions and updates of the statistical packages occur more rapidly than we can revise this book. In fact, by the time the 1990 edition came out, SPSSPC had already moved to a Windows version and what we were telling you was not accurate for that version. Thus, we have decided not to attempt to offer computer commands and sample statistical runs with printouts here. Instead, we are going to describe how students and faculty might use computers in their research and scholarly work. We divide this section into three parts:

- Using personal computers in statistical analysis and scholarly writing
- Using statistical packages on larger mainframe computers
- Using computers to control experiments and collect data

Using Personal Computers in Statistical Analysis and Scholarly Writing

With today's technology, nearly all students and faculty have access to a relatively powerful personal computer. These computers typically have a point-and-click environment (e.g., Windows for IBM or compatibles, Macintosh) that allow the use of several programs simultaneously and the exporting and importing of data among programs. This permits the user to input research data (either manually or from computer storage) for statistical analysis, complete the analysis, export the data to a graphics program to produce figures and tables, and export the figures and tables to a word-processing program where the scholarly manuscript is being written. We have selected a sample of these three types of processes (statistical analysis—Statistical Package for the Social Sciences PC, graphics—Power Point, and word-processing—WordPerfect) that can be used in a compatible environment, and we will describe how they work. Each of these packages is compatible and can be used under a Windows environment (point-and-click) for IBM or compatible personal computers (at least a 386 and preferably a 486 machine). Both SPSSPC and Power Point also have versions for

Macintosh that can be used with a word-processing package like Word in the Macintosh's point-and-click environment. These programs have understandable manuals, and most have tutorials that take you through the types of things the programs will do. The commercial software packages named here are certainly not the only ones that are useful and available. It is just software that we have used and that works well in this circumstance.

Statistical Package for the Social Sciences—Personal Computer

This package is available for both personal computers and mainframe computers (large central computers at computer centers in the college or university). Increasingly as colleges and universities are moving to distributed computing and local area networks (LANs), the SPSSPC version is becoming more popular. With the increased level of power and technology of personal computers, even the multivariate statistical techniques are available for IBM and Macintosh. Only when researchers have very large data sets are the mainframe computers needed.

SPSSPC will allow you to input data and run jobs in an interactive mode (see page 450 for an example of how to get started): The computer lets you know at each step if you have made a mistake. SPSSPC offers a number of options to deal with your data once it is entered such as transformations, selection of cases, weighting and ordering cases, and restructuring files. It also offers procedure for describing and evaluating your data such as tabulation, frequencies, plots, means, standard deviations, ranges, skewness, kurtosis, cross-tabulations, and measures of association (e.g, r). Many sophisticated correlational techniques are available including multiple correlation, canonical correlation, factor analysis, and structural modeling. Procedures for estimating differences among groups include t tests, analysis of variance and covariance (simple and factorial), discriminant analysis, multivariate analysis of variance and covariance, and repeated measures designs. Also, many nonparametric procedures are available.

These programs are relatively easy to learn, and use menus and point-and-click procedures to simplify the tasks. Outputs for the analyses are effectively labeled for understanding. You can use the data from the problems in chapter 6, 7, and 8 (where you know the answers) to experiment with these programs.

Power Point (from Microsoft)

Power Point allows you to import data from SPSSPC (and other packages) for use in developing figures and tables. These figures and tables can be set up as slides or overhead, printed as hard copy, or exported into a word-processing program. Power Point has a variety of shapes, lines, and other design elements you can draw freehand, and you can use clip art. You have control over the fonts, type size, and colors you want to use. Power Point uses point-and-click technology within Windows.

WordPerfect

WordPerfect is just one of many word-processing programs, but it is a good one and quite popular. It offers many features that are useful in preparing manuscripts, both theses and dissertations, class papers, and journal papers. WordPerfect includes all the options we have come to expect in word-processing programs—editing, search and replace, spell checkers, thesaurus, flexible layouts, graphics, etc. You can set up tables in WordPerfect, or you can import tables and figures you have developed in a graphics program (e.g., Power Point). WordPerfect uses a point-and-click procedure in Windows.

Using Statistical Packages on Larger Mainframe Computers

SAS (Statistical Analysis System)

SAS Institute (1982). *SAS Users Guide: Statistics.* Cary, NC: SAS Institute

SAS is an acronym for Statistical Analysis System, which has developed into an all-purpose data analysis system that provides tools for information storage and retrieval, data modification and programming, report writing, statistical analysis, and file handling. However, in this book we are mainly concerned with the part of SAS that analyzes statistics.

The SAS statistical manual is divided into sections: Regression, Analysis of Variance, Categorical Data Analysis, Multivariate Methods, Discriminant Analysis, Clustering, Scoring, and MATRIX. Within each major section, an introductory chapter describes the procedures. Then, each procedure is explained in a separate chapter. Each chapter is divided into abstract, introduction, specifications, details, examples, and references.

The section on regression serves as a good example. The first chapter, "Introduction to SAS Regression Procedures," is followed by separate chapters:

NLIN—builds nonlinear regression models

REG—performs general purpose regression with many diagnostics and input/output capabilities

RSQUARE—builds models and shows fitness measures for all possible models

RSREG—builds quadratic response-surface regression models

STEPWISE—implements several stepping methods for selecting models

SAS runs interactively (communicates back and forth with a terminal) or in batch (all programming and data read in without stopping). The data can be input from cards, disks, or tape and organized into an SAS data set. Of course, all options may not be available at all computer centers.

SPSS (Statistical Package for the Social Sciences)

SPSS Inc. (1983). *SPSS User's Guide* . Chicago: SPSS Inc.

SPSS is an acronym for Statistical Package for the Social Sciences. Although older editions were not as flexible as SAS, the latest edition is quite flexible and usable. SPSS has features that allow you to verify and update data and to develop tables, reports, graphics, and comprehensive statistical procedures.

The SPSS manual is divided by sections according to statistical procedures. Suggested statistical guides and bibliographies are also included to aid the user in appropriate application. The statistical sections include the following:

Frequency Distributions and Descriptive Statistics

Relationships Between Two or More Variables (CROSSTABS)

Correlation Coefficients and Scatterplots

Multiple Regression Analysis

Factor Analysis

Discriminant Analysis

Survival Analysis

Analysis of Additive Scales

Nonparametric Statistics

Loglinear Models

Box-Jenkins Analysis of Time Series Data

Again to use regression as an example, SPSS allows six equation-building methods, including the following:

FORWARD—forward entry of variables with an entry criterion

BACKWARD—backward elimination of variables with removal criterion

STEPWISE—stepwise selection with both entry and removal criteria

ENTER—an option to control the order of entering variables

REMOVE—an option to force the order of variables removed

TEST—a means of testing specific subsets of variables for the maximum R^2

SPSS may be used interactively or through the batch mode if your computer center is set up for both.

BIMED (Biomedical Computer Programs, P-Series)(BMDP)

Dixon, W.J., & Brown, M.B. (1981). *BMDP Statistical Software 1981 Manual.* Berkeley, CA: University of California Press.

BMDP (or BIMED) is an acronym for Biomedical Computer Programs, P-Series. BIMED is one of the oldest (begun in 1961) and probably the most widely used mainframe statistical package. Although the programs have their own internal control language (which is consistent across programs), BMDP also allows user-specified FORTRAN (a popular computer language) statements.

The BMDP manual has seven introductory chapters to teach the use of the system, followed by the statistical section (each containing chapters for the various techniques):

Data Description

Data Into Groups

Plots and Histograms

Frequency Tables

Missing Values

Regression

Nonlinear Regression (maximum likelihood estimation)

Analysis of Variance and Covariance

Nonparametric Analysis

Survival Analysis

Time Series

Again using the regression section as an example, BMDP has five techniques for developing regression equations:

P1R—multiple linear regression using all the predictor variables

P2R—stepwise regression using either forward or backward stepping with specified criteria

P4R—regression on the principal components derived from the set of predictor variables

P5R—used when the criterion variable has nonlinear relationship to the predictors

P9R—regression using all possible subsets of predictor variables

Although BMDP is not as flexible for data management as SAS, the newer version is much improved. BMDP may be used interactively or in batch, depending on the capabilities of your computer center.

Using Computers in Measuring Movement

Whereas any type of computer can be used in measuring movement, microcomputers are the most common. These computers may be used in controlling data collection and recording data.

Controlling the Data-Collection Situation

Programs are frequently written for microcomputers that either partially or completely control the testing session. In a motor behavior experiment, the task might be to make either a long or a short movement when a stimulus light appears. A computer program can be written that works as follows:

1. The experimenter loads the program into the microcomputer before the subject arrives in the testing situation.
2. When the subject arrives, the experimenter enters his or her name, I.D. number, and any other pertinent characteristics, such as age, gender, handedness, and group.
3. The computer then displays a picture of the task and written instructions concerning how the subject is to perform.
4. The computer provides a set number of practice trials. After each trial, the subject is told his or her reaction time and movement time.
5. The computer controls all aspects of the experimental testing session, including flashing the warning light, flashing the movement signal, randomizing the interval between the warning and movement signals, controlling the interval between trials, providing results at a precise point between trials, and even retesting a trial if a reaction or movement time is outside a specified range.

Computers are typically used in exercise physiology laboratories for regulating the conditions of the exercise (e.g., speed and elevation of the treadmill) and controlling the time intervals for the various measurements that are taken during the exercise bout.

Recording and Reducing the Data

In the previously described situation, the microcomputer is also used to record the data after each trial.

Sometimes, however, the micro might be used to record data but not to control the data-collection situation. For example, an observer could enter data directly into a micro while observing a physical education class. If a program were written to handle data for the ALT-PE coding instrument (Siedentop et al., 1979; 1982), the data could be entered into a micro as easily as it could be written on a code sheet.

Computers may be used in reducing the data to usable form. For example, biomechanists often use high-speed video to record a subject's movement. This video is then used with computer software to reduce this movement to quantifiable units. The x, y, and z coordinates of a joint center (e.g., elbow) during each frame of the video can be digitized to provide data to determine accelerations and velocities to use in analyses.

Limitations

The limitations in using microcomputers are easily observed. First, micros cost money. Second, once the micro is obtained, it must be interfaced with the equipment, and programs must be written to control the experimental situation and reduce the data. Because these programs may be unique to the experiment being conducted, they may not be available commercially. Thus, technical support must be obtained. Finally, micros are not maintenance free; they require supplies such as disks, and eventually they may need additional hardware and more advanced programs to work effectively.

SPSS for Windows: Getting Started

1. The SPSS Windows screen will have three boxes or windows:

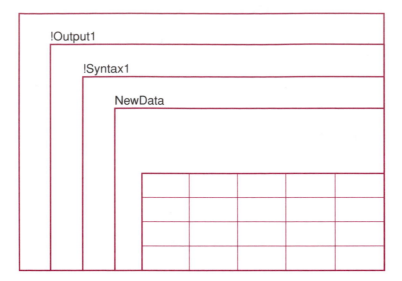

2. SPSS operates when you click the mouse (left button) once or twice. To start a new problem (or enter data for a new data set) you will click in the upper left corner of the NEWDATA window. A menu will give you choices; select **Maximize** and the screen will fill with the NEWDATA window. The top row has VAR over each column. The cursor will be blinking in a blank box above the row called VAR. You will need to do two things, which can be done in either order.

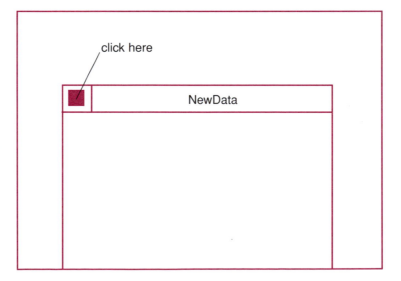

a. **Type in data:** Type the numbers (or letters) for a variable, then hit enter. SPSS automatically moves the number from the box into the row and column that is highlighted in bold. You can move the bold column by putting the crosshairs (the circle with a vertical and horizontal line through) and clicking, or by using the arrows to move the bold box. If your cursor is not at the top of the screen in the box above the VAR row, you can move it there and click the mouse button to begin.

b. **Define the variables:** At the top of the screen, above the NEWDATA window is a list of words (FILE, EDIT, DATA, TRANSFORM, STATISTICS, GRAPHS, etc.). Move the crosshairs to the top, until they become an arrow, place the arrow in DATA, and click. A menu will drop down. You can hit enter, since DEFINE VARIABLE will already be highlighted, or use the mouse to select DEFINE VARIABLE. A new screen will appear which allows you to
  • name the variable (currently VAR001),
  • label the variable (give a longer name or description—this is especially important for thesis data),
  • change or give other characteristics (e.g., if it is a word or letter select string), and
  • give value labels (1=experimental, 2=control).

3. **To save your data set**, click on FILE, then SAVE. For a data set you must save the file with a name (up to six letters followed by .sav). This is very important. If you want to save to a disk, be sure to use the appropriate prefix (e.g., a: or b:).

Sample: resmet.sav

You could stop now and begin again by asking for your data set. To do that see step 6.

4. To **analyze** your data set you will select the STATISTICS button on the top row. The drop-down menu has many choices. Click on one and GO FOR IT!

5. Your analysis will be shown on your screen in the **!OUTPUT1** window. If you want to see further down the page or to the side, click on the arrows on the bottom or left side of the screen. To print, you can click on **FILE** and then **PRINT** in the drop-down menu. You can also use edit to copy the output to a word-processing file. The advantage of this is that you can cut the output to fit a page. The print function from OUTPUT does not always look neat because it doesn't end at the end of a page of paper. You can save your output in either an output file or a word-processing file. Nothing in your data set is damaged if you don't save your output. However, if you fail to save your data set, you are in BIG trouble!

6. Now, suppose you need to get back into a data set for corrections or more analysis. From the opening windows cascade (as in step 1) you click on **FILE** and from the drop-down menu select **OPEN** by clicking. A side menu will appear. Select **DATA**. You can either type in your file name or click on your file if it appears in the box. Click on **OKAY**. Your data set should appear.

Sample Consent Forms

Sample Form D.1

LOG #HS-_____

Application for the Conduct of Research Involving Human Subjects
Arizona State University
University Human Subjects Research Review Committee

The Arizona State University Human Subjects Research Review Committee reviews all requests to conduct research involving human subjects. In completing the following application, be advised that the persons reviewing it may be entirely unfamiliar with the field of study involved. Present the request in typewritten form and in nontechnical terms understandable to the committee. It is the investigator's responsibility to give information about research procedure that is most likely to entail risk *but not to express judgment about the risk*. Please submit a copy of your complete proposal, an informed-consent/assent form as subjects will view it, and a curriculum vita or biographical sketch.

Principal investigator/director:	Department/center:	Date of request:

Type of review: New ☐   Renewal ☐   Continuation ☐
  Exempt ☐   Identify by numbers that apply (see page 2) _____
  Expedite ☐   Identify by numbers that apply (see page 4) _____
  If Renewal or Continuation, are there any substantive changes? Yes ☐ No ☐

Project title:

Agency submitted to:	Submission date:	Location of project:

1. General purpose of the research:

2. Data obtained by: Mail ☐   Telephone ☐   Interview ☐
          Observation ☐   Experiment ☐   Secondary Source ☐
          Other (explain) _____

3. Project description: The committee must have sufficient information, nontechnical and detailed, about what will happen with/to subjects to evaluate/estimate the risks. Assurance from the investigator, no matter how strong, will not substitute for a description of the transaction between investigator and subject. *If a questionnaire is used, attach a copy.*

Sample Form D.1   *(continued)*

When visual or auditory stimuli, chemical substances, or other measures might affect the health of subjects, a statement from a qualified person or other appropriate documentation will aid in evaluating the nature of any risk created. In questionable cases, the committee will require such documentation.

---

4. Subject selection: Will subjects be less than 18 years of age?   Yes ☐   No ☐

How many subjects will participate? _____   Male ☐   Female ☐   Age ____ to _____

Will subjects be students at Arizona State University?   Yes ☐   No ☐

Source: _____

---

5. How will subjects be selected, enlisted, or recruited?

---

6. How will subjects be informed of procedures, intent of the study, and potential risks to them?

---

7. What steps will be taken to allow subjects to withdraw at any time without prejudice?

---

8. How will subjects' privacy be maintained and confidentiality guaranteed?

Attachments: Please indicate those items we can expect to find as attachments.

Complete proposal   ☐   Informed-consent form (as subjects will view it)   ☐

Questionnaire   ☐   Assent form (as child will view it)   ☐

Other instrumentation   ☐   Curriculum vita or biographical sketch   ☐

Other documentation _____

In making this application, I certify that I have read and understand the *Policies and Procedures for Projects that Involve Human Subjects*, and that I intend to comply with the letter and spirit of the university policy. Significant changes in the protocol will be submitted to the committee for written approval prior to these changes being put into practice. Informed-consent/assent records of the subjects will be kept for at least (3) years after the completion of the research.

| Signatures: *Principal investigator (faculty)* | *Department chair* | Date |

This application has been reviewed by the Arizona State University IRB:

Full Board Review ☐   Exempt ☐   Expedite ☐   Categories: _____

Approved ☐   Deferred ☐   Disapproved ☐

Project requires review more often than annual ☐   every _____ months.

Renewal or continuation ☐   Approved with no substantive changes ☐

Disapproved ☐   Approved with changes attached ☐

Third-party verification sought ☐

Comments, modification/conditions for approval, or reason for disapproval:

Signature:

Chair of the University Committee   Date

Sample Form D.2

Informed-Consent Form for Adults

Read and address each numbered element of this model form in developing an informed-consent form for the proposed human research study. The items numbered and in quotations are to be included in the consent form. PLEASE NUMBER THE CONSENT FORM FOR SUBMISSION TO THE COMMITTEE. You may request the numbering be waived during data collection. The consent form must be written in lay language and must be typewritten. The language may be further simplified to meet the needs of a specific population. Add additional statements when appropriate.

1. *"Investigator's name*, who is *title/position*, has requested my participation in a research study at this institution. The title of the research is *title of research*."* [Place title of project at top of all pages of consent form.]

2. "I have been informed that the purpose of the research is to . . ." [Describe the justification for the research. If appropriate, include the number of subjects involved and why the subject is included.]

3. "My participation will involve . . ." [Describe the subject's participation and identify those aspects of participation that are experimental. Indicate the expected duration of the subject's participation.]

4. "I understand there are foreseeable risks or discomforts to me if I agree to participate in the study. The possible risks are . . ." "Possible discomforts include . . ." [Any foreseeable risks or discomforts are to be explained/described.]

   OR

   "There are no foreseeable risks or discomforts."

5. "I understand that there are alternative procedures available. Alternative procedures include . . ." [Describe any alternative procedures to be included in language the subject can understand.]

   OR

   "There are no feasible alternative procedures available for this study."

6. "I understand that the possible benefits of my participation in the research are . . ." [Describe the benefits of participation, or lack of benefits, to the individual subject as well as to society.]

7. "I understand that the results of the research study may be published but that my name or identify will not be revealed. In order to maintain confidentiality of my records, *name of investigator* will . . ." [Indicate specifically how the investigator will keep the names of the subjects confidential, the use of subject codes, how this information will be secured, and who will have access to the confidential information. "Confidentiality will be maintained" is not acceptable.]

8. "I understand that in case of injury I can expect to receive the following treatment or care which will be provided at my expense:" [If *more* than minimal risk of foreseeable injury is anticipated, describe the facilities, medical treatment, or services that will be made available in the event of injury or illness to a subject. Description may include on- and off-campus services.]

   OR

   "I have been advised that the research in which I will be participating does not involve more than minimal risk." [If the research will *not* involve more than minimal risk, briefly explain how or why the investigator determined that the subject would be exposed to no more than minimal risk.]

9. "I have been informed that I will be compensated for my participation as follows:" [If compensation is to be provided to subject, include amount of compensation, method of payment, and schedule for payment including whether payment will be made in increments or in one lump sum.]

   OR

   "I have been informed that I will not be compensated for my participation."

Sample Form D.2   *(continued)*

10. "I have been informed that any questions I have concerning the research study or my participation in it, before or after my consent, will be answered by *name of individual, address, and telephone number*." [This refers to the principal investigator. In the event the investigator is a student, the name of the doctoral or thesis advisor (responsible faculty member) must be included.]

11. "I understand that in case of injury, if I have questions about my rights as a subject/participant in this research, or if I feel I have been placed at risk, I can contact the Chair of the Human Subjects Research Review Committee." [This information must be included in all consent forms.]

12. "I have read the above information. The nature, demands, risks, and benefits of the project have been explained to me. I knowingly assume the risks involved, and understand that I may withdraw my consent and discontinue participation at any time without penalty or loss of benefit to myself. In signing this consent form, I am not waiving any legal claims, rights, or remedies. A copy of this consent form will be given to me."

Subject's signature _____ Date _____

Other signature (if appropriate) _____ Date _____

13. "I certify that I have explained to the above individual the nature and purpose, the potential benefits, and possible risks associated with participation in this research study, have answered any questions that have been raised, and have witnessed the above signature."

14. "These elements of informed consent conform to the Assurance given by Arizona State University to the Department of Health and Human Services to protect the rights of human subjects."

15. "I have provided the subject/participant a copy of this signed consent document."

Signature of investigator _____ Date _____

Sample Form D.3

Informed–Consent Form for Minors

The elements of the informed-consent form for adults are used with the following variations:

1. *"Investigator's name,* who is *title/position* at Arizona State University, has requested my minor child's (ward's) participation in a research study at this institution. The title of the research is *title of research."*
2. [same as adult]
3. "My child's (ward's) participation will involve . . ."
4. [same as adult]
5. [same as adult]
6. "I understand that the possible benefits of my child's (ward's) participation in the research are . . ."
7. "I understand that the results of the research study may be published but that my child's (ward's) name or identity will not be revealed. In order to maintain confidentiality of my child's (ward's) records, *name of investigator* will . . ."
8. "I understand that in case of injury I can expect the following treatment or care to be provided at my expense . . ."

   OR

   "I have been advised that the research in which my child (ward) will be participating does not involve more than minimal risk."
9. "I have been informed that compensation for participation is as follows: . . ."

   OR

   "I have been informed that I will not be compensated for my child's (ward's) participation."
10. [same as adult]
11. [same as adult]
12. [same as adult]

Subject's signatur _____   Date _____
(father, mother, legal guardian, or legally authorized official)

Other signature _____   Date _____

13. [same as adult]
14. [same as adult]
15. [same as adult]

Sample Form D.4

Child Assent Form

Language must be simplified as appropriate for the age-group used as subjects, such as:

I, _____, understand that my parents (mom and dad) have given

permission (said it's okay) for me to take part in a project about _____

_____

done by _____

    I am taking part because I want to, and I have been told that I can stop at any time I want to and I won't get in trouble (nothing bad will happen to me if I want to stop).

_____

Signature

OR

I, _____, understand that my parents have given permission for me

to participate in a study concerning _____

_____

under the direction of _____

    My involvement in this project is voluntary, and I have been told that I may withdraw from participation in this study at any time without penalty and loss of benefit to myself.

_____

Signature

Sample Form D.5

Date filed: _____   Project no.: _____

Animal Protocol Review
Arizona State University Animal Care and Use Committee

Please read "Instructions for Completing Animal Protocol Review."

I. A. A single member of the university faculty and/or principal investigator is considered the responsible individual.

   Name: _____   Campus phone: _____

   B. University position and department: _____

   C. Project/program title: _____

   _____

   D. ___ Nonfunded research   ___ Teaching   ___ Grant/contract

   E. Protocol type: New ___   Renewal ___   Revision ___   Previous no. ___

   F. Research (see 1, 2, 3, and 4 below): ___

   Teaching (see 5 and 6 below): ___

   1. Granting agency: _____   Deadline: _____

   2. Coinvestigator(s): _____

   3. Graduate student: _____   Phone: _____

   4. Thesis/research degree program: _____

   _____

   5. Course title, schedule: _____

   6. Teaching assistant/laboratory instructor(s): _____

   _____

II. A. List species:

   B. Where will you prefer animals be housed? _____

   C. Does project require a waiver of provision(s) of PHS policy?

   No ___ Yes ___   (If yes, attach a Request of Waiver statement justifying the need for the waiver.)

   Review date(s): _____   Approval date: _____

   Signature, Chair: _____

III. A. *Abstract of planned use of animals.* Write a brief yet complete description of the planned use of animals. (Use additional pages if necessary.) Use language understandable to a layperson. One complete copy of a grant proposal or graduate student research proposal must be attached to the original.

   B. *Rationale for involving animals and the appropriateness of the species and number used* (include potential contribution the species may generate and state briefly why living vertebrates are required rather than some alternate model).

Sample Form D.5 *(continued)*

IV. Animals to be used:

    A. Species (give both scientific and common names for unusual species):
       Is this a threatened or endangered species? Yes ____ No ____

    B. Estimated number: Per year _____ Entire study _____
       Are these estimated number of animals maximum for the entire study?
                      Yes ____   No ____

    C. Sex and age (or weight range): _____

    D. Source (e.g., purchased, institutional breed, transferred from another study, donated, captured from wild):

       _____

    E. Will animals stay in investigator's lab at any time?   Yes ____   No ____
       If so, how long? _____
       If greater than 24 hours, state justification: _____

       _____

    All facilities or laboratories that house animals for longer than 24 hours must be inspected and approved according to DHEW policy.

V.   Major categories of use:

    Please check those applicable and attach appropriate sections concerning methodology from your grant proposal or a brief description of the methodology to be used in nonfunded project or course.

Yes   No

____   ____   a. Harvest tissue, blood, etc.

____   ____   b. Immunization for antibody production; describe antigen adjuvant used, route of immunization, method of obtaining blood.

____   ____   c. Physiologic measurements; if surgery is necessary, see "n."

____   ____   d. Dietary manipulations (e.g., caloric restrictions, specific constituent restriction).

____   ____   e. Pharmacologic/toxicologic material used, route of administration, etc.

____   ____   f. Immunologic studies.

____   ____   g. Behavioral studies.

____   ____   h. Irradiation; include Radioisotope Approval Form.

____   ____   i. Biohazardous materials (carcinogens, chemicals, etc.); include Biohazard Approval Form.

____   ____   j. Infectious agents; include Biohazard Approval Form.

____   ____   k. *Trauma, injury, burning, freezing, electric shock.

____   ____   l. *Environmental stress (e.g., temperature, long-term restraint, forced exercise, nutritional distress).

____   ____   m. Other: _____

____   ____   n. Surgery: *If "Yes," complete Item VI below.*

               *Submit necessary justifications(s).

(continued)

Sample Form D.5 *(continued)*

VI. Surgical procedures:

A. Survival* _____   Nonsurvival _____
*All survival surgery will be performed under aseptic conditions.

B. Where is surgery to be performed?

C. Person performing surgery; person's qualifications: _____
_____

D. Anesthetic regimen:

Drug: _____   Dose: _____

Route: _____   Duration: _____

Monitoring procedures:

Who will administer/monitor anesthesia, and what are their qualifications?
_____

If anesthetics are not used, justify: _____
_____

E. Postoperative pain or distress:

Is postoperative pain or distress anticipated?   Yes ___   No ___

Will analgesics/tranquilizers be used?   Yes ___   No ___

Drug: _____   Dose: _____

Route: _____   Duration: _____

If pain/distress are anticipated but analgesics/tranquilizers will not be used, attach Justification of Pain or Distress statement.
_____

F. Postoperative care:

Intensive care required?   Yes ___   No ___

What time period? _____

Who will provide care? _____

Postoperative routine:

Who will provide? _____

What monitoring will be performed? _____

What drugs administered? _____

Antibiotics (type/dosage/frequency)? _____

Special care to be provided: _____
_____

Person(s) to contact in case of emergency:
_____

Phone: Office _____   Home _____

What postoperative complications may be expected? _____
_____

Method of treatment: _____
_____

Sample Form D.5 *(continued)*

    G. Multiple surgical procedures: Will individual animals be subjected to more than one surgical procedure? ___ Yes ___ No

       If yes, provide justification.

    H. Have all personnel on this protocol been certified in the federal mandated training requirement? ___ Yes ___ No

VII. Euthanasia

    A. What is (are) method(s) of euthanasia?

       Chemical/gas: Agent _____ Dose _____

                  Agent _____ Dose _____

       Physical: ___ Cervical dislocation (mice, immature rats)

              ___ Decapitation (rodents)

              ___ Captive bolt

              ___ Exsanguination under anesthesia

              ___ Other* _____

              ___ *Scientific justification (references if possible):

                  _____

    B. Name any qualifications of person(s) performing euthanasia:

       _____

       _____

VIII. Assurance:

The information contained herein is accurate to the best of my knowledge. Procedures involving animals will be carried out humanely, and all procedures will be performed by or under the direction of trained or experienced persons. Any revisions to animal care and use in this project will be promptly forwarded to the Animal Care and Use Committee for review. *Revised protocols will not be used until committee clearance is received. The use of alternatives to animal models has been considered and found to be unacceptable at this time.*

_____   _____

Signature (individual listed on I.A. and graduate student,   Date
if applicable)

IX. Additional approval:

    The department chair and the college dean must sign the protocol after approval by the Animal Care and Use Committee.

_____   _____

Chair   Date

_____   _____

Dean   Date

References

Adams, J.A. (1971). A closed-loop theory of motor learning. *Journal of Motor Behavior*, **3**, 111-150.

Adelman, M.L. (1983, spring). "Academicians and American athletics: A decade of progress," *Journal of Sport History*, **10**, 80-106.

Adelman, M.L. (1986). *A sporting time: New York City and the rise of modern athletics, 1820-1870*. Urbana: University of Illinois Press.

Agar, M.H. (1986). *Speaking of ethnography*. Beverly Hills, CA: Sage.

American Alliance for Health, Physical Education, Recreation and Dance. (1980). *AAHPERD health related physical fitness test manual*. Reston, VA: Author.

American Association for Health, Physical Education and Recreation. (1958). *AAHPER youth fitness test manual*. Washington, DC: Author.

American Psychological Association. (1959). *Graduate education in psychology*. Washington, DC: Author.

American Psychological Association. (1994). *Publication manual of the American Psychological Association* (4th ed.). Washington, DC: Author.

Anon. (1835, June). The great foot race. *American Turf Register and Sporting Magazine*, **6**, 518-520.

Anshel, M.H., & Marisi, D.Q. (1978). Effects of music and rhythm on physical performance. *Research Quarterly*, **49**, 109-115.

Appleby, J. (1978). Modernization theory and the formation of modern social theories in England and America. *Comparative Studies in Society and History*, **20**, 261.

Appleby, J., Hunt, L., & Jacob, M. (1994). *Telling the truth about history*. New York.

Arlin, M. (1977). One-study publishing typifies educational inquiry. *Educational Researcher*, **6**(9), 11-15.

Atkinson, R.F. (1978). *Knowledge and explanation in history*. Ithaca: Cornell University Press.

Bain, L.L. (1989). Interpretive and critical research in sport and physical education. *Research Quarterly for Exercise and Sport*, **60**, 21-24.

Barnes, B. (1982). *T.S. Kuhn and social science*. New York: Columbia University Press.

Barnett, V., & Lewis, T. (1978). *Outliers in statistical data*. New York: Wiley.

Barzun, J., & Graff, H.F. (1977). *The modern researcher* (3rd ed.). New York.

Baumgartner, T.A. (1989). Norm-referenced measurement: Reliability. In M.J. Safrit & T.M. Wood (Eds.), *Measurement concepts in physical education and exercise science* (pp. 45-72). Champaign, IL: Human Kinetics.

Baumgartner, T.A., & Jackson, A.S. (1991). *Measurement for evaluation in physical education* (4th ed.). Dubuque, IA: Wm. C. Brown.

Baxter, N. (1993-94, winter). Is there another degree in your future? Choosing among professional and graduate schools. *Occupational Outlook Quarterly*, pp. 19-49.

Behnke, A.R., & Wilmore, J.H. (1974). *Evaluation and regulation of body build and composition*. Englewood Cliffs, NJ: Prentice Hall.

Bender, T. (1986, June). Wholes and parts: The need for synthesis in American history. *Journal of American History*, **73**, 120-136.

Bentham, J. (1970). *Introduction to the principles of morals and legislation*. London: Athalone Press.

Berelson, B. (1960). *Graduate education in the United States*. New York: McGraw-Hill.

Berryman, J.W., & Park, R.J. (Eds.) (1992). *Sport and exercise science: Essays in the history of sports medicine*. Urbana: University of Illinois Press.

Betz, N.E. (1987). Use of discriminant analysis in counseling psychology research. *Journal of Counseling Psychology*, **34**, 393-403.

Blair, S.N. (1993). Physical activity, physical fitness, and health (1993 C.H. McCloy Research Lecture). *Research Quarterly for Exercise and Sport*, **64**, 365-376.

Bogdan, R.C., & Biklen, S.K. (1992). *Qualitative research for education: An introduction to theory and methods*. Boston: Allyn & Bacon.

Boorman, M.A. (1990). *Effect of age and menopausal status on cardiorespiratory fitness in masters women endurance athletes*. M.S. thesis, Arizona State University, Tempe.

Borg, G.A. (1962). *Physical performance and perceived exertion*. Lund, Sweden: Gleerup.

Borg, W.R., & Gall, M.D. (1989). *Educational research* (5th ed.). New York: Longman.

Bouchard, C., Shepard, R.J., & Stephens, T. (Eds.). (1994). *Physical activity, fitness, and health*. Champaign, IL: Human Kinetics.

Boyer, C.J. (1973). *The doctoral dissertation as an informational source: A study of scientific information flow*. Metuchen, NJ: Scarecrow Press.

Braudel, F. (1980). *On history* (Sarah Matthews, Trans.) (pp. 25-54). Chicago: University of Chicago Press.

Brown, J.A.C. (1954). *The social psychology of industry*. Middlesex, England: Penguin.

Burgess, R.G. (Ed.) (1982). *Field research: A source book and field manual*. London: G. Allen & Unwin.

Burke, P. (1980). *Sociology and history*. London: G. Allen & Unwin.

Butsch, R. (Ed.). (1990). *For fun and profit: The transformation of leisure into consumption*. Philadelphia: Temple University Press.

Callinicos, A. (1988). *Making history*. Ithaca: Cornell University Press.

Carlberg, C.C., Johnson, D.W., Johnson, R., Maruyama, G., Kavale, K., Kulik, C., Kulik, J.A., Lysakowski, R.S., Pflaum, S.W., & Walberg, H. (1984). Meta-analysis in education: A reply to Slavin. *Educational Researcher*, **13**(4), 16-23.

Carron, A.V., Widmeyer, W.N., & Brawley, L.R. (1985). The development of an instrument to assess cohesion in sport teams: The group environment questionnaire. *Journal of Sport Psychology*, **7**, 244-266.

Cartmell, M. (1993). *A view to a death in the morning: Hunting and nature through history*. Cambridge: Harvard University Press.

Cheffers, J.T.F. (1973). The validation of an instrument design to expand the Flanders' system of interaction analysis to describe nonverbal interaction, different varieties of teacher behavior and pupil responses (Doctoral dissertation, Temple University, Philadelphia, 1972). *Dissertation Abstracts International*, **34**, 1674a.

Chien, I. (1981). Appendix: An introduction to sampling. In L.H. Kidder (Ed.), *Selltiz, Wrightsman, and Cook's research methods in social relations* (4th ed.). New York: Holt, Rinehart & Winston.

Christina, R.W. (1989). Whatever happened to applied research in motor learning? In J.S. Skinner et al. (Eds.), *Future directions in exercise and sport science research* (pp. 411-422). Champaign, IL: Human Kinetics.

Chronicle of Higher Education. (1983, September 14). APA Statement on authorship of research papers. *Chronicle of Higher Education*, **27**, 7.

Clarke, H.H. (Ed.) (1968, December). *Physical Fitness Newsletter*, **14**(4).

Clarke, H.H., & Clarke, D.H. (1970). *Research processes in physical education, recreation, and health*. Englewood Cliffs, NJ: Prentice Hall.

Cohen, J. (1969). *Statistical power analysis for the behavioral sciences* (2nd ed.). New York: Academic Press.

Cohen, J. (1990). Things I have learned (so far). *American Psychologist*, **45**, 1304-1312.

Cohen, J., & Cohen, P. (1983). *Applied multiple regression in behavioral research*. New York: Holt, Rinehart & Winston.

Conover, W.J. (1971). *Practical nonparametric statistics*. New York: Wiley.

Cook, T.D., & Campbell, D.T. (1979). *Quasi-experimentation: Design and analysis issues for field settings*. Chicago: Rand-McNally.

Cooper, H., & Hedges, L.V. (Eds.) (1994). *The handbook of research synthesis*. New York: Sage Foundation.

Coorough, C., & Nelson, J.K. (in press). The dissertation in education from 1950 to 1990. *Educational Research Quarterly for Exercise and Sport*.

Costill, D.L. (1985). Practical problems in exercise physiology research. *Research Quarterly for Exercise and Sport*, **56**, 378-384.

Crase, D., & Rosato, F.D. (1992). Single versus multiple authorship in professional journals. *Journal of Physical Education, Recreation & Dance*, **63**(7), 28-31.

Creswell, J.W. (1994). *Research design: Qualitative and quantitative approaches.* Thousand Oaks, CA: Sage.

Crews, D.J., & Landers, D.M. (1987). A meta-analytic review of aerobic fitness and reactivity to psychosocial stressors. *Medicine and Science in Sports and Exercise*, **19** (suppl. 5), 120-144.

Cronbach, L. (1951). Coefficient alpha and the internal structure of tests. *Psychometrika*, **16**, 297-334.

Davidson, M.L. (1972). Univariate versus multivariate tests in repeated-measures experiments. *Psychological Bulletin*, **77**, 446-452.

Day, R.D. (1983). *How to write and publish a scientific paper* (2nd ed.). Philadelphia: ISI Press.

Day, R.D. (1988). *How to write and publish a scientific paper* (3rd ed.). Phoenix: Oryx Press.

Denton, J.J., & Tsai, C. (1991). Two investigations into the influence of incentives and subject characteristics on mail survey responses in teacher education. *Journal of Experimental Education*, **59**, 352-366.

Dillman, D.A. (1978). *Mail and telephone survey: The total design method.* New York: Wiley.

Dolgener, F.A., Hensley, L.D., Marsh, J.J., & Fjelstul, J.K. (1994). Validation of the Rockport Fitness Walking Test in college males and females. *Research Quarterly for Exercise and Sport*, **65**, 152-158.

Drowatzky, J.N. (1993). Ethics, codes, and behavior. *Quest*, **45**, 22-31.

Edwards, A.L. (1957). *Techniques of attitude and scale construction.* New York: Appleton-Century-Crofts.

Erickson, F. (1986). Qualitative methods in research on teaching. In M.C. Wittrock (Ed.), *Handbook of research on teaching* (3rd ed.) (pp. 119-161). New York: Macmillan.

Fabian, A. (1990). *Card sharps, dream books, and bucket shops: Gambling in 19th-century America.* Ithaca: Cornell University Press.

Fahlberg, L.L., & Fahlberg, L.A. (1994). A human science for the study of movement: An integration of multiple ways of knowing. *Research Quarterly for Exercise and Sport*, **65**, 100-109.

Falk, J.D. (1989, May/June). OCLC and RLIN: research libraries at the scholar's fingertips. *American Historical Association Newsletter Perspectives*, **27**, 1, 11-13, 17.

Farquhar, A.B., & Farquhar, H. (1891). *Economic and industrial delusions: A discourse of the case for protection.* New York: Putnam.

Fassinger, R.E. (1987). Use of structural equation modeling in counseling psychology research. *Journal of Counseling Psychology*, **34**, 425-436.

Feltz, D.L., & Landers, D.M. (1983). The effects of mental practice on motor skill learning and performance: A meta-analysis. *Journal of Sport Psychology*, **5**, 25-57.

Fielding, N.G., & Fielding, J.L. (1986). *Linking data.* Beverly Hills, CA: Sage.

Fine, M.A., & Kurdek, L.A. (1993). Reflections on determining authorship credit and authorship order on faculty-student collaborations. *American Psychologist*, **48**, 1141-1147.

Firestone, W.A. (1987). Meaning in method: The rhetoric of quantitative and qualitative research. *Educational Researcher*, **16**(7), 16-21.

Flanders, N.A. (1970). *Analyzing teaching behavior.* Reading, MA: Addison-Wesley.

Fowler, F.J., Jr. (1988). *Survey research methods.* Newbury Park, CA: Sage.

Fowler, H.W., & Fowler, F.G. (1954). *The king's English.* Oxford: Oxford University Press.

Fraleigh, W. (1984). *Right actions in sport: Ethics for contestants.* Champaign, IL: Human Kinetics.

Franks, B.D., & Huck, S.W. (1986). Why does everyone use the .05 significance level? *Research Quarterly for Exercise and Sport*, **57**, 245-249.

French, K.E. (1985). *The relation of knowledge development to children's basketball performance.* Unpublished doctoral dissertation, Louisiana State University, Baton Rouge.

French, K.E., & Thomas, J.R. (1987). The relation of knowledge development to children's basketball performance. *Journal of Sport Psychology*, **9**, 15-32.

Gagan, D.P., George, P.J., & Oksanen, E.H. (1986, winter). On regression models with observation-specific dummy variables. *Historical Methods*, **19**, 5-8.

Garcia, C. (1994). Gender differences in young children's interactions when learning fundamental motor skills. *Research Quarterly for Exercise and Sport*, **65**, 213-225.

Giddens, A. (1984). *The constitution of society.* Berkeley: University of California.

Giddens, A. (1987). *Sociology: A brief but critical introduction* (pp. 11-12). New York.

Gill, D.L., & Deeter, T.E. (1988). Development of the Sport Orientation Questionnaire. *Research Quarterly for Exercise and Sport*, **59**, 191-202.

Glaser, B.G., & Strauss, A.L. (1967). *The discovery of grounded theory.* Chicago: Aldine.

Glass, G.V. (1976). Primary, secondary, and meta-analysis. *Educational Researcher*, **5**, 3-8.

Glass, G.V. (1977). Integrating findings: The meta-analysis of research. *Review of Research in Education*, **5**, 351-379.

Glass, G.V., McGaw, B., & Smith, M. (1981). *Meta-analysis in social research*. Beverly Hills, CA: Sage.

Glass, G.V., & Smith, M.L. (1979). Meta-analysis of research on the relationship of class-size and achievement. *Evaluation and Policy Analysis, 1*, 2-16.

Glassford, R.G. (1987). Methodological reconsideration: The shifting paradigms. *Quest, 39*, 295-312.

Goetz, J.P., & LeCompte, M.D. (1984). *Ethnography and qualitative design in educational research*. Orlando, FL: Academic Press.

Goodrich, J.E., & Roland, C.G. (1977). Accuracy of published medical reference citations. *Journal of Technical Writing and Communication, 7*, 15-19.

Gorn, E. (1986). *The manly art: Bare-knuckle prize fighting in America*. Ithaca: Cornell University Press.

Grabe, S.A., & Widule, C.J. (1988). Comparative biomechanics of the jerk in Olympic weight lifting. *Research Quarterly for Exercise and Sport, 59*, 1-8.

Graves, R.M., & Kahn, R.L. (1979). *Surveys by telephone: A national comparison with personal interviews*. New York: Academic Press.

Green, K.E. (1991). Reluctant respondents: Differences between early, late, and nonresponders to a mail survey. *Journal of Experimental Education, 59*, 268-276.

Green, S.B. (1991). How many subjects does it take to do a regression analysis? *Multivariate Behavioral Research, 26*, 499-510.

Greenockle, K.M., Lee, A.M., & Lomax, R. (1990). The relation between selected student characteristics and activity patterns in required high school physical education class. *Research Quarterly for Exercise and Sport, 61*, 59-69.

Griffin, P., & Templin, T.J. (1989). An overview of qualitative research. In P.W. Darst, D.B. Zakrajsek, & V.H. Mancini (Eds.), *Analyzing physical education and sport instruction* (2nd ed.) (pp. 399-410). Champaign, IL: Human Kinetics.

Grover, K. (Ed.) (1989). *Fitness in American culture: Images of health, sport, and the body, 1830-1940*. Amherst: University of Massachusetts Press.

Gruneau, R. (1983). *Class, sports, and social development*. Amherst, MA: University of Massachusetts Press.

Guba, E.G., & Lincoln, Y.S. (1981). *Effective evaluation*. San Francisco: Jossey-Bass.

Guttmann, A. (1978). *From ritual to record: The nature of modern sport*. New York: Columbia University Press.

Haase, R.F., & Ellis, M.V. (1987). Multivariate analysis of variance. *Journal of Counseling Psychology, 34*, 404-413.

Hackensmith, C.W. (1966). *History of physical education*. New York: Harper & Row.

Hall, J.R. (1984, fall). Temporality, social action, and the problem of quantification in historical analysis, *Historical Methods, 17*, 206-218.

Halverson, L.E., Roberton, M.A., & Langendorfer, S. (1982). Development of the overarm throw: Movement and ball velocity changes by seventh grade. *Research Quarterly for Exercise and Sport, 53*, 198-205.

Hambleton, R.K., & Novick, M.R. (1973). Toward an integration of theory and method for criterion-referenced tests. *Journal of Educational Measurement, 10*, 159-170.

Hamlyn, D.W. (1990). *In and out of the black box*. Oxford: Basil Blackwell.

Hammersley, M., & Atkinson, P. (1983). *Ethnography: Principles in practice*. London: Tavistock.

Handlin, O. (1979). *Truth in history* (p. 120). Cambridge, MA: Belknap Press.

Hardy, C.J. (1983). *The mediational role of social influence in the perception of exertion*. Unpublished doctoral dissertation, Louisiana State University, Baton Rouge.

Hardy, S., & Ingham, A. (1983, winter). Games, structures, and agency: Historians on the American play movement, *Journal of Social History, 17*, 285-301.

Harper, W.A. (1972, February). Taking and giving in sport. Essay presented at the Symposium on the Philosophy of Sport, Brockport, NY.

Harris, C. (1963). *Problems in measuring change*. Madison: University of Wisconsin Press.

Harris, R.J. (1985). *A primer of multivariate statistics* (2nd ed.). Orlando, FL: Academic Press.

Harwell, M.R. (1990). A general approach to hypothesis testing for nonparametric tests. *Journal of Experimental Education, 58*, 143-156.

Hedges, L.V. (1981). Distribution theory for Glass's estimator of effect size and related estimators. *Journal of Educational Statistics, 6*, 107-128.

Hedges, L.V. (1982a). Fitting categorical models to effect sizes from a series of experiments. *Journal of Educational Statistics, 7*, 119-137.

Hedges, L.V. (1982b). Estimation of effect size from a series of independent experiments. *Psychological Bulletin, 92*, 490-499.

Hedges, L.V. (1984). Estimation of effect size under nonrandom sampling: The effects of censoring studies yielding statistically insignificant mean differences. *Journal of Educational Statistics, 9*, 61-85.

Hedges, L.V., & Olkin, I. (1980). Vote counting methods in research synthesis. *Psychological Bulletin, 88*, 359-369.

Hedges, L., & Olkin, I. (1983). Regression models in research synthesis. *American Statistician*, **37**, 137-140.

Hedges, L.V., & Olkin, I. (1985). *Statistical methods for meta-analysis*. New York: Academic Press.

Helmstadter, G.C. (1970). *Research concepts in human behavior*. New York: Appleton-Century-Crofts.

Henderson, J. (1990, March 1). When scientists fake it. *American Way*, 56-62, 100-101.

Herkowitz, J. (1984). Developmentally engineered equipment and playgrounds. In J.R. Thomas (Ed.), *Motor development during childhood and adolescence*. Minneapolis: Burgess.

Hollinger, D. (1973, April). T.S. Kuhn's theory of science and its implications for history, *American Historical Review*, **78**, 370-393.

Humphrey, S.R. (1980). The historian, his documents, and elementary modes of historical thought, *History and Theory*, **19**, 1-20.

Hunter, J.E., & Schmidt, F.L. (1990). *Methods of meta-analysis: Correcting error and bias in research findings*. Newbury Park, CA: Sage.

Husserl, E. (1962). *Ideas: General introduction to pure phenomenology* (W.R. Boyce, Trans.). New York: Collier Books.

Hyde, J.S. (1981). How large are cognitive gender differences? A meta-analysis using ω^2 and *d*. *American Psychologist*, **36**, 892-901.

Hyland, D. (1990). *Philosophy of sport*. New York: Paragon House.

Jacks, P., Chubin, D.E., Porter, A.L., & Connally, T. (1983). The ABCs of ABDs: An interview study of incomplete doctorates. *Improving College and University Teaching*, **31**, 74-81.

Jackson, A.W. (1978). *The twelve-minute swim as a test for aerobic endurance in swimming*. Unpublished doctoral dissertation, University of Houston.

Jacob, E. (1987). Qualitative research traditions: A review. *Review of Educational Research*, **57**(1), 1-50.

Jacob, E. (1988). Clarifying qualitative research: A focus on tradition. *Educational Researcher*, **17**, 16-19, 22-24.

Jarausch, K.H., & Hardy, K.A. (1991). *Quantitative methods for historians: A guide to research, data, and statistics*. Chapel Hill: University of North Carolina Press.

Johnson, B.L., & Nelson, J.K. (1986). *Practical measurements for evaluation in physical education* (4th ed.). Minneapolis: Burgess.

Johnson, R.L. (1979). *The effects of various levels of fatigue on the speed and accuracy of visual recognition*. Unpublished doctoral dissertation, Louisiana State University, Baton Rouge.

Jones, E.R. (1988, winter). Philosophical tension in a scientific discipline: So what else is new? *NASPSPA Newsletter*, **14**(1), 10-16.

Joynt, C.B., & Rescher, N. (1961). The problem of uniqueness in history. *History and Theory*, **2**, 150-162.

Kavale, K., & Mattson, P.D. (1983). One jumped off the balance beam: Meta-analysis of perceptual-motor training. *Journal of Learning Disabilities*, **16**, 165-173.

Kendall, M.G. (1959). Hiawatha designs an experiment. *American Statistician*, **13**, 23-24.

Kennedy, J.J. (1983). *Analyzing qualitative data: Introductory loglinear analysis for behavioral research*. New York: Praeger.

Kennedy, M.M. (1979). Generalizing from single case studies. *Evaluation Quarterly*, **3**, 661-679.

Kirk, D. (1992). *Defining physical education: The social construction of a school subject in postwar Britain*. London: Faimer Press.

Kirk, J., & Miller, M.L. (1986). *Reliability and validity in qualitative research*. Newbury Park, CA: Sage.

Kirk, R.E. (1982). *Experimental design: Procedures for the behavioral sciences* (2nd ed.). Belmont, CA: Brooks/Cole.

Kleinman, S. (1968, May). Toward a non-theory of sport. *Quest*, **10**, 29-34.

Kraemer, H.C., & Thiemann, S. (1987). *How many subjects?* Newbury Park, CA: Sage.

Kraus, H., & Hirschland, R.P. (1954). Minimum muscular fitness tests in school children. *Research Quarterly*, **25**, 177-188.

Kretchmar, R.S. (1994). *Practical philosophy of sport*. Champaign, IL: Human Kinetics.

Kroll, W.P. (1971). *Perspectives in physical education*. New York: Academic Press.

Kruskal, W., & Mosteller, F. (1979). Representative sampling, III: The current statistical literature. *International Statistical Review*, **47**, 245-265.

Kuhn, T.S. (1962, 1970). *The structure of scientific revolutions*. Chicago: University of Chicago Press.

Kuklick, B. (1991). *To every thing a season: Shibe Park in urban Philadelphia, 1909-1976*. Princeton: Princeton University Press.

Lane, K.R. (1983). *Comparison of skinfold profiles of black and white boys and girls ages 11-13*. Unpublished master's thesis, Louisiana State University, Baton Rouge.

Lawson, H.A. (1993). After the regulated life. *Quest*, **45**, 523-545.

Lee, M. (1983). *A history of physical education and sports in the U.S.A.* New York: Wiley.

Lee, T.D. (1982). *On the locus of contextual interference in motor skill acquisition*. Unpublished doctoral dissertation, Louisiana State University, Baton Rouge.

Leonard, F.G., & Affleck, G.B. (1947). *A guide to the history of physical education* (3rd ed.). Philadelphia: Lea & Febiger.

Levine, R.V. (1990, September/October). The pace of life. *American Scientist*, **78**, 450-459.

Lincoln, Y.S., & Guba, E.G. (1985). *Naturalistic inquiry*. Newbury Park, CA: Sage.

Linn, R.L. (1986). Quantitative methods in research on teaching. In M.C. Wittrock (Ed.), *Handbook of research on teaching* (3rd ed.) (pp. 92-118). New York: Macmillan.

Lipsey, M.W. (1990). *Design sensitivity: Statistical power for experimental research*. Thousand Oaks, CA: Sage.

Locke, L.F. (1987). The question of quality in qualitative research. In J.K. Nelson (Ed.), *Proceedings of the fifth measurement and evaluation symposium* (pp. 31-36). Baton Rouge: Louisiana State University Press.

Locke, L.F. (1989). Qualitative research as a form of scientific inquiry in sport and physical education. *Research Quarterly for Exercise and Sport*, **60**, 1-20.

Locke, L.F., Spirduso, W.W., & Silverman, S.J. (1993). *Proposals that work: A guide for planning dissertations and grant proposals* (3rd ed.). Newbury Park, CA: Sage.

Loehle, C. (1990). A guide to increased creativity in research—Inspiration or perspiration? *Bioscience*, **40**, 123-129.

Looney, M.A. (1989). Criterion-referenced measurement: Reliability. In M.J. Safrit & T.M. Wood (Eds.), *Measurement concepts in physical education and exercise science* (pp. 137-152). Champaign, IL: Human Kinetics.

Looney, M.A., Feltz, C.S., & VanVleet, C.N. (1994). The reporting and analysis of research findings for within subjects designs: Methodological issues for meta-analysis. *Research Quarterly for Exercise and Sport*, **65**, 363-366.

Lord, F.M. (1969). Statistical adjustments when comparing preexisting groups. *Psychological Bulletin*, **72**, 336-337.

Lottinville, S. (1976). *The rhetoric of history*. Norman: University of Oklahoma Press.

Mabley, J. (1963, January 22). Mabley's report. *Chicago American*, p. 62.

Mandelbaum, M. (1977). *The anatomy of historical knowledge*. Baltimore: Johns Hopkins University Press.

Mangan, J. A., & Walvin, J. (Eds.) (1987). *Manliness and morality: Middle-class masculinity in Britain and America, 1800-1940*. New York: St. Martin's Press.

Marascuilo, L.A., & McSweeney, M. (1977). *Nonparametric and distribution-free methods for the social sciences*. Monterey, CA: Brooks/Cole.

Margerison, T. (1965, January 3). Review of *writing technical reports* (by B.M. Copper). *Sunday Times*. In R.L. Weber (Compiler) & E. Mendoza (Ed.), *A random walk in science* (p. 49). New York: Crane, Russak.

Marrou, H-I. (1967). *The meaning of history* (Robert J. Olsen, Trans.) (pp. 76-77). Baltimore: Johns Hopkins University Press.

Marshall, C., & Rossman, G.B. (1989). *Designing qualitative research*. Newbury Park, CA: Sage.

Martens, R. (1973, June). People errors in people experiments. *Quest*, **20**, 16-20.

Martens, R. (1977). *Sport competition anxiety test*. Champaign, IL: Human Kinetics.

Martens, R. (1979). About smocks and jocks. *Journal of Sport Psychology*, **1**, 94-99.

Martens, R. (1987). Science, knowledge, and sport psychology. *Sport Psychologist*, **1**, 29-55.

Massengale, J.D., & Swanson, R.A. (Eds.) (1996). *History of exercise and sport sciences*. Champaign, IL: Human Kinetics.

Matt, K.S. (1993). Ethical issues in animal research. *Quest*, **45**, 45-51.

Matthews, P.R. (1979). The frequency with which the mentally retarded participate in recreation activities. *Research Quarterly*, **50**, 71-79.

Mattson, D.E. (1981). *Statistics: Difficult concepts, understandable explanations*. St. Louis: C.V. Mosby.

McPherson, S.L. (1987). *The development of children's expertise in tennis: Knowledge structure and sport performance*. Unpublished doctoral dissertation, Louisiana State University, Baton Rouge, LA.

McPherson, S.L., & Thomas, J.R. (1989). Relation of knowledge and performance in boys' tennis: Age and expertise. *Journal of Experimental Child Psychology*, **48**, 190-211.

McPhie, W.E. (1960). Factors affecting the value of dissertations. *Social Education*, **24**, 375-377, 385.

Megill, A. (1989, June). Recounting the past: 'Description,' explanation, and narrative in historiography. *American Historical Review*, **94**, 627-653.

Meier, K.V. (1980). An affair of flutes: An appreciation of play. *Journal of the Philosophy of Sport*, **7**, 24-45.

Merleau-Ponty, M. (1964). *The primacy of perception*. Evanston: Northwestern University Press.

Merriam, S.B. (1988). *Case study research in education*. San Francisco: Jossey-Bass.

Merriam-Webster. (1989). *Webster's ninth new collegiate dictionary.* Springfield, MA: Merriam-Webster.

Metheny, E. (1968). *Movement and meaning.* New York: McGraw-Hill.

Micceri, T. (1989). The unicorn, the normal curve, and other improbable creatures. *Psychological Bulletin,* **105,** 156-166.

Miles, M.B., & Huberman, A.M. (1994). *Qualitative data analysis: A sourcebook of new methods* (2nd ed.) Thousand Oaks, CA: Sage.

Milligan, John D. (1979). The treatment of an historical source. *History and Theory,* **18,** 177-196.

Monkkonen, Eric. (1984, summer). The Challenge of Quantitative History. *Historical Methods,* **17,** 89-90.

Mood, D.P. (1989). Measurement methodology for knowledge tests. In M.J. Safrit & T.M. Wood (Eds.), *Measurement concepts in physical education and exercise science* (pp. 251-270). Champaign, IL: Human Kinetics.

Morgan, D.L. (1988). *Focus groups as qualitative research.* Thousand Oaks, CA: Sage.

Morgan, W.J. (1994). *Leftist theories of sport.* Urbana: University of Illinois Press.

Morgenstern, N.L. (1983). Cogito ergo sum: Murphy's refutation of Descartes. In G.H. Scherr (Ed.), *The best of The Journal of Irreproducible Results* (p. 112). New York: Workman Press.

Morland, R.B. (1958). A philosophical interpretation of the educational views held by leaders in American physical education (Unpublished doctoral dissertation, New York University). *Health, Physical Education and Recreation Microform Publications,* **1,** October 1949-March 1965, PE394.

Morrow, J.R., Jr. (1989). Generalizability theory. In M.J. Safrit & T.M. Wood (Eds.), *Measurement concepts in physical education and exercise science* (pp. 73-96). Champaign, IL: Human Kinetics.

Morrow, J.R., Jr., Bray, M.S., Fulton, J.E., & Thomas, J.R. (1992). Interrater reliability of 1987-1991 *Research Quarterly for Exercise and Sport* reviews. *Research Quarterly for Exercise and Sport,* **63,** 200-204.

Morrow, J.R., & Frankiewicz, R.G. (1979). Strategies for the analysis of repeated and multiple measure designs. *Research Quarterly,* **50,** 297-304.

National Children and Youth Fitness Study. (1985). *Journal of Physical Education, Recreation & Dance,* **56**(1), 44-90.

National Children and Youth Fitness Study II. (1987). *Journal of Physical Education, Recreation & Dance,* **56**(9), 147-167.

Nelson, J.K. (1988, March). Some thoughts on research, measurement, and other obscure topics. LAHPERD Scholar Lecture presented at the LAHPERD Convention, New Orleans.

Nelson, J.K. (1989). Measurement methodology for affective tests. In M.J. Safrit & T.M. Wood (Eds.), *Measurement concepts in physical education and exercise science* (pp. 229-248). Champaign, IL: Human Kinetics.

Nelson, K.R. (1988). *Thinking processes, management routines, and student perceptions of expert and novice physical education teachers.* Unpublished doctoral dissertation, Louisiana State University.

Newell, K.M. (1987). On masters and apprentices in physical education. *Quest,* **39,** 88-96.

Newell, K.M., & Hancock, P.A. (1984). Forgotten moments: A note on skewness and kurtosis as influential factors in inferences extrapolated from response distributions. *Journal of Motor Behavior,* **16,** 320-335.

Nietzsche, F. (1967). *The will to power.* (W. Kaufmann & R. Hollingdale, Trans.). New York: Vintage Books.

Nunnaly, J.C. (1978). *Psychometric theory* (2nd ed.). New York: McGraw-Hill.

Oakman, R.L. (1984). *Computer methods for literary research.* Athens: University of Georgia Press.

Ornstein, M.D. (1983, summer). Discrete multivariate analysis: An example from the 1871 Canadian census. *Historical Methods,* **16,** 101-108.

Park, R.J. (1980). The *Research Quarterly* and its antecedents. *Research Quarterly for Exercise and Sport,* **51,** 1-22.

Park, R.J. (1983, June). Research and scholarship in the history of physical education and sport, *Research Quarterly for Exercise and Sport,* **54,** 93-103.

Park, R.J. (1986, spring). Hermeneutics, semiotics, and the nineteenth-century quest for a corporeal self, *Quest,* **38,** 33-49.

Patterson, P. (1989). The use of validity generalization in exercise science. In M.J. Safrit & T.M. Wood (Eds.), *Measurement concepts in physical education and exercise science* (pp. 97-115). Champaign, IL: Human Kinetics.

Patton, M.Q. (1987). *How to use qualitative methods in evaluation.* Newbury Park, CA: Sage.

Payne, V.G., & Morrow, J.R., Jr. (1993). Exercise and $\dot{V}O_2$max in children: A meta-analysis. *Research Quarterly for Exercise and Sport,* **64,** 305-313.

Pedhazur, E.J. (1982). *Multiple regression in behavioral research: Explanation and prediction* (2nd ed.). New York: Holt, Rinehart & Winston.

Peshkin, A. (1993). The goodness of qualitative research. *Educational Researcher*, **22**(2), 23-29.

Polanyi, M. (1958). *Person knowledge: Toward a post-critical philosophy*. Chicago: University of Chicago Press.

Porter, A.C., & Raudenbush, S.W. (1987). Analysis of covariance: Its model and use in psychological research. *Journal of Counseling Psychology*, **34**, 383-392.

Porter, A.L., Chubin, D.E., Rossini, F.A., Boeckmann, M.E., & Connally, T. (1982, September/October). The role of the dissertation in scientific careers. *American Scientist*, pp. 475-481.

Porter, A.L., & Wolfe, D. (1975). Utility of the doctoral dissertation. *American Psychologist*, **30**, 1054-1061.

Porter, D.H. (1975). History as process. *History and Theory*, **14**, 297-313.

Porter, D.H. (1981). *The emergence of the past: A theory of historical explanation*. Chicago: University of Chicago Press.

Powell, K.E., Kohl, H.W., Caspersen, C.J., & Blair, S.N. (1986). An epidemiological perspective on the causes of running injuries. *Physician and Sportsmedicine*, **14**(6).

Punch, M. (1986). *The politics and ethics of fieldwork*. Beverly Hills, CA: Sage.

Puri, M.L., & Sen, P.K. (1969). A class of rank order tests for a general linear hypothesis. *Annals of Mathematical Statistics*, **40**, 1325-1343.

Puri, M.L., & Sen, P.K. (1985). *Nonparametric methods in general linear models*. New York: Wiley.

Realist, B.A. [G. Benford]. (1982, March). How to write a scientific paper. *Omni*, p. 130.

Roberts, G.C. (1993). Ethics in professional advising and academic counseling of graduate students. *Quest*, **45**, 78-87.

Rogers, J.L., Howard, K.I., & Vessey, J.T. (1993). Using significance tests to evaluate equivalence between two experimental groups. *Psychological Bulletin*, **113**, 553-565.

Rosen, S. (1989). *The ancients and the moderns: Rethinking modernity*. New Haven: Yale University Press.

Rosenau, P.M. (1992). *Post-modernism and the social sciences: Insights, inroads, and intrusions*. Princeton: Princeton University Press.

Rosenthal, R. (1966). Sport, art, and particularity: The best equivocation. *Journal of the Philosophy of Sport*, **13**, 49-63.

Rosenthal, R. (1979). The file-drawer problem and tolerance for null results. *Psychological Bulletin*, **86**, 638-641.

Rosenthal, R. (1991). Cumulating psychology: An appreciation of Donald T. Campbell. *Psychological Science*, **2**, 213, 217-221.

Rosnow, R.L., & Rosenthal, R. (1989). Statistical procedures and the justification of knowledge in psychological science. *American Psychologist*, **44**, 1276-1284.

Rovegno, I. (1994). Teaching within a curricular zone of safety: School culture and the situated nature of student teachers' pedagogical content knowledge. *Research Quarterly for Exercise and Sport*, **65**, 269-279.

Rudy, W. (1962). Higher education in the United States, 1862-1962. In W.W. Brickman & S. Lehrer (Eds.), *A century of higher education: Classical citadel to collegiate colossus* (pp. 20-21). New York: Society for the Advancement of Education.

Ryan, E.D. (1970). The cathartic effect of vigorous motor activity on aggressive behavior. *Research Quarterly*, **41**, 542-551.

Safrit, M.J. (1989). Criterion-referenced measurement: Validity. In M.J. Safrit & T.M. Wood (Eds.), *Measurement concepts in physical education and exercise science* (pp. 119-135). Champaign, IL: Human Kinetics.

Safrit, M.J. (Ed.) (1980). *Research Quarterly for Exercise and Sport*, **51**(1).

Safrit, M.J. (Ed.) (1976). *Reliability theory*. Washington, DC: American Alliance for Health, Physical Education and Recreation.

Safrit, M.J., Cohen, A.S., & Costa, M.G. (1989). Item response theory and the measurement of motor behavior. *Research Quarterly for Exercise and Sport*, **60**, 325-335.

Safrit, M.J., & Wood, T.M. (1983). The health-related fitness test opinionnaire: A pilot survey. *Research Quarterly for Exercise and Sport*, **54**, 204-207.

Sage, G.H. (1989). A commentary on qualitative research as a form of inquiry in sport and physical education. *Research Quarterly for Exercise and Sport*, **60**, 25-29.

Schein, E.H. (1987). *The clinical perspective in fieldwork*. Newbury Park, CA: Sage.

Scheffé, H. (1953). A method for judging all contrasts in analysis of variance. *Biometrika*, **40**, 87-104.

Scherr, G.H. (Ed.) (1983). *The best of the Journal of Irreproducible Results* (p. 152). New York: Workman Press.

Schmidt, A. (1981). *History and structure* Jeffrey Herf, Trans.). Cambridge: Harvard University Press.

Schmidt, F.L., Hunter, J.E., & Urry, V.W. (1976). Statistical power in criterion-related validation studies. *Journal of Applied Psychology*, **61**, 473-485.

Schmidt, R.A. (1975). A schema theory of discrete motor skill learning. *Psychological Review*, **82**, 225-260.

Schmidt, R.A. (1988). *Motor control and learning*. Champaign, IL: Human Kinetics.

Schutz, R.W. (1989). Qualitative research: Comments and controversies. *Research Quarterly for Exercise and Sport*, **60**, 30-35.

Schutz, R.W., & Gessaroli, M.E. (1987). The analysis of repeated measures designs involving multiple dependent variables. *Research Quarterly for Exercise and Sport*, **58**, 132-149.

Serlin, R.C. (1987). Hypothesis testing, theory building, and the philosophy of science. *Journal of Counseling Psychology*, **34**, 365-371.

Shafer, R. (1980). *A guide to historical method* (3rd ed.). Homewood, IL.

Shammas, C. (1981, winter). Dealing with dichotomous dependent variables, *Historical Methods*, **14**, 47-51.

Shore, E.G. (1991, February). *Analysis of a multi-institutional series of completed cases*. Paper presented at Scientific Integrity symposium. Harvard Medical School, Boston.

Siedentop, D. (1980). Two cheers for Rainer. *Journal of Sport Psychology*, **2**, 2-4.

Siedentop, D. (1989). Do the lockers really smell? *Research Quarterly for Exercise and Sport*, **60**, 36-41.

Siedentop, D., Birdwell, D., & Metzler, M. (1979, March). *A process approach to measuring teaching effectiveness in physical education*. Paper presented at the American Alliance for Health, Physical Education, Recreation and Dance national convention, New Orleans.

Siedentop, D., Trousignant, M., & Parker, M. (1982). *Academic learning time—Physical education: 1982 coding manual*. Columbus: Ohio State University, School of Health, Physical Education, and Recreation.

Siegel, S. (1956). *Nonparametric statistics for the behavioral sciences*. New York: McGraw-Hill.

Simon, R. (1991). *Fair play: Sports, values, and society*. Englewood Cliffs, NJ: Prentice Hall.

Singer, R.N., Murphey, M., & Tennant, L.K. (Eds.) (1993). *Handbook of research on sport psychology*. New York: Macmillian.

Slavin, R.E. (1984a). Meta-analysis in education: How it has been used. *Educational Researcher*, **13**(4), 6-15.

Slavin, R.E. (1984b). A rejoinder to Carlberg et al. *Educational Researcher*, **13**(4), 24-27.

Smith, M.L. (1980). Sex bias in counseling and psychotherapy. *Psychological Bulletin*, **87**, 392-407.

Smith, R.A. (1988). *Sports and freedom: The rise of big-time college athletics*. New York.

Snyder, C.W., Jr., & Abernethy, B. (Eds.) (1992). *The creative side of experimentation*. Champaign, IL: Human Kinetics.

Sparling, P.B. (1980). A meta-analysis of studies comparing maximal oxygen uptake in men and women. *Research Quarterly for Exercise and Sport*, **51**, 542-552.

Spray, J.A. (1987). Recent developments in measurement and possible applications to the measurement of psychomotor behavior. *Research Quarterly for Exercise and Sport*, **58**, 203-209.

Spray, J.A. (1989). New approaches to solving measurement problems. In M.J. Safrit & T.M. Wood (Eds.), *Measurement concepts in physical education and exercise science* (pp. 229-248). Champaign, IL: Human Kinetics.

Stamm, C.L., & Safrit, M.J. (1975). Comparison of significance tests for repeated measures ANOVA design. *Research Quarterly*, **46**, 403-409.

Starkes, J.L., & Allard, F. (Eds.) (1993). *Cognitive issues in motor expertise*. Amsterdam: North Holland.

Stearns, P.N. (1980, winter). Modernization and social history: Some suggestions and a muted cheer, *Journal of Social History*, **14**, 189-210.

Stock, W.A. (1994). Systematic coding for research synthesis. In H. Cooper & L.V. Hedges (Eds.), *The handbook of research synthesis*. New York: Sage Foundation.

Struna, N.L. (1985, June). In 'glorious disarray': The literature of American sport history, *Research Quarterly for Exercise and Sport*, **56**, 151-160.

Struna, N.L. (1986, spring). E.P. Thompson's notion of 'context' and the writing of physical education and sport history, *Quest*, **38**, 24-27.

Struna, N.L. (1988, December). Sport and society in early America, *International Journal of the History of Sport*, **5**, 292-311.

Struna, N.L. (1996). Sport history, in John Massengale and Richard Swanson (Eds.), *History of exercise and sport science* (chap. 9). Urbana: University of Illinois Press.

Stull, G.A., Christina, R.W., and Quinn, S.A. (1991). Accuracy of references in the *Research Quarterly for Exercise and Sport*. *Research Quarterly for Exercise and Sport*, **62**, 245-248.

Suits, B. (1978). *The grasshopper: Games, life, and utopia*. Toronto: University of Toronto Press.

Taylor, S.J., & Bogdan, R. (1984). *Introduction to qualitative research methods* (2nd ed.). New York: Wiley.

Tew, J. (1988). *Construction of a sport specific mental imagery assessment instrument using item response and classical test theory methodology.* Unpublished doctoral dissertation, Louisiana State University, Baton Rouge.

Tew, J., & Wood, M. (1980). *Proposed model for predicting probable success in football players.* Houston: Rice University Press.

Thomas, J.R. (Spring 1989). An abstract for all seasons. *NASPSPA Newsletter*, **14**(2), 4-5.

Thomas, J.R. (1977). A note concerning analysis of error scores from motor-memory research. *Journal of Motor Behavior*, **9**, 251-253.

Thomas, J.R. (1980). Half a cheer for Rainer and Daryl. *Journal of Sport Psychology*, **2**, 266-267.

Thomas, J.R. (Ed.) (1984). *Motor development during childhood and adolescence*. Minneapolis: Burgess.

Thomas, J.R. (Ed.) (1983). Publication guidelines. *Research Quarterly for Exercise and Sport*, **54**, 219-221.

Thomas, J.R. (Ed.) (1986). Editor's viewpoint: Research notes. *Research Quarterly for Exercise and Sport*, **57**, iv-v.

Thomas, J.R., & French, K.E. (1985). Gender differences across age in motor performance: A meta-analysis. *Psychological Bulletin*, **98**, 260-282.

Thomas, J.R., & French, K.E. (1986). The use of meta-analysis in exercise and sport: A tutorial. *Research Quarterly for Exercise and Sport*, **57**, 196-204.

Thomas, J.R., French, K.E., & Humphries, C.A. (1986). Knowledge development and sport skill performance: Directions for motor behavior research. *Journal of Sport Psychology*, **8**, 259-272.

Thomas, J.R., & Gill, D.L. (Eds.) (1993). The Academy Papers: Ethics in the study of physical activity [special issue]. *Quest*, **45**(1).

Thomas, J.R., Nelson, J.K., & Magill, R.A. (1986). A case for an alternative format for the thesis/dissertation. *Quest*, **38**, 116-124.

Thomas, J.R., Salazar, W., & Landers, D.M. (1991). What is missing in $p < .05$? Effect size. *Research Quarterly for Exercise and Sport*, **62**, 344-348.

Thomas, J.R., Thomas, K.T., Lee, A.M., Testerman, E., & Ashy, M. (1983). Age differences in use of strategy for recall of movement in a large scale environment. *Research Quarterly for Exercise and Sport*, **54**, 264-272.

Thompson, B. (1991). Methods, plainly speaking: A primer on the logic and use of canonical correlation analysis. *Measurement and Evaluation in Counseling and Development*, **24**, 80-95.

Thompson, E.P. (1972, spring). Anthropology and the discipline of historical context. *Midland History*, **3**, 41-55.

Thompson, E.P. (1978). *The poverty of theory and other essays* (pp. 28-29). New York.

Tinberg, C.M. (1993). *The relation of practice time to coaches' objectives, players' improvement, and level of expertise* (Unpublished master's thesis, Arizona State University, Tempe).

Tinsley, H.E., & Tinsley, D.J. (1987). Uses of factor analysis in counseling psychology research. *Journal of Counseling Psychology*, **34**, 414-424.

Tolson, H. (1980). An adjustment to statistical significance: ω^2. *Research Quarterly for Exercise and Sport*, **51**, 580-584.

Toothaker, L.E. (1991). *Multiple comparisons for researchers*. Newbury Park, CA: Sage.

Tran, Z.V., Weltman, A., Glass, G.V., & Mood, D.P. (1983). The effects of exercise on blood lipids and lipoproteins: A meta-analysis. *Medicine and Science in Sports and Exercise*, **15**, 393-402.

Tuckman, B.W. (1978). *Conducting educational research* (2nd ed.). New York: Harcourt Brace Jovanovich.

University of Chicago Press. (1993). *The Chicago manual of style* (14th ed.). Chicago: Author.

Van Dalen, D.B., & Bennett, B.L. (1971). *A history of physical education* (2nd ed.). Englewood Cliffs, NJ: Prentice Hall.

Vealey, R.S. (1986). The conceptualization of sport-confidence and competitive orientation: Preliminary investigation and instrument development. *Journal of Sport Psychology*, **8**, 221-246.

Verducci, F.M. (1980). *Measurement concepts in physical education*. St. Louis: C.V. Mosby.

Vertinsky, P. (1990). *The eternally wounded woman: Women, exercise, and doctors in the late nineteenth century*. Manchester: Manchester University Press.

Vockell, E.L. (1983). *Educational research*. New York: Macmillan.

Wainer, H. (1992). Understanding graphs and tables. *Educational Researcher*, **21**(1), 14-23.

Webb, E.J., Campbell, D.T., Schwartz, R.D., & Sechrest, L. (1966). *Unobtrusive measures: Nonreactive research in the social sciences*. Chicago: Rand-McNally.

Weiss, M.R., Bredemeier, B.J., & Shewchuk, R.M. (1985). An intrinsic/extrinsic motivation scale for the youth sport setting: A confirmatory factor analysis. *Journal of Sport Psychology, 7,* 75-91.

Weiss, P. (1969). *Sport: A philosophic inquiry.* Carbondale: Southern Illinois University Press.

Werner, P., & Rink, J. (1989). Case studies of teacher effectiveness in physical education. *Journal of Teaching in Physical Education, 8,* 280-297.

Westlake, W.J. (1981). Bioequivalence testing—A need to rethink. *Biometrics, 37,* 591-593.

White, P.A. (1990). Ideas about causation in philosophy and psychology. *Psychological Bulletin, 108,* 3-18.

Wilson, A. (1981, summer). Inferring attitudes from behavior. *Historical Methods, 14,* 143-144.

Wood, G.S. (1979). Intellectual history and the social sciences. In John Higham & Paul Conkin (Eds.), *New directions in American intellectual history.* Baltimore: Johns Hopkins University Press.

Wood, T.M., & Safrit, M.J. (1987). A comparison of three multivariate models for estimating test battery reliability. *Research Quarterly for Exercise and Sport, 58,* 150-159.

Yin, R.K. (1984). *Case study research: Design and methods.* Newbury Park, CA: Sage.

Zelaznik, H.N. (1993). Ethical issues in conducting and reporting research: A reaction to Kroll, Matt, and Safrit. *Quest, 45,* 62-68.

Ziv, A. (1988). Teaching and learning with humor: Experiment and replication. *Journal of Experimental Education, 57,* 5-15.

Author Index

Subject Index

About the Contributors

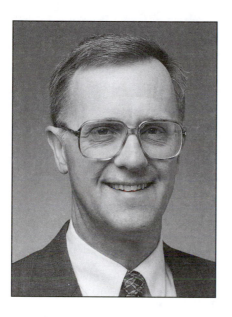

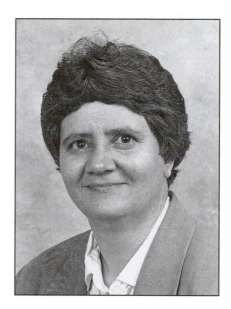

R. Scott Kretchmar, PhD, is widely regarded as one of the leading sport philosophers in the United States. He not only has taught philosophy of sport for over 25 years but also has played a key role in making it a legitimate field of scholarship and study. Dr. Kretchmar, a founding member and past president of the Philosophic Society for the Study of Sport, is also a past president of the Philosophy Academy of the National Association for Sport and Physical Education.

Kretchmar earned a bachelor's degree from Oberlin College in 1966 and a doctorate in physical education from the University of Southern California in 1971. He is a professor in Penn State University's Department of Exercise and Sport Science where he served as department head from 1984 to 1989. He is also an assistant editor for the *Journal of the Philosophy of Sport* and an editor of the Fair Play column in *Strategies*. In 1989 Dr. Kretchmar was elected a Fellow in the American Academy of Kinesiology and Physical Education.

Nancy L. Struna, PhD, has been an associate professor in the Department of Kinesiology and an affiliate associate professor in the Department of History at the University of Maryland since 1988. She is also director of the Department of Kinesiology Honors Program. She earned a bachelor's degree from the University of Wisconsin, Madison, in 1972 and a doctorate from the University of Maryland, College Park, in 1979.

A member of several historical organizations, Dr. Struna is serving a two-year term as president of the North American Society for Sport History. She is the author of *People of Prowess: Sport, Leisure and Labor in Early Anglo-America* and of a forthcoming book on the social history of sports in America. She serves on the editorial board of the *Journal of Sport History* and is a reviewer for other scholarly publications. In 1992 Dr. Struna became a Fellow in the American Academy of Kinesiology and Physical Education and received the Distinguished Scholar Award from the National Association for Physical Education in Higher Education.

Related titles from Human Kinetics

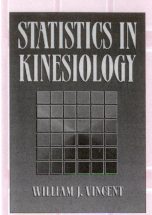

William J. Vincent, EdD
1995 • Paper • 272 pp
Item BVIN0699
ISBN 0-87322-699-2
$25.00 ($37.50 Canadian)

Statistics in Kinesiology is proof that statistics need not be complicated! From its logical organization to its simplified formula notation, this book presents information in a way that is both easy to read and easy to comprehend. Geared toward students without advanced math skills, the text examines many statistical techniques commonly used in the various professions and disciplines of physical education, exercise science, and leisure studies/recreation.

This text uses examples exclusively from kinesiology and related fields to present statistical concepts and procedures. Students find it easier to understand these concepts because the examples are relevant to their field. They are able to work with data and variables similar to what they will encounter in their careers, making the learning process more applicable and enjoyable.

Several other features add to the book's appeal. It leads readers through a series of statistical concepts that build logically on one another. The easy-to-understand symbols used for the formulas let students concentrate on the concepts and their meanings rather than on confusing details and notations. A flowchart helps students determine the correct statistical procedure for the data they want to analyze. And sample problems at the end of each chapter give students an opportunity to test their knowledge.

Statistics in Kinesiology is an outstanding main text for undergraduate statistics courses and an excellent supplemental text for undergraduate tests and measurements courses. It is also a user-friendly desk reference for researchers and practitioners in the physical activity sciences.

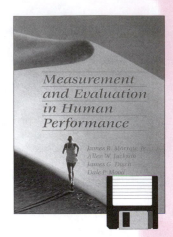

James R. Morrow, Jr., PhD, Allen W. Jackson, EdD, James G. Disch, PED, and Dale P. Mood, PhD

Book with Windows software • 1995
416 pp • 3-1/2" disk
Item BMOR0731
ISBN 0-87322-731-X
$49.00 ($73.50 Canadian)

Audiences: *Text for undergraduate exercise and sport science courses. Reference for professionals in the human performance field.*

A comprehensive text and software package, this unique textbook includes the powerful MYSTAT, the graphic and data management program that helps students apply important concepts hands-on.

Measurement and Evaluation in Human Performance is more than a textbook of concepts and formulae. It not only explains the theories and principles of measurement, it also takes the undergraduate student on a fascinating journey through computer applications and practical physical education science problems and solutions. Students can use MYSTAT to conduct the tasks assigned in the text as well as create and analyse their own real and hypothetical data sets.

The book also includes special features that help bring this topic to life and guide students through the content: summary tables, figures and graphs, highlighted key words and sentences, running glossary, controversial and issue-oriented topics, index, side bars and photos.

The 164 Mastery Items emphasise important principles and challenge students to apply concepts and solve problems.

Instructor Guide Software
Windows Item BMOR0645
Macintosh Item BMOR0647
1996 • 3 1/2" disk • FREE to course adopters.
See order form for special instructions.

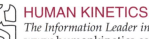

Thomas, Jerry R.
Research methods in physical
activity